The American Psychiatric Association Publishing

TEXTBOOK OF
PERSONALITY DISORDERS

THIRD EDITION

The American Psychiatric Association Publishing

TEXTBOOK OF

PERSONALITY DISORDERS

THIRD EDITION

EDITED BY

Andrew E. Skodol, M.D.
John M. Oldham, M.D., M.S.

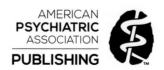

AMERICAN
PSYCHIATRIC
ASSOCIATION
PUBLISHING

Manufactured in the United States of America on acid-free paper
25 24 23 22 21   5 4 3 2 1

American Psychiatric Association Publishing
800 Maine Avenue SW
Suite 900
Washington, DC 20024-2812
www.appi.org

Library of Congress Cataloging-in-Publication Data
Names: Skodol, Andrew E., editor. | Oldham, John M., editor. | American Psychiatric
   Association Publishing, issuing body.
Title: The American Psychiatric Association Publishing textbook of personality disorders /
   edited by Andrew E. Skodol, John M. Oldham.
Other titles: American Psychiatric Publishing textbook of personality disorders | Textbook of
   personality disorders
Description: Third edition. | Washington, DC : American Psychiatric Association Publishing,
   [2021] | Preceded by American Psychiatric Publishing textbook of personality disorders /
   edited by John M. Oldham, Andrew E. Skodol, Donna S. Bender. Second edition. 2014. |
Includes bibliographical references and index.
Identifiers: LCCN 2020055937 (print) | LCCN 2020055938 (ebook) | ISBN 9781615373390
   (hardcover) | ISBN 9781615373741 (ebook)
Subjects: MESH: Personality Disorders—therapy | Personality Disorders—etiology |
   Personality Disorders—diagnosis
Classification: LCC RC554 (print) | LCC RC554 (ebook) | NLM WM 190 | DDC
616.85/81—dc23
LC record available at https://lccn.loc.gov/2020055937
LC ebook record available at https://lccn.loc.gov/2020055938

British Library Cataloguing in Publication Data
A CIP record is available from the British Library.

To our families, who have supported us.
To our colleagues, who have helped us.
To our patients, who have taught us.
And to our friendship that has enriched our work together.

Contents

PART II
Risk Factors, Etiology, and Impact

PART III
Treatment

PART V
Future Directions

  Christian Schmahl, M.D.
  Sabine C. Herpertz, M.D.

APPENDIX

Contributors

Anthony W. Bateman, M.A., FRCPsych
University College London, United Kingdom

Donna S. Bender, Ph.D., FIPA
Director, Tulane University Counseling Center; Adjunct Professor of Psychiatry and Behavioral Sciences, Tulane School of Medicine, New Orleans, Louisiana

David M. Benedek, M.D., Col., M.C., U.S.A.
Professor and Chair, Department of Psychiatry, Uniformed Services University School of Medicine, Bethesda, Maryland

Donald W. Black, M.D.
Professor Emeritus of Psychiatry, University of Iowa Roy J. and Lucille A. Carver College of Medicine, Iowa City, Iowa

Nancee S. Blum, M.S.W.
Instructor Emeritus of Clinical Psychiatry, University of Iowa Roy J. and Lucille A. Carver College of Medicine, Iowa City, Iowa

Philippe Boursiquot, M.D., FRCPC
Assistant Clinical Professor, Department of Psychiatry and Behavioural Neurosciences, Michael G. DeGroote School of Medicine, McMaster University, Hamilton, Ontario, Canada

Beth S. Brodsky, Ph.D.
Associate Clinical Professor of Medical Psychology, Columbia University Irving Medical Center; Associate Director, Suicide Prevention Training, Implementation and Evaluation Program, New York State Psychiatric Institute, New York, New York

Chloe Campbell, Ph.D.
University College London, United Kingdom

Andrew M. Chanen, M.B.B.S., Ph.D., FRANZCP
Head, Personality Disorder Research and Director of Clinical Programs and Services Orygen, Melbourne, Australia; Professorial Fellow, Centre for Youth Mental Health, The University of Melbourne, Australia

Lois W. Choi-Kain, M.D., M.Ed.
Assistant Professor of Psychiatry, Harvard Medical School; Director, Gunderson Personality Disorders Institute, McLean Hospital, Belmont, Massachusetts

John F. Clarkin, Ph.D.
Clinical Professor of Psychology in Psychiatry and Co-Director of the Personality Disorders Institute, Weill Cornell Medical College, New York, New York

Jennifer C. Elliott, Ph.D.
Assistant Professor of Clinical Psychology, Department of Psychiatry, Columbia University; Research Scientist, New York State Psychiatric Institute, New York, New York

Peter Fonagy, Ph.D.
University College London, United Kingdom

J. Christopher Fowler, Ph.D.
Professor, Houston Methodist Academic Institute, Houston, Texas

Sharely Fred Torres, M.D.
Resident Physician, Icahn School of Medicine at Mount Sinai, New York, New York

Lauren R. Gorfinkel, M.P.H.
Department of Epidemiology, Columbia University, New York, New York

Ilana Gratch, B.A.
Research Assistant, Division of Molecular Imaging and Neuropathology, New York State Psychiatric Institute, New York, New York

Carlos M. Grilo, Ph.D.
Professor of Psychiatry, Yale University School of Medicine; Professor of Psychology, Yale University, New Haven, Connecticut

Thomas G. Gutheil, M.D.
Professor of Psychiatry, Department of Psychiatry, Beth Israel-Deaconess Medical Center; Co-founder, Program in Psychiatry and the Law, Massachusetts Mental Health Center, Harvard Medical School, Boston, Massachusetts

John M. Hart, Ph.D.
Clinical Consultant, Houston Methodist Behavioral Health, Houston, Texas

Deborah S. Hasin, Ph.D.
Professor of Epidemiology, Columbia University, New York, New York

Sabine C. Herpertz, M.D.
Department of General Psychiatry, University of Heidelberg, Heidelberg, Germany

Richard Hersh, M.D.
Special Lecturer, Department of Psychiatry, Columbia University College of Physicians and Surgeons, New York, New York

Christian Hicks, M.D.
Clinical Fellow in Consultation-Liaison Psychiatry, Department of Psychiatry, Columbia University Irving Medical Center/New York State Psychiatric Institute, New York, New York

David Kealy, Ph.D.
Assistant Professor, Department of Psychiatry, University of British Columbia, Vancouver, British Columbia, Canada

Amy R. Kegley, Ph.D.
Private Practice, Lexington, Massachusetts

Sophie Kerr, B.A.
Doctoral Student, Department of Psychology, University of Houston, Houston, Texas

Harold W. Koenigsberg, M.D.
Professor and Director of the Mood and Personality Disorders Program, Department of Psychiatry, Icahn School of Medicine at Mount Sinai, New York, New York

Jay L. Lebow, Ph.D.
Senior Scholar and Senior Therapist, Clinical Professor of Psychology, The Family Institute at Northwestern, Evanston, Illinois

Kenneth N. Levy, Ph.D.
Associate Professor, Department of Psychology, The Pennsylvania State University, University Park, Pennsylvania

Madison Links, M.D.
Resident, Department of Pediatrics, Schulich School of Medicine & Dentistry, Western University, London, Ontario, Canada

Paul S. Links, M.D., FRCPC
Professor, Department of Psychiatry and Behavioural Neurosciences, Michael G. DeGroote School of Medicine, McMaster University, Hamilton, Ontario, Canada

Nicolas Lorenzini, Ph.D.
University College London, United Kingdom; International Psychoanalytic University Berlin, Germany

Patrick Luyten, Ph.D.
KU Leuven, Belgium, and University College London, United Kingdom

Ricky D. Malone, M.D., Col. (Ret.), M.C., U.S.A.
Assistant Professor, Department of Psychiatry, Uniformed Services University School of Medicine, Bethesda, Maryland

Jacquelyn L. Meyers, Ph.D.
Assistant Professor of Psychiatry and Behavioral Sciences, State University of New York Downstate Medical Center, Brooklyn, New York

Leslie C. Morey, Ph.D.
Abell Professor of Liberal Arts, Department of Psychological and Brain Sciences, Texas A&M University, College Station, Texas

Philip R. Muskin, M.D., M.A., DLFAPA, LFACLP
Professor of Psychiatry, Columbia University Irving Medical Center; Senior Consultant in Consultation-Liaison Psychiatry, New York-Presbyterian Hospital/Columbia University Irving Medical Center, New York, New York

Sara Siris Nash, M.D., FACLP, FAPA
Assistant Professor of Psychiatry, Columbia University Irving Medical Center; Director, Fellowship Program in Consultation-Liaison Psychiatry, Consultation-Liaison Psychiatry Service, New York-Presbyterian Hospital/Columbia University Irving Medical Center, New York, New York

Katharine J. Nelson, M.D.
Associate Professor of Psychiatry and Behavioral Sciences, University of Minnesota Medical School, Minneapolis, Minnesota

Antonia S. New, M.D.
Professor, Residency Training Director, and Vice Chair for Education, Department of Psychiatry, Icahn School of Medicine at Mount Sinai, New York, New York

John S. Ogrodniczuk, Ph.D.
Professor and Director of Psychotherapy Program, Department of Psychiatry, University of British Columbia, Vancouver, British Columbia, Canada

John M. Oldham, M.D., M.S.
Distinguished Emeritus Professor, Baylor College of Medicine, Houston, Texas

William H. Orme, Ph.D.
Assistant Professor, Houston Methodist Behavioral Health, Houston, Texas

M. Mercedes Perez-Rodriguez, M.D., Ph.D.
Assistant Professor and Assistant Training Director for Research, Department of Psychiatry, Icahn School of Medicine at Mount Sinai, New York, New York

Seth J. Prins, Ph.D., M.P.H.
Assistant Professor of Epidemiology and Sociomedical Sciences, Columbia University, New York, New York

Daniel R. Rosell, M.D., Ph.D.
Assistant Professor, Department of Psychiatry, Icahn School of Medicine at Mount Sinai, New York, New York

Abigail B. Schlesinger, M.D.
Chief, Child & Adolescent Psychiatry and Integrated Care, Western Psychiatric Hospital and Children's Hospital of Pittsburgh; Associate Professor of Psychiatry and Pediatrics, University of Pittsburgh School of Medicine, Pittsburgh, Pennsylvania

Christian Schmahl, M.D.
Department of Psychosomatic Medicine and Psychotherapy, Central Institute of Mental Health, Mannheim, Germany

Carla Sharp, Ph.D.
Professor and Interim Dean for Faculty and Research, Department of Psychology, College of Liberal Arts and Social Sciences, University of Houston, Houston, Texas

Andrew E. Skodol, M.D.
Research Professor of Psychiatry, University of Arizona College of Medicine, Tucson, Arizona

Jennifer Sotsky, M.D.
Clinical Fellow in Consultation-Liaison Psychiatry, Department of Psychiatry, Columbia University Irving Medical Center/New York State Psychiatric Institute, New York, New York

Barbara Stanley, Ph.D.
Professor of Medical Psychology, Department of Psychiatry, Columbia University Irving Medical Center; Director, Suicide Prevention Training, Implementation and Evaluation, New York State Psychiatric Institute, New York, New York

Svenn Torgersen, Ph.D.
Professor, Department of Psychology, University of Oslo, Oslo, Norway

Sherab Tsheringla, M.D.
Resident Physician, Department of Psychiatry, Yale School of Medicine, New Haven, Connecticut

Amanda A. Uliaszek, Ph.D.
Assistant Professor, Departments of Psychology and Psychological Clinical Science, University of Toronto, Toronto, Ontario, Canada

Drew Westen, Ph.D.
Professor of Psychology, Department of Psychology and Department of Psychiatry and Behavioral Sciences, Emory University, Atlanta, Georgia

Victoria Winkeller, M.D.
Medical Director, Children's Community Pediatrics Behavioral Health; Assistant Professor of Psychiatry, University of Pittsburgh School of Medicine, Pittsburgh, Pennsylvania

Frank E. Yeomans, M.D.
Clinical Associate Professor of Psychiatry, Weill Cornell Medical College; Adjunct Associate Professor of Psychiatry, Columbia University Center for Psychoanalytic Training and Research, New York, New York

Disclosure of Competing Interests

The following contributors to this book have indicated a financial interest in or other affiliation with a commercial supporter, a manufacturer of a commercial product, a provider of a commercial service, a nongovernmental organization, and/or a government agency, as listed below:

Anthony W. Bateman, M.A., FRCPsych—*Honoraria:* trainings in mentalization-based treatment; *Royalties:* various books on mentalizing

Donna S. Bender, Ph.D., FIPA—*Royalties:* American Psychiatric Association Publishing; Wolters Kluwer (UpToDate)

Donald W. Black, M.D.—*Consultant:* Otsuka

Nancee S. Blum, M.S.W.—*Royalties:* American Psychiatric Association Publishing (SIDP)

Peter Fonagy, Ph.D.—*Honoraria:* trainings in mentalization-based treatment; *Royalties:* various books on mentalizing

Carlos M. Grilo, Ph.D.—*Consultant:* Sunovion; Weight Watchers; *Honoraria:* lectures, CME activities, and presentations at scientific conferences and universities; *Royalties:* Guilford Press; Taylor & Francis

Patrick Luyten, Ph.D.—The author has been involved in the training, evaluation, and dissemination of mentalization-based therapy

Katharine J. Nelson, M.D.—*Grant support:* American Board of Psychiatry and Neurology; *Royalties:* Wolters Kluwer (UpToDate); Oxford University Press

John M. Oldham, M.D., M.S.—*Joint Editor: Journal of Personality Disorders* (Guilford); *Joint Editor-in-Chief: Borderline Personality Disorders and Emotion Dysregulation,* BioMed Central; *Co-owner:* Npsp25.com, LLC

Andrew E. Skodol, M.D.—*Royalties:* Merck (Merck Manual); Wolters Kluwer (UpToDate)

The following contributors have indicated that they have no financial interests or other affiliations that represent or could appear to represent a competing interest with the contributions to this book:

David M. Benedek, M.D., Col, M.C., U.S.A.
Philippe Boursiquot, M.D., FRCPC
Beth S. Brodsky, Ph.D.
Chloe Campbell, Ph.D.
Andrew M. Chanen, M.B.B.S., Ph.D., FRANZCP
Lois W. Choi-Kain, M.D., M.Ed.
John F. Clarkin, Ph.D.
Jennifer C. Elliott, Ph.D.
J. Christopher Fowler, Ph.D.
Sharely Fred Torres, M.D.
Lauren R. Gorfinkel, M.P.H.
Ilana Gratch, B.A.
Thomas G. Gutheil, M.D.
John M. Hart, Ph.D.
Deborah S. Hasin, Ph.D.
Sabine C. Herpertz, M.D.
Richard Hersh, M.D.
Christian Hicks, M.D.
David Kealy, Ph.D.
Amy R. Kegley, Ph.D.
Sophie Kerr, B.A.
Harold W. Koenigsberg, M.D.
Jay L. Lebow, Ph.D.
Kenneth N. Levy, Ph.D.

Madison Links, M.D.
Paul S. Links, M.D., FRCPC
Nicolas Lorenzini, Ph.D.
Ricky D. Malone, M.D., Col (Ret.) M.C., U.S.A.
Jacquelyn L. Meyers, Ph.D.
Leslie C. Morey, Ph.D.
Philip R. Muskin, M.D., M.A.
Sara Siris Nash, M.D., FACLP, FAPA
Antonia S. New, M.D.
John S. Ogrodniczuk, Ph.D.
William H. Orme, Ph.D.
Seth J. Prins, Ph.D., M.P.H.
Daniel R. Rosell, M.D., Ph.D.
Abigail B. Schlesinger, M.D.
Christian Schmahl, M.D.
Carla Sharp, Ph.D.
Jennifer Sotsky, M.D.
Barbara Stanley, Ph.D.
Svenn Torgersen, Ph.D.
Sherab Tsheringla, M.D.
Amanda A. Uliaszek, Ph.D.
Drew Westen, Ph.D.
Victoria Winkeller, M.D.
Frank E. Yeomans, M.D.

Preface

There is a vast and rich literature in science, medicine, philosophy, and the arts reflecting worldwide fascination with the subject of personality—what makes each of us unique and different from each other, and what determines the ways in which we are alike. The traditional mandate of medicine, however, is to understand illness— how to identify it, how to treat it, and how to prevent it. This new edition of *The American Psychiatric Association Publishing Textbook of Personality Disorders* brings to its pages the wisdom and guidance of some of the world's experts, and the energy and vision of a new generation of scientists, to teach us about the illnesses we call personality disorders. Particularly in the realm of personality, there are not clear categorical distinctions differentiating individuals with "normal" personalities from those who suffer from impairments in personality functioning. Personality functioning and personality traits exist along continuous spectra, from healthy to unhealthy and from adaptive to maladaptive. There are variations in the degree of disturbance in a person's sense of self and in interpersonal relationships (central defining aspects of personality disorders), but significant impairment in these areas of functioning plus the prevalence of pathological traits can impede a person's effective navigation in the world.

For decades, it was widely thought that some severely disturbed individuals just seemed to have been "born that way," a view resulting from cases with significant genetic loading or risk. We know, of course, that environments in early life are also critically important—these range from health-promoting, highly nurturing environments to stressful, abusive, or neglectful environments from which only the most resilient emerge unscathed. We are steadily learning more about complex polygenic risk factors that confer vulnerability to the development of most psychiatric disorders. The importance of epigenetics is increasingly recognized, clarifying the capacity of stressful environmental experiences to activate risk genes and launch a cascade of events resulting in the emergence of psychopathology, including personality pathology.

With the advent of standardized diagnostic systems, empirical and clinical research on the personality disorders has expanded. Semi-structured research interviews are being used to study clinical and community-based populations to provide better data about the epidemiology of these disorders. Overall, personality disorders occur in 11%–12% of the general population, and their public health significance has been well documented, reflecting sometimes extreme impairment in functioning and high health care utilization. As clinical populations are becoming better defined, new and more rigorous treatment studies are being carried out, with increasingly promising results. In addition, longitudinal naturalistic studies have shown surprising patterns of improvement in patients with selected personality disorders, challenging the assumption that these disorders are almost always "stable and enduring" over time. Genetic and neurobiological studies have clarified that the personality disorders, like other psychiatric disorders, emerge developmentally based on the combination of heritable risk factors and environmental stress.

Fundamental challenges remain, such as clarifying the relationship between normal personality and personality disorders themselves. A strong consensus has developed among personality experts that the personality disorders are best conceptualized dimensionally, and Section III, "Emerging Measures and Models," of DSM-5 contains an alternative model for the personality disorders, a hybrid dimensional and categorical model that is extensively referenced and discussed in this volume (see particularly Chapter 4, "The Alternative DSM-5 Model for Personality Disorders," and Chapter 5, "Manifestations, Assessment, Diagnosis, and Differential Diagnosis").

In light of the continuing and increased activity and progress in the field of personality studies and personality disorders, we judged the time to be right to develop this new edition of the *Textbook of Personality Disorders*, with an emphasis on updating information we believe to be essential to clinicians. Dozens of comprehensive tables and illustrative figures serve to succinctly summarize the vast data that continue to accumulate on personality pathology and to provide clinical guidance, and many real-life case examples further ensure the clinical relevance of the material.

The new volume is organized into five parts as detailed below.

Part I: Clinical Concepts

The first section of this textbook might be thought of as the foundation for the parts that follow. First, in Chapter 1 ("Personality Disorders: Recent History and New Directions"), Oldham presents a brief overview of the recent history of the personality disorders, along with a summary look at the evolution of the personality disorders component in successive editions of DSM, including the shift toward more dimensional representations of personality pathology. In Chapter 2 ("Theories of Personality and Personality Disorders"), Westen and Kegley review major theories that have influenced thinking about the nature of personality and personality disorders, including psychodynamic, cognitive-social, trait, and integrative theories. The next chapter (Chapter 3, "Articulating a Core Dimension of Personality Pathology"), by Morey and Bender, follows naturally from the previous one, emphasizing the fundamental roles of self and interpersonal functioning as core components of personality and as defining features of impairment in personality disorders. These concepts are central components of the Alternative DSM-5 Model for Personality Disorders (AMPD), described in more detail in Chapters 4 and 5. In Chapter 4, Skodol, Bender, and Oldham summarize current controversies about and present a detailed chronicle of the evidence supporting the AMPD, and the complex process of its development. In Chapter 5, Skodol reviews the defining features of DSM-5 Section II and Section III personality disorder assessment models, discusses complementary approaches to the clinical assessment of a patient with possible personality psychopathology, provides guidance on general problems encountered in the routine clinical evaluation, and outlines processes of diagnosis and guidelines for differential diagnosis according to the AMPD. Throughout,

Skodol provides expert guidance to introduce readers to the new model, clarifying the differences in the application of this innovative dimensional-categorical hybrid system compared with the traditional DSM-IV (and now DSM-5 Section II) categorical approach.

Part II: Risk Factors, Etiology, and Impact

Part II begins with data on prevalence, sociodemographics, and levels of functional impairment associated with personality disorders, described by Torgersen in Chapter 6 ("Prevalence, Sociodemographics, and Functional Impairment"). Although there are relatively few well-designed population-based studies, Torgersen reviews important contributions, including his own Norwegian study, and he tabulates prevalence ranges and averages for individual DSM-defined personality disorders as well as for all personality disorders taken together. Fonagy and colleagues, in Chapter 7 (Development, Attachment, and Childhood Experiences: A Mentalizing Perspective"), then present a developmental perspective, stressing the importance of healthy attachment experiences as building blocks for effective adult personality functioning. Disruptions in attachment, conversely, set the stage for future impairment, and they correlate strongly with the development of the neurobiological dysregulation that is present in many patients with personality disorders, described in Chapter 8 ("Genetics and Neurobiology") by Fred Torres and colleagues. In Chapter 9 ("Longitudinal Course and Outcomes"), Grilo and Skodol provide an overview of the clinical course and symptomatic and functional outcomes of personality disorders, synthesizing the empirical literature on the long-term course of personality disorder psychopathology, including the importance of comorbidity and continuity of psychopathology over time in understanding personality stability and change.

Part III: Treatment

Chapters 10–19 offer a range of treatment options and clinical considerations that cut across therapeutic modalities. In a new, cutting-edge chapter for the third edition of this textbook, Sharp and colleagues, in Chapter 10 ("Early Identification and Prevention of Personality Pathology: An AMPD-Informed Model of Clinical Staging"), argue for the early identification of borderline psychopathology in children and young adolescents, in an effort to prevent the development of the full-blown disorder later in life. The authors describe how the DSM-5 AMPD provides a framework for understanding why the transition from childhood to adulthood appears to be a sensitive period for the development of personality pathology, and a developmentally sensitive clinical staging approach to prevention of and early intervention for personality pathology. The treatment section continues with Chapter 11 ("Therapeutic Alliance"), in which Bender underscores the necessity of explicitly considering aspects of alliance building with various styles of personality psychopathology across all treatment modalities. Yeomans and colleagues, in Chapter 12 ("Psychodynamic Psychotherapies"), summarize the salient features of psychodynamic psychotherapies—both traditional and eclectic therapies—including discussions of mechanisms of change and of empirical validation, as applied to patients with personality pathology. In Chapter 13 ("Dialectical Behavioral Therapy"), Stanley and colleagues review the essentials of dialectical behavior therapy (DBT). In Chapter 14 ("Cognitive-Behavioral Therapy"), Fowler and colleagues summarize several specific cognitive-behavioral therapy strategies, including traditional cognitive-behavioral therapy itself, schema-focused therapy, and DBT, as applied in working with patients with personality disorders. In another new chapter for this edition, Chapter 15 ("Good Psychiatric Management: Generalist Treatments and Stepped Care for Borderline Personality Disorder"), Choi-Kain and Hersch detail the essentials of "Good Psychiatric Management," a treatment that can be used successfully by "generalists" in various mental health settings and in primary care, thus addressing a critical public health need caused by the shortage of therapists trained in "brand name," evidence-based treatments, such as DBT.

Apart from the realm of individual treatments, there are other venues for therapeutic interventions. In Chapter 16 ("Group, Family, and Couples Therapies"), Ogrodniczuk and colleagues demonstrate the application of group, family, and couples therapies to personality disorders, emphasizing the unique aspects of each type of therapy that can facilitate treatment of personality pathology. Nelson and Tsheringla then take up the issue, in Chapter 17 ("Pharmacological Management"), of pharmacotherapy, because many patients with personality disorders may benefit from complementing their psychosocial treatments with evidence-based, symptom-targeted adjunctive medications. Winkeller and Schlesinger, in Chapter 18 ("Collaborative Treatment"), provide recommendations about the best ways of negotiating collaborative treatments, because many patients with personality disorders are engaged in several treatment modalities with several clinicians at the same time. In the final chapter in this section (Chapter 19, "Boundary Issues"), Gutheil sagely cautions practitioners about dynamics that can lead to boundary violations when working with certain patients with personality disorders.

Part IV: Special Problems, Populations, and Settings

In recognition of the fact that patients with personality disorders can be particularly challenging, we have included five chapters devoted to special issues and populations. Of prime importance is the risk for suicide. In Chapter 20 ("Assessing and Managing Suicide Risk"), Links and colleagues provide evidence on the association of suicidal behavior and personality disorders, examine modifiable risk factors, and discuss clinical approaches to the assessment and management of suicide risk. In Chapter 21 ("Co-occurring Substance Use Disorders"), Gorfinkel and colleagues focus on pathways to co-occurring substance abuse in patients with personality disorders, and they discuss issues of differential diagnosis and treatment. Substance use and abuse is common in many patients with personality disorders, perhaps particularly in patients with antisocial personality disorder. Black and Blum, in Chapter 22 ("Antisocial Personality Disorder and Other Antisocial Behavior"), present the latest findings regarding antisocial behavior. Of the personality disorders, antisocial personality disorder is one of the costliest to society, and it can be associated with serious personal consequences. Unfortunately, far too little is available to offer at this point in terms of effective treatment, and many of these individuals end up in correctional and forensic settings.

In Chapter 23 ("Personality Disorders in the Medical Setting"), Nash and colleagues provide a new take on presentations of personality pathology in general medical settings, and how to manage them, since physical conditions frequently coexist with and are complicated by personality pathology and patients with personality disorders often seek treatment from primary care or family medicine practitioners. In the final chapter in this section, Chapter 24 ("Personality Disorders in the Military Operational Environment"), Malone and Benedek focus on an important population that often gets overlooked: soldiers on active duty in the U.S. military. In military settings, personality disorders can be masked or unrecognized but can eventually lead to significant impairment in functioning. The armed services are increasingly alert to the accurate recognition of personality disorders within their ranks, and to the not uncommon co-occurrence of PTSD, traumatic brain injury, major depression, and suicide risk.

Part V: Future Directions

In the final chapter of this textbook (Chapter 25, "Translational Research in Borderline Personality Disorder"), Schmahl and Herpertz focus on the increasing usefulness of translational research to deepen understanding of the biopsychosocial nature of the personality disorders, particularly borderline personality disorder. They discuss recent research on dysfunctions of social interaction and the role of oxytocin, and on perceptual alterations, including pain processing and dissociation, believed to be central to borderline pathology.

We are grateful to all of the chapter authors for their careful and thoughtful contributions, and we hope that we have succeeded in providing a current, definitive review of the field.

Andrew E. Skodol, M.D.
John M. Oldham, M.D., M.S.

PART I

Clinical Concepts

CHAPTER 1

Personality Disorders

Recent History and New Directions

John M. Oldham, M.D., M.S.

Personality Types and Personality Disorders

People are different, and what makes us different from one another has a lot to do with something called personality, the phenotypic patterns of thoughts, feelings, and behaviors that uniquely define each of us. In many important ways, we are what we do. At a school reunion, for example, recognition of classmates not seen for decades derives as much from familiar behavior as from physical appearance. To varying degrees, heritable temperaments that differ widely from one individual to another determine an amazing range of human behavior. Even in the newborn nursery, one can see strikingly different infants, ranging from cranky babies to placid ones. Throughout life, each individual's temperament remains a key component of that person's developing personality, added to by the shaping and molding influences of family, caregivers, and environmental experiences. This process is also bidirectional, so that the "inborn" behavior of the infant can elicit behavior in parents or caregivers that can, in turn, reinforce infant behavior: placid, happy babies may elicit warm and nurturing behaviors; irritable babies may elicit impatient and neglectful behaviors.

But even-tempered, easy-to-care-for infants can have bad luck and land in a nonsupportive or even abusive environment, which may set the stage for a personality disorder (PD), and difficult-to-care-for infants can have good luck, protected from future personality pathology by specially talented and attentive caregivers. Once these highly individualized dynamics have had their main effects and an individual has reached late adolescence or young adulthood, his or her personality often will have been pretty well established. This is not an ironclad rule, however; there are "late bloomers," and high-impact life events can derail or reroute any of us. How much we can change if we need to and want to is variable, but change is possible. How we define the differences between personality styles and PDs, how the two relate to each other, what systems best capture the magnificent variety of nonpathological human behavior, and how we think about and deal with extremes of thoughts, feelings, and behaviors that we call PDs are spelled out in great detail in the chapters that follow in this textbook. In this first chapter, I briefly describe how the American Psychiatric Association (APA) has approached the definition and classification of the PDs, building on broader international concepts and theories of psychopathology.

Although personality pathology has been well known for centuries, it is often thought to reflect weakness of character or willfully offensive behavior, produced by faulty upbringing, rather than to be a type of "legitimate" psychopathology. In spite of these common attitudes, clinicians have long recognized that patients with personality problems experience significant emotional distress, often accompanied by disabling levels of impairment in social or occupational functioning. General clinical wisdom has guided treatment recommendations for these patients, at least for those who seek treatment, plus evidence-based treatment guidelines have been developed for patients with borderline PD. Patients with paranoid, schizoid, or antisocial patterns of thinking and behaving often do not seek treatment. Others, however, seek help for problems ranging from self-destructive behavior to anxious social isolation to just plain chronic misery, and many of these patients have specific or mixed PDs, often coexisting with other conditions such as mood or anxiety disorders.

The DSM System

Contrary to assumptions commonly encountered, PDs have been included in every edition of the APA's *Diagnostic and Statistical Manual of Mental Disorders* (DSM). Largely driven by the need for standardized psychiatric diagnoses in the context of World War II, the U.S. War Department, in 1943, developed a document labeled Technical Bulletin 203, representing a psychoanalytically oriented system of terminology for classifying mental illness precipitated by stress (Barton 1987). The APA charged its Committee on Nomenclature and Statistics to solicit expert opinion and to develop a diagnostic manual that would codify and standardize psychiatric diagnoses. This diagnostic system became the framework for the first edition of DSM (American Psychiatric Association 1952). This manual has subsequently been revised on several occasions, leading to new editions: DSM-II (American Psychiatric Association 1968), DSM-III (American Psychiatric Association 1980), DSM-III-R (American Psychiatric Association 1987), DSM-IV (American Psychiatric Association 1994), DSM-IV-TR (American Psychiatric Association 2000), and DSM-5 (American Psychiatric Association 2013).

Figure 1–1 portrays the ontogeny of diagnostic terms relevant to the PDs, from the first edition of DSM through DSM-5 (Skodol 1997). DSM-IV-TR involved only text revisions but retained the same diagnostic terms as DSM-IV, and DSM-5 (in its main diagnostic component, Section II, "Diagnostic Criteria and Codes") includes the same PD diagnoses as DSM-IV except that the two provisional diagnoses, passive-aggressive and depressive, listed in DSM-IV Appendix B, "Criteria Sets and Axes Provided for Further Study," have been deleted. Additionally, Section III, "Emerging Measures and Models," of DSM-5 includes the Alternative DSM-5 Model for Personality Disorders, which is reviewed extensively throughout this book.

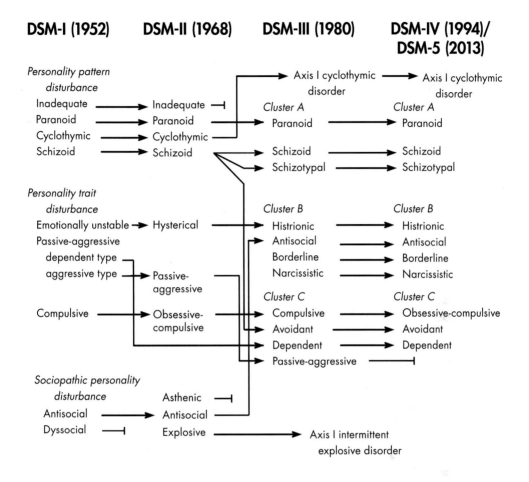

DSM-I (1952)	DSM-II (1968)	DSM-III (1980)	DSM-IV (1994)/ DSM-5 (2013)

Personality pattern disturbance
Inadequate → Inadequate ⊣
Paranoid → Paranoid →
Cyclothymic → Cyclothymic ⌐
Schizoid → Schizoid

→ Axis I cyclothymic disorder → Axis I cyclothymic disorder

Cluster A
Paranoid →

Cluster A
Paranoid →

Schizoid → Schizoid
Schizotypal → Schizotypal

Personality trait disturbance
Emotionally unstable → Hysterical →
Passive-aggressive
 dependent type ⌐
 aggressive type → Passive-aggressive

Cluster B
Histrionic → Histrionic
Antisocial → Antisocial
Borderline → Borderline
Narcissistic → Narcissistic

Cluster B

Compulsive → Obsessive-compulsive →

Cluster C
Compulsive → Obsessive-compulsive
Avoidant → Avoidant
Dependent → Dependent
Passive-aggressive ⊣

Cluster C

Sociopathic personality disturbance
 Asthenic ⊣
Antisocial → Antisocial ⊣
Dyssocial ⊣ Explosive → Axis I intermittent explosive disorder

⊣ Indicates that category was discontinued.

FIGURE 1–1. Ontogeny of personality disorder classification.

No changes were made to the personality disorder classification in DSM-III-R except for the inclusion of self-defeating and sadistic personality disorders in Appendix A. These two categories were not included in DSM-IV, DSM-IV-TR, or DSM-5. Passive-aggressive and depressive personality disorders were present in Appendix B of DSM-IV and DSM-IV-TR but have been removed from DSM-5. An Alternative DSM-5 Model for Personality Disorders (not shown here) is included in Section III, "Emerging Measures and Models," of DSM-5.

Source.   Modified from Skodol 1997.

Although not explicit in the narrative text, the first edition of DSM reflected the general view of PDs at the time, elements of which persist to the present. Generally, PDs were viewed as more or less permanent patterns of behavior and human interaction that were established by early adulthood and were unlikely to change throughout the life cycle. Thorny issues such as how to differentiate PDs from personality styles or traits, which remain actively debated today, were clearly identified.

In the first edition of DSM, PDs were generally viewed as deficit conditions, reflecting partial developmental arrests, or distortions in development secondary to inadequate or pathological early caregiving. The PDs were grouped primarily into *personality pattern disturbances*, *personality trait disturbances*, and *sociopathic personality*. Personality pattern disturbances were viewed as the most entrenched conditions, likely to be recalcitrant to change, even with treatment; these conditions included inadequate personality, schizoid personality, cyclothymic personality, and paranoid personality. Personality trait disturbances were thought to be less pervasive and disabling, so in the absence of stress these patients could function relatively well. If under significant stress, however, patients with emotionally unstable, passive-aggressive, or compulsive personalities were thought to show emotional distress and deterioration in functioning, and they were variably motivated for and amenable to treatment. The category of sociopathic personality reflected what were generally seen as types of social deviance; it included antisocial reaction, dyssocial reaction, sexual deviation, and addiction (subcategorized into alcoholism and drug addiction).

The primary stimulus leading to the development of a new, second edition of DSM was the publication of the eighth revision of the *International Classification of Diseases* (World Health Organization 1967) and the wish of the APA to reconcile its diagnostic terminology with this international system. In the DSM revision process, an effort was made to move away from theory-derived diagnoses and to reach consensus on the main constellations of personality that were observable, measurable, enduring, and consistent over time. The earlier view that patients with PDs did not experience emotional distress was discarded, as were the subcategories described in the previous paragraph. One new PD was added, called asthenic PD, only to be deleted in the next edition of DSM.

By the mid-1970s, greater emphasis was placed on increasing the reliability of all diagnoses. DSM-III defined PDs (and all other disorders) by explicit diagnostic criteria and introduced a multiaxial evaluation system. Disorders classified on Axis I included those generally seen as episodic "symptom disorders" characterized by exacerbations and remissions, such as psychoses, mood disorders, and anxiety disorders. Axis II was established to include the PDs as well as specific developmental disorders; both groups were seen as being composed of early-onset, persistent conditions, but the specific developmental disorders were understood to be "biological" in origin, in contrast to the PDs, which were generally regarded as "psychological" in origin. The decision to place the PDs on Axis II led to greater recognition of the PDs and stimulated extensive research and progress in our understanding of these conditions. (New data, however, have called into question the rationale to conceptualize the PDs as fundamentally different from other types of psychopathology, such as mood or anxiety disorders, and in any event the multiaxial system of DSM-III and DSM-IV has been removed in DSM-5.)

As shown in Figure 1–1, the DSM-II diagnoses of inadequate PD and asthenic PD were discontinued in DSM-III. Also in DSM-III, the DSM-II diagnosis of explosive PD was changed to intermittent explosive disorder, cyclothymic PD was renamed cyclothymic disorder, and both of these diagnoses were moved to Axis I. Schizoid PD was thought to be too broad a category in DSM-II and therefore was recrafted into three PDs: schizoid PD, reflecting "loners" who are uninterested in close personal relationships; schizotypal PD, understood to be on the schizophrenia spectrum of disorders and characterized by eccentric beliefs and nontraditional behavior; and avoidant PD, typified by self-imposed interpersonal isolation driven by self-consciousness and anxiety. Two new PD diagnoses were added in DSM-III: borderline PD and narcissistic PD. In contrast to initial notions that patients called "borderline" were on the border between the psychoses and the neuroses, the criteria defining borderline PD in DSM-III emphasized emotion dysregulation, unstable interpersonal relationships, and loss of impulse control more than persistent cognitive distortions and marginal reality testing, which were more characteristic of schizotypal PD. Among many scholars whose work greatly influenced and shaped the conceptualization of borderline pathology introduced in DSM-III were Kernberg (1975) and Gunderson (1984). Although concepts of narcissism had been described by Sigmund Freud, Wilhelm Reich, and others, the essence of the current views of narcissistic PD emerged from the work of Millon (1969), Kohut (1971), and Kernberg (1975).

DSM-III-R was published in 1987 after an intensive process to revise DSM-III, involving widely solicited input from researchers and clinicians and following similar principles to those articulated in DSM-III, such as ensuring reliable diagnostic categories that were clinically useful and consistent with research findings, thus minimizing reliance on theory. In DSM-III-R, no changes were made in diagnostic categories of PDs, although some adjustments were made in certain criteria sets—for example, they were made uniformly polythetic instead of defining some PDs with monothetic criteria sets (i.e., with all criteria required), such as for dependent PD, and others with polythetic criteria sets (i.e., with some minimum number, but not all criteria, required), such as for borderline PD. In addition, on the basis of previous clinical recommendations to the DSM-III-R PD subcommittee, two PDs were included in DSM-III-R in Appendix A, "Proposed Diagnostic Categories Needing Further Study": self-defeating PD and sadistic PD. These diagnoses were considered provisional.

DSM-IV was developed after an extensive process of literature review, data analysis, field trials, and feedback from the profession. Because of the increase in research stimulated by the criteria-based multiaxial system of DSM-III, more evidence existed to guide the DSM-IV process. As a result, the threshold for approval of revisions for DSM-IV was a higher one than that used in DSM-III or DSM-III-R. DSM-IV introduced, for the first time, a set of general diagnostic criteria for any PD, underscoring qualities such as early onset, long duration, inflexibility, and pervasiveness. These general criteria, however, were developed by expert consensus and were not derived empirically. Diagnostic categories and dimensional organization of the PDs into clusters remained the same in DSM-IV as in DSM-III-R, with the exception of the relocation of passive-aggressive PD from the "official" diagnostic list to Appendix B, "Criteria Sets and Axes Provided for Further Study." Passive-aggressive PD, as defined by DSM-III and DSM-III-R, was thought to be too unidimensional and generic; it was tentatively retitled "negativistic PD," and the criteria were revised. In addition, the two provisional Axis II diagnoses in DSM-III-R, self-defeating PD and sadistic PD, were dropped because of insufficient research data and clinical consensus to support their retention. One other PD, depressive PD, was proposed and added to Appendix B. Although substantially controversial, this provisional diagnosis was proposed as a pessimistic cognitive style, presumably distinct from passive-aggressive PD or dysthymic disorder.

The diagnostic terms and criteria of DSM-IV were not changed in DSM-IV-TR, published in 2000. The intent of DSM-IV-TR was to revise the descriptive, narrative text accompanying each diagnosis where it seemed indicated and to update the information provided. Only minimal revisions were made in the text material accompanying the PDs.

Since the publication of DSM-IV, new knowledge has rapidly accumulated about the PDs, and discussions about controversial areas have intensified. Although DSM-IV had an increased empirical basis compared with previous versions of DSM, some limitations of the categorical approach were apparent, and many unanswered questions remained. Are the PDs fundamentally different from other categories of major mental illness such as mood disorders or anxiety disorders? What is the relationship of normal personality to PD? Are the PDs best conceptualized dimensionally or categorically? What are the pros and cons of polythetic criteria sets, and what should determine the appropriate number of criteria (i.e., threshold) required for each diagnosis? Which PD categories have construct validity? Which dimensions best cover the full scope of normal and abnormal personality? Many of these discussions overlap with and inform one another.

Among these controversies, one stands out with particular prominence: whether a dimensional approach or a categorical one is preferred to classify the PDs. Much of the literature poses this topic as a debate or competition, as if one must choose sides. Dimensional structure implies continuity, whereas categorical structure implies discontinuity. For example, being pregnant is a categorical concept, whereas height might be better conceptualized dimensionally because there is no exact definition of "tall" or "short," notions of tallness or shortness may vary among different cultures, and all gradations of height exist along a continuum.

We know, of course, that the DSM system is referred to as categorical and is contrasted with any number of systems referred to as dimensional, such as the interpersonal circumplex (Benjamin 1993; Kiesler 1983; Wiggins 1982), the three-factor model (Eysenck and Eysenck 1975), several four-factor models (Clark et al. 1996; Livesley et al. 1993, 1998; Watson et al. 1994; Widiger 1998), the "Big Five" model (Costa and McCrae 1992), and the seven-factor model (Cloninger et al. 1993). How fundamental is the difference between the two types of systems? Elements of dimensionality already exist in the traditional DSM categorical system, represented by the organization of the PDs into Cluster A (odd or eccentric), Cluster B (dramatic, emotional, or erratic), and Cluster C (anxious or fearful). (This cluster system was based on descriptive patterns, grouping the PDs according to prominent cognitive symptoms [A], prominent mood symptoms [B], and prominent anxiety symptoms [C]. However, a persuasive empirical basis to validate these clusters has not been demonstrated [e.g., Bastiaansen et al. 2011; O'Connor 2005]). In addition, a patient can just meet the threshold for a PD or can have all of the criteria, presumably a more extreme version of the disorder. Certainly, if a patient is one criterion short of receiving a PD diagnosis, clinicians do not necessarily assume that no element of the disorder is present; instead, prudent clinicians would understand that features of the disorder need to be recognized if present and may need attention. Busy clinicians, however, often think categorically, deciding what disorder or disorders a patient "officially" has. In practice, when a patient is thought to have a PD, clinicians generally assign only one PD diagnosis, whereas systematic studies of clinical populations that use semistructured interviews show that patients with personality psychopathology generally have multiple PD diagnoses (Oldham et al. 1992; Shedler and Westen 2004; Skodol et al. 1988; Widiger et al. 1991).

In the early 2000s, the APA convened, in collaboration with the National Institute of Mental Health, a series of research conferences to develop an agenda for DSM-5, the proceedings of which were subsequently published. In an introductory monograph (Kupfer et al. 2002), a chapter was devoted to personality and relational disorders, in which First et al. (2002) stated that "the classification scheme offered by the DSM-IV for both of these domains is woefully inadequate in meeting the goals of facilitating communication among clinicians and researchers or in enhancing the clinical management of those conditions" (p. 179). In that same volume, in a chapter on basic nomenclature issues, Rounsaville et al. (2002) argued that "well-informed clinicians and researchers have suggested that variation in psychiatric symptomatology may be better represented by dimensions than by a set of categories, especially in the area of personality traits" (p. 12). Subsequently, an entire monograph, "Dimensional Models of Personality Disorders: Refining the Research Agenda for DSM-V" (Widiger et al. 2006), was published, with in-depth analyses of dimensional approaches for the PDs. Shortly thereafter, a Work Group on Personality and Personality Disorders was established by the APA, and efforts were launched to develop a dimensional proposal for the PDs for DSM-5. This process is described in detail in this volume (Chapter 4, "The Alternative DSM-5 Model for Personality Disorders"). It was challenging for the work group to reach a consensus in support of a single dimensional model for the PDs to be used in clinical practice, just as it had been difficult for the field. In the end, a hybrid dimensional and categorical model was proposed, and this model was approved by the APA as an alternative model and placed in Section III of DSM-5, whereas the DSM-IV criteria-defined categorical system was retained in Section II of the manual, for continued use. The alternative model includes six specific PDs, plus a seventh diagnosis of *personality disorder—trait specified* that allows description of individual trait profiles of patients with PDs who do not have any of the six specified disorders. In addition, the alternative model involves assignment of level of impairment in functioning, an important additional element of dimensionality when making PD diagnoses. As described in Chapter 5, "Manifestations, Assessment, Diagnosis, and Differential Diagnosis," the alternative model also presents a coherent core definition of all PDs, as moderate or greater impairment in self and interpersonal functioning, along with five pathological trait domains, each of which is characterized by a set of trait facets.

Questions have been raised about the stability of the PDs over time, even though their enduring nature is one of the generic defining features of the PDs in DSM-5 Section II. Personality pathology is often activated or intensified by circumstance, such as the loss of a job or the end of a meaningful relationship. In the ongoing findings of the Collaborative Longitudinal Personality Disorders Study (CLPS), for example, stability of DSM-IV–defined PD diagnoses reflected sustained pathology at or above the diagnostic threshold, but substantial percentages of patients showed fluctuation over time, sometimes being above and sometimes below the diagnostic threshold (Gunderson et al. 2011). In the CLPS, which used a stringent definition of remission (the presence of no more than two criteria for at least 1 year), 85% of patients with DSM-IV–defined borderline PD at intake showed remission at the 10-year follow-up point. However, impairment in functioning was much slower to remit, perhaps consistent with more recent evidence indicating that trait-defined PDs are more persistent over time than DSM-IV–defined PDs (Hopwood et al. 2013).

Finally, it is interesting to note the substantial revision in the classification of PDs in ICD-11. This new edition was released in June 2018 and was adopted by the World

Health Assembly in May 2019 (Pull and Janca 2020). ICD-11 removes all but one of the ICD-10 categorical PD syndromes and replaces them with one primary diagnosis of PD, adding one subcategory, as a borderline PD qualifier. ICD-11 also specifies five trait domains that, for the most part, align remarkably well with the trait domains of the Alternative DSM-5 Model for Personality Disorders. In addition, the ICD-11 system requires assessment of the level of severity of impairment resulting from the PD (Bach et al. 2020; Bagby and Widiger 2020). Overall, there is a growing convergence in the field toward more dimensional approaches to our understanding of the PDs.

Conclusion

This brief review of the history of the classification of personality pathology serves as a window on the progress in our field and in our understanding of the PDs. Increasingly, a stress/diathesis framework seems applicable in medicine in general, as a unifying model of illness—a model that can easily apply to the PDs. Variable genetic vulnerabilities predispose us all to potential future illness, which may or may not develop depending on the balance of specific stressors and protective factors.

The PDs can be thought of as maladaptive exaggerations of nonpathological personality styles, resulting from predisposing temperaments combined with stressful circumstances. Neurobiological abnormalities have been identified in at least some PDs, as is the case in many other psychiatric disorders. Our challenge for the future is to better characterize variations in personality psychopathology and determine whether and how PDs are different from other classes of psychiatric disorders. As we learn more about the etiologies and pathology of the PDs, it will no longer be necessary, or even desirable, to limit our diagnostic schemes to atheoretical, descriptive phenomena, and we can look forward to an enriched understanding of personality pathology, better treatments, and guidance for prevention.

References

American Psychiatric Association: Diagnostic and Statistical Manual: Mental Disorders. Washington, DC, American Psychiatric Association, 1952

American Psychiatric Association: Diagnostic and Statistical Manual of Mental Disorders, 2nd Edition. Washington, DC, American Psychiatric Association, 1968

American Psychiatric Association: Diagnostic and Statistical Manual of Mental Disorders, 3rd Edition. Washington, DC, American Psychiatric Association, 1980

American Psychiatric Association: Diagnostic and Statistical Manual of Mental Disorders, 3rd Edition, Revised. Washington, DC, American Psychiatric Association, 1987

American Psychiatric Association: Diagnostic and Statistical Manual of Mental Disorders, 4th Edition. Washington, DC, American Psychiatric Association, 1994

American Psychiatric Association: Diagnostic and Statistical Manual of Mental Disorders, 4th Edition, Text Revision. Washington, DC, American Psychiatric Association, 2000

American Psychiatric Association: Diagnostic and Statistical Manual of Mental Disorders, 5th Edition. Arlington, VA, American Psychiatric Association, 2013

Bach B, Kerber A, Aluja A, et al: International assessment of DSM-5 and ICD-11 personality disorder traits: toward a common nosology in DSM-5.1. Psychopathology 53(3–4):179–188, 2020.

Bagby RM, Widiger TA: Assessment of the ICD-11 dimensional trait model: an introduction to the special section. Psychol Assess 32:1–7, 2020

Barton WE: The History and Influence of the American Psychiatric Association. Washington, DC, American Psychiatric Press, 1987

Bastiaansen L, Rossi G, Schotte C, DeFruyt F: The structure of personality disorders: comparing DSM-IV-TR Axis II classification with the five-factor model framework using structural equation modeling. J Pers Disord 25:378–396, 2011

Benjamin LS: Interpersonal Diagnosis and Treatment of Personality Disorders. New York, Guilford, 1993

Clark LA, Livesley WJ, Schroeder ML, et al: Convergence of two systems for assessing specific traits of personality disorder. Psychol Assess 8:294–303, 1996

Cloninger CR, Svrakic DM, Przybeck TR: A psychobiological model of temperament and character. Arch Gen Psychiatry 50:975–990, 1993

Costa PT, McCrae RR: The five-factor model of personality and its relevance to personality disorders. J Pers Disord 6:343–359, 1992

Eysenck HJ, Eysenck SBG: Manual of the Eysenck Personality Questionnaire. San Diego, CA, Educational and Industrial Testing Service, 1975

First MB, Bell CC, Cuthbert B, et al: Personality disorders and relational disorders: a research agenda for addressing crucial gaps in DSM, in A Research Agenda for DSM-V. Edited by Kupfer DJ, First MB, Regier DA. Washington, DC, American Psychiatric Association, 2002, pp 123–199

Gunderson JG: Borderline Personality Disorder. Washington, DC, American Psychiatric Press, 1984

Gunderson JG, Stout RL, McGlashan TH, et al: Ten-year course of borderline personality disorder: psychopathology and function from the Collaborative Longitudinal Personality Disorders Study. Arch Gen Psychiatry 68:827–837, 2011

Hopwood CJ, Morey LC, Donnellan MB, et al: Ten-year rank-order stability of personality traits and disorders in a clinical sample. J Pers 81:335–344, 2013

Kernberg O: Borderline Conditions and Pathological Narcissism. New York, Jason Aronson, 1975

Kiesler DJ: The 1982 interpersonal circle: a taxonomy for complementarity in human transactions. Psychological Review 90:185–214, 1983

Kohut H: The Analysis of the Self: A Systematic Approach to the Psychoanalytic Treatment of Narcissistic Personality Disorders. New York, International Universities Press, 1971

Kupfer DJ, First MB, Regier DA (eds): A Research Agenda for DSM-V. Washington, DC, American Psychiatric Association, 2002

Livesley WJ, Jang KL, Jackson DN, et al: Genetic and environmental contributions to dimensions of personality disorder. Am J Psychiatry 150:1826–1831, 1993

Livesley WJ, Jang KL, Vernon PA: Phenotypic and genetic structure of traits delineating personality disorder. Arch Gen Psychiatry 55:941–948, 1998

Millon T: Modern Psychopathology: A Biosocial Approach to Maladaptive Learning and Functioning. Philadelphia, PA, WB Saunders, 1969

O'Connor BP: A search for consensus on the dimensional structure of personality disorders. J Clin Psychol 61:323–345, 2005

Oldham JM, Skodol AE, Kellman HD, et al: Diagnosis of DSM-III-R personality disorders by two structured interviews: patterns of comorbidity. Am J Psychiatry 149:213–220, 1992

Pull CB, Janca A: Arrangement for personality disorder in the 11th Revision of the International Classification of Diseases. Curr Opin Psychiatry 33:43–44, 2020

Rounsaville BJ, Alarcón RD, Andrews G, et al: Basic nomenclature issues for DSM-V, in A Research Agenda for DSM-V. Edited by Kupfer DJ, First MB, Regier DA. Washington, DC, American Psychiatric Association, 2002, pp 1–30

Shedler J, Westen D: Refining personality disorder diagnosis: integrating science and practice. Am J Psychiatry 161:1350–1365, 2004

Skodol AE: Classification, assessment, and differential diagnosis of personality disorders. J Pract Psychiatry Behav Health 3:261–274, 1997

Skodol AE, Rosnick L, Kellman D, et al: Validating structured DSM-III-R personality disorder assessments with longitudinal data. Am J Psychiatry 145:1297–1299, 1988

Watson D, Clark LA, Harkness AR: Structures of personality and their relevance to psychopathology. J Abnorm Psychol 103:18–31, 1994

Widiger TA: Four out of five ain't bad (commentary). Arch Gen Psychiatry 55:865–866, 1998

Widiger TA, Frances AJ, Harris M, et al: Comorbidity among Axis II disorders, in Personality Disorders: New Perspectives on Diagnostic Validity. Edited by Oldham JM. Washington, DC, American Psychiatric Press, 1991, pp 163–194

Widiger TA, Simonsen E, Sirovatka PJ, et al (eds): Dimensional Models of Personality Disorders: Refining the Research Agenda for DSM-V. Arlington, VA, American Psychiatric Association, 2006

Wiggins J: Circumplex models of interpersonal behavior in clinical psychology, in Handbook of Research Methods in Clinical Psychology. Edited by Kendall P, Butcher J. New York, Wiley, 1982, pp 183–221

World Health Organization: International Classification of Diseases, 8th Revision. Geneva, World Health Organization, 1967

CHAPTER 2

Theories of Personality and Personality Disorders

Drew Westen, Ph.D.

Amy R. Kegley, Ph.D.

Personality refers to enduring patterns of thought, feeling, motivation, self-regulation, and behavior that are activated over time and across situations or in interpersonally or adaptively significant situations (see Mischel and Shoda 1995; Westen 1995). In one sense, this is a minimalist, intentionally descriptive definition that most personality psychologists would accept, despite their widely differing theories. However, it underscores several key aspects of personality and explains why personality plays such an important role, on the one hand, in life satisfaction and adaptation and, on the other, as a key diathesis for (i.e., a source of vulnerability to) virtually every form of pathology in DSM-5 (American Psychiatric Association 2013)—from personality disorders (PDs) themselves to anxiety, mood, and other disorders.

That is why assessing personality is so essential for both clinical work and research, despite the failure to assess it comprehensively in initial clinical interviews in many forms of treatment and in the vast majority of studies of disorders for which research has found personality to be a primary diathesis. Those disorders range from what are generally considered *internalizing disorders,* such as anxiety and depressive disorders, to *externalizing disorders,* such as disruptive, impulse-control, and conduct disorders and many substance-related and addictive disorders (although internalizing personality characteristics such as anxiety and depression can lead to self-medication), to disorders that are not so readily classified or have elements of both, such as trauma-

Preparation of the manuscript for this chapter was supported in part by National Institute of Mental Health grants MH59685 and MH60892.

and stressor-related disorders, dissociative disorders, and feeding and eating disorders (Kotov et al. 2017; Krueger et al. 1998; Westen et al. 2006).

Personality and Personality Pathology

Among the implications of that definition, first, personality encompasses the major functional domains in human life and social interaction, which is why it is or should be correlated with and predictive of both adaptive functioning and psychopathology. It is not limited to one or another domain (e.g., cognition or affect). It refers to all of these domains and the ways they can interact. Key to both adaptation and pathology are how clearly and creatively we think and under what circumstances our thought can become disrupted by external circumstances or "internal circumstances," such as strong affect. Equally key to adaptation and pathology are what we can and cannot feel or allow ourselves to feel; what we feel too intensely or not intensely enough; what we wish for, fear, and value; and how we regulate our thoughts, feelings, motives, and behavior, both consciously and unconsciously (or explicitly and implicitly, depending on which theoretical language one prefers). Perhaps most important for adaptation and pathology are the ways we habitually behave, particularly interpersonally (which reflects the ways we experience ourselves, important people in our lives, and relationships, cognitively, affectively, and motivationally), and the extent to which we can adjust our behavior depending on the situation (which depends on personality domains such as awareness and adaptive use of our affects and how well and in what ways we regulate our affects and impulses). All of these functions are among those described by personality theorists since the early twentieth century, when the field of personality began.

As importantly, these domains, and the myriad ways in which they interact, can create problems at any level of severity. At the milder end of the spectrum of *personality pathology* (the broader term for personality problems, which may or may not rise to the level of PDs) are the kinds of enduring patterns that simply make people's lives more complicated or lead to mild or episodic but temporary distress in themselves or the people around them. For example, a person may be self-critical or overly critical of others (empirically, the two tend to correlate more strongly than one might suppose), prone to shame or guilt, or prone to turning anger into sadness, but these habitual ways of responding do not substantially interfere with the ability to form good relationships, to work effectively, or to enjoy life (the three primary components of psychological health—adding the third to Sigmund Freud's famous dictum that psychological health is the capacity to love and to work).

At the other end of the spectrum are severe PDs, which typically involve dysfunction across several or all of the domains of functioning outlined earlier. Schizotypal PD, for example, is characterized first and foremost by peculiarities of thinking, but it also includes flat or peculiar emotions, disturbances in motivation, difficulty regulating thought and emotion, and peculiar interpersonal behavior. Borderline PD (BPD) is characterized by disturbances in thinking when strong affect is aroused, particularly in attachment relationships; substantial deficits in affect regulation, not only strong negative affects but more broadly with difficulty regulating affects, impulses, and cognition when emotions become powerful; and a range of interpersonal problems in close relationships, associated with problematic ways of viewing the self and others and regulating behavior, particularly in intimate relationships but also often in work situations, which require consistency of behavior that cannot depend on the person's mood.

Second, irrespective of the severity or the degree to which personality characteristics disrupt adaptive functioning, they are enduring over time. Some forms of pathology, such as the tendency to experience anxiety or depression or to be angry or aggressive or lack empathy for other people, may be consistent over time, beginning as early as the preschool years. Aggressive preschoolers, anxious children, and borderline adolescents often grow into aggressive, anxious, or borderline adults. But consistency over time can be far more complex. Aggression in preschool (e.g., pushing other kids) may look very different from aggression in adulthood (e.g., repeatedly driving subordinates to tears with explosive behaviors in meetings or criticism). Alternatively, a child who has trouble forming friendships when young may grow out of it, may develop a stably avoidant attachment style, may develop peculiar thinking as part of a neurodevelopmental disorder, or may get involved with aggressive or otherwise externalizing teenagers as a way of "belonging" in adolescence. Nevertheless, if an underlying personality disposition (e.g., difficulty relating to other people, tendency to be rejected or neglected by peers) persists but takes different forms at different times, it is still an enduring aspect of personality.

Similarly, internalizing and externalizing tendencies in childhood may predict very different forms of pathology in adulthood, such as the tendency to be anxious or depressed versus psychopathic or substance abusing. However, these broad dimensions tend to be highly correlated in childhood and may have genetic and environmental variance in common (Mikolajewski et al. 2013). Thus, a child who expressed distress through disruptive or delinquent behavior in childhood may continue to experience distress as an adult but express it instead as anxiety, depression, or avoidance or, more broadly, in anxious, depressive, or detached personality pathology. Empirically, personality pathology in childhood or adolescence is as likely to manifest in symptoms such as major depression as it is in a PD in adulthood, because it may create a vulnerability to a range of symptoms or personality constellations (see Cohen et al. 2005; Stringaris et al. 2015; Venta et al. 2014).

Third, although personality pathology may be more readily recognizable to the extent that aspects of personality are so rigid or generalized that they appear cross-situationally (e.g., inability to regulate aggression that prevents a person from maintaining both jobs and relationships), the enduring ways of responding that characterize personality need not be broadly generalized to be aspects of personality or to lead to distress or dysfunction. Many personality processes are triggered by specific situations, activating thoughts, feelings, motives, and unconscious networks of associations that trigger automatized reactions or bring to the fore feelings that seem to other people or the person himself or herself inappropriate to the situation. For example, a tendency to bristle and respond with opposition, anger, or passive resistance to perceived demands of male authority figures, stemming from a difficult relationship with a harsh, critical father, may or may not be present with female authorities, peers, lovers, colleagues or coworkers, or subordinates. Nevertheless, this tendency can reflect enduring patterns of thought, feeling, motivation, emotion, self-regulation, or behavior that can lead to distress or dysfunction.

Psychosocial Versus Biological Approaches to Personality Disorders: Descartes' Other Error

Of the dozens of approaches to personality advanced over the past century, we focus here on the two most widely used in clinical practice—psychodynamic and cognitive-social or cognitive-behavioral—and one widely used in guiding research: trait approaches. We then focus on two integrative approaches.

In previous editions of this chapter, we included a "Biological Perspectives" section, which included behavioral genetic and neural systems approaches. That seemed appropriate at the time for multiple reasons. Perhaps first and foremost, biological perspectives have influenced the understanding and classification of PDs from the start, reflected in the first two and all subsequent editions of the DSM, beginning with the observations of the pioneering psychiatric taxonomists in the early twentieth century. Bleuler (1911/1950), Kraepelin (1896/1919), and others noticed that the relatives of patients with schizophrenia (or what today we would call, more broadly, psychotic disorders) sometimes appeared to have attenuated symptoms of the disorder that never crossed a threshold for psychosis but reflected enduring aspects of their personalities. In particular, they noted both cognitive and interpersonal peculiarities that today we would consider attenuated versions of positive and negative symptoms, respectively. They similarly noted that the relatives of severely depressed patients often showed stably "melancholic" features at a low level or that relatives of "manic-depressive" patients often had subthreshold symptoms that appeared to be enduring aspects of personality.

Including a section called "Biological Perspectives" also, however, reflected an implicit acceptance of the mind-body, mind-brain, and nature-nurture distinctions that have been central to Western philosophy[1] for millennia and were equally central to theoretical arguments in psychiatry and psychology throughout the twentieth century. Those included arguments as to whether personality and PDs were "psychological" or "biological" phenomena. Today, however, particularly in light of developments in genetics, epigenetics, and neuroimaging, the separation of "biological" from "psychosocial" disorders or approaches is no longer tenable for three reasons that are crucial to any theoretical understanding of personality and its pathology.

First, for decades psychologists, psychiatrists, and other professionals concerned with mental health asked the question, "Which is more important, nature or nurture?" In different eras, they arrived at different conclusions. In the 1920s, the hyperbolic behaviorist (who no doubt learned his flair for drama environmentally) John Watson declared that he could turn anyone into anything by simply shaping environmental conditions. A less extreme but nonetheless strongly envirocentric view dominated the 1960s, an era of both prosperity and "social engineering," in which changing social conditions did, in fact, produce substantial alterations in personality, as witnessed, for ex-

---

[1]Descartes, for example, tried to solve this problem by locating the region in which the mind and body-brain converge in the pineal gland. We do not, of course, mean to disparage a genius whose insights were central to the development of modern science, mathematics, and philosophy, who brought us, among things, Cartesian coordinates—an achievement we unfortunately are not in a position to match, despite the advantage of a few extra centuries.

ample, in changing norms, values, and behaviors caused by the women's movement and efforts to combat racism, which allowed people of color to express aspects of themselves that had been suppressed for centuries in the United States. With the development of behavioral genetics, however, the pendulum swung in the opposite direction by the 1970s and 1980s, with results seeming to show strong heritability and weak shared environmental effects for virtually every cognitive and personality trait studied. That fueled an intensity in the nature-nurture debate.

Today, we have, at long last, an answer to the nature-nurture and mind-body debate: we have been asking the wrong question. Research in genetics, epigenetics, and developmental psychopathology has made it amply clear, beginning perhaps most dramatically with the work of Caspi, Moffitt, and colleagues in their longitudinal analyses of their population sample in Dunedin, New Zealand, that whether a particular allele is of etiological significance to personality and psychopathology, such as antisocial behavior, suicidality, or depression, frequently depends on the presence or absence of specific developmental experiences, such as childhood sexual or physical abuse (Caspi et al. 2002, 2010).

Research in behavioral genetics, although not an alternative theory of personality pathology, remains highly relevant to understanding its etiology (see Chapter 8, "Genetics and Neurobiology," in this volume). It is also now widely used, in combination with the latest techniques for aggregating multivariate data, to derive and validate empirically based taxonomies (Krueger et al. 1998; Livesley 2011; see also Kendler et al. 2011; Wichers et al. 2013). Behavioral genetic studies have shown moderate to large heritability (30%–60%) for a range of personality traits (Livesley et al. 1993; Plomin and Caspi 1999) of relevance to PDs. The most frequently studied traits—extraversion and neuroticism—have produced heritability estimates of 54%–74% and 42%–64%, respectively (Eysenck 1990).

As we have known for decades, however, environmental and genetic influences can be extremely difficult to pull apart, in large samples or in a given patient, for a range of reasons (Turkheimer et al. 2014). For example, adolescents and adults select their environments based on aspects of their personality that have been shaped by a range of genetic and environmental influences, which can set off a cascade of mixed causes of future events and influences on personality development. Similarly, the environmental effect of having an alcoholic parent can be substantial but appears to be nonexistent when treated in behavioral genetic analysis as "shared environmental variance" because siblings can have *nonshared responses to shared experiences* that are opposites of each other. When the same circumstance can elicit substantial, but substantially different, environmental effects in two siblings, the apparent effect on personality will be masked, producing estimates of "environmental effects" hovering near zero, because their responses will cancel each other out. For example, some adolescents respond to having an abusive alcoholic parent by following in the parent's footsteps, whereas others eschew alcohol and any form of externalizing behavior and often become workaholics instead (Hinrichs et al. 2011). Although their shared environment may play a decisive role in their personality development, their divergent responses will cancel each other out and can be detected only by examining variance in correlations between personality characteristics of children and their parents, not mean correlations, which will appear to be near zero, depending on the percentage of children who respond one way or the other (or not at all).

Complicating matters further in identifying "biogenic" versus "psychogenic" disorders, as perhaps most dramatically demonstrated by Turkheimer's work on the heritability of IQ, we know that heritability coefficients in every domain are highly dependent on population characteristics (Turkheimer et al. 2003). Middle-class environments, for example, tend to provide what the psychoanalyst Heinz Hartmann (1951) called an "average expectable environment," which provides input our brains evolved to "expect." That minimizes coefficients that capture environmental effects and maximizes the apparent influence of genes. Put another way, if we hold environmental influences relatively constant by providing children with "good-enough parenting," as the psychoanalyst Michael Balint (1969) might have put it, and "good-enough financial resources," the only effects left will be genetic. Conversely, impoverished environments tend to provide much more environmental variability, which can minimize heritability coefficients.

If research in developmental psychopathology and behavioral genetics did not shake our faith in the viability of the nature-nurture distinction, research in epigenetics certainly did (Gescher et al. 2018; Ressler 2016). Research by Ressler and colleagues, for example, showing the cross-generational transmission of environmental events in cross-fostered rodents over multiple generations made clear that Jean-Baptiste Lamarck had more going for him than we ever imagined (Dias and Ressler 2014). Not only the genome, the roughly three billion pairs of genetic material that define an individual's unique genetic instructions, but also the epigenome, the chemicals that interact with that DNA to "turn genes on or off," which are affected by environmental events, can be transmitted intergenerationally (Manuck and McCaffery 2014; Toyokawa et al. 2012). That renders any simple distinction between "biological" and "psychosocial" influences on or approaches to personality or psychopathology impossible to sustain (e.g., Cicchetti 2016; Ressler 2016).

An amassing body of research on changes in gene expression related to environmental events, particularly trauma, has documented that these processes are as germane to the etiology of PDs as any other forms of pathology (Cattane et al. 2017; Gescher et al. 2018). Patients with severe PDs often experience severe traumatic events in childhood, which may have direct effects; effects moderated by specific sets of genes; or, commonly, both. Even seemingly innocuous environmental events, however, such as duration of exposure to breastfeeding, may influence the etiology of the most severe forms of personality pathology, such as psychopathic behavior, depending on the presence or absence of genes such as *5HTTLPR* (Jackson and Beaver 2016).

For all of these reasons, conceptually, viewing "biological approaches" as somehow distinct theoretical perspectives no longer seems tenable. The second reason we have eliminated "biological approaches" is less conceptual than methodological. Researchers from every theoretical approach are increasingly relying on multiple sources of data to test hypotheses and develop knowledge from their own theoretical standpoints, and biological methods are part of the methodological arsenal that can be, and are, used by researchers of every persuasion. Attachment theory, for example, emerged from the work of the psychoanalyst John Bowlby (1969, 1973) and remains a quintessentially psychodynamic theory, with its focus on internal working models of relationships (mental representations), unconscious forms of affect regulation (i.e., defensive process, as opposed to coping, which refers to conscious coping strategies) (Westen and Blagov 2007), and styles of relating in intimate relationships. Yet attachment researchers are intensely interested in the neural circuitry of attachment that has evolved over 100,000 years in humans and in the millions of years before the emergence of Homo sapiens. Of particular interest are the ways those circuits may vary with different attachment styles or developmental experiences that can affect attachment or in questions such as how attachment status in infancy and early childhood can affect health years later (e.g., Moutsiana et al. 2015; Puig et al. 2013).

Trait approaches are today as thoroughly grounded in genetics as they once were in psychometrics, and researchers have been studying their neural bases and correlates for decades. Eysenck's work a half-century ago (e.g., Eysenck 1967) was as pathbreaking as it was counterintuitive in its consideration of the possibility that, for example, extraverts might seek activity and interaction not because their brains were active but because they needed to supplement their brains' resting activity with environmental stimulation. Trait psychology also lent itself to behavioral genetic analyses, whether historically or conceptually (Krueger 1999; Wichers et al. 2013), more so than other approaches, but its primary focus on discrete dimensions such as neuroticism or negative affectivity also renders it particularly conducive to both genome-wide association studies and neuroimaging studies examining the neural networks involved in negative or positive affectivity (Hsu et al. 2018).

Third, although evolutionary psychology and psychiatry have not yet produced a robust enough literature to render them candidates for a section of this chapter (and may never, for reasons similar to the first two), as with other "biological perspectives," every approach to personality is conceptually infused, at least indirectly, with evolutionary thinking, and any theory that is not is not likely viable (e.g., Bowlby 1969; Millon 1990, 2016; Millon and Davis 1996). Humans would not have evolved most personality functions if they did not have adaptive significance, and like other animals, they are intensely attuned to the extent to which conspecifics have personality features that bear on their fitness as mating partners, coalition partners, potential enemies, "cheaters" who do not pull their weight or reciprocate other people's altruism, and the like (e.g., Buss 2009, 2016, 2017; Buss and Schmitt 2019).

Freud was born at the same time as *The Evolution of Species*, and his thinking was thoroughly infused with it. Had he not changed to the dual-instinct theory for which he is known—sex and aggression—he would have been known instead for his first, and prescient, dual-instinct theory—self-interest/survival and sex/reproduction—which foreshadowed contemporary thinking about survival and reproduction as the two key elements of "reproductive success" in evolutionary psychology. Behaviorist theory, at least as developed by Skinner, was moored in evolutionary thinking, as was classic work stemming back 50 years on how animals are "prepared" to make certain associations and less likely to make others, such as the natural tendency to associate tastes and smells with subsequent nausea (e.g., Garcia and Koelling 1966). Skinner described operant conditioning as picking up where evolution left off, as an evolved capacity, like classical conditioning, that allows animals to learn and respond flexibly to their environments. As he described it, operant conditioning is nothing but the natural selection of behaviors, which typically foster an organism's adaptation to the environment. That he and other behaviorists used terms such as *extinction* is not accidental. Although cognitive theories have attended less to evolutionary thinking than other approaches, in their most recent theorizing, Beck and Haigh (2014) have begun integrating neurobiological systems into their model of emotional disorders as they appear to be developing a theory of personality to undergird their theory of symptoms.

Psychodynamic Theories

Psychoanalytic theorists were the first to generate a concept of PD (also called *character disorder*, reflecting the idea that PDs involve character problems not isolated to a specific symptom or set of independent symptoms). PDs began to draw considerable theoretical attention in psychoanalysis by the middle of the twentieth century (e.g., Fairbairn 1952; Reich 1933/1978), in part because they were common and difficult to treat and in part because they defied understanding using the psychoanalytic models prevalent at the time.

For years, analysts had understood psychological problems in terms of conflict and defense using Freud's topographic model (conscious, preconscious, unconscious) or structural model (id, ego, superego). In classical psychoanalytic terms, most symptoms reflect maladaptive compromises forged outside of awareness among conflicting wishes, fears, and moral standards. For example, a patient with anorexia nervosa who is uncomfortable with her impulses and who fears losing control over them may begin to starve herself as a way of demonstrating that she can control even the most persistent of desires, hunger. From this standpoint, and empirically, fear of developing into a sexually mature female is a prominent characteristic in anorexia nervosa. Some of the PDs identified in Section II of DSM-5 (American Psychiatric Association 2013) have their roots in early psychoanalytic theorizing about conflict—notably, dependent, obsessive-compulsive, and histrionic PD (originally called *hysterical* in DSM-I and DSM-II [American Psychiatric Association 1952, 1968])—presumed to reflect fixations at the oral, anal, and phallic stages, respectively.

Although personality pathology at every level of severity is infused with conflict, because nothing in our brains prevents us from forming positive and negative emotional and motivational associations with the same person or thing (e.g., through loving and angry interactions with anyone who means much to us), by the 1930s through the 1970s, most psychoanalytic theorists had turned to ego psychology, object relations theory, self psychology, and more recent versions of these theories called relational theories to help them understand patients with PDs. According to these approaches, the problems seen in patients with character disorders run deeper than maladaptive compromises among conflicting motives and indicate derailments in personality development reflecting temperament, early attachment experiences, and their interaction (e.g., Balint 1969; Kernberg 1975b). Many of the DSM-5 PDs, notably schizoid, borderline, and narcissistic, have roots in these later approaches. With the emergence of these theories to explain more severe forms of personality disturbance, psychodynamic theorists came to recognize that deficits in various domains of ego functioning (e.g., attention or impulse regulation) or object relations (e.g., problematic ways of representing other people) could cause problems in personality functioning that did not approach the degree of severity required to be considered PDs and were in fact common in most patients.

Psychoanalytic ego psychology focuses on the psychological functions (e.g., skills, procedures, and processes involved in self-regulation) that must be in place for people to function adaptively, attain their goals, and meet external demands (see Bellak et al. 1973; Blanck and Blanck 1974; Redl and Wineman 1951). From this perspective, patients with PDs have various deficits in functioning, such as poor impulse control, difficulty regulating their affects, and deficits in the capacity for self-reflection. These deficits may render them incapable of behaving consistently in their own best interest or of taking the interests of others appropriately into account (e.g., lashing out aggressively without forethought, cutting themselves when they become upset).

Object relations theories identified interpersonal deficits, such as distorted representations of the self and others, difficulty maintaining consistent views of the self and others in different emotional states (e.g., when feeling disappointed or rejected, often misattributing others' intentions), and difficulty regulating affects in relationships with others, as common to patients with PDs (e.g., Greenberg and Mitchell 1983; Westen 1991b). In the same tradition followed attachment theory (Bowlby 1969, 1973; Obsuth et al. 2014; Shaver and Mikulincer 2005), self psychology (Kohut 1971, 1977), and relational theories (e.g., Aron 1996; Aron and Starr 2013; Mitchell 1988).

Although many psychoanalysts have been drawn to self-psychological and relational theories, the latter being more current than earlier object-relations theories, only object relations and attachment theory have generated empirical literatures that can guide research and practice. The primary exception is Lorna Benjamin's interpersonal theory, called Structural Analysis of Social Behavior (Benjamin 1993, 1996a, 1996b), which emerged before relational approaches but has always had a strong empirical and psychometric basis. Influenced by Sullivan's (1953) interpersonal theory of psychiatry, object relations approaches, and research using the interpersonal circumplex (e.g., Kiesler 1983; Leary 1957; Schaefer 1965), the Structural Analysis of Social Behavior is a sophisticated three-dimensional circumplex model with three "surfaces," focusing on actions directed at another person (e.g., abuse by a parent toward the patient); the person's response to real or perceived actions by the other (e.g., recoiling from the abusive parent); and the person's actions toward himself or herself (e.g., self-abuse).

From the point of view of object relations theories and their intellectual progeny, patients with PDs show several difficulties that cannot be readily accounted for by conflict or ego psychology models (for empirical reviews, see Stein and Slavin-Mulford 2018; Westen 1991b, 1998; see also Mullin et al. 2018; Richardson et al. 2018; Stein and Siefert 2018). First, internalization of attitudes of hostile, abusive, critical, inconsistent, or neglectful parents may leave patients with PDs vulnerable to fears of abandonment, self-hatred, a tendency to treat themselves as their parents treated them, or a tendency to mistreat others (Benjamin 1996a, 1996b; Masterson 1976; McWilliams 2011). Second, patients with PDs often fail to develop mature, constant, multifaceted representations of the self and others. As a result, they may be vulnerable to emotional swings when significant others are momentarily disappointing, and they may have difficulty understanding or imagining what might be in the minds of the people with whom they interact (Fonagy and Target 1997; Fonagy et al. 1991, 2003, 2018). Third, patients with PDs often appear to have difficulty forming a realistic, balanced view of the self that can weather momentary failures or criticisms and a corresponding inability to activate procedures (hypothesized to be based on loving, soothing experiences with early caregivers) that would be useful for self-soothing in the face of loss, failure, or threats to safety or self-esteem (see, e.g., Adler and Buie 1979). A substantial body of research supports many of these propositions, particularly with regard to BPD, the most extensively studied PD (e.g., Baker et al. 1992; Gunderson 2001; Westen 1990a, 1991a).

From a psychodynamic point of view, perhaps the most important features of PDs are the following: 1) they represent constellations of psychological processes, not distinct symptoms that can be understood in isolation; 2) they can be located on a continuum of personality pathology from relative health to relative sickness; 3) they can be characterized in terms of character style, which is orthogonal to level of disturbance (e.g., a patient can have a narcissistic or an obsessive personality style but be relatively sick or relatively healthy); 4) they involve both unconscious and conscious (implicit and explicit) personality processes, only some of which are available to introspection (and thus amenable to self-report); and 5) they reflect processes that are deeply ingrained in personality, which often serve multiple functions and have become associated with regulation of affects and hence are resistant to change.

The most comprehensive theory that embodies these principles is the theory of personality structure, or organization, developed by Otto Kernberg (1975a, 1984, 1996). For Kernberg, personality *organization* refers to levels of functioning or severity of disturbance, defined by the ability to think clearly without thought disturbance, regulate emotions effectively, and form meaningful relationships. Kernberg proposed a continuum of pathology, from chronically psychotic, through what he called borderline personality *organization* (or what today we would call severe PDs), through neurotic to normal functioning. Although his theory is more complex, in speaking of "borderline" as a level of functioning, Kernberg was following the psychiatric and psychoanalytic nomenclature of the 1950s and 1960s, describing a level of severity of pathology between the "lower border" of psychotic functioning and the "higher border" of neurotic to normal functioning. Nevertheless, his more theory-rich construct of borderline personality organization (Kernberg 1984, 1996; Lenzenweger et al. 2001) shaped many of the features of the diagnosis of BPD in DSM.[2]

Although many of Kernberg's major contributions have been in the understanding of borderline phenomena, his theory of narcissistic disturbance contributed substantially to the development of the diagnosis of narcissistic PD in DSM-III (American Psychiatric Association 1980), just as it did to the development of the BPD diagnosis. According to Kernberg, whereas patients with BPD lack an integrated identity, patients with narcissistic PD are typically developmentally more advanced, in that they have been able to develop a coherent (if distorted) view of themselves. Narcissistic phenomena, in Kernberg's view, lie on a continuum from normal (characterized by adequate self-esteem regulation) to pathological (narcissistic PD) (Kernberg 1984, 1998). Individuals with narcissistic PD need to construct a grossly inflated view of

---

[2]Borderline personality organization is a broader construct than BPD that is used to describe patients not only with DSM-5 BPD but also with severe variants of other DSM-5 PDs. In Kernberg's view, patients with borderline personality organization, or severe PDs, are distinguished from people whose personality is organized at a psychotic level by their relatively intact reality testing (e.g., absence of hallucinations, delusions) and ability to distinguish between their own thoughts and feelings and those of others (e.g., the absence of beliefs that their thoughts are being broadcast on the radio, or their recognition, although sometimes less than complete, that the persecutory thoughts they may hear inside their head are voices from the past rather than true hallucinations). They are distinguished from people "north of the border," who have "neurotic" (i.e., healthier) character structures, by 1) more maladaptive modes of regulating their emotions, through immature, reality-distorting defenses such as denial and projection (e.g., refusing to recognize the part they play in generating some of the hostility they engender from others), and 2) difficulty forming mature, multifaceted representations of themselves and significant others (e.g., believing that a person they once loved is really all bad, with no redeeming features, and is motivated only by the desire to hurt them).

themselves to maintain self-esteem, and they may appear grandiose, sensitive to the slightest attacks on their self-esteem (and hence vulnerable to rage or depression), or both. Not only are the conscious self representations of patients with narcissistic PD inflated, but so, too, are the representations that constitute their ideal self. Actual and ideal self representations stand in dynamic relation to one another. Thus, one reason that patients with narcissistic PD must maintain an idealized view of self is that they have a correspondingly grandiose view of who they should be, divergence from which leads to tremendous feelings of shame, failure, and humiliation.

The concept of a grandiose self is central to the self psychology of Heinz Kohut, a major theorist of narcissistic personality pathology, whose ideas, like those of Kernberg, contributed to the development of the narcissistic PD diagnosis in DSM-III (Goldstein 1985), which, like most diagnoses, remains largely intact in Section II of DSM-5, with some empirical tinkering between DSM-III, DSM-III-R (American Psychiatric Association 1987), and DSM-IV (American Psychiatric Association 1994). Kohut's theory grew out of his own and others' clinical experiences with patients whose problems (e.g., feelings of emptiness or unstable self-esteem) did not respond well to existing (psychoanalytic) models. Pathology, according to Kohut, results from faulty self development. The "self," in its particular Kohutian meaning, refers to the nucleus of a person's central ambitions and ideals and the talents and skills used to actualize them (Kohut 1971, 1977; Wolf 1988). It develops through two pathways (in Kohut's language, "poles"), which provide the basis for self-esteem.

The first pole is what Kohut calls the *grandiose self*—an idealized representation of self that emerges in children through empathic mirroring by their parents ("Mommy, watch!") and provides the nucleus for later ambitions and strivings. The second pole he calls the *idealized parent imago*—an idealized representation of the parents, which provides the foundation for ideals and standards for the self. Parental mirroring allows the child to see his or her reflection in the eyes of a loving and admiring parent. Idealizing parents allows the child to identify with and become like them. In the absence of adequate experiences with parents who can mirror the child or serve as appropriate targets of the child's idealization (e.g., when the parents are self-involved or abusive), the child's self structure cannot develop, preventing the achievement of cohesion, vigor, and normal self-esteem (which Kohut describes as "healthy narcissism"). As a result, the child develops a disorder of the self, of which pathological narcissism is a prototypical example. Empirically informed theorizing on narcissism has developed substantially since the seminal contributions by Kernberg and Kohut on narcissism in the 1960s and 1970s (e.g., Gabbard and Crisp-Han 2018), as has empirical work, for example, on subtypes of narcissistic PD long held to exist by clinicians (Russ et al. 2008).

Although clinical theorizing continues to develop in self psychology and relational psychoanalysis, neither has built much of an empirical literature. Spurred by demands for manualized treatments and randomized controlled trials, however, Kernberg and colleagues (Caligor et al. 2018; Levy et al. 2017; Yeomans et al. 2015) have tested a treatment focused on exploring the relationship between the patient and the therapist called transference-focused psychotherapy (TFP), and Fonagy and Bateman have developed a psychodynamic treatment similarly focused on patients' mental representations of themselves and others called mentalization-based therapy (MBT) (Fonagy et al. 2018). Both manualized treatments (in the broadest sense, principle-based descriptions of treatments, often in plainer, more understandable language than previous work) started with BPD but have since branched out to the range of PDs and personality pathology more generally (Caligor et al. 2018; Fonagy et al. 2018; Levy et al. 2017; Yeomans et al. 2015). A meta-analysis in *JAMA Psychiatry* showed that both TFP and MBT produced similar effect sizes and effects of the same magnitude as dialectical behavior therapy, which is widely described, erroneously, in the treatment literature taught to trainees and experienced clinicians in continuing education workshops as the only evidence-based treatment for BPD (Cristea et al. 2017). Although TFP and MBT differ substantially in many ways theoretically and pragmatically, they both match the prototype of psychodynamic approaches to PDs described earlier (e.g., with their focus on unconscious processes, mental representations of people, and relationships). (See Chapter 12, "Psychodynamic Psychotherapies," in this volume for a more detailed discussion of TFP and MBT.)

Cognitive-Social Theories

Cognitive-social theories (Bandura 1986; Mischel 1973, 1979) offered the first comprehensive alternative to psychodynamic approaches to personality. First developed in the 1960s, these approaches are sometimes called social learning theory and cognitive-social learning theory. In more clinical settings, their shared ancestor in behaviorism led to some links with cognitive-behavioral therapy (CBT). Although CBT began as a symptom-focused treatment, over time it has expanded into the treatment of PDs, although it has yet to offer a comprehensive theory of personality. Here we treat cognitive-social and cognitive-behavioral approaches together, because their principles are similar, and when combined, they provide an alternative approach that can be useful in case formulation, treatment, and research.

Cognitive-social theories developed from behaviorist and cognitive roots. From a behaviorist perspective, personality consists of learned behaviors and emotional reactions that tend to be relatively specific (rather than highly generalized) and tied to particular environmental contingencies. Cognitive-social theories share the behaviorist beliefs that learning is the basis of personality and that personality dispositions tend to be relatively specific and shaped by their consequences. These theories share the cognitive view that the way people encode, transform, and retrieve information, particularly about themselves and others, is central to personality. From a cognitive-social perspective, personality reflects a constant interplay between environmental demands and the way the individual processes information about the self and the world (Bandura 1986).

Cognitive-social theorists rarely dipped into the waters of PDs. Nor did CBT theorists until the 1990s (e.g., Beck et al. 2004; Linehan 1993b; Pretzer and Beck 1996; Young 1990), although that has now changed substantially (e.g., Barazandeh et al. 2016; Beck and Haigh 2014; Cristea et al. 2017). In large part, this relatively late arrival to the PD discourse reflected the assumption, initially inherited from behaviorism, that personality comprises relatively discrete, learned processes that are more malleable and situation specific than is implied by the concept of PD. Over time, however, that changed, in part because of longitudinal studies showing much more stability over time than cognitive-social theorists such as Walter Mischel recognized and in part because of the clinical observation and both basic and applied research findings, now common to all theories (and underlying "transdiagnostic" manuals), that many of the diatheses for psychiatric problems such as depression, anxiety, and addictions are shared across many disorders and reflect enduring dimensions of personality.

In fact, despite their origins in theoretical assumptions that minimized the role of enduring personality patterns, cognitive-social theories focus on several variables of substantial relevance to understanding PDs and personality pathology more broadly, including schemas, expectancies, goals, skills and competencies, and self-regulation (Bandura 1986, 1999; Cantor and Kihlstrom 1987; Mischel 1973, 1979; Mischel and Shoda 1995). A comprehensive cognitive-social account of PDs would likely address more basic processes of maladaptive learning at the level of conditioned emotional responses to people and maladaptive operant conditioning, such as learning that getting the attention of significant others requires behaviors such as cutting, through variables such as the schemas involved in encoding and processing information about the self and others (Beck et al. 2004).

For example, patients with PDs have dysfunctional schemas that lead them to misinterpret information (such as when patients with BPD misread and misattribute people's intentions), attend to and encode information in biased ways (such as when patients with paranoid PD maintain vigilance for perceived slights or attacks), or view themselves as bad or incompetent (pathological self-schemas). Related to these schemas are problematic expectancies, such as pessimistic expectations about the world, beliefs about the malevolence of others, and fears of being mocked. Patients with PDs may have pathological self-efficacy expectancies, such as the dependent patient's belief that he cannot survive on his own, the avoidant patient's belief that she is likely to fail in social circumstances, or the narcissistic patient's grandiose expectations about what he can accomplish. Equally important are competencies—that is, skills and abilities used for solving problems. In social-cognitive terms, social intelligence includes a variety of competencies that help people navigate interpersonal waters (Cantor and Harlow 1994; Cantor and Kihlstrom 1987), and patients with PDs tend to be notoriously poor interpersonal problem solvers.

Of particular relevance to severe PDs is self-regulation, which refers to the process of setting goals and subgoals, evaluating one's performance in meeting these goals, and adjusting one's behavior to achieve these goals in the context of ongoing feedback (Bandura 1986; Mischel 1990). Problems in self-regulation, including a deficit in specific skills, form a central aspect of Linehan's approach to treatment of BPD (Linehan 1993a, 1993b, 2020), which is now being applied to a wide range of disorders. Although Linehan's treatment includes modules that address numerous personality functions, she regards emotion dysregulation as perhaps the essential feature of BPD. The key characteristics of emotion dysregulation include difficulty 1) inhibiting inappropriate behavior related to intense affect, 2) organizing oneself to meet behavioral goals, 3) regulating physiological arousal associated with intense emotional arousal, and 4) refocusing attention when emotionally stimulated (Linehan 1993a). Many of the behavioral manifestations of BPD (e.g., impulsivity) can be viewed as consequences of emotion dysregulation. Deficits in emotion regulation lead to other problems, such as difficulties with interpersonal functioning and the development of a stable sense of self.

According to another cognitive-behavioral approach, Beck's cognitive theory (Beck 1999; Beck et al. 2004; Pretzer and Beck 1996), dysfunctional beliefs constitute the primary pathology involved in the PDs (Beck et al. 2001, 2015), which are viewed as "pervasive, self-perpetuating cognitive-interpersonal cycles" (Pretzer and Beck 1996, p. 55). Beck's theory highlights three aspects of cognition: automatic thoughts (beliefs and assumptions about the world, the self, and others), interpersonal strategies, and cognitive distortions (systematic errors in rational thinking). Beck and colleagues have described a unique cognitive profile characteristic of each of the DSM-IV PDs. For example, an individual diagnosed with schizoid PD would have a view of himself as a self-sufficient loner, a view of others as unrewarding and intrusive, and a view of relationships as messy and undesirable, and his primary interpersonal strategy would involve keeping his distance from other people (Pretzer and Beck 1996). He would use cognitive distortions that minimize his recognition of ways relationships with others can be sources of pleasure. Studies of dysfunctional beliefs have shown some support for the link between particular beliefs and the DSM-IV PDs (Beck et al. 2001; Bhar et al. 2012). More recently, Beck has attempted to build what began as a theory and treatment for changing dysfunctional beliefs leading to depression into a theory of personality, impressively integrating even neurobiological systems and unconscious "deep schemas" into his model to explain and treat the range of disorders, from a tendency to experience depression or anxiety to psychotic disorders (Beck and Haigh 2014).

Building on Beck's cognitive theory, and leading to its more recent development into a more thorough approach to personality and psychopathology, Young and colleagues (Young and Gluhoski 1996; Young and Kellogg 2006; Young and Lindemann 2002; Young et al. 2003) added early maladaptive schemas, defined as "broad and pervasive themes regarding oneself and one's relationships with others, developed during childhood and elaborated throughout one's life" (Young and Lindemann 2002, p. 95). Young and colleagues distinguish these from automatic thoughts and underlying assumptions, noting that early maladaptive schemas are associated with greater levels of affect, are more pervasive, and involve a strong interpersonal aspect. Young and colleagues have identified 18 early maladaptive schemas, each comprising cognitive, affective, and behavioral components (Young and Kellogg 2006; Young et al. 2003). They also propose three cognitive processes involving schemas that define key features of PDs: 1) schema maintenance, which refers to the processes by which maladaptive schemas are rigidly upheld (e.g., cognitive distortions, self-defeating behaviors); 2) schema avoidance, which refers to the cognitive, affective, and behavioral ways individuals avoid the negative affect associated with the schema; and 3) schema compensation, which refers to ways of overcompensating for the early maladaptive schema (e.g., workaholism in response to an early maladaptive schema of self as failure).

Young and colleagues (Young and Kellogg 2006; Young et al. 2003) subsequently incorporated psychodynamic and attachment theories, as well as some strategies from emotion-focused approaches, resulting in a more integrative conceptualization and treatment of PDs. One feature of this revised approach has been the development of the concept of "modes" as central to PDs, especially to what Young and colleagues refer to as the more severe PDs (borderline, narcissistic, and antisocial). For example, harkening back to the psychodynamic theorizing of James Masterson (1976) and to the interpersonal theory of Lorna Benjamin (1996b), Young describes five modes, or "aspects of self," as central to BPD: the abandoned and abused child, the angry and impulsive child, the detached protector, the punitive parent, and the healthy adult. Treatment strategies were designed to target each mode via four "mechanisms of healing and change": limited reparenting, emotion-focused work, cognitive restructuring and education, and behavioral pattern breaking. Research examining the effectiveness of schema therapy has largely focused on BPD and provides some support for the model (e.g., Lobbestael et al. 2005; Nadort et al. 2009).

Mischel and Shoda (1995) have offered a compelling social-cognitive account of personality that focuses on *if-then* contingencies—that is, conditions that activate particular thoughts, feelings, and behaviors. Although Mischel and Shoda have not linked this model to PDs, one could view PDs as involving a host of rigid, maladaptive if-then contingencies. For example, for some patients, the first hints of trouble in a relationship may activate concerns about abandonment. These may elicit anxiety or rage, to which the person with a PD responds with desperate attempts to lure the other person back (e.g., through manipulative statements and suicidal gestures) that often backfire. From an integrative psychodynamic-cognitive viewpoint, Horowitz (1988, 1998) has offered a model that focuses on the conditions under which certain states of mind become active, which he has tied more directly to a model of PDs. Similarly, Wachtel (1977, 1997) has described *cyclical psychodynamics*, in which people manage to elicit from others precisely the kinds of reactions of which they are the most afraid.

Trait Theories

Trait psychology has not developed approaches to treatment in the same way that psychodynamic and cognitive-behavioral approaches have, in large measure because it did not emerge from the clinic, but it has been highly generative of research and has proven most conducive to genetic and behavioral genetic analyses. *Traits* are emotional, cognitive, and behavioral tendencies on which individuals vary (e.g., the tendency to experience negative emotions).

As originally understood by Gordon Allport (1937), who pioneered the trait approach to personality, the concept of *trait* has two separate but complementary meanings. On the one hand, a trait is an observed tendency to behave in a particular way. On the other hand, a trait is an inferred, underlying personality disposition that generates this behavioral tendency. Allport thus would have been comfortable with the concept that is now culturally widespread of an "introverted extrovert"—that is, someone who behaves like an extrovert because doing so is more socially valued in many circumstances but feels like an introvert on the inside. The distinction, in that sense, between a "genuine" extrovert—someone who both appears and is temperamentally extroverted—and someone who "plays the role" of an extrovert because he or she can, and doing so is socially valued, is that a person who is extroverted in both senses ends an evening of social engagement energized, whereas an introverted extrovert feels drained, having had to work hard to put on the skills and maintain the "face" of an extrovert for a considerable length of time.

In many respects, the perceived lack of clinical utility of many contemporary trait approaches reflects the trade-off between the theoretical complexity of Allport's dual conceptualization of traits and the psychometric advantages of focusing primarily on behavioral tendencies, which are readily subjected to factor analysis from self-report questionnaires. In the empirical literature, traits have largely been defined operationally, as the average of a set of self-report items designed to assess them. Although it is theoretically possible to assess both the outward experience of appearing extroverted and the inward experience of feeling drained after social contact, it is unlikely that the two would load on the same factor. Even if researchers were to measure the outward appearance of extroversion and the inward experience of feeling drained by social interaction, however, and if the latter were to constitute a lower-order dimension or "facet" of introversion-extroversion, the higher-order factor score, and genetic or behavioral genetic analyses using it, could not readily distinguish between a person who is moderately extroverted and one who is highly extroverted "on the outside" but highly introverted "on the inside."

From a clinical standpoint, the same is true of virtually every significant trait. In his hit single "Tears of a Clown," Motown superstar Smokey Robinson described the experience of a person who can express outward pleasure, and even feel it while putting it on, but who underneath is deeply depressed. Comics often describe themselves as turning to comedy to escape their pain or conflict and feeling alive, excited, and even happily engaged onstage but deflated the moment the club closes down. Whether they obtain pleasure in adulation that can be captured in another, lower-level or subordinate trait such as "low humility" or simply experience pleasure only to the extent that they can escape pain onstage differs by the person, but those individual differences are precisely what was readily captured by Allport, who was more psychodynamic in his thinking, but not readily captured by contemporary trait theories. The same is true of the "masked depression" described for years in the literature on adolescent boys, who often express depression with outwardly externalizing behaviors, such as aggression, oppositionality, or rage, because to them, it is more comfortable than sadness or admitting grief, self-criticism, or rejection. The Alternative DSM-5 Model for Personality Disorders (AMPD), discussed later in this chapter, has begun to grapple with this limitation of factor analytically derived trait models, for example, in its inclusion of "covert grandiosity" as a trait characteristic of narcissistic PD.

Contemporary models of traits do, however, reflect another important aspect of Allport's thinking about traits—namely, what is called the *lexical hypothesis of personality*, that important personality attributes will gradually emerge and be used in everyday language. The lexical hypothesis is solid not only from a sociolinguistic standpoint but also from an evolutionary one: in a linguistic species such as ours, just as other animals, particularly primates, recognize socially significant attributes of conspecifics, every language is likely to develop words over time that describe salient aspects of personality of adaptive significance, such as those that bear on another person's capacity to enter into committed romantic and parenting relationships, enter into coalitions, work diligently, behave altruistically, treat other people well, and parent in ways conducive to adaptation given environmental circumstances. That led Allport to look for personality in an unlikely place: in adjectival descriptions of personality from *Webster's Unabridged Dictionary* (Allport and Odbert 1936). By factor analyzing those descriptions, Allport did not identify the current most widely accepted trait models of personality, but by winnowing those descriptions down in various ways, over time, personality researchers have largely converged on what is generally considered the most comprehensive trait model of personality, the five-factor model of personality (FFM; Kajonius and Mac Giolla 2017; McCrae and Costa 1997; Widiger 2000; Widiger and Costa 1994; Widiger et al. 2019).

The FFM is a description of the way adjectival and other brief personality descriptors tend to covary in ways that provide a comprehensive roadmap that can be identified via factor analysis as comprising the latent factors or underlying dimensions of personality. Numerous studies, including cross-cultural investigations, have found that when people are asked to rate themselves on dozens or hundreds of adjectives or brief sentences derived from everyday language, the pattern of their self-descriptions often can be reduced to five overarching constructs: neuroticism, extraversion, conscientiousness, agreeableness, and openness to experience (Costa and McCrae 1997; Goldberg 1993). McCrae and Costa (1990, 1997) have proposed a set of lower-order traits, or *facets*, within each of these broadband traits, which can allow a more discriminating portrait of personality. Thus, neuroticism includes facets that assess the extent to which individuals tend to experience negative affects such as anxiety and depression and to express hostility, and the extent to which they are vulnerable to stress. Extraversion comprises facets such as the extent to which the individual tends to experience positive affect and to be gregarious, assertive, and high in energy. Conscientiousness includes facets that assess the extent to which the person tends to be careful and deliberate, dutiful, and orderly. Agreeableness reflects their tendency to get along with others and to be compassionate, altruistic, and complaint. Openness to experience comprises the extent to which the individual is likely to be open to emotional, aesthetic, and intellectual experiences. Thus, an individual's personality profile is represented by 35 dimensions, one score for each of the five factors and one for each of six lower-order facets or subfactors within each of these broader constructs, providing a picture of personality with finer resolution than five adjectives. To be high on neuroticism, for example, an individual might show elevations on some combination of its facets but not necessarily all of them. For example, a patient could be high on the neuroticism facets of anxiety, depression, self-consciousness (shyness or social anxiety), and vulnerability (susceptibility to stress) but moderate on hostility and impulsivity.

In principle, one could classify personality pathology in one of three ways using the FFM. The first, championed by Widiger and colleagues (2019), is to view the FFM as adequate to the task of characterizing both nonpathological and pathological variants of personality. In this view, PDs simply reflect extreme versions of nonpathological personality traits, so the same system can be used for diagnosing nonpathological and pathological personality. This approach is most consistent with the theoretical and psychometric tradition within which the FFM developed, because it should not, theoretically, require new items or instruments, although it could expand the item pool to include more descriptors at the pathological poles of each factor and facet. From this standpoint, extreme values on each of the five factors (and at least some of their facets) represent personality pathology. This is well illustrated by neuroticism, in which extremely high scores on both the factor and its facets—anxiety, hostility, depression, self-consciousness, impulsiveness, and vulnerability—all clearly represent aspects of personality pathology.

Matters of debate, however, are whether this strategy is appropriate for all factors and facets and when to consider extreme responses on one or both poles of a dimension to be pathological. Extreme extraversion, for example, may or may not be pathological, depending on the social milieu and the person's other traits. Similarly, extreme openness to experience could imply a genuinely open attitude toward emotions, art, and so forth, in keeping with the original name of the factor when first identified factor analytically long before the FFM came into vogue, when Warren Norman (1963), who proposed what he called the "Big Five" personality traits, labeled it "culture." Alternatively, it could reflect an affectively shallow, peculiar, more schizotypal cognitive style. How to distinguish those two types of "extreme openness," however, raises psychometric problems that require a revision of the items and the model. Just as one might ask, "How open is too open?," one might similarly wonder how humble (a facet of agreeableness) is too humble. Is Archbishop Desmond Tutu pathological in his humility? Was Martin Luther King abnormal (beyond statistically abnormal) in his ability to set aside legitimate "angry hostility" in a Birmingham jail?

The advantage of this approach, however, is that it integrates the understanding and assessment of nonpathological and pathological personality and establishes dimensions of personality pathology using well-understood empirical procedures (factor analysis), although it likely requires a substantial number of additional items to flesh out the pathological poles, which may or may not lead to a five-factor model or to facets resembling those that may be useful for assessing personality. A useful analogy is intelligence testing; outside two standard deviations, the test has little meaning, so that when laypeople think they are geniuses because someone tells them that they have an IQ of 155, they do not realize that the derivation samples do not have enough people in the upper one percentile for us to know what differences among IQs higher than 130 mean, if anything. It may well be, for example, that above an IQ of 130, the interaction with other intellectual traits, such as creativity, or with personality traits, such as emotional intelligence, is a much better predictor of success than simply racking up extra IQ points.

Because clinicians have generally found the FFM unwieldy and lacking in clinical utility, a second way Widiger and colleagues suggested using the FFM as derived from factor analysis was to translate the clinically derived categories that have been relatively stable from DSM-III-R through DSM-5 into five-factor language (Coker et al. 2002; Lynam and Widiger 2001; Widiger and Costa 1994; Widiger et al. 2002). For example, Widiger and colleagues (2002) describe antisocial PD as combining low agreeableness with low conscientiousness. Because analysis at the level of five factors often lacks the specificity to characterize complex disorders such as BPD (high neuroticism plus high extraversion), proponents of the FFM have often moved to the facet level. Thus, whereas all six neuroticism facets (anxiety, hostility, depression, self-consciousness, impulsivity, and vulnerability) are characteristic of patients with BPD, patients with avoidant PD are characterized by only four of these facets (anxiety, depression, self-consciousness, and vulnerability).

Similarly, Widiger and colleagues (2002) described obsessive-compulsive PD as primarily an extreme, maladaptive variant of conscientiousness. They add, however, that patients with obsessive-compulsive PD tend to be low on the compliance and altruism facets of agreeableness (i.e., they are oppositional and stingy) and low on some of the facets of openness to experience, as reflected in being closed to feelings and closed to values (i.e., morally inflexible). Numerous studies have shown predicted links between DSM-IV Axis II disorders and FFM factors and facets (Axelrod et al. 1997; Ross et al. 2002; Trull et al. 2001), although other studies have found substantial overlap among the FFM profiles of patients with very different PDs (e.g., borderline and obsessive-compulsive) using major FFM self-report inventories (Morey et al. 2002).

A third approach, which retained a version of the FFM, was the one selected by the Personality and Personality Disorders Work Group for DSM-5 but was ultimately placed in Section III of DSM-5 ("Emerging Measures and Models") (Skodol et al. 2013). This approach, spearheaded by Krueger and colleagues (2012), started with the FFM but made substantial revisions to the factors, facets, and items used to assess them. The goal was to "pathologize" a version of the FFM so that it would have greater clinical utility and clinical acceptance (Hopwood et al. 2012; Kerber et al. 2019). That, in turn, required the development of an alternative to the most widely used and accepted FFM measure, the NEO Personality Inventory–Revised, which the authors called the Personality Inventory for DSM-5 (PID-5).

In a first step, the researchers redefined each of the first four dimensions—neuroticism, extraversion, conscientiousness, and agreeableness—by its negative pole. Thus, neuroticism stayed neurotic (called negative affectivity in the AMPD), but extraversion was transformed into detachment (its pathological pole); conscientiousness became disinhibition; and agreeableness became antagonism. That still left all the problems of the FFM for clinical practice, requiring the second step—namely, the development of a different measure, with different items and facets as well as factors—to make them more clinically relevant and rationally consistent rather than, strictly speaking, true to the FFM. The item set required substantial changes to capture more severe personality pathology than most people encounter in everyday life and thus in everyday adjectives, the basis of the lexical hypothesis and the factors derived from it. Furthermore, analysis of the subordinate-level dimensions (facets) shows some rearrangement to address conceptual problems with the facet structure of the FFM, such as its inclusion of hostility and impulsivity in the neuroticism factor, when those would be better included within an externalizing dimension, which includes antagonism and disinhibition.

Those changes still do not fully address item overlap (cross-correlations of subordinate facets with the wrong superordinate factors), such as the anger in hostility, which can be an aspect of neuroticism (and is often considered part of a highly correlated factor in the PID-5 and other personality instruments, negative affectivity, or internalizing pathology, but also of externalizing traits such as antagonism), but it improved on the facets of the FFM vis-à-vis psychopathology. Finally, "openness" was never a particularly robust factor in the FFM, for example, across cultures, and it was not useful in a psychopathology measure or diagnostic system. It also failed to capture schizotypal thinking or more serious forms of thought disorder, which would be necessary to cover, so it was replaced with a genuine "psychoticism" dimension. Although that took the PID-5 even further from the FFM on which it was modeled, it rendered its five factors much more useful in predicting a broader range of psychopathology, now including psychotic disorders as well as depression, anxiety, impulse-regulation disorders, and the gamut of disorders its authors hoped to be able to explain using a personality instrument, aligning personality more closely with psychopathology (Krueger et al. 2018).

Thus, in developing the PID-5, which assesses these new, quasi-FFM, pathological personality traits, the FFM is no longer really the FFM psychologists know and love. Conversely, clinicians did not know and love the FFM, which consistently was rated the lowest of all PD systems in research when comparing it with alternative systems on measures of clinical utility (e.g., Rottman et al. 2009). In retrospect, that makes sense, based on the lexical hypothesis: the language that evolved to describe everyday personality used by laypeople is not the language that evolved to describe clinically important personality pathology among experienced, trained clinicians any more than oncologists can be expected to find "big lump" or "funny color" to be more than a useful first description from a layperson of a problem he or she noticed that brought him or her to see a physician. Thus, the trait model that constitutes Criterion B of the AMPD, based on the PID-5, is not your grandfather's FFM, but for purposes of modeling psychopathology, it has a smoother ride, with its 5 maladaptive factors and 25 subordinate facets (see DSM-5, Table 3, pp. 779–781).

Finally, before leaving trait theories, it is important to note that although the FFM (and, increasingly, its pathological cousin, the trait model in the AMPD) is the most widely accepted trait model of personality, it is not the only one, for several reasons. First, different factor solutions may be useful for different purposes. Caspi and Moffitt (2018) have argued for a psychopathological analog to the "g" factor in intelligence testing of "general intelligence," by extracting one factor from data on psychopathology: general pathology, which predicts multiple forms of pathology. One of the virtues of the PID-5, and the AMPD in which it is embedded, is that it has intelligible factor solutions beginning with a two-factor solution, and conceptually, the factors make clinical and empirical sense irrespective of the number of factors. If a data analyst extracts just two factors from its item set—that is, decides to "lump" all the items into two "bins" of items (factors), in which items tend to correlate strongly with each other within one factor but not with the other factor—the result will be an intelligible two-factor solution: internalizing and externalizing pathology. That finding is consistent with work years earlier by Krueger (1999) and colleagues, before they were trying to adapt the FFM to psychopathology. In several samples, they and others found that broadband internalizing and externalizing personality factors account for much of the variance in many common symptom disorders (e.g., mood, anxiety, substance use), and that genetic and environmental sources of variance in twin samples are associated with many of both the higher- and the lower-order factors they identified. Importantly, these are the same broadband factors found for decades in child and adolescent samples, suggesting continuity in pathological trait structure beginning in early childhood and continuing through adulthood.

If a data analyst extracts three factors from the PID-5, the internalizing factor splits into two sets of items (factors)—detachment and negative affect—and the externalizing factor remains as it was at the two-factor solution. Once again, converging data from other samples support these findings. Fifty years earlier, Hans Eysenck (1967, 1981) proposed perhaps the primary alternative to the FFM identified through factor analysis in both nonpathological and pathological samples, a three-factor solution, with scales he labeled neuroticism, extraversion, and psychoticism (although his psychoticism scale had nothing to do with psychosis; it was closer to impulsivity, disinhibition, or, more broadly, externalizing pathology). Tellegen's Multidimensional Personality Questionnaire, originally developed to assess nonpathological personality, but which Krueger has used extensively across multiple studies on internalizing and externalizing pathology, similarly produces a three-factor structure: positive emotionality, negative emotionality, and constraint (Tellegen and Waller 1993).

When four factors are extracted from the PID-5, detachment and negative affect do not change, but externalizing breaks into two factors (antagonism and disinhibition), equivalents to low agreeableness and low conscientiousness. This solution is also broadly consistent with data from a different self-report personality pathology instrument developed years earlier by Livesley et al. (2003), who, like Krueger, argued that behavioral genetic data can help address the persistent lack of consensus among trait psychologists regarding which traits to study by examining the causes of trait covariation as opposed to simply describing it. Establishing congruence between a proposed phenotypic model of personality traits and the genetic structure underlying it would support the validity of a proposed factor model. The same holds true for models of PDs. To test this approach, Livesley et al. (1998) administered the Dimensional Assessment of Personality Pathology—Basic Questionnaire (DAPP-BQ) to a large sample of individuals with and without PDs, including twin pairs. Factor analysis indicated a four-factor solution that is not identical to but certainly resembles the four-factor solution in the PID-5 (reordering the factors to match the PID-5 four-factor solution: inhibition, emotional dysregulation, dissocial behavior, and compulsivity, the opposite pole of which is impulsivity). Results showed high congruence for all four factors between the phenotypic and the behavioral genetic analyses, indicating strong support for the proposed factor solution. Later, Livesley (2011) identified a dimensional model of PDs based on the DAPP-BQ, which again produced four factors not identical to but highly similar to the PID-5 four-factor solution (once again reordering them for clarity: social avoidance, emotional dysregulation, dissocial behavior, and compulsivity).[3]

Finally, extracting five factors from the PID-5 leaves detachment, negative affect, antagonism, and disinhibition intact but splits off a psychoticism factor. That is less interesting, however, because the instrument was designed to produce that result, which leads to another reason that factor analysis can produce differing solutions: what one puts into it determines what comes out of it. For example, Cloninger developed a trait theory of PDs based on a neurobiological model of personality (Cloninger 1998; Cloninger et al. 1993), identifying what he called four "temperament" dimensions, each theoretically linked to particular neurotransmitter systems: 1) novelty seeking (exploration, extravagance, impulsivity), associated with dopamine; 2) harm avoidance (characterized by pessimism, fear, timidity), associated with serotonin and γ-aminobutyric acid; 3) reward dependence (sentimentality, social attachment, openness), associated with norepinephrine and serotonin; and 4) persistence (industriousness, determination, ambitiousness, perfectionism), associated with glutamate and serotonin (Cloninger 1998, p. 70). He then added items designed to capture three character dimensions, which are more idiosyncratic: 1) self-directedness (responsibility, purposefulness, self-acceptance), considered the "major determinant of the presence or absence of personality disorder" (Cloninger et al. 1993, p. 979); 2) cooperativeness (empathy, compassion, helpfulness); and 3) self-transcendence (spirituality, idealism, enlightenment). Cloninger (1998) proposed that all PDs are low on the character dimensions of self-directedness and cooperativeness but that the Cluster A, B, and C (in the language of DSM-IV) PDs can be distinguished on the basis of the temperament dimensions. He later amended his model and measure in ways that are more difficult to follow (Cloninger 2004, 2008).

What all of the models and measures described thus far share, however, is what psychometricians call significant *method variance*, a methodological feature that can-

---

[3]Where all of these trait models differ, however, is at the subordinate levels (e.g., FFM facets). Livesley's model, for example, includes 30 personality traits thought to underlie the four dimensions. For example, the subordinate traits attributed to the social avoidance domain include low affiliation, avoidant attachment, restricted emotional expression, self-constraint, inhibited sexuality, and attachment need (Livesley 2011). Livesley views the four higher-order dimensions and 30 primary traits as the genetic "architecture" of personality.

not be readily disentangled from *true variance,* or the dimensions that exist in nature. In this case, that shared method variance relates to the use of self-reports to identify factor structure and ultimately the system of classification of personality pathology. Westen and colleagues have argued that the lexical hypothesis does not support the use of self-reports or any other form of lay reports as a primary source of data for taxonomic work. Rather, it would support the use of everyday clinical language, as used by clinically trained observers. For example, structured interviews such as the gold standard measure in psychiatric diagnosis research, the Structured Clinical Interview for DSM-5, rely on language about signs and symptoms that evolved over a century of psychiatric observation and classification, not the language of laypeople describing what they believe about their own personalities using lay language. Just as laypeople use lay language to understand people, clinicians, whether they are general radiologists, thoracic surgeons, or psychiatrists, use the language of experts to understand patients. Thus, to be maximally useful to clinicians, an instrument might be developed instead for clinicians, with straightforward clinical language without theory-specific jargon, so that it can be used by clinicians irrespective of their theoretical orientation (Westen and Weinberger 2004). These researchers also note that self-reports of PDs require laypeople to possess knowledge they are not trained to have and that they may also lack because of the limits of self-awareness, especially in patients with PDs (Westen et al. 2014b [see source for references]):

> Both meta-analytic investigations (Klonsky, Oltmanns, & Turkheimer, 2002) and data from recent large-N studies (Clifton, Turkheimer, & Oltmanns, 2005) have shown that self-reported pathological personality traits correlate only moderately (in meta-analytic research, r = .36) with the same traits assessed by lay informants and weakly with longitudinal evaluation by experts using all available data (Klein, Ouimette, Kelly, Ferro, & Riso 1994; Pilkonis, Heape, Ruddy, & Serrao, 1991). By contrast, both traits and dimensional personality disorder diagnoses derived from data provided by experienced clinicians using a systematic clinical research interview correlate in the range of r = .50 to .70 with the same variables as assessed by treating clinicians (Westen & Muderrisoglu, 2003, 2006; Westen et al., 2012). Similarly, research on "illusory mental health" (Shedler, Mayman, & Manis, 1993) demonstrates that self-report measures of neuroticism (or negative affectivity) cannot distinguish psychologically healthy individuals from psychologically distressed individuals who lack self-awareness. (Westen et al. 2014b, p. 283)

Westen and colleagues (2014b) thus designed a 200-item instrument developed over multiple iterations for use by experienced clinicians and applied it to data on one patient each from the practices of 1,201 clinicians in North America. As in a similar study with a sample of 950 adolescents that used an adolescent version of the same instrument, they could not recover anything like a four- or five-factor structure. Rather, they identified a 14-factor structure that included a mix of traits that resemble FFM traits or facets and dimensions that resemble PDs: psychopathy, psychological health, obsessionality, schizotypy, emotional avoidance, emotional dysregulation, narcissism, anxious somatization, sexual conflict, depression, social anxiety/avoidance, unstable commitments, histrionic sexualization, and hostility. Ongoing work involves examining the extent to which different measures, models, and informants produce data with better antecedent, concurrent, and predictive validity, in correlating with variables such as adaptive functioning, psychopathology, aggregated informant reports, follow-up data at 18–24 months, implicit personality measurement, and etiologically relevant variables (e.g., genes, family history, and measures of childhood trauma), using a sample of approximately 250 patients interviewed by multiple doctoral-level interviewers.

Integrative Approaches

We conclude by addressing two integrative approaches: the Alternative DSM-5 Model for Personality Disorders and Westen's functional domains model. The two have many features in common. Both combine functional with descriptive diagnosis and assessment, dimensional and categorical diagnosis, and measures of personality health-sickness (on a range from severe PD to relatively healthy functioning). These features reflect the same goal—namely, to render them maximally grounded in, and useful for, both clinical practice and research.

The AMPD (included in Section III of DSM-5) includes an assessment of the patient's interpersonal functioning and self-relatedness, which simultaneously serves as a measure of severity; a psychometrically derived trait taxonomy, developed to extend the most widely accepted trait approach used in studies of nonpathological personality to psychopathology; and six of the categorical PDs included in DSM-5.

The functional domains model also includes a functional assessment focusing on three domains: the patient's wishes, fears, and values and the ways he or she resolves conflicts among them; cognitive, emotional, and self-regulatory capacities, such as range of affect and ways of regulating affect; and experience of self and others and capacity for interpersonal relatedness. Like the AMPD, it includes a psychometrically derived, dimensional classification of personality pathology but focuses more on personality constellations derived from the three domains, which are more similar to the DSM PDs.

Alternative DSM-5 Model for Personality Disorders

Because this model is covered elsewhere in this textbook (see Chapter 4, "Alternative DSM-5 Model for Personality Disorders," and the appendix to this textbook), and we have already described the trait model in detail that constitutes one of the two novel aspects of it, we will be somewhat telegraphic here. The AMPD includes multiple steps (Skodol et al. 2015). The first is a five-point assessment of level of severity of pathology, grounded in two aspects of self, called *identity* and *self-direction*, and two aspects of interpersonal relatedness, called *empathy* and *intimacy*. The second step is an assessment of the pathological traits modified from the FFM traits measured and derived from the PID-5. The third step is an application of the severity index and traits to the six categorical diagnoses retained from among the 10 PDs in DSM-IV. That entails a determination of whether each of the disorders, to the extent present, is severe enough to warrant further consideration and has enough of the relevant traits to warrant one or more categorical PD diagnoses. Regardless of whether the patient meets criteria for any of the disorders at that point, the clinician can still determine whether the patient merits specification of any other pathological traits, which is an advantage over a purely categorical descriptive diagnosis using one of the six DSM-IV/DSM-5 Section II categories retained in the model.

Finally, as in standard DSM differential diagnosis, the clinician rules out better explanations for any observed pathology, such as substance abuse or depression. Although not specified as a step in the model, another advantage is the attempt of this model to blend personality diagnosis with diagnosis of other DSM-5 disorders. Aside from other disorders just serving as rule-outs for a PD, the personality traits are themselves diatheses for those disorders, which the trait model was designed to explain (Kotov et al. 2017).

Westen's Functional Domains Model: An Alternative to an Alternative?

Westen (Westen 1995, 1996, 1998, 2012; Westen and Heim 2005; Westen et al. 2012, 2014a) has described a model of domains of personality functioning and descriptive diagnosis that draws substantially on multiple clinical, theoretical, and empirical approaches. For purposes of exposition, we draw here the most significant distinctions between this model and the AMPD.

Like the DSM-5 model, the functional domains model includes a model of functional assessment, but it casts a broader net, attempting to provide a comprehensive functional account of the patient's motives and conflicts, cognitive strengths and difficulties, affect and affect regulation, impulse regulation, and self and interpersonal functioning. It does not assume the primacy of any of those domains or that one or another alone would define level of severity, although they tend to be highly correlated in the personality health-sickness ratings they produce. For example, we have spent more than 30 years developing 5- to 7-point dimensional ratings of level of interpersonal and self functioning that empirically predict adaptive functioning, developmental history of abuse, changes that occur, progress in psychotherapy, and other relevant variables (e.g., DeFife et al. 2010, 2013a, 2013b; Mullin et al. 2018; Stein and Siefert 2018; Westen 1991b). We do not assume the primacy of any single domain in determining level of functioning, although clearly interpersonal and self-functioning are crucial to psychological health–pathology.

The model suggests that a systematic personality case formulation must answer three questions, each composed of a series of subquestions that require assessment:

1. What does the person wish for, fear, and value, and to what extent are these motives conscious or unconscious, collaborating or conflicting?
2. What psychological resources—including cognitive processes (e.g., intelligence, memory, intactness of thinking processes, attention [and under what circumstances]), affects, affect regulation strategies (conscious coping strategies and unconscious defenses), and behavioral skills—does the person have at his or her disposal to meet internal and external demands?
3. What is the person's experience of the self and others, and how able is the individual—cognitively, emotionally, motivationally, and behaviorally—to sustain meaningful and mutually satisfying relationships?

From a psychodynamic perspective, these questions correspond roughly to the issues raised by classical theories of motivation and conflict early in the development of dynamic thinking but brought forward to the twenty-first century; ego-psychological approaches to adaptive functioning; and theory and research in object relations and attachment, which address people's experience of self, others, and relationships. Each of these questions and subdimensions, however, is also associated with several other research traditions in personality, clinical, cognitive, and developmental psychology (e.g., on the development of children's representations of self, representations of others, moral judgment and intuition, ability to tell coherent narratives) (Damon and Hart 1988; Fonagy et al. 2002; Harter 1999; Livesley and Bromley 1973; Main 1995; Westen 1990a, 1990b, 1991b, 1994). Westen and colleagues (2012, 2014b) used this model with adolescents and adults as a rough theoretical guide to ensure comprehensive coverage of personality domains in developing items for a personality pathology instrument for use by experienced clinicians or with a systematic clinical research interview (Westen and Muderrisoglu 2003, 2006).

From this point of view, individuals with particular PDs are likely to be characterized by distinct constellations of motives and conflicts; specific deficits in cognition, emotion, emotion regulation, and impulse regulation; and specific deficits in self-experience and interpersonal thought, feeling, and behavior. Patients with BPD, for example, tend to have 1) chronic worries about abandonment; 2) impaired thinking under severe stress, difficulty regulating affect (Linehan 1993b, 2015; Westen 1991a), and poor impulse control under stress; and 3) a propensity to form simplistic, one-dimensional representations; to misunderstand why people (including themselves) behave as they do; and to expect malevolence from other people. Like the AMPD, the same model that applies to PDs applies to people at any level of personality pathology. Individuals who are relatively healthy, for example, may still have conflicts; chronic ways of over- or underregulating affect that cause them trouble (e.g., refusing to take responsibility for their mistakes); trouble with overregulation of their impulses, as in many high-functioning restricting anorexic patients; and problems with self-esteem or interpersonal relatedness, such as repeatedly picking romantic partners who are bad for them but match prototypes of relationships from their past.

In this model, a person's level of personality health-sickness can be assessed reliably in multiple ways. One is a personality health prototype developed empirically, which assesses each of these functional domains (Westen et al. 2012). A second is a measure of domains of social cognition and object relations, such as complexity of representations of people, affective quality of representations (from malevolent to realistic and benevolent), and coherence of identity, which has been used in nonpathological and pathological samples of children, adolescents, and adults (e.g., Stein and Siefert 2018; Stein and Slavin-Mulford 2018; Westen 1991a, 1991b, 1998; Westen et al. 1991). Still another involves simple five-point ratings of personality pathology derived from Kernberg's conceptualization of levels of severity and similar ratings of quality of relationships, social support, and work functioning, which can be aggregated, along with Global Assessment of Functioning scores, to produce global measures of personality health disturbance with high reliability and validity (e.g., DeFife et al. 2010; Nakash et al. 2018).

Finally, we developed two measures, the Shedler-Westen Assessment Procedure–II (SWAP-II) and an adolescent version of the instrument (SWAP II-A), with item sets that assess both these sets of functions and these three questions; descriptive signs and symptoms of different forms and levels of severity of personality pathology, including versions of all the criteria from the last three DSM editions before DSM-5; as well as empirical research on personality and clinical writing on personality, "character," and personality pathology. Our goal was thus to derive dimensional descriptive diagnoses from a functional assessment, not to separate the processes. For both adolescents and adults, we used these instruments much like the PID-5 to derive dimensions empirically, including both trait dimensions and constellational dimensions (personality styles that resemble DSM PDs). To identify traits, we used traditional factor analysis. To identify personality constellations, we used a form of factor analysis that groups people based on their similarity across the 200 items of the instruments rather than grouping items based on their correlations across people. We are uncertain as to which form of dimensional diagnosis will prove more useful for research or whether they might be useful for different purposes or in combination, although as described earlier, multiple research groups have found that clinicians tend to find dimensional diagnosis of personality styles (e.g., PDs) to be more useful than dimensional diagnosis of traits.

We did not find any overarching or hierarchical trait structure in either adolescent or adult samples, but we did find a hierarchical structure in both adolescents and adults when empirically deriving dimensional PD diagnoses. The PD clusters that emerged empirically showed a striking convergence with Krueger's data on internalizing and externalizing pathology, which is exciting, given the difference in methods, observers, and items. We believe the DSM-5 Section II PD clusters that emerged empirically are more sensible than the DSM-IV Clusters A, B, and C. The first two of three clusters of personality styles in both adolescents and adults were internalizing and externalizing. In the adult sample, the internalizing cluster includes depressive, anxious, dependent–self-defeating, and schizoid PDs. The externalizing cluster includes narcissistic, psychopathic, and paranoid PDs. The third cluster is borderline/emotionally dysregulated. (With both the adults and the adolescents, we also identified an obsessional "neurotic style," but it was not pathological enough to be considered a PD.) The superordinate adolescent clusters were the same, with some minor variations from the adult data at the level of specific disorders (e.g., dependent–self-defeating emerged as a subtype of borderline/emotionally dysregulated rather than internalizing).

Conclusion

To what extent any of the five approaches reviewed here will prove more useful, or whether different approaches will prove useful for different purposes, remains unclear. The only way to answer those questions is to place them in head-to-head comparisons with different criterion variables. We believe that the stars would have to be in an unusual alignment if one approach turned out to be superior for all purposes, particularly with these two alternative approaches, which derive from multiple theoretical and psychometric perspectives.

References

Adler G, Buie D: Aloneness and borderline psychopathology: the possible relevance of child development issues. Int J Psychoanal 60:83–96, 1979

Allport G: Personality: A Psychological Interpretation. New York, Henry Holt, 1937

Allport G, Odbert H: Trait-Names: A Psycho-Lexical Study (Psychological Monographs, Vol 47). Princeton, NJ, Psychological Review Company, 1936

American Psychiatric Association: Diagnostic and Statistical Manual: Mental Disorders. Washington, DC, American Psychiatric Association, 1952

American Psychiatric Association: Diagnostic and Statistical Manual of Mental Disorders, 2nd Edition. Washington, DC, American Psychiatric Association, 1968

American Psychiatric Association: Diagnostic and Statistical Manual of Mental Disorders, 3rd Edition. Washington, DC, American Psychiatric Association, 1980

American Psychiatric Association: Diagnostic and Statistical Manual of Mental Disorders, 3rd Edition, Revised. Washington, DC, American Psychiatric Association, 1987

American Psychiatric Association: Diagnostic and Statistical Manual of Mental Disorders, 4th Edition. Washington, DC, American Psychiatric Association, 1994

American Psychiatric Association: Diagnostic and Statistical Manual of Mental Disorders, 5th Edition. Arlington, VA, American Psychiatric Association, 2013

Aron L: A Meeting of Minds: Mutuality in Psychoanalysis. New York, Analytic Press, 1996

Aron L, Starr K: A Psychotherapy for the People: Toward a Progressive Psychoanalysis. New York, Routledge, 2013

Axelrod SR, Widiger TA, Trull TJ, et al: Relations of five-factor model antagonism facets with personality disorder symptomatology. J Pers Assess 69:297–313, 1997

Baker L, Silk KR, Westen D, et al: Malevolence, splitting, and parental ratings by borderlines. J Nerv Ment Dis 180:258–264, 1992

Balint M: The Basic Fault: Therapeutic Aspects of Regression. Evanston, IL, Northwestern University Press, 1969

Bandura A: Social Foundations of Thought and Action. Englewood Cliffs, NJ, Prentice-Hall, 1986

Bandura A: Social cognitive theory of personality, in Handbook of Personality: Theory and Research, 2nd Edition. Edited by Pervin L, John O. New York, Guilford, 1999, pp 154–196

Barazandeh H, Kissane DW, Saeedi N, Gordon M: A systematic review of the relationship between early maladaptive schemas and borderline personality disorder/traits. Pers Individ Dif 94:130–139, 2016

Beck A: Cognitive aspects of personality disorders and their relation to syndromal disorders: a psychoevolutionary approach, in Personality and Psychopathology. Edited by Cloninger CR. Washington, DC, American Psychiatric Association, 1999, pp 411–429

Beck AT, Haigh EAP: Advances in cognitive theory and therapy: the generic cognitive model. Annu Rev Clin Psychol 10:1–24, 2014

Beck A, Butler A, Brown G, et al: Dysfunctional beliefs discriminate personality disorders. Behav Res Ther 39:1213–1225, 2001

Beck A, Freeman A, Davis D: Cognitive Therapy of Personality Disorders, 2nd Edition. New York, Guilford, 2004

Beck AT, Davis D, Freeman A: Cognitive Therapy of Personality Disorders, 3rd Edition. New York, Guilford, 2015

Bellak L, Chassan JB, Gediman HK, et al: Ego function assessment of analytic psychotherapy combined with drug therapy. J Nerv Ment Dis 157:465–469, 1973

Benjamin L: Interpersonal Diagnosis and Treatment of Personality Disorders. New York, Guilford, 1993

Benjamin LS: Interpersonal Diagnosis and Treatment of Personality Disorders, 2nd Edition. New York, Guilford, 1996a

Benjamin LS: An interpersonal theory of personality disorders, in Major Theories of Personality Disorder. Edited by Clarkin JF, Lenzenweger MF. New York, Guilford, 1996b, pp 141–220

Bhar S, Beck A, Butler A: Beliefs and personality disorders: an overview of the personality beliefs questionnaire. J Clin Psychol 68:88–100, 2012

Blanck G, Blanck R: Ego Psychology: Theory and Practice. New York, Columbia University Press, 1974

Bleuler E: Dementia Praecox or the Group of Schizophrenias (1911). New York, International Universities Press, 1950

Bowlby J: Attachment and Loss, Vol 1: Attachment. New York, Basic Books, 1969

Bowlby J: Attachment and Loss, Vol 2: Separation. New York, Basic Books, 1973

Buss DM: The great struggles of life: Darwin and the emergence of evolutionary psychology. Am Psychol 64:140–148, 2009

Buss DM (ed): Handbook of Evolutionary Psychology, 2nd Edition. New York, Wiley, 2016

Buss DM: Sexual conflict in human mating. Curr Dir Psychol Sci 26:307–313, 2017

Buss DM, Schmitt DP: Mate preferences and their behavioral manifestations. Annu Rev Psychol 70:77–110, 2019

Caligor E, Kernberg OF, Clarkin JF, Yeomans FE: Psychodynamic Therapy for Personality Pathology: Treating Self and Interpersonal Functioning. Washington, DC, American Psychiatric Association Publishing, 2018

Cantor N, Harlow RE: Personality, strategic behavior, and daily life problem solving. Curr Dir Psychol Sci 3:169–172, 1994

Cantor N, Kihlstrom JF: Personality and Social Intelligence. Englewood Cliffs, NJ, Prentice-Hall, 1987

Caspi A, Moffitt TE: All for one and one for all: mental disorders in one dimension. Am J Psychiatry 175:831–844, 2018

Caspi A, McClay J, Moffitt TE, et al: Role of genotype in the cycle of violence in maltreated children. Science 297:851–854, 2002

Caspi A, Hariri AR, Holmes A, et al: Genetic sensitivity to the environment: the case of the serotonin transporter gene and its implications for studying complex diseases and traits. Am J Psychiatry 167:509–527, 2010

Cattane N, Rossi R, Lanfredi M, Cattaneo A: Borderline personality disorder and childhood trauma: exploring the affected biological systems and mechanisms. BMC Psychiatry 17:221, 2017

Cicchetti D: Socioemotional, personality, and biological development: illustrations from a multilevel developmental psychopathology perspective on child maltreatment. Annu Rev Psychol 67:187–211, 2016

Cloninger CR: The genetics and psychobiology of the seven-factor model of personality, in Biology of Personality Disorders. Edited by Silk KR (Review of Psychiatry Series, Vol 17; Oldham JM, Riba MB, series eds). Washington, DC, American Psychiatric Press, 1998, pp 63–92

Cloninger CR: Feeling Good: The Science of Well-Being. New York, Oxford University Press, 2004

Cloninger CR: The psychobiological theory of temperament and character: comment on Farmer and Goldberg (2008). Psychol Assess 20:292–299, 2008

Cloninger CR, Svrakic DM, Przybeck TR: A psychobiological model of temperament and character. Arch Gen Psychiatry 50:975–990, 1993

Cohen P, Crawford TN, Johnson JG, Kasen S: The Children in the Community study of developmental course of personality disorder. J Pers Disord 19:466–486, 2005

Coker L, Samuel D, Widiger T: Maladaptive personality functioning within the Big Five and the five-factor model. J Pers Disord 16:385–401, 2002

Costa P, McCrae R: Longitudinal stability of adult personality, in Handbook of Personality Psychology. Edited by Hogan R, Johnson J. San Diego, CA, Academic Press, 1997, pp 269–290

Cristea IA, Gentili C, Cotet CD, et al: Efficacy of psychotherapies for borderline personality disorder: a systematic review and meta-analysis. JAMA Psychiatry 74:319–328, 2017

Damon W, Hart D: Self-Understanding in Childhood and Adolescence. New York, Cambridge University Press, 1988

DeFife JA, Drill R, Nakash O, Westen D: Agreement between clinician and patient ratings of adaptive functioning and developmental history. Am J Psychiatry 167(12):1472–1478, 2010

DeFife JA, Goldberg M, Westen D: Dimensional assessment of self- and interpersonal functioning in adolescents: implications for DSM-5's general definition of personality disorder. J Pers Disord 27:1–12, 2013a

DeFife JA, Peart J, Bradley B, et al: Validity of prototype diagnosis for mood and anxiety disorders. JAMA Psychiatry 70:140–148, 2013b

Dias BG, Ressler KJ: Parental olfactory experience influences behavior and neural structure in subsequent generations. Nat Neurosci 17:89–96, 2014

Eysenck H: The Biological Basis of Personality. Springfield, IL, Charles C Thomas, 1967

Eysenck H: A Model for Personality. New York, Springer-Verlag, 1981

Eysenck HJ: Biological dimensions of personality, in Handbook of Personality: Theory and Research. Edited by Pervin LA. New York, Guilford, 1990, pp 244–276

Fairbairn WR: Psychoanalytic Studies of the Personality. London, Tavistock, 1952

Fonagy P, Target M: Attachment and reflective function: their role in self-organization. Dev Psychopathol 9:679–700, 1997

Fonagy P, Steele H, Steele M: Maternal representations of attachment during pregnancy predict the organization of infant-mother attachment at one year of age. Child Dev 62:891–905, 1991

Fonagy P, Gergely G, Jurist EL, et al: Affect Regulation, Mentalization, and the Development of the Self. New York, Other Press, 2002

Fonagy P, Target M, Gergely G, et al: The developmental roots of borderline personality disorder in early attachment relationships: a theory and some evidence. Psychoanalytic Inquiry 23:412–459, 2003

Fonagy P, Target M, Bateman A: The mentalization based approach to psychotherapy for borderline personality disorder, in The Psychoanalytic Therapy of Severe Disturbance. Edited by Williams P. New York, Routledge, 2018, pp 35–80

Gabbard GO, Crisp-Han H: Narcissism and Its Discontents: Diagnostic Dilemmas and Treatment Strategies With Narcissistic Patients. Washington, DC, American Psychiatric Association Publishing, 2018

Garcia J, Koelling RA: Relation of cue to consequence in avoidance learning. Psychonomic Science 4:123–124, 1966

Gescher DM, Kahl KG, Hillemacher T, et al: Epigenetics in personality disorders: today's insights. Front Psychiatry 9:579, 2018

Goldberg L: The structure of phenotypic personality traits. Am Psychol 48:26–34, 1993

Goldstein W: DSM-III and the narcissistic personality. Am J Psychother 39:4–16, 1985

Greenberg JR, Mitchell S: Object Relations in Psychoanalytic Theory. Cambridge, MA, Harvard University Press, 1983

Gunderson JG: Borderline Personality Disorder: A Clinical Guide. Washington, DC, American Psychiatric Publishing, 2001

Harter S: The Construction of the Self: A Developmental Perspective. New York, Guilford, 1999

Hartmann H: Ego psychology and the problem of adaptation, in Organization and Pathology of Thought: Selected Sources. Edited by Rapaport D. New York, Columbia University Press, 1951, pp 362–396

Hinrichs J, DeFife JA, Westen D: Personality subtypes in adolescent and adult children of alcoholics: a two-part study. J Nerv Ment Dis 199:487–498, 2011

Hopwood CJ, Thomas KM, Markon KE, et al: DSM-5 personality traits and DSM-IV personality disorders. J Abnorm Psychol 121:424–432, 2012

Horowitz M: Introduction to Psychodynamics: A Synthesis. New York, Basic Books, 1988

Horowitz M: Cognitive Psychodynamics: From Conflict to Character. New York, Wiley, 1998

Hsu W-T, Rosenberg MD, Scheinost D, et al: Resting-state functional connectivity predicts neuroticism and extraversion in novel individuals. Soc Cogn Affect Neurosci 13:224–232, 2018

Jackson DB, Beaver KM: The association between breastfeeding exposure and duration, neuropsychological deficits, and psychopathic personality traits in offspring: the moderating role of 5HTTLPR. Psychiatr Q 87:107–127, 2016

Kajonius P, Mac Giolla E: Personality traits across countries: support for similarities rather than differences. PLoS One 12:e0179646, 2017

Kendler KS, Myers JM, Maes HH, et al: The relationship between the genetic and environmental influences on common internalizing psychiatric disorders and mental well-being. Behav Genet 41:641–650, 2011

Kerber A, Schultze M, Müller S, et al: Development of a short and ICD-11 compatible measure for DSM-5 maladaptive personality traits using ant colony optimization algorithms. November 17, 2019. Available at: https://psyarxiv.com/rsw54. Accessed March 24, 2020

Kernberg O: Borderline Conditions and Pathological Narcissism. Northvale, NJ, Jason Aronson, 1975a

Kernberg O: Transference and countertransference in the treatment of borderline patients. J Natl Assoc Priv Psychiatr Hosp 7:14–24, 1975b

Kernberg O: Severe Personality Disorders. New Haven, CT, Yale University Press, 1984

Kernberg O: A psychoanalytic theory of personality disorders, in Major Theories of Personality Disorder. Edited by Clarkin J, Lenzenweger M. New York, Guilford, 1996, pp 106–140

Kernberg O: Pathological narcissism and narcissistic personality disorder: theoretical background and diagnostic classification, in Disorders of Narcissism: Diagnostic, Clinical, and Empirical Implications. Edited by Ronningstam E. Washington, DC, American Psychiatric Association, 1998, pp 29–51

Kiesler D: The 1982 interpersonal circle: a taxonomy for complementarity in human transactions. Psychol Rev 90:185–214, 1983

Kohut H: The Analysis of the Self: A Systematic Approach to the Treatment of Narcissistic Personality Disorders. New York, International Universities Press, 1971

Kohut H: The Restoration of the Self. Madison, WI, International Universities Press, 1977

Kotov R, Krueger RF, Watson D, et al: The hierarchical taxonomy of psychopathology (HiTOP): a dimensional alternative to traditional nosologies. J Abnorm Psychol 126:454–477, 2017

Kraepelin E: Dementia Praecox and Paraphrenia (1896). Chicago, IL, Chicago Medical Book Company, 1919

Krueger RF: The structure of common mental disorders. Arch Gen Psychiatry 56:921–926, 1999

Krueger RF, Caspi A, Moffitt TE, Silva PA: The structure and stability of common mental disorders (DSM-III-R): a longitudinal-epidemiological study. J Abnorm Psychol 107:216–227, 1998

Krueger RF, Derringer J, Markon KE, et al: Initial construction of a maladaptive personality trait model and inventory for DSM-5. Psychol Med 42:1879–1890, 2012

Krueger RF, Kotov R, Watson D, et al: Progress in achieving quantitative classification of psychopathology. World Psychiatry 17(3):282–293, 2018

Leary T: Interpersonal Diagnosis of Personality: A Functional Theory and Methodology for Personality Evaluation. Oxford, UK, Ronald Press, 1957

Lenzenweger MF, Clarkin JF, Kernberg OF, Foelsch PA: The Inventory of Personality Organization: psychometric properties, factorial composition, and criterion relations with affect, aggressive dyscontrol, psychosis proneness, and self-domains in a nonclinical sample. Psychol Assess 13:577–591, 2001

Levy KN, Meehan KB, Clouthier TL, et al: Transference-focused psychotherapy for adult borderline personality disorder, in Case Studies Within Psychotherapy Trials: Integrating Qualitative and Quantitative Methods. Edited by Fishman DB, Messer SB, Edwards DJA, Dattilio FM. New York, Oxford University Press, 2017, pp 190–245

Linehan M: Cognitive-Behavioral Treatment of Borderline Personality Disorder. New York, Guilford, 1993a

Linehan M: Skills-Training Manual for Treatment of Borderline Personality Disorder. New York, Guilford, 1993b

Linehan M: DBT Skills Training Manual, 2nd Edition. New York, Guilford, 2015

Linehan M: Building a Life Worth Living: A Memoir. New York, Random House, 2020

Livesley WJ: An empirically-based classification of personality disorders. J Pers Disord 25:397–420, 2011

Livesley WJ, Bromley DB: Person Perception in Childhood and Adolescence. London, Wiley, 1973

Livesley WJ, Jang K, Jackson D, et al: Genetic and environmental contributions to dimensions of personality disorder. Am J Psychiatry 150:1826–1831, 1993

Livesley WJ, Jang KL, Vernon PA: Phenotypic and genetic structure of traits delineating personality disorder. Arch Gen Psychiatry 55:941–948, 1998

Livesley WJ, Jang K, Vernon P: Genetic basis of personality structure, in Handbook of Psychology: Personality and Social Psychology, Vol 5. Edited by Millon T, Lerner M. New York, Wiley, 2003, pp 59–83

Lobbestael J, Arntz A, Sieswerda S: Schema modes and childhood abuse in borderline and antisocial personality disorders. J Behav Ther Exp Psychiatry 36:240–253, 2005

Lynam DR, Widiger TA: Using the five-factor model to represent the DSM-IV personality disorders: an expert consensus approach. J Abnorm Psychol 110:401–412, 2001

Main M: Recent studies in attachment: overview, with selected implications for clinical work, in Attachment Theory: Social, Developmental, and Clinical Perspectives. Edited by Goldberg S, Muir R, Kerr J. Hillsdale, NJ, Analytic Press, 1995, pp 407–474

Manuck S, McCaffery J: Gene-environment interaction. Annu Rev Psychol 65:41–70, 2014

Masterson J: Psychotherapy of the Borderline Adult: A Developmental Approach. New York, Brunner/Mazel, 1976

McCrae R, Costa P: Personality in Adulthood. New York, Guilford, 1990

McCrae RR, Costa PT Jr: Personality trait structure as a human universal. Am Psychol 52:509–516, 1997

McWilliams N: Psychoanalytic Diagnosis: Understanding Personality Structure in the Clinical Process, 2nd Edition. New York, Guilford, 2011

Mikolajewski AJ, Allan NP, Hart SA, et al: Negative affect shares genetic and environmental influences with symptoms of childhood internalizing and externalizing disorders. J Abnorm Child Psychol 41:411–423, 2013

Millon T: Toward a New Psychology. New York, Wiley, 1990

Millon T: What is a personality disorder? J Pers Disord 30:289–306, 2016

Millon T, Davis R: An evolutionary theory of personality disorders, in Major Theories of Personality Disorder. Edited by Clarkin J, Lenzenweger M. New York, Guilford, 1996, pp 221–346

Mischel W: Toward a cognitive social learning reconceptualization of personality. Psychol Rev 39:351–364, 1973

Mischel W: On the interface of cognition and personality: beyond the person-situation debate. Am Psychol 34:740–754, 1979

Mischel W: Personality dispositions revisited and revised: a view after three decades, in Handbook of Personality: Theory and Research. Edited by Pervin L. New York, Guilford, 1990, pp 111–134

Mischel W, Shoda Y: A cognitive-affective system theory of personality: reconceptualizing situations, dispositions, dynamics, and invariance in personality structure. Psychol Rev 102:246–268, 1995

Mitchell SA: Relational Concepts in Psychoanalysis: An Integration. Cambridge, MA, Harvard University Press, 1988

Morey L, Gunderson J, Quigley B, et al: The representation of borderline, avoidant, obsessive-compulsive, and schizotypal personality disorders by the five-factor model. J Pers Disord 16:215–234, 2002

Moutsiana C, Johnstone T, Murray L, et al: Insecure attachment during infancy predicts greater amygdala volumes in early adulthood. J Child Psychol Psychiatry 56:540–548, 2015

Mullin ASJ, Hilsenroth MJ, Gold J, Farber BA: Facets of object representation: process and outcome over the course of psychodynamic psychotherapy. J Pers Assess 100:145–155, 2018

Nadort M, Arntz A, Smit JH, et al: Implementation of outpatient schema therapy for borderline personality disorder with versus without crisis support by the therapist outside office hours: a randomized trial. Behav Res Ther 47:961–973, 2009

Nakash O, Nagar M, Westen D: Agreement between clinician, patient, and independent interviewer ratings of adaptive functioning and developmental history. J Nerv Ment Dis 206:116–121, 2018

Norman WT: Toward an adequate taxonomy of personality attributes: replicated factors structure in peer nomination personality ratings. J Abnorm Soc Psychol 66:574–583, 1963

Obsuth I, Hennighausen K, Brumariu LE, Lyons-Ruth K: Disorganized behavior in adolescent–parent interaction: relations to attachment state of mind, partner abuse, and psychopathology. Child Dev 85:370–387, 2014

Plomin R, Caspi A: Behavioral Genetics and Personality. New York, Guilford, 1999

Pretzer JL, Beck AT: A cognitive theory of personality disorders, in Major Theories of Personality Disorder. Edited by Clarkin J, Lenzenweger M. New York, Guilford, 1996, pp 36–105

Puig J, Englund MM, Simpson JA, Collins WA: Predicting adult physical illness from infant attachment: a prospective longitudinal study. Health Psychol 32:409–417, 2013

Redl F, Wineman D: Children Who Hate: The Disorganization and Breakdown of Behavior Controls. Glencoe, IL, Free Press, 1951

Reich W: Character Analysis, 3rd Edition (1933). New York, Simon & Schuster, 1978

Ressler KJ: The intersection of environment and the genome in posttraumatic stress disorder. JAMA Psychiatry 73:653–654, 2016

Richardson LA, Porcerelli JH, Dauphin VB, et al: The use of the Social Cognition and Object Relations Scale in a primary care setting. J Pers Assess 100:156–165, 2018

Ross S, Lutz C, Bailley S: Positive and negative symptoms of schizotypy and the five-factor model: a domain and facet level analysis. J Pers Assess 79:53–72, 2002

Rottman B, Ahn W, Sanislow C, Kim N: Can clinicians recognize DSM-IV personality disorders from five-factor model descriptions of patient cases? Am J Psychiatry 166:427–433, 2009

Russ E, Shedler J, Bradley R, Westen D: Refining the construct of narcissistic personality disorder: diagnostic criteria and subtypes. Am J Psychiatry 165:1473–1481, 2008

Schaefer E: Configurational analysis of children's reports of parent behavior. J Consult Psychol 29:552–557, 1965

Shaver PR, Mikulincer M: Attachment theory and research: resurrection of the psychodynamic approach to personality. J Res Pers 39:22–45, 2005

Skodol AE, Morey LC, Bender DS, Oldham JM: The ironic fate of the personality disorders in DSM-5. Personal Disord 4(4):342–349, 2013

Skodol A, Morey L, Bender D, Oldham J: The Alternative DSM-5 Model for Personality Disorders: a clinical application. Am J Psychiatry 172:607–613, 2015

Stein MB, Siefert CJ: Introduction to the special section on the Social Cognition and Object Relations Scale–Global Rating Method: from research to practice. J Pers Assess 100:117–121, 2018

Stein MB, Slavin-Mulford J: Social Cognition and Object Relations Global Rating Method (SCORS-G): A Comprehensive Guide for Clinicians and Researchers. New York, Routledge, 2018

Stringaris A, Vidal-Ribas Belil P, Artiges E, et al: The brain's response to reward anticipation and depression in adolescence: dimensionality, specificity, and longitudinal predictions in a community-based sample. Am J Psychiatry 172:1215–1223, 2015

Sullivan HS: The Interpersonal Theory of Psychiatry. New York, WW Norton, 1953

Tellegen A, Waller NG: Exploring personality through test construction: development of the Multidimensional Personality Questionnaire, in Personality Measures: Development and Evaluation, Vol 1. Edited by Briggs SR, Cheeks JM. Greenwich, CT, JAI Press, 1993

Toyokawa S, Uddin M, Koenen KC, Galea S: How does the social environment "get into the mind"? Epigenetics at the intersection of social and psychiatric epidemiology. Soc Sci Med 74(1):67–74, 2012

Trull T, Widiger T, Burr R: A structured interview for the assessment of the five-factor model of personality: facet-level relations to the Axis II personality disorders. J Pers 69:175–198, 2001

Turkheimer E, Haley A, Waldron M, et al: Socioeconomic status modifies heritability of IQ in young children. Psychol Sci 14:623–628, 2003

Turkheimer E, Pettersson E, Horn EE: A phenotypic null hypothesis for the genetics of personality. Annu Rev Psychol 65:515–540, 2014

Venta A, Herzhoff K, Cohen P, Sharp C: The longitudinal course of borderline personality disorder in youth, in Handbook of Borderline Personality Disorder in Children and Adolescents. Edited by Sharp C, Tackett JL. New York, Springer Science + Business Media, 2014, pp 229–245

Wachtel P: Psychoanalysis and Behavior Therapy. New York, Basic Books, 1977

Wachtel P: Psychoanalysis, Behavior Therapy, and the Relational World. Washington, DC, American Psychological Association, 1997

Westen D: The relations among narcissism, egocentrism, self-concept, and self-esteem: experimental, clinical and theoretical considerations. Psychoanalysis and Contemporary Thought 13:183–239, 1990a

Westen D: Towards a revised theory of borderline object relations: contributions of empirical research. Int J Psychoanal 71:661–693, 1990b

Westen D: Cognitive-behavioral interventions in the psychoanalytic psychotherapy of borderline personality disorders. Clin Psychol Rev 11:211–230, 1991a

Westen D: Social cognition and object relations. Psychol Bull 109:429–455, 1991b

Westen D: Toward an integrative model of affect regulation: applications to social-psychological research. J Pers 62:641–667, 1994

Westen D: A clinical-empirical model of personality: life after the Mischelian ice age and the NEO-lithic era. J Pers 63:495–524, 1995

Westen D: A model and a method for uncovering the nomothetic from the idiographic: an alternative to the five-factor model? J Res Pers 30:400–413, 1996

Westen D: Case formulation and personality diagnosis: two processes or one? in Making Diagnosis Meaningful: Enhancing Evaluation and Treatment of Psychological Disorders. Edited by Barron JW. Washington, DC, American Psychological Association, 1998, pp 111–138

Westen D: Prototype diagnosis of psychiatric syndromes. World Psychiatry 11:16–21, 2012

Westen D, Blagov P: A clinical-empirical model of emotion regulation: from defenses and motivated reasoning to emotional constraint satisfaction, in Handbook of Emotion Regulation. Edited by Gross J. New York, Guilford, 2007, pp 373–392

Westen D, Heim A: Theories of personality and personality disorders, in The American Psychiatric Publishing Textbook of Personality Disorders. Edited by Oldham JM, Skodol AE, Bender DS. Washington, DC, American Psychiatric Publishing, 2005, pp 17–34

Westen D, Muderrisoglu S: Assessing personality disorders using a systematic clinical interview: evaluation of an alternative to structured interviews. J Pers Disord 17:351–369, 2003

Westen D, Muderrisoglu S: Clinical assessment of pathological personality traits. Am J Psychiatry 163:1285–1297, 2006

Westen D, Weinberger J: When clinical description becomes statistical prediction. Am Psychol 59:595–613, 2004

Westen D, Klepser J, Ruffins S, et al: Object relations in childhood and adolescence: the development of working representations. J Consult Clin Psychol 59:400–409, 1991

Westen D, Shedler J, Bradley R: A prototype approach to personality disorder diagnosis. Am J Psychiatry 163:846–856, 2006

Westen D, Shedler J, Bradley B, DeFife JA: An empirically derived taxonomy for personality diagnosis: bridging science and practice in conceptualizing personality. Am J Psychiatry 169:273–284, 2012

Westen D, DeFife J, Malone J, Dilallo J: An empirically derived classification of adolescent personality disorders. J Am Acad Child Adolesc Psychiatry 53:528–549, 2014a

Westen D, Waller N, Shedler J, Blagov P: Dimensions of personality and personality pathology: factor structure of the Shedler–Westen Assessment Procedure–II (SWAP-II). J Pers Disord 28:281–318, 2014b

Wichers M, Gardner C, Maes HH, et al: Genetic innovation and stability in externalizing problem behavior across development: a multi-informant twin study. Behav Genet 43:191–201, 2013

Widiger T: Personality disorders in the 21st century. J Pers Disord 14:3–16, 2000

Widiger T, Costa P: Personality and personality disorders. J Abnorm Psychol 103:78–91, 1994

Widiger T, Trull T, Clarkin J, et al: A description of the DSM-IV personality disorders with the five-factor model of personality, in Personality Disorders and the Five-Factor Model of Personality, 2nd Edition. Edited by Costa P, Widiger T. Washington, DC, American Psychological Association, 2002, pp 89–99

Widiger TA, Sellbom M, Chmielewski M, et al: Personality in a hierarchical model of psychopathology. Clin Psychol Sci 7:77–92, 2019

Wolf E: Treating the Self: Elements of Clinical Self Psychology. New York, Guilford, 1988

Yeomans FE, Clarkin JF, Kernberg OF: Transference-Focused Psychotherapy for Borderline Personality Disorder: A Clinical Guide. Washington, DC, American Psychiatric Association Publishing, 2015

Young J: Cognitive Therapy for Personality Disorders: A Schema-Focused Approach. Sarasota, FL, Professional Resource Exchange, 1990

Young J, Gluhoski V: Schema-focused diagnosis for personality disorders, in Handbook of Relational Diagnosis and Dysfunctional Family Patterns. Edited by Kaslow F. Oxford, UK, Wiley, 1996, pp 300–321

Young J, Kellogg S: Schema therapy for borderline personality disorder. J Clin Psychol 62:445–458, 2006

Young J, Lindemann M: An integrative schema-focused model for personality disorders, in Clinical Advances in Cognitive Psychotherapy: Theory and Application. Edited by Leahy R, Dowd T. New York, Springer, 2002, pp 93–109

Young J, Klosko J, Weishaar M: Schema therapy for borderline personality disorder, in Schema Therapy: A Practitioner's Guide. New York, Guilford, 2003

CHAPTER 3

Articulating a Core Dimension of Personality Pathology

Leslie C. Morey, Ph.D.
Donna S. Bender, Ph.D., FIPA

Problems with the categorical approach to personality disorders (PDs) presented in DSM-III (American Psychiatric Association 1980), DSM-IV (American Psychiatric Association 1994), and the DSM-5 (American Psychiatric Association 2013) Section II PD classification (which is virtually identical to DSM-IV) have been well documented. Among the issues of greatest concern is the extensive co-occurrence of PDs, such that most patients who receive a PD diagnosis meet criteria for more than one (e.g., Grant et al. 2005; Morey 1988; Oldham et al. 1992; Zimmerman et al. 2005). Another concern is the relatively poor convergent validity of PD criteria sets, apparent when considering that patient groups diagnosed by different methods may be only weakly related to one another (Clark 2007; Hyler et al. 1989; Pilkonis et al. 1995). This unfortunate situation results in manifestations of putatively different "personality diagnoses" that are more highly associated than different phenotypic variations within the same "personality diagnosis" (e.g., Morey and Levine 1988).

Although extensive co-occurrence is perhaps the most consistently replicated result in the field of PDs, the various editions of DSM, including PDs in DSM-5 Section II ("Diagnostic Criteria and Codes"), have yet to offer any representation of PD that accounts for this phenomenon or provide a compelling explanation as to why it is so reliably found. At the outset of work on DSM-5, the Personality and Personality Disorders (P&PD) Work Group was charged with developing a new approach to the "Personality Disorders" section of DSM-5 that would begin to rectify the comorbidity problem (Kupfer et al. 2002; Rounsaville et al. 2002). As part of these deliberations, the work group sought to provide some representation of PD that would delineate the essential similarities, apparently shared by most, if not all, DSM PD categories, that were driving the remarkable comorbidity among these disorders. The DSM-IV (and DSM-5) general criteria for a PD indicate that an enduring pattern of inner experience and behavior is manifest in two or more of the following areas: cognition, affectivity, interpersonal functioning, and impulse control. These very broad criteria do not appear to be very specific for PDs, nor are they always consistent with the specific criteria for individual PDs in DSM, creating possible confusion about whether individual PDs always meet the general criteria. Finally, it is important to understand that these general PD criteria were introduced in DSM-IV without justification or any empirical basis— there is no mention of them in the PD chapters of the *DSM-IV Sourcebook* (Gunderson 1996; Widiger et al. 1996) or in articles that described the development of the revised classification (Frances et al. 1990, 1991; Pincus et al. 1992; Widiger et al. 1991). Consequently, the general criteria for PD in DSM have commonly been ignored in clinical practice and research, and they fail to provide any insight into the shared elements that are common to PDs and that differentiate them from other forms of mental disorder.

Many of the significant shortcomings of the DSM PD categories were addressed by the P&PD Work Group, who developed the Alternative DSM-5 Model for Personality Disorders (AMPD) found in DSM-5 Section III, "Emerging Measures and Models" (American Psychiatric Association 2013). The AMPD consists of dimensional assessments of shared core impairments in personality functioning common to all PDs, as well as dimensional assessments of pathological personality traits that may be found to varying degrees across different patients. When combined with other DSM-IV-like inclusion and exclusion criteria, this combination of core impairments and pathological traits yields diagnoses that bear substantial empirical similarity to DSM-IV PDs (Morey and Skodol 2013) but have a clear conceptual structure that maps out the elemental "traits" that are present to an unusual degree and also provides an essential assessment structure of the core features of personality dysfunction.

In this chapter, we provide an overview of the notion of "core dysfunction" in PD, describing the history of such a concept and the instantiation of the concept in the DSM-5 Section III model. We also review research that helps articulate the concept and demonstrates its potential validity and utility, along with clinical illustrations of its utility.

Historical Background

It is somewhat ironic that there was a significant subgroup of PD experts opposing the DSM-5 Section III model on the grounds that it is a substantial departure from precedent, given that the notion of a unitary construct of personality disturbance greatly predates the DSM-III/DSM-IV representation of discrete PD categories. In fact, in 1963, Menninger surveyed 2,000 years of the history of classification in psychiatry and identified "a steady trend toward simplification and reduction of the categories from thousands to hundreds to dozens to a mere four or five" (Menninger 1963, p. 9). Menninger thus proposed a revolutionary psychiatric classification that comprised a single class—a unitary conception of what he called "personality dysorganization," in contrast to "disorganization," in that personality organization has not been lost but only impaired to various degrees. This "dysorganization" was manifest at five different levels of severity of impairment in adaptive control, impulse management, and ego failures.

Menninger's early views and observations by others (e.g., Rushton and Irwing 2011) have pointed out that the history of the study of personality is replete with such unitary, dimensional severity models. Sir Francis Galton (1887) described a general factor of personality in his paper "Good and Bad Temper in English Families," using ratings from family members across generations to group 15 adjectives indicative of "good temper" (e.g., self-controlled) and 46 markers of "bad temper" (e.g., proud, uncertain, vindictive) that could be arrayed along a single dimension. Although there were about three times as many markers of "bad" personality as "good," he believed that the ratio of the number of these markers present was distributed in a bell-shaped fashion, with comparable numbers of individuals at each extreme (identified by Galton as those manifesting a 2:1 ratio of these adjectives, in either direction). In this description, Galton was echoing in many ways James Cowles Prichard's (1835) concept of *moral insanity*, which Prichard described as "a morbid perversion of the natural feelings, affections, inclinations, temper, habits, moral dispositions, and natural impulses, without any remarkable disorder or defect of the intellect or knowing and reasoning faculties, and particularly without any insane illusion or hallucination" (p. 24). Prichard acknowledged that this single class of mental disorder could take many forms, stating that "the varieties of moral insanity are perhaps as numerous as the modifications of feeling or passion in the human mind" (Prichard 1835, p. 24). These different forms could involve extremes in emotion (despondency or excitement), impulses, hostility, eccentricity, or "decay of social affection," but Rushton and Irwing (2011) noted that the common denominator to moral insanity was self-control ("will-power"), a lack of which could cause harm to oneself or to others.

In contrast to the taxonomic work of psychiatric writers such as Emil Kraepelin (1902), who delineated classes of disorder such as manic-depression and dementia praecox that were presented as qualitatively different phenomena, many personality-oriented writers continued to emphasize a more unitary approach that identified critical differences as existing between points along a single continuum. In many accounts, this continuum was thought to reflect a developmental process, and individuals could be grouped according to various "stages" in this process. Whereas Freud's models of development, including psychosexual stages (Freud 1905/1953) and the evolution of narcissism to object-love (Freud 1914/1957), were of considerable heuristic influence, many other theorists described stage models with considerable overlap in the indicators of placement along this continuum. Theorists such as Piaget (1932), Kohlberg (1963), Erikson (1950), and Loevinger (1976) all denoted developmental sequences that with maturation resulted in greater self-control and increased prosocial behavior.

Although Menninger (1963) obviously misread the trend that produced the explosion of diagnostic entities in DSM-III that descended from a Kraepelinian rather than a unitary tradition (Blashfield 1984), Menninger's overview of the historical evolution of this model provides a compelling reminder that the significance of a severity gradient in evaluating personality problems has been described for far longer than the specific personality entities introduced in DSM-III. For example, in the long history of personality assessment research, the specter of a single, overarching dimension of personality dysfunction has repeatedly emerged in various empirical approaches to the study of personality. Early personality inventories such as the Minnesota Multiphasic

Personality Inventory (Hathaway and McKinley 1943) were seemingly saturated with a large single source of variability, with repeated efforts to "eliminate" the contributions of this large component as an undesirable artifact (e.g., Meehl 1945; Tellegen et al. 2003) rather than as a personality characteristic of substantive significance. The "lexical" tradition of factor analysis of personality adjectives, pioneered by Norman (1963) and Digman (1990) and culminating in the five-factor model (FFM), began with a set of personality descriptors that purposefully sought to remove "evaluative" (i.e., good vs. bad) descriptors of personality as a basis for the resulting dimensional structure, presumably because of the compelling influence such a dimension had on subsequent factor analyses (Block 1995). Despite those efforts, it appears that a unitary dimension of dysfunction may underlie even putatively orthogonal factor structures such as the FFM. For example, research studying the different DSM PDs consistently finds that the various disorders display quite similar configurations on the FFM (Morey et al. 2000, 2002; Saulsman and Page 2004; Zweig-Frank and Paris 1995), a configuration particularly characterized by high neuroticism and low conscientiousness and agreeableness. Several studies have concluded that the five factors themselves are subsumed under higher-order factors, such as the "Big Two" factors, labeled *alpha* and *beta* by Digman (1997) or *stability* and *plasticity* by DeYoung et al. (2002). However, evidence supports the contention that even these two super factors are themselves subsumed by a higher-order dimension. In two meta-analyses of Big Five interscale correlations, Rushton and Irwing (2008) and Van der Linden et al. (2010) concluded that there was strong evidence of what Rushton and Irwing described as a single "general factor of personality"; these meta-analyses included the data sets that Digman (1997) had used to establish the "alpha" and "beta" factors. Additional analyses found very poor fit of a model specifying that the Big Two were uncorrelated.

In addition to results from factor analysis studies, theoretical accounts support the contention of a super factor of personality functioning. Block (2010) provided the interesting observation that the Big Two components of stability and plasticity, as two presumably desirable elements of personality, have important theoretical parallels to Piaget's (1932) notions of assimilation and accommodation, fundamental processes in the development of the child. Piaget identified these as the core principles by which the child constructs and modifies internal representations of objects and actions, allowing him or her to achieve equilibrium as well as adapt to the world. As Block (2010) noted, assimilation and accommodation represent manifestations of a single, central developmental process that continues to influence behavior throughout the life span, and research on social cognition supports the conclusion that these processes play a foundational role in shaping interactions with others. For example, Anderson and Cole (1990) demonstrated that when a new acquaintance is assimilated into a category of "significant other representations," perceivers are quick to inappropriately apply preconceived notions that are, in some instances, quite inaccurate. Thus, maturation (or the failure thereof) of these representational processes has a powerful influence on one's view of self and of others.

Kernberg (1967) was one of the first contemporary writers to formulate a classification of character pathology that encompasses different forms of personality problems arrayed along a severity continuum reflecting what he terms different levels of "personality organization." Central to this concept was the notion of *identity*, comprising the various ways in which individuals experience themselves in relation to others

(Kernberg 1984). Normal identity involves a self-view that is realistic and integrated, with a correspondingly realistic and stable experience of others. With increasingly problematic personality organization, identity becomes more diffuse, inflexible, unstable, and poorly integrated. Kernberg and Caligor (2005) offered an ordering of the different DSM categories of PD, as they could be arrayed along this continuum of personality organization severity.

Contemporary Status of Global Concept of Personality Impairment

Efforts to identify core elements of PD are found in numerous measures and scales designed to identify personality problems. In the process of attempting to identify these core impairments in personality functioning, Bender et al. (2011) reviewed several reliable and valid clinician-administered measures for assessing personality functioning and psychopathology and demonstrated that content relevant to representations of self and other permeates such instruments and that these instruments have solid empirical bases and significant clinical utility. For example, numerous studies using measures of self and interpersonal functioning have demonstrated their utility for determining the existence, type, and severity of personality pathology. These measures include clinician-completed rating scales or interviews, as well as patient self-report measures. Among the clinician instruments reviewed were measures such as the Social Cognition and Object Relations Scale (M. Hilsenroth, M. Stein, and J. Pinsker, "Social Cognition and Object Relations Scale: Global Method [SCORS-G]," unpublished manuscript, The Derner Institute of Advanced Psychological Studies, Adelphi University, Garden City, NY, 2004; Westen et al. 1990) and the Structured Interview of Personality Organization (Stern et al. 2010). The review by Bender et al. (2011) found that all such measures sampled content pertaining to distorted and maladaptive thinking about oneself and others. A synthesis of these common elements suggested that the components most central to effective personality functioning fall under the rubrics of *identity*, *self-direction*, *empathy*, and *intimacy*, with reliability estimates for existing measures of these constructs typically exceeding 0.75.

Such concepts appeared to merit consideration as common mechanisms that may underlie all PDs. The existence of such core impairments is suggested by the high rates of co-occurring PD diagnoses based on DSM criteria (e.g., Morey 1988). The idea that all PDs may be arrayed along a common dimension reflecting PD severity was also supported by the finding that efforts to make the DSM diagnostic rules more restrictive (by narrowing the diagnostic rules to include only the most "prototypical" cases) had the seemingly paradoxical effect of increasing rather than decreasing PD comorbidity. An early effort by Morey (2005) examined three different data sets that each included information about every DSM-defined PD criterion. In these data sets, a score was calculated for each patient that reflected the summed count of all PD criteria present in that patient. In these three data sets, the coefficient alpha values were 0.81, 0.96, and 0.94, suggesting that the problematic behaviors and characteristics listed in the criteria for the various DSM PDs form an internally consistent dimension that cuts across virtually all of the disorders. Given the nature of the DSM decision rules, it was apparent that higher "scores" on this single dimension would account for the widely observed comorbidity because the presence of additional symptom features would by definition increase the likelihood of any particular disorder. However, the high internal consistency values indicated that this was not simply a computational artifact but rather the operation of a substantive construct. The conclusion from this study was that failures in empathic relatedness, including the inability to accurately understand the perspective of others in shaping the self-concept, were present in varying degrees in all PDs. Furthermore, more severe and pervasive empathy problems are linked to the presence of more and diverse PD features and hence to assignment of multiple PD diagnoses to such patients.

Our work with the Collaborative Longitudinal Personality Disorders Study (CLPS) (Gunderson et al. 2000; Skodol et al. 2005) provided an important opportunity to better understand the correlates and implications of this putative global personality pathology dimension. The CLPS was a 10-year prospective, repeated-measures study that included patients with one of four specific DSM-IV-TR (American Psychiatric Association 2000) PDs (schizotypal, borderline, avoidant, or obsessive-compulsive) or patients with major depressive disorder in the absence of PD as a comparison group. Participants in the CLPS were assessed with interview and questionnaire measures of PD symptoms, traits, and functioning regularly throughout the course of the study. In a set of CLPS analyses reported by Hopwood et al. (2011), we sought to disentangle elements of global personality severity from the stylistic expression of these problems, because these were confounded in the DSM-III and DSM-IV conceptualization of PD. Thus, that study had four aims: 1) to identify which DSM PD features constitute the best markers of "severity"; 2) to isolate elements of personality style that are independent of general severity; 3) to examine whether the severity and stylistic elements of PD should be assessed in parallel; and 4) to determine whether each element provides incremental information about impairment, longitudinal course, and outcomes of patients.

As in the various data sets described by Morey (2005), the severity composite representing the sum of all DSM-IV PD criteria was highly internally consistent (coefficient $\alpha=0.90$). The PD criteria that had the largest item-total correlations with this severity composite consistently demonstrated problems in self (e.g., avoidant: "feelings of inadequacy"; borderline: "identity disturbance") or interpersonal (e.g., avoidant: "social ineptness" or "preoccupation with being rejected"; schizotypal: "paranoid ideation") domains. The analyses of the predictive validity of this composite suggested that generalized personality pathology severity was the strongest predictor of concurrent and prospective dysfunction, although stylistic elements of personality pathology symptom expression proved incrementally useful for predicting specific kinds of dysfunction. Interestingly, most pathological personality traits and even those normative (i.e., FFM) traits thought to be most related to PD tended to be strongly related to global severity rather than to specific styles of dysfunction. Given that the global severity score accounted for most of the valid variance provided by PD concepts in predicting patient outcome, Hopwood et al. (2011, p. 317) offered the following recommendation for DSM-5:

> PD severity should be represented in the DSM-5 by a single quantitative dimension that accommodates a diverse array of elements, including dysfunction in social, emotional, and identity-related functioning, analogous to the GAF [Global Assessment of Functioning] score for general functioning but specifically linked to personality systems.

The DSM-5 P&PD Work Group explicitly attempted to follow through on these recommendations by reviewing relevant literature (Bender et al. 2011) and by analyzing additional existing data sets to further elaborate this dimension (Morey et al. 2011). Specifically, Morey et al. (2011) sought to identify items reflective of the core impairments in self and other representation described by the DSM-5 P&PD Work Group (Bender et al. 2011), with the aim of characterizing the manifestations of this impairment continuum at different levels of severity using item response theory (Lord 1980). The study derived a composite dimension of severity that was significantly associated with 1) the probability of being assigned any DSM-IV PD diagnosis, 2) the total number of DSM-IV PD features manifested, and 3) the probability of being assigned multiple DSM-IV PD diagnoses. The key markers of this dimension involved important functions related to self (e.g., identity integration, integrity of self-concept) and interpersonal (e.g., capacity for empathy and intimacy) relatedness—features that, as reviewed by Bender et al. (2011), play a prominent role in influential theoretical conceptualizations of core personality pathology (Kernberg and Caligor 2005; Kohut 1971; Livesley 2003). The patterning of markers along the putative severity continuum demonstrated some interesting features. Self-related features such as identity issues, low self-worth, and impaired self-direction appear to be central characteristics of milder levels of personality pathology, whereas interpersonal issues (in addition to self pathology) become discriminating at the more severe levels of personality pathology. Such a finding is consistent with the view of Kernberg (e.g., Kernberg 1984) and others that identity issues play a foundational role in driving the characteristic interpersonal dysfunction noted in PDs.

Taking findings from these and other studies into account, the DSM-5 P&PD Work Group sought to synthesize various concepts across self-other models to form a foundation for rating personality functioning on a continuum, with the goal of creating a severity scale that could be easily applied by clinicians. This rating scale was refined through a focus on elements that could be assessed reliably in previous research (Bender et al. 2011) and that also emerged in various studies as discriminating markers of this dimension. The resulting scale, titled the Level of Personality Functioning Scale (LPFS; American Psychiatric Association 2013), was thus designed to serve as a basis for determining global level of impairment in personality functioning in DSM-5. This rating represents a single-item composite evaluation of impairment in the four self-other areas described in Table 3–1. The LPFS provides anchor points describing characteristics of five impairment levels (little or none, some, moderate, severe, and extreme). (The LPFS is provided in its entirety in the Appendix to this volume. See also Chapter 4, "The Alternative DSM-5 Model for Personality Disorders," in this volume for a more complete discussion of the AMPD.)

Measures of DSM-5 Personality Functioning

In the AMPD, the assessment of PD core impairment is presented as a rating scale, with a clinician applying the LPFS to provide a rating on a five-point scale of severity ranging from healthy functioning (level=0) to extreme impairment (level=4). Although the LPFS has been criticized as potentially being too difficult for clinicians to use without extensive training, which would result in poor reliability (e.g., Pilkonis

TABLE 3–1.   **Four self-other areas of personality functioning typically impaired in personality disorder**

Self

Identity: Experience of oneself as unique, with clear boundaries between self and others; stability of self-esteem and accuracy of self-appraisal; capacity for, and ability to regulate, a range of emotional experience.

Self-direction: Pursuit of coherent and meaningful short-term and life goals; utilization of constructive and prosocial internal standards of behavior; ability to self-reflect productively.

Interpersonal

Empathy: Comprehension and appreciation of others' experiences and motivations; tolerance of differing perspectives; understanding of the effects of one's own behavior on others.

Intimacy: Depth and duration of positive connection with others; desire and capacity for closeness; mutuality of regard reflected in interpersonal behavior.

et al. 2011), studies have found that speculation to be unsubstantiated and indicated that, in fact, it can be used with adequate reliability. For example, Morey (2019) had 123 clinicians rate AMPD constructs on 12 clinical vignettes. The interrater reliability for the LPFS total score had an intraclass correlation of 0.50 for a single rater and 0.98 when aggregated across the multiple raters, values that were larger than those attained for any of the DSM-IV categorical PD diagnoses. Other studies have reported that even lay raters can achieve adequate interrater reliability on the LPFS. For example, Zimmermann et al. (2014) had undergraduate psychology students view recorded clinician interviews and provide LPFS ratings of personality functioning. The median internal consistency/coefficient alpha for the aggregated LPFS markers was greater than 0.75 for both domain and total scores, and the interrater reliability for the LPFS total score had an intraclass correlation of 0.51 for a single rater and 0.96 when aggregated across the multiple raters, values that are virtually identical to those obtained by Morey (2019) in his study of experienced clinicians. In a different study, Morey (2018) determined that undergraduate students were able to use the LPFS indicators with very high internal consistency, and the indicators aligned well with their lay concepts of a disordered personality. As such, it appears that concerns about the difficulty of applying the LPFS in standard practice are unwarranted.

In addition to the clinical use of the LPFS as a rating scale, a variety of formal assessment techniques for measuring this core impairment dimension have been developed since the introduction of the AMPD, including both structured clinical interviews and self-report questionnaires. Structured interviews for this purpose include the Semi-Structured Interview for Personality Functioning DSM-5 (STiP-5.1; Hutsebaut et al. 2017), Clinical Assessment of the LPFS (CALF; Thylstrup et al. 2016), and Structured Clinical Interview for the Level of Personality Functioning Scale (SCID-5-AMPD Module I; Bender et al. 2018). Use of these structured techniques may lead to even greater interrater reliability for the LPFS than with the unstructured use described earlier; for example, Hutsebaut et al. (2017) described an intraclass interrater correlation of 0.89 for the STiP total score when applied to a clinical sample, whereas Buer Christensen et al. (2018) obtained an intraclass reliability with the SCID-5-AMPD Module I of 0.96 for the total LPFS score. However, Thylstrup et al. (2016) obtained a somewhat lower interrater reliability value of 0.65 for the total score when they used the CALF in their total sample, which they attributed to the relatively higher level of inference required in using that interview.

A variety of self-report questionnaires to measure the AMPD core impairment dimension also have been developed, including the LPFS—Self-Report (LPFS-SR; Morey 2017), the LPFS—Brief Form (LPFS-BF; Hutsebaut et al. 2016), the DSM-5 Levels of Personality Functioning Questionnaire (DLOPFQ; Huprich et al. 2018), the Self and Interpersonal Functioning Scale (Gamache et al. 2019), and a questionnaire designed for use with adolescents, the Levels of Personality Functioning Questionnaire (LoPF-Q 12–18; Goth et al. 2018). Each of these self-report questionnaires has certain advantages and disadvantages. The LPFS-BF is a very brief measure involving three items targeting each of the four content areas of the LPFS, resulting in a total of 12 items. It has shown expected associations with indicators of problem severity and well-being and incremental prediction of problems over and above measures of problematic personality traits (Bach and Hutsebaut 2018). However, because of its brevity, the LFPS-BF has a limited ability to sample problems that might manifest across different levels of personality dysfunction. In contrast, the LPFS-SR includes 80 items written to capture each specific indicator described in the LPFS table (see Appendix) and is thus particularly well suited for studying the conceptual organization of these features. The LPFS-SR has been found to correlate substantially with a wide range of problematic personality traits, PD constructs, and interpersonal problems, while showing discriminant validity with other indicators of personality with less relationship to distress and dysfunction (Hopwood et al. 2018). However, at 80 items, the LPFS-SR is appreciably longer than the 12-item LPFS-BF. Finally, the DLOPFQ has 132 items that assess levels of functioning across work or school and close relationships. The DLOPFQ scales have demonstrated incremental prediction over and above problematic traits on several criterion measures (Huprich et al. 2018), although its correspondence with provider ratings of LPFS constructs is limited (Nelson et al. 2018). With 132 items, the DLOPFQ is lengthy, and the items have less clear correspondence to the DSM-5 LPFS concepts than the preceding instruments.

As would be expected in a unidimensional construct representing a core impairment dimension, the internal consistency of these questionnaires tends to be quite high, in excess of 0.90 for most instruments. Although test-retest reliability has received less research attention to date, the LPFS-SR also had test-retest correlations of 0.91 for the total score over short-term periods (Hopwood et al. 2018). As such, these questionnaires represent efficient and reliable ways to estimate an individual's level of personality dysfunction.

Research on Level of Personality Functioning Scale Core Dimensionality and Utility

Researchers have increasingly been exploring whether the LPFS does indeed capture a unitary construct at the heart of personality functioning across a spectrum and how useful this approach is in clinical work and in characterizing dysfunction.

To ascertain both the utility and the validity of clinician judgments when using the LPFS, Morey et al. (2013a) examined clinician-rated LPFS scores as applied to a broad sample of patients with and without prominent PD features. This study had three important aspects. First, it was assumed that LPFS ratings should be related to DSM-IV PD diagnoses, given the assumption that all PDs reflect impairment in this core self-other dimension and that this rating would differentiate those receiving such diagnoses from those not diagnosed with PD. Second, the study explored whether LPFS ratings were significantly related to critical clinical judgments, such as estimates of broad adaptive functioning, risk for harm to self or others, long-term prognosis, and clinical appraisals of needed treatment intensity. Finally, the study sought to determine whether mental health professionals would view the LPFS ratings as clinically useful—whether conceptualizing their patient in this way would be seen as relevant for patient description and treatment decision making. These questions were addressed in a national sample of 337 clinicians providing complete PD diagnostic information about a patient with whom they were familiar, which involved a full formulation of both DSM-IV and DSM-5 AMPD diagnostic judgments.

The results of the Morey et al. (2013a) study demonstrated that, consistent with the assumption that these personality functioning deficits underlie all PDs, the single-item LPFS showed solid sensitivity (0.846) and specificity (0.727) for identifying the presence or absence of DSM-IV PDs. Furthermore, the scale was also related to DSM-IV PD comorbidity, with those individuals receiving multiple DSM-IV diagnoses obtaining more severe ratings on the LPFS. Furthermore, analyses were conducted to compare the incremental validity of the DSM-5 LPFS rating with that of DSM-IV PD diagnoses with respect to their ability to predict clinical judgments of psychosocial functioning, short-term risk, estimated prognosis, and optimal level of treatment intensity. All predictive validity correlations for both LPFS ratings and DSM-IV diagnoses were statistically significant. However, for three of the four validity variables, the single-item DSM-5 LPFS rating yielded adjusted multiple correlations that were larger than those provided when considering all 10 DSM-IV PD diagnoses. In the areas of functioning, prognosis, and treatment intensity needs, the DSM-5 LPFS successfully captured an appreciable part of the valid variance contributed by DSM-IV PD diagnoses and significantly incremented that information as well. Only in the area of risk assessment did information about the specific PD diagnoses prove useful as a supplement to the LPFS rating of impairment in personality functioning.

In addition to the results described earlier, a separate investigation by these researchers (Morey et al. 2013b) examined clinicians' perceptions of the clinical utility of the LPFS and other PD diagnostic constructs. Following completion of ratings for DSM-IV criteria and the LPFS rating, clinicians were asked six questions about the perceived clinical utility of each set of information provided. Compared with the DSM-5 LPFS rating, DSM-IV was seen as easier to use and more useful for communication with other professionals. However, in every other respect—for treatment planning, patient description, and communicating to the patient—the DSM-5 LPFS had higher mean usefulness ratings than DSM-IV. Thus, clinicians perceived the single-item DSM-5 LPFS rating as being generally more useful in several important ways than the entire set of 79 DSM-IV PD criteria. This is in spite of these clinicians' greater presumed familiarity with DSM-IV over the previous 18 years and their having no experience with the DSM-5 Section III proposal at the time of the study.

Research on validity, latent structure, and internal consistency of the LPFS has continued to evolve. For example, high internal consistency, unidimensionality, and concurrent validity were demonstrated in two investigations of the LPFS-SR by Morey

(2017, 2018). The 2017 study showed an internal consistency alpha estimate of 0.969 for the LPFS-SR total score and alphas ranging from 0.816 to 0.891 for the four subcomponents. A single component representing more than 85% of the variance among the four subscales was yielded by a principal components process, supporting the notion that the LPFS represents a single dimension in structure. Analysis of relevant measures in exploring concurrent validity indicated that the LPFS had correlations often exceeding 0.80 for the overall total score. Morey (2018) replicated the internal consistency finding in a study that also showed that undergraduate students were able to easily and effectively apply the LPFS.

The structure of the LPFS dimension was assessed in another study that yielded two highly correlated factors (Zimmermann et al. 2015). In addition, a principal components analysis by Cruitt et al. (2019) supported a single underlying LPFS dimension. Hopwood et al. (2018) used multiple measures to explore the validity of the LPFS-SR and suggested: "Data further support that identity, self-direction, intimacy, and empathy components of the LPFS–SR can be characterized by a single factor and have similar correlations with criterion variables, consistent with the hypothesis that DSM-5 Criterion A is a relatively homogeneous construct" (p. 650).

Other studies have also explored the validity of the LPFS and its utility as a measure of functional capacities of clinical importance. Several self-report measures have shown convergence with personality functioning and severity of personality psychopathology assessment instruments (Bach and Anderson 2020; Gamache et al. 2019; Hopwood et al. 2018; Hutsebaut et al. 2016; Morey 2017; Oltmanns and Widiger 2019; Sleep et al. 2019; Weekers et al. 2019) such as the Severity Indices of Personality Problems (Verheul et al. 2008), the Personality Assessment Inventory (Morey 2007), and the General Assessment of Personality Disorder (Hentschel and Livesley 2013). Presence of DSM-5 Section II PDs (Cruitt et al. 2019; Dereboy et al. 2018; Hutsebaut et al. 2017; Preti et al. 2018; Zimmermann et al. 2014), number of PD symptoms and prognosis (Few et al. 2013; Hutsebaut et al. 2017; Morey et al. 2013a), maladaptive traits (Hopwood et al. 2018; Morey 2018; Oltmanns and Widiger 2019), and interpersonal dysfunction (Dowgwillo et al. 2018; Hopwood et al. 2018; Roche et al. 2018) also have been found to be significantly related to the core construct measured by the LPFS. In addition, the dimensions of a self-other functioning scale developed by Gamache et al. (2019) yielded significant associations with poor self-esteem, identity diffusion, negative emotions, and interpersonal distress. Overall low levels of well-being also were shown to be correlated with personality functioning in several studies (Gamache et al. 2019; Huprich et al. 2018; Nelson et al. 2018). Similarly, Cruitt et al. (2019) noted that the personality functioning ratings were useful in predicting clinical outcome, and strong clinical utility ratings were reported by Zimmermann et al. (2014).

Level of Personality Functioning Case Illustrations

To demonstrate the enhanced utility of the DSM-5 Section III LPFS over the DSM-IV/ DSM-5 Section II categorical approach to PDs, we offer a case comparison. As mentioned earlier, one of the problems with the categorical polythetic criteria approach to PDs is that there can be significant variations within the same diagnosis, causing important clinical information to be lost if one does not look beyond the limited information conveyed by a categorical diagnostic label. The following two clinical case examples show the importance of assessing the core LPFS elements of personality functioning.

Case Example 1

Madison is an intelligent, funny, talkative, attractive, age 20-something woman who sought psychotherapy because she was determined to build a better life for herself than her family, particularly her emotionally volatile mother and sister, had managed. She also has been "too stressed out" at her job. Madison had done very well academically in college and succeeded in obtaining a good position with a large consulting firm. She works long hours but is often concerned that she is not doing her projects "perfectly," which makes her very anxious at times. Her perfectionism causes her to spend excessive effort trying to be completely thorough, adding unnecessary additional time at the office. She also refuses to take help from colleagues because she is sure they will make mistakes or not have high enough standards. In spite of her worries, she has gotten very positive reviews from her supervisors, but she does not derive much reassurance from that. She also attends a demanding master's program during the evenings and weekends, so most of her time is devoted to work, with little left for socializing.

Madison also impresses one as determined to be an engaged and productive "good patient." She talks in excessive detail and in a highly intellectualized manner, but strong emotions are very difficult for her to tolerate and talk about. She can explain very well how she thinks about things but has trouble considering how she feels. She described one occasion when it was apparent that she had a panic attack rather than let herself know how angry she was at her colleagues. Although she is able to consider others' perspectives, she has little tolerance for those who do not agree with her or live up to her standards. These attitudes lead to additional stress and frustration for Madison in the workplace.

Madison has a close group of women friends she has known since the beginning of college, but she is sometimes critical of some of their life choices. She obviously values these friends and does what she can to socialize with them, given her overloaded schedule. She also has a boyfriend but is having some difficulty getting close to him and is inhibited in expressing her affection. She is jealous of other women as well, with likely unwarranted worries that her boyfriend will be unfaithful, but she does not understand why he finds it troublesome to be distrusted in that way.

Given her excessive devotion to work, perfectionism, overconscientious approach to tasks, and refusal to delegate tasks to others, Madison meets criteria for DSM-IV/DSM-5 Section II obsessive-compulsive PD. Looking more closely at her inner life and personality functioning with the LPFS, Madison's profile fits with level 1, some impairment. She has a relatively intact sense of self but has some difficulty handling strong emotions (identity); she is overly intellectualizing, is excessively goal-directed, and has unrealistically high standards (self-direction); she is resistant to appreciating others' perspectives, although she can, and does not quite understand why her jealousy bothers her boyfriend (empathy); and she has solid and enduring relationships, but they are somewhat compromised by her inhibitions in emotional expression and excessively high standards for others (intimacy).

Case Example 2

Ryan presented with a similar style to Madison's. He is a married, well-educated, highly intelligent, and verbal 28-year-old engineer. Ryan greatly values his career and is proud of working for a prestigious firm. His presenting complaint was difficulty with completing work effectively, due to perfectionism that generates excessive anxiety. Ryan puts in long hours at his job attempting to make progress on his projects but often dwells on fairly insignificant points for days on end. He also experiences some friction at times with his coworkers because of his insistence that his opinions and approach to tasks are most correct. Ryan also reported that he is very active in his church, at least on Sundays, the only day he does not work. He seemingly derives satisfaction from that community, with his and his wife's social life centering on their relationships there. However, Ryan has been very upset that his suggestions to the church leadership for changing procedures have not been accepted unconditionally. He is considering leaving the congregation because of this, but his wife has managed to convince him to stay thus far.

Like Madison, Ryan's perfectionism interferes with task completion, and he is excessively devoted to work. He is stubborn and rigid in his collaborations with others and becomes too preoccupied with the small details of his projects. Given these characteristics, Ryan also meets criteria for obsessive-compulsive PD.

However, if one stopped the clinical interview of Ryan at this point, a great deal of very important information would be lost, and an inadequate treatment plan may be formulated. By probing about the LPFS areas of identity, self-direction, empathy, and intimacy, one discovers important differences between Madison and Ryan. Ryan reported that he often feels terrible about himself and has an ongoing terror of being criticized. He constantly seeks approval from his boss and feels miserable if he is not praised for his work. He sees himself as particularly gifted and entitled to special recognition and as much smarter than his colleagues. Similarly, his anger at his church for not taking his suggestions makes him feel "invisible" and indignant. "I have an Ivy League degree, and those dullards can't seem to appreciate what I have to offer." Clearly, he has some issues with regulating self-esteem and looks to others for ongoing approval (identity). It is also apparent that Ryan's slavish devotion to work is not motivated only by an internal set of high standards but is primarily a means to try to gain external approval (self-direction).

In the area of empathy, Ryan does not have a very good sense of how his stubborn, opinionated behavior might affect others, nor does he seem to care very much. He longs for praise and acceptance at work and at church, but he seems to lack the ability to consider why others might have a different opinion, and he has trouble having dialogues. When asked about his marriage and friendships, Ryan says his relationships often disappoint him because people do not appreciate him enough (intimacy). Not surprisingly, he is having some marital problems.

As can be seen in the comparison of these two cases, it is important to clinically explore the core components of personality functioning to get beyond surface behaviors and attitudes. Both of these patients meet criteria for obsessive-compulsive PD under the DSM-5 Section II criteria, but the significant differences in their character structures are identified by the LPFS assessment. Whereas Madison showed personality difficulties rated at level 1, indicating some impairment, Ryan had more marked problems, which would be scored as level 2, for moderate impairment. In addition, as assessed with the new Section III model, Madison would not meet full criteria for a PD because an LPFS level of 2 or greater is required for disorder status to be assigned. As a clinician, one would likely take a different approach with Madison, because her self-structure is more intact, than with Ryan, who has more vulnerable self-esteem. Furthermore, with the greater severity of Ryan's central personality issues, we begin to see indications of other PD diagnoses (such as attributes of narcissistic PD), which in DSM-IV/DSM-5 Section II would be portrayed as "comorbidity," leading to possible confusion and contradictions when considering the criteria of multiple categories. However, the LPFS more effectively represents these phenomena simply as increased impairment in the core components.

Conclusion

In contrast with any "official" representation of PD provided in various editions of DSM, the DSM-5 AMPD diagnostic system delineates a specific continuum of core personality functioning that captures features underlying all PDs. This continuum is represented in the new system with a single-item rating of the LPFS that Morey et al. (2013a, 2013b) found to bear strong relationships to PD diagnosis and to important clinical judgments. The lack of a conceptualization of PD severity in the DSM-IV taxonomy (a lack that continues to pertain to DSM-5 Section II) represents a significant failure of an antiquated diagnostic system to adequately capture a primary source of variance in virtually all markers of clinical validity. Availability of such a PD-specific severity measure not only may assist in identifying central aspects of personality pathology but also will help guide treatment decisions and help stimulate research on the fundamental nature of PD. It is hoped that in future revisions, DSM will provide the field with official recognition of the importance of such an assessment.

References

American Psychiatric Association: Diagnostic and Statistical Manual of Mental Disorders, 3rd Edition. Washington, DC, American Psychiatric Association, 1980

American Psychiatric Association: Diagnostic and Statistical Manual of Mental Disorders, 4th Edition. Washington, DC, American Psychiatric Association, 1994

American Psychiatric Association: Diagnostic and Statistical Manual of Mental Disorders, 4th Edition, Text Revision. Washington, DC, American Psychiatric Association, 2000

American Psychiatric Association: Diagnostic and Statistical Manual of Mental Disorders, 5th Edition. Arlington, VA, American Psychiatric Association, 2013

Anderson SM, Cole SW: "Do I know you?" The role of significant others in general social perception. J Pers Soc Psychol 59:384–399, 1990

Bach B, Anderson JL: Patient-reported ICD-11 personality disorder severity and DSM-5 level of personality functioning. J Pers Disord 34:231–249, 2020

Bach B, Hutsebaut J: Level of Personality Functioning Scale—Brief Form 2.0: utility in capturing personality problems in psychiatric outpatients and incarcerated addicts. J Pers Assess 100:660–670, 2018

Bender DS, Morey LC, Skodol AE: Toward a model for assessing level of personality functioning in DSM-5, part I: a review of theory and methods. J Pers Assess 93:332–346, 2011

Bender DS, Skodol AE, First MB, et al: Module I: structured clinical interview for the level of personality functioning scale, in Structured Clinical Interview for the DSM-5 Alternative Model for Personality Disorders (SCID-AMPD). Washington, DC, American Psychiatric Association Publishing, 2018

Blashfield RK: The Classification of Psychopathology: Neo-Kraepelinian and Quantitative Approaches. New York, Plenum, 1984

Block J: A contrarian view of the five-factor approach to personality description. Psychol Bull 117:187–215, 1995

Block J: The five-factor framing of personality and beyond: some ruminations. Psychological Inquiry 21:2–25, 2010

Buer Christensen T, Paap MC, Arnesen M, et al: Interrater reliability of the structured clinical interview for the DSM–5 alternative model of personality disorders module I: Level of Personality Functioning Scale. J Pers Assess 100:630–641, 2018

Clark LA: Assessment and diagnosis of personality disorder: perennial issues and an emerging reconceptualization. Annu Rev Psychol 58:227–257, 2007

Cruitt PJ, Boudreaux MJ, King HR, et al: Examining Criterion A: DSM–5 level of personality functioning as assessed through life story interviews. Personal Disord 10:224–234, 2019

Dereboy F, Dereboy Ç, Eskin M: Validation of the DSM-5 alternative model personality disorder diagnoses in Turkey, part 1: LEAD validity and reliability of the personality functioning ratings. J Pers Assess 100:603–611, 2018

DeYoung CG, Peterson JB, Higgins DM: Higher order factors of the Big Five predict conformity: are there neuroses of health? Pers Individ Dif 33:533–552, 2002

Digman JM: Personality structure: emergence of the five-factor model. Annu Rev Psychol 50:116–123, 1990

Digman JM: Higher-order factors of the Big Five. J Pers Soc Psychol 73:1246–1256, 1997

Dowgwillo EA, Roche MJ, Pincus AL: Examining the interpersonal nature of Criterion A of the DSM-5 Section III alternative model for personality disorders using bootstrapped confidence intervals for the interpersonal circumplex. J Pers Assess 100:581–592, 2018

Erikson EH: Childhood and Society. New York, WW Norton, 1950

Few LR, Miller JD, Rothbaum AO, et al: Examination of the Section III DSM-5 diagnostic system for personality disorders in an outpatient clinical sample. J Abnorm Psychol 122:1057–1069, 2013

Frances A, Pincus HA, Widiger TA, et al: DSM-IV: work in progress. Am J Psychiatry 147:1439–1448, 1990

Frances AJ, First MB, Widiger TA, et al: An A to Z guide to DSM-IV conundrums. J Abnorm Psychol 100:407–412, 1991

Freud S: Three essays on the theory of sexuality (1905), in The Standard Edition of the Complete Psychological Works of Sigmund Freud, Vol 12. Translated by Strachey J. London, Hogarth Press, 1953, pp 135–243

Freud S: On narcissism: an introduction (1914), in The Standard Edition of the Complete Psychological Works of Sigmund Freud, Vol 14. Translated by Strachey J. London, Hogarth Press, 1957, pp 73–102

Galton F: Good and bad temper in English families. Fortnightly Review 42:21–30, 1887

Gamache D, Savard C, Leclerc P, et al: Introducing a short self-report for the assessment of DSM-5 level of personality functioning for personality disorders: the Self and Interpersonal Functioning Scale. Personal Disord 10:438–447, 2019

Goth K, Birkhölzer M, Schmeck K: Assessment of personality functioning in adolescents with the LoPF-Q 12-18 self-report questionnaire. J Pers Assess 100:680–690, 2018

Grant BF, Stinson FS, Dawson DA, et al: Co-occurrence of DSM-IV personality disorders in the United States: results from the National Epidemiologic Survey on Alcohol and Related Conditions. Compr Psychiatry 46:1–5, 2005

Gunderson JG: Introduction to Section IV: personality disorders, in DSM-IV Sourcebook, Vol 2. Edited by Widiger TA, Frances AJ, Pincus HA, et al. Washington, DC, American Psychiatric Association, 1996, pp 647–664

Gunderson JG, Shea T, Skodol AE, et al: The Collaborative Longitudinal Personality Disorders Study: development, aims, design, and sample characteristics. J Pers Disord 14:300–315, 2000

Hathaway SR, McKinley JC: Manual for the Minnesota Multiphasic Personality Inventory. New York, Psychological Corporation, 1943

Hentschel AG, Livesley WJ: The General Assessment of Personality Disorder (GAPD): factor structure, incremental validity of self-pathology, and relations to DSM-IV personality disorders. J Pers Assess 95:479–485, 2013

Hopwood CJ, Malone JC, Ansell EB, et al: Personality assessment in DSM-V: empirical support for rating severity, style, and traits. J Pers Disord 25:305–320, 2011

Hopwood CJ, Good EW, Morey LC: Validity of the DSM-5 Levels of Personality Functioning Scale—Self Report. J Pers Assess 100:650–659, 2018

Huprich SK, Nelson SM, Meehan KB, et al: Introduction of the DSM-5 Levels of Personality Functioning Questionnaire. Personal Disord 9:553–563, 2018

Hutsebaut J, Feenstra DJ, Kamphuis JH: Development and preliminary psychometric evaluation of a brief self-report questionnaire for the assessment of the DSM-5 Level of Personality Functioning Scale: the LPFS Brief Form (LPFS-BF). Personal Disord 7:192–197, 2016

Hutsebaut J, Kamphuis JH, Feenstra DJ, et al: Assessing DSM-5-oriented level of personality functioning: development and psychometric evaluation of the Semi-Structured Interview for Personality Functioning DSM-5 (STiP-5.1). Personal Disord 8:94–101, 2017

Hyler SE, Rieder RO, Williams JB, et al: A comparison of clinical and self-report diagnoses of DSM-III personality disorders in 552 patients. Compr Psychiatry 30:170–178, 1989

Kernberg OF: Borderline personality organization. J Am Psychoanal Assoc 15:641–685, 1967

Kernberg OF: Severe Personality Disorders: Psychotherapeutic Strategies. New Haven, CT, Yale University Press, 1984

Kernberg OF, Caligor E: A psychoanalytic theory of personality disorders, in Major Theories of Personality Disorder. Edited by Clarkin JF, Lenzenweger MF. New York, Guilford, 2005, pp 114–156

Kohlberg L: The development of children's orientations towards a moral order, I: sequence in the development of moral thought. Vita Hum Int Z Lebensalterforsch 6:11–33, 1963

Kohut H: The Analysis of the Self: A Systematic Approach to the Psychoanalytic Treatment of Narcissistic Personality Disorders. New York, International Universities Press, 1971

Kraepelin E: Clinical Psychiatry: A Textbook for Students and Physicians, 6th Edition. Translated by Diefendorf AR. London, Macmillan, 1902

Kupfer DJ, First MB, Regier DA: A Research Agenda for DSM-V. Washington, DC, American Psychiatric Association, 2002

Livesley WJ: Diagnostic dilemmas in classifying personality disorder, in Advancing DSM: Dilemmas in Psychiatric Diagnosis. Edited by Phillips KA, First MB, Pincus HA. Washington, DC, American Psychiatric Publishing, 2003, pp 153–189

Loevinger J: Ego Development. San Francisco, CA, Jossey-Bass, 1976

Lord FM: Applications of Item Response Theory to Practical Testing Problems. Hillsdale, NJ, Erlbaum, 1980

Meehl PE: An investigation of a general normality or control factor in personality testing. Psychological Monographs 59:i–62, 1945

Menninger K: The Vital Balance. New York, Viking Press, 1963

Morey LC: Personality disorders under DSM-III and DSM-III-R: an examination of convergence, coverage, and internal consistency. Am J Psychiatry 145:573–577, 1988

Morey LC: Personality pathology as pathological narcissism, in Personality Disorders. WPA Series: Evidence and Experience in Psychiatry, Vol 8. Edited by Maj M, Akiskal HS, Mezzich JE, Okasha A. Chichester, West Sussex, England, Wiley, 2005, pp 328–331

Morey LC: Personality Assessment Inventory Professional Manual, 2nd Edition. Odessa, FL, Psychological Assessment Resources, 2007

Morey LC: Development and initial evaluation of a self-report form of the DSM-5 Level of Personality Functioning Scale. Psychol Assess 29:1302–1308, 2017

Morey LC: Application of the DSM-5 Level of Personality Functioning Scale by lay raters. Personal Disord 32:709–720, 2018

Morey LC: Interdiagnostician reliability of the DSM-5 Section II and Section III Alternative Model criteria for Borderline Personality Disorder. J Pers Disord 33:721–735, 2019

Morey LC, Levine DJ: A multitrait multimethod examination of Minnesota Multiphasic Personality Inventory (MMPI) and Millon Clinical Multiaxial Inventory (MCMI). J Psychopathol Behav Assess 10:333–344, 1988

Morey LC, Skodol AE: Convergence between DSM-IV-TR and DSM-5 diagnostic models for personality disorder: evaluation of strategies for establishing diagnostic thresholds. J Psychiatr Pract 19:179–193, 2013

Morey LC, Gunderson JG, Quigley BA, et al: Dimensions and categories: the "Big Five" factors and the DSM personality disorders. Assessment 7:203–216, 2000

Morey LC, Gunderson JG, Quigley BD, et al: The representation of borderline, avoidant, obsessive-compulsive and schizotypal personality disorders by the five-factor model. J Pers Disord 16:215–234, 2002

Morey LC, Berghuis H, Bender DS, et al: Toward a model for assessing level of personality functioning in DSM-5, part II: empirical articulation of a core dimension of personality pathology. J Pers Assess 93:347–353, 2011

Morey LC, Bender DS, Skodol AE: Validating the proposed DSM-5 severity indicator for personality disorder. J Nerv Ment Dis 201:729–735, 2013a

Morey LC, Skodol AE, Oldham JM: Clinician judgments of clinical utility: a comparison of DSM-IV-TR personality disorders and the alternative model for DSM-5 personality disorders. J Abnorm Psychol 123:398–405, 2013b

Nelson SM, Huprich SK, Meehan KB, et al: Convergent and discriminant validity and utility of the DSM-5 Levels of Personality Functioning Questionnaire (DLOPFQ): associations with medical health care provider ratings and measures of physical health. J Pers Assess 100:671–679, 2018

Norman WT: Toward an adequate taxonomy of personality attributes: replicated factor structure in peer nomination personality ratings. J Abnorm Soc Psychol 66:574–583, 1963

Oldham JM, Skodol AE, Kellman HD, et al: Diagnosis of DSM-III-R personality disorders by two structured interviews: patterns of comorbidity. Am J Psychiatry 149:213–220, 1992

Oltmanns JR, Widiger TA: Evaluating the assessment of the ICD-11 personality disorder diagnostic system. Psychol Assess 31:674–684, 2019

Piaget J: The Moral Judgment of the Child. New York, Free Press, 1932

Pilkonis PA, Heape CL, Proietti JM, et al: The reliability and validity of two structured diagnostic interviews for personality disorders. Arch Gen Psychiatry 52:1025–1033, 1995

Pilkonis PA, Hallquist MN, Morse JQ, et al: Striking the (im)proper balance between scientific advances and clinical utility: commentary on the DSM-5 proposal for personality disorders. Personal Disord 2:68–82, 2011

Pincus HA, Frances A, Davis WW, et al: DSM-IV and new diagnostic categories: holding the line on proliferation. Am J Psychiatry 149:112–117, 1992

Preti E, Di Pierro R, Costantini G, et al: Using the Structured Interview of Personality Organization for DSM-5 Level of Personality Functioning rating performed by inexperienced raters. J Pers Assess 100:621–629, 2018

Prichard JC: A treatise on insanity and other disorders affecting the mind. London, Sherwood, Gilbert & Piper, 1835

Roche MJ, Jacobson NC, Phillips JJ: Expanding the validity of the Level of Personality Functioning Scale observer report and self-report versions across psychodynamic and interpersonal paradigms. J Pers Assess 100:571–580, 2018

Rounsaville BJ, Alarcon RD, Andrews G, et al: Basic nomenclature issues for DSM-V, in A Research Agenda for DSM-V. Edited by Kupfer DJ, First MB, Regier DA. Washington, DC, American Psychiatric Association, 2002, pp 1–29

Rushton JP, Irwing P: A general factor of personality (GFP) from two meta-analyses of the Big Five: Digman (1997) and Mount, Barrick, Scullen, and Rounds (2005). Pers Individ Dif 45:679–683, 2008

Rushton JP, Irwing P: The general factor of personality, in The Wiley-Blackwell Handbook of Individual Differences. Edited by Chamorro-Premuzic T, von Stumm S, Furnham A. Oxford, UK, Wiley-Blackwell, 2011, pp 132–161

Saulsman LM, Page AC: The five-factor model and personality disorder empirical literature: a meta-analytic review. Clin Psychol Rev 23:1055–1085, 2004

Skodol AE, Gunderson JG, Shea MT, et al: The Collaborative Longitudinal Personality Disorders Study (CLPS): overview and implications. J Pers Disord 19:487–504, 2005

Sleep CE, Lynam DR, Widiger TA, et al: An evaluation of DSM-5 Section III personality disorder Criterion A (impairment) in accounting for psychopathology. Psychol Assess 31:1181–1191, 2019

Stern BL, Caligor E, Clarkin JF, et al: Structured Interview of Personality Organization (STIPO): preliminary psychometrics in a clinical sample. J Pers Assess 92:35–44, 2010

Tellegen A, Ben-Porath YS, McNulty JL, et al: MMPI-2 Restructured Clinical (RC) Scales: Development, Validation, and Interpretation. Minneapolis, University of Minnesota Press, 2003

Thylstrup B, Simonsen S, Nemery C, et al: Assessment of personality-related levels of functioning: a pilot study of clinical assessment of the DSM-5 level of personality functioning based on a semi-structured interview. BMC Psychiatry 16:298, 2016

Van der Linden D, te Nijenhuis J, Bakker AB: The general factor of personality: a meta-analysis of Big Five intercorrelations and a criterion-related validity study. J Res Pers 44:315–327, 2010

Verheul R, Andrea H, Berghout C, et al: Severity Indices of Personality Problems (SIPP–118): development, factor structure, reliability, and validity. Psychol Assess 20:23–34, 2008

Weekers LC, Hutsebaut J, Kamphuis JH: The Level of Personality Functioning Scale—Brief Form 2.0: update of a brief instrument for assessing level of personality functioning. Personal Ment Health 13:3–14, 2019

Westen D, Lohr N, Silk K, et al: Object relations and social cognition in borderlines, major depressives, and normals: a Thematic Apperception Test analysis. Psychol Assess 2:355–364, 1990

Widiger TA, Frances AJ, Pincus HA, et al: Toward an empirical classification for the DSM-IV. J Abnorm Psychol 100:280–288, 1991

Widiger TA, Frances AJ, Pincus HA, et al (eds): DSM-IV Sourcebook, Vol 2. Washington, DC, American Psychiatric Association, 1996

Zimmermann J, Benecke C, Bender DS, et al: Assessing DSM-5 level of personality functioning from videotaped clinical interviews: a pilot study with untrained and clinically inexperienced students. J Pers Assess 96:397–409, 2014

Zimmermann J, Böhnke JR, Eschstruth R, et al: The latent structure of personality functioning: investigating Criterion A from the alternative model for personality disorders in DSM-5. J Abnorm Psychol 124:532–534, 2015

Zimmerman M, Rothchild L, Chelminski I: The prevalence of DSM-IV personality disorders in psychiatric outpatients. Am J Psychiatry 162:1911–1918, 2005

Zweig-Frank H, Paris J: The five-factor model of personality in borderline and nonborderline personality disorders. Can J Psychiatry 40:523–526, 1995

CHAPTER 4

The Alternative DSM-5 Model for Personality Disorders

Andrew E. Skodol, M.D.

Donna S. Bender, Ph.D., FIPA

John M. Oldham, M.D., M.S.

The diagnosis of personality disorders (PDs) according to explicit criteria and their placement on Axis II of the multiaxial diagnostic system of DSM-III (American Psychiatric Association 1980) have had beneficial effects on this often confusing and poorly understood area of psychopathology. Since the innovations of DSM-III, assessment methods have been developed and refined, and sound research on PDs has increased dramatically. Axis II provided a framework with which to determine the independent consequences of personality psychopathology for the individual and for society and the impact of PDs on the course and outcomes of other forms of psychopathology. It is now generally understood that PDs are prevalent in both clinical and community settings. They are associated with high rates of social and occupational impairment and predict slower recovery, more likely relapse, and a more chronic course for a host of other mental disorders. These broad effects of personality psychopathology have costly implications for both individual well-being and society.

Critiques of DSM's approach to the diagnosis of PD, however, appeared almost immediately after the publication of DSM-III (Frances 1980, 1982). DSM's exclusively categorical approach has resulted in well-documented problems: extensive co-occurrence

The authors would like to thank the members of the DSM-5 Personality and Personality Disorders Work Group, and especially Robert F. Krueger, Ph.D., Lee Anna Clark, Ph.D., and Leslie C. Morey, Ph.D., for their contributions to this chapter.

of PDs, such that most patients receiving a PD diagnosis have personality features that meet criteria for more than one PD (e.g., Grant et al. 2005; Oldham et al. 1992; Zimmerman et al. 2005); extreme heterogeneity among patients with the same PD diagnosis, meaning that two patients with a particular disorder may share very few features (Johansen et al. 2004); temporal instability of PD diagnoses, occurring at rates incompatible with the basic definition of a PD (Gunderson et al. 2011; Zanarini et al. 2012); arbitrary diagnostic thresholds in polythetic criteria sets with little or no empirical basis, resulting in the reification of disorders as present or absent with variable levels of underlying pathology (Balsis et al. 2011) and limited validity and clinical utility (Hyman 2010; Morey et al. 2007, 2012); poor coverage of personality pathology, such that the diagnosis of PD not otherwise specified (PDNOS) has been the most commonly diagnosed PD (Verheul and Widiger 2004); and poor convergent validity of PD criteria sets, such that patient groups diagnosed by different methods may be only weakly related to one another (Clark et al. 1997). None of these problems was successfully addressed in the ensuing iterations of DSM, including DSM-IV (American Psychiatric Association 1994).

As a consequence of these myriad problems, DSM-IV PD diagnoses often were not used (e.g., "Diagnosis Deferred on Axis II"), were underused (e.g., PDNOS), or were erroneously used (e.g., diagnoses made on the basis of too few of the required criteria). Despite these long-recognized and significant shortcomings, however, the criteria for PDs in DSM-5 (American Psychiatric Association 2013) Section II, "Diagnostic Criteria and Codes," did not change from those in DSM-IV.

The Personality and Personality Disorders (P&PD) Work Group for DSM-5 was charged with developing a new approach to the PD section that would begin to rectify some of these problems (Kupfer et al. 2002; Rounsaville et al. 2002). When the work group began its deliberations, a study endorsed by influential North American (Association for Research on Personality Disorders) and international (International Society for the Study of Personality Disorders) PD research organizations surveyed PD experts and found that 74% thought that the DSM-IV categorical approach to PDs should be replaced, 87% stated that personality pathology was dimensional in nature, and 70% supported a mixed dimensional-categorical approach to PD diagnosis as the most desirable alternative to DSM-IV (Bernstein et al. 2007). Hybrid models combining elements of dimensions and categories have been suggested by PD experts since before the publication of DSM-IV (Benjamin 1993; Blashfield 1993).

Such a dimensional-categorical hybrid had been developed in a DSM-5 planning meeting (Krueger et al. 2007), which preceded the formation of the P&PD Work Group and the start of work group discussions. A mixed approach improves on the DSM-IV system by striking a balance between introducing new elements called for by the field (e.g., dimensional elements) and maintaining continuity (e.g., preservation of PD categories)—an approach that takes into account research developments since the time of DSM-III, while still aiming to be minimally disruptive to clinical practice and research.

The alternative model for PDs in DSM-5 Section III, "Emerging Measures and Models" (American Psychiatric Association 2013), consists of assessments of the following: 1) new general criteria for PDs, 2) impairments in personality functioning, 3) pathological personality traits, and 4) criteria for six specific PDs. Impairments in personality functioning and the descriptiveness of pathological personality traits are fundamentally dimensional in nature and, when combined with other DSM-IV-like inclusion and exclusion criteria, yield categorical diagnoses of six PDs and a category called personality disorder–trait specified (PD-TS) for all other PD presentations. All six of these PDs were included in DSM-IV, but in the new model they are more consistently and coherently represented by impairment and trait manifestations. In this chapter, we review the rationale behind the alternative, hybrid model and discuss future research needs relevant to the possible inclusion of the model in the main section of the next revision of DSM.

General Criteria for Personality Disorder

The DSM-IV general criteria for a PD (GCPD) describe an enduring pattern of inner experience and behavior that is manifest in two or more of the following areas: cognition, affectivity, interpersonal functioning, and impulse control. These general criteria were introduced without justification or indication of an empirical basis. There is no mention of the GCPD in the PD chapters of the *DSM-IV Sourcebook* (Gunderson 1996; Widiger et al. 1996) or in articles that described the development of the revised classification (Frances et al. 1990, 1991; Pincus et al. 1992; Widiger et al. 1991). The DSM-IV GCPD do not appear to be specific for PDs; other chronic mental disorders seem likely to also meet the GCPD, leading to problems in differential diagnosis. Furthermore, the specific criteria for individual PDs in DSM-IV are often inconsistent with the GCPD, creating additional possible confusion.

In the DSM-5 Section III GCPD (see the Appendix to this textbook), the DSM-IV A criterion is divided into two criteria: the new Criterion A requires moderate or greater impairment in personality functioning, and the new Criterion B requires the presence of pathological personality traits. All PDs in Section III include specific, typical expressions of these A and B criteria, and PD-TS includes the GCPD A and B criteria themselves, making all PD diagnoses in DSM-5 Section III consistent with the GCPD.

Impairment in Personality (Self and Interpersonal) Functioning

Self and interpersonal impairments are at the core of personality psychopathology. Hopwood et al. (2011) demonstrated empirically that the DSM-IV PD criteria most strongly related to a PD severity dimension (based on a count of all criteria) were preoccupation with social rejection, fear of social ineptness, feelings of inadequacy, anger, identity disturbance, and paranoid ideation. The nature and importance of these criteria are consistent with the proposition that at the core of PDs of all types is a disturbance in how one views one's self and other people. Previously, Morey (2005) showed that difficulties in empathic capacity, at varying levels, can be found at the core of all types of personality psychopathology (for a detailed discussion of this self-other core of personality psychopathology, see Chapter 3, "Articulating a Core Dimension of Personality Pathology," in this volume).

DSM-IV (and DSM-5 Section II) PD criteria are heavily oriented toward self and interpersonal difficulties. In the DSM-IV GCPD, the "cognition" area under Criterion A gives "ways of perceiving and interpreting self, other people, and events" as a definition. The "interpersonal" criterion refers to "interpersonal functioning" (American

Psychiatric Association 1994). Thus, the centrality of self and interpersonal issues in PDs was recognized in DSM-IV but was not represented systematically or consistently. Hundreds of studies have been conducted on the relations between self and interpersonal constructs and personality psychopathology. The inclusion of impairment in self and interpersonal functioning in the GCPD of the DSM-5 Section III model, and as core elements of the Level of Personality Functioning Scale (LPFS; see the following subsection) and the Section III PDs, is an explicit extension of what was implicit in DSM-IV and has been well supported empirically.

The process of formulating the core impairments in personality functioning that are central to PDs began with a literature review (Bender et al. 2011) that considered several reliable and valid clinician-administered measures for assessing personality functioning and psychopathology. The review found that a self-other dimensional perspective has an empirical basis and significant clinical utility. Numerous studies using measures of self and interpersonal functioning have shown that a self-other approach is informative in determining the existence, type, and severity of personality pathology. For example, Salvatore et al. (2005) illustrated that patients with paranoid PD (PPD) typically see themselves as weak and inadequate and view others as hostile and deceitful. Patients with narcissistic PD (NPD) have been found to have dominant states of mind pervaded by distrust toward others and feelings of either being excluded or being harmed (Dimaggio et al. 2008). Jovev and Jackson (2004) reported that individuals with avoidant PD (AVPD) use maladaptive schemas centering on a self that is defective and shame-ridden, expecting to be abandoned because of their shortcomings, and that persons with obsessive-compulsive PD (OCPD) are burdened by a schema of self-imposed, unrelenting standards. Eikenaes et al. (2013) found that patients with AVPD could be distinguished from patients with social phobia on the basis of having more problems with self-esteem, identity, and relationships. Several studies have found the representations of self and others of patients with borderline PD (BPD) to be more elaborated and complex than those of other types of patients, but also more distorted and biased toward hostile attributions (e.g., Stuart et al. 1990; Westen et al. 1990). For example, patients with BPD are significantly more likely to assign negative attributes and emotions to the picture of a face with a neutral expression (Donegan et al. 2003; Wagner and Linehan 1999).

Reliable ratings can be made on a broad range of self-other constructs, such as identity and identity integration, agency, self-control, sense of relatedness, capacity for emotional investment in and maturity of relationships with others, responsibility, and social concordance. The most reliable (intraclass correlation coefficient [ICC]≥0.75) dimensions found in the clinician-administered measures considered in the review by Bender et al. (2011) were *identity, self-direction, empathy,* and *intimacy.* These were retained for the definition of personality functioning in the Alternative DSM-5 Model for Personality Disorders (AMPD). Definitions of these four elements are presented in Table 4–1.

Self-other constructs have shown robust reliability and validity in characterizing PDs. Criterion-level reliability studies have found that criteria related to self (e.g., chronic emptiness, identity disturbance) and interpersonal (e.g., unstable or stormy relationships) functioning are rated as having reliability equal to or greater than other BPD criteria (e.g., affective instability, physically self-damaging acts), with no significant differences between self and interpersonal criteria (Frances et al. 1984; Grilo et al. 2004, 2007; Gunderson et al. 1981; Zanarini et al. 2002a, 2003). A two-item self-report

TABLE 4–1.   **Elements of personality functioning**

Self:

1. *Identity:* Experience of oneself as unique, with clear boundaries between self and others; stability of self-esteem and accuracy of self-appraisal; capacity for, and ability to regulate, a range of emotional experience.

2. *Self-direction:* Pursuit of coherent and meaningful short-term and life goals; utilization of constructive and prosocial internal standards of behavior; ability to self-reflect productively.

Interpersonal:

1. *Empathy:* Comprehension and appreciation of others' experiences and motivations; tolerance of differing perspectives; understanding of the effects of one's own behavior on others.

2. *Intimacy:* Depth and duration of connection with others; desire and capacity for closeness; mutuality of regard reflected in interpersonal behavior.

measure of personality functioning (one self item, one interpersonal item) had good test-retest reliability across four DSM-5 academic center field trial sites (pooled ICC = 0.69) (Narrow et al. 2013).

Verheul et al. (2008) assessed core components of personality functioning in 2,730 patients and community members in the Netherlands with the Severity Indices of Personality Problems (SIPP-118), a self-report questionnaire. Twelve of 16 facets of personality functioning distinguished patients with PDs from *both* psychiatrically healthy comparison subjects and patients with other mental disorders, with a median effect size of 0.92 (moderate to large) for the differences between PD and healthy samples. The 16 facets factored into five higher-order domains: self-control, identity integration, relational capacities, social concordance, and responsibility. Each of the five domains distinguished patients with no PDs from those with one PD and those with one PD from those with two or more PDs. These results were replicated in a sample of 767 adolescent patients and comparison subjects by Feenstra et al. (2011), who found that all 16 SIPP-118 personality functioning facets reflected greater impairments in patients with PDs. Patients with the most PD traits (criteria) had the most impairment in the five domains of the SIPP-118, with self-control and identity integration showing the largest differences. Berghuis et al. (2012) assessed personality functioning with the General Assessment of Personality Disorder (GAPD) and the SIPP-118, PDs with the Structured Clinical Interview for DSM-IV Axis II Personality Disorders (SCID-II), and personality traits with the NEO Personality Inventory—Revised (NEO-PI-R) in 424 patients. Principal components analysis clearly distinguished general personality dysfunction from personality traits. The general personality dysfunction model consisted of three factors: self-identity dysfunction, relational dysfunction, and prosocial functioning. These three studies, involving almost 4,000 patients and control subjects, lent strong support for the inclusion of impairment in personality functioning (both self and interpersonal) in Criterion A of the GCPD.

Morey et al. (2011) conducted secondary analyses of data from two of the previously mentioned studies in the Netherlands (Berghuis et al. 2012; Verheul et al. 2008) with more than 2,000 patients and community subjects who had completed the self-report measures of personality functioning and had received semistructured interview assessments of DSM-IV PDs. Approximately 44% of patients in the Berghuis sample and 52% in the Verheul sample met criteria for a DSM-IV PD. Item Response Theory analyses characterized the types of self and interpersonal problems associated with different levels of impairment as represented by the LPFS in DSM-5 Section III (see the following subsection). The results delineated a coherent global dimension of impairment in personality functioning that was related to the likelihood of receiving any PD diagnosis, two or more PD diagnoses, and one of the more severe PDs (e.g., BPD, schizotypal PD [STPD], antisocial PD [ASPD]) (Morey et al. 2011). Research with the GAPD has indicated that self-pathology adds incremental validity over interpersonal pathology in predicting overall severity of personality pathology (Hentschel and Livesley 2013), which also supports the AMPD definition of personality functioning.

Impairment in self and interpersonal functioning is consistent with multiple theories of PD and their research bases, including cognitive-behavioral, interpersonal, psychodynamic, attachment, developmental, social-cognitive, and evolutionary theories, and has been viewed as a key aspect of personality pathology in need of clinical attention (e.g., Bender 2013, 2019; Herpertz and Bertsch 2014; Hopwood et al. 2013b; Luyten and Blatt 2011, 2013; Mulay et al. 2018; Pincus 2011; Waugh et al. 2017). A factor-analytic study of existing measures of psychosocial functioning found "self-mastery" and "interpersonal and social relationships" to be two of four major factors (Ro and Clark 2009). Furthermore, personality functioning constructs align well with the National Institute of Mental Health Research Domain Criterion of "social processes" (Sanislow et al. 2010), in which "perception and understanding of self" and "perception and understanding of others" are core constructs. The interpersonal dimension of personality pathology has been related to attachment and affiliative systems regulated by neuropeptides (Herpertz and Bertsch 2015; Stanley and Siever 2010), and variation in the encoding of receptors for these neuropeptides may contribute to variation in complex human social behavior and social cognition, such as trust, altruism, social bonding, and the ability to infer the emotional state of others (Donaldson and Young 2008). Neural instantiations of the "self" and of empathy for others also have been linked to the medial prefrontal cortex and other cortical midline structures—the sites of the brain's so-called default network (Fair et al. 2008; Northoff 2016; Northoff et al. 2006; Preston et al. 2007; Qin and Northoff 2011; Scalabrini et al. 2018).

Impairment in personality functioning exists on a continuum, and empirical analyses determined the level at which a "disorder" is diagnosed. Moderate impairment in personality functioning is required by the revised Criterion A. Moderate impairment is indicated by a rating of 2 or greater on the LPFS. Moderate impairment in personality functioning had a sensitivity of 0.85, a specificity of 0.73, and an area under the ROC (receiver operating characteristic) curve of 0.83 for a DSM-IV PD in a study of 337 clinician-rated patients conducted by Morey et al. (2013a). Requiring only mild impairment increased sensitivity (99%) but decreased specificity dramatically (15%). From the clinician's point of view, therefore, a single-item rating on the LPFS constitutes a highly efficient and effective screen for the possible presence of a PD.

Level of Personality Functioning Scale

Research indicates that generalized severity is the most important single predictor of concurrent and prospective dysfunction in assessing personality psychopathology (Hopwood et al. 2011). Furthermore, PDs are optimally characterized by a generalized personality severity continuum with additional stylistic elements derived from both PD symptom constellations (e.g., peculiarity) and personality traits. There is wide consensus (e.g., Crawford et al. 2011; Parker et al. 2002; Pulay et al. 2008; Tyrer 2005; Wakefield 2008) that severity assessment is essential to any dimensional system for personality psychopathology. Moreover, the ICD-11 PD Work Group has proposed severity as the central element of PD (Tyrer et al. 2011, 2015) (see "Conclusion and Future Directions" below and Chapter 1, "Personality Disorders: Recent History and New Directions," in this volume). Thus, the DSM-5 P&PD Work Group determined that a personality dysfunction severity scale would be a necessary improvement to PD assessment for DSM-5 and included the LPFS in the Section III model (see the Appendix to this textbook).

The LPFS uses each of the elements of personality functioning that are incorporated into Criterion A of the alternative model—identity, self-direction, empathy, and intimacy—to differentiate five levels of impairment on a continuum of severity ranging from little or no impairment (Level 0) to extreme impairment (Level 4). The Appendix to this textbook provides the full LPFS with definitions for every level of functioning. In the DSM-5 academic center field trials, the LPFS was rated with adequate test-retest reliability overall (ICC=0.42) by untrained but experienced clinicians and rated with higher reliability than several other DSM-5 dimensional measures.

With respect to utility, self and interpersonal problems such as insecure attachment and maladaptive schemas have been shown to be associated significantly with PD psychopathology and impairments in psychosocial functioning, as well as to affect clinical outcome (e.g., Bender et al. 1997; Fonagy et al. 1996; Jovev and Jackson 2004; Levy et al. 2006). Self-other dimensions have discriminated different types of PD pathology, predicted various areas of psychosocial functioning, and been shown to be moderators of treatment alliance and outcome (e.g., DeFife et al. 2015; Diguer et al. 2004; Feenstra et al. 2011; Peters et al. 2006; Piper et al. 2004; Verheul et al. 2008).

For example, in a sample of 90 patients in outpatient treatment, a Social Cognitions and Object Relations Scale (SCORS) composite was significantly correlated with psychosocial functioning measured by the Global Assessment of Functioning (GAF), the Global Assessment of Relational Functioning, and the Social and Occupational Functioning Assessment Scale (Peters et al. 2006). The correlation was strongest (0.53, large effect) for relational functioning. In a sample of 294 adolescent patients, the composite self-other variables from the SCORS predicted global functioning, school functioning, externalizing behavior, and past hospitalization (DeFife et al. 2015). In this study, the SCORS composite significantly predicted variance in the domains of adaptive functioning above and beyond age and DSM-IV PD diagnosis. In another sample of 378 adolescent patients and 389 community adolescents (Feenstra et al. 2011), the total amount of PD pathology, as represented by the number of diagnostic criteria met, was significantly related to the amount of impairment in the domains of self-control, identity integration, relational capacities, social concordance, and responsibility, as measured by the SIPP-118. These studies support the clinical significance of measuring severity of impairment in personality functioning on a continuum.

The severity of impairment in self and interpersonal functioning also has predicted empirically important factors such as treatment use and treatment course and outcome (e.g., Ackerman et al. 2000; Bateman and Fonagy 2008; Feenstra et al. 2011; Harpaz-Rotem and Blatt 2009; Piper et al. 2004; Verheul et al. 2008; Vermote et al. 2010).

The degree of impairment in personality functioning shows short-term stability but is sensitive to change. For example, in a sample of university students, 14- to 21-day test-retest reliabilities of SIPP-118 domains were very good to excellent, with correlations ranging from 0.87 for social concordance to 0.95 for self-control (median=0.93) (Verheul et al. 2008). In 60 patients in that study who were treated for an average of 11+ months as outpatients or in a day hospital and followed up after 2 years, SIPP-118 domains of self-control, identity integration, and responsibility gradually improved over time; relational capacities improved over the first year; and social concordance improved during the second year. In a subsample of 53 adolescents in the Feenstra et al. (2011) study who were treated as inpatients, 14 of 16 facets of the SIPP-118 showed significant improvement after 1 year, with effect sizes ranging from 0.37 to 1.24, indicating small to very large effects. In a study of interpretative treatment in 72 outpatients, level of the quality of object relations predicted outcome measured by general symptomatology and dysfunction (including self-esteem and interpersonal distress) and by social and sexual maladjustment (Piper et al. 2004). These studies illustrate that the self-other dimension is not subject to brief changes in clinical state but can reflect adaptive change, for example, as a result of treatment. Thus, the LPFS provides a useful dimensional severity assessment capability to the realm of DSM PDs.

In summary, self-other dimensions historically have discriminated different types of PD pathology, predicted impairment in various areas of psychosocial functioning, and been shown to be moderators of treatment alliance and outcome. More recently, in a survey of clinicians (Morey and Benson 2016; Morey et al. 2013a), the single-item LPFS rating predicted variance in clinician ratings of psychosocial functioning, prognosis, and treatment needs over and above that predicted by all 10 DSM-IV PD diagnoses combined (i.e., diagnoses based on 79 adult criteria). Specific self and interpersonal problems, such as insecure attachment and maladaptive schemas, have been shown to be associated significantly with PD psychopathology and with impairments in psychosocial functioning, as well as to affect clinical outcome (Skodol et al. 2014).

In the large Collaborative Longitudinal Personality Disorders Study (CLPS) patient sample, general PD features representing "disorder" severity had less stability over 10 years of follow-up than did specific features representing "style," consistent with the notion that personality functioning is the more dynamic and changeable aspect of personality pathology, whereas personality traits are more stable (Wright et al. 2016). However, general PD features were most strongly related to broad markers of psychosocial functioning, concurrently and longitudinally, supporting their validity as the core of personality pathology. In another sample of 628 patients, a general PD factor related meaningfully to multiple indices of psychosocial impairment and particularly predicted interpersonal dysfunction (Williams et al. 2018).

In a community sample of 306 individuals, items from the LPFS–Self Report (Morey 2017) measuring the four domains of the LPFS showed high internal consistency, were highly related to one another—supporting the unidimensionality of personality dysfunction—and had high correlations to concurrent validators. In three other large community samples, the LPFS–Self Report was highly reliable across a brief retest interval and correlated substantially with a wide range of maladaptive personality traits, PD constructs, and interpersonal problems (Hopwood et al. 2018). The LPFS–Brief Form version 2.0 scored on a four-point response scale of descriptiveness showed a two-factor structure, adequate internal consistency, and construct validity in relation to associations with PD criteria counts and SIPP-118 domains and was sensitive to change after 3 months of inpatient treatment (Weekers et al. 2019). Version 2.0 was also found to incrementally predict reduced healthy adult functioning, fulfillment, and well-being over and above DSM-5 personality traits (Bach and Hutsebaut 2018), as measured by the Personality Inventory for DSM-5 (PID-5; Krueger et al. 2012).

Necessary training and experience.   When the LPFS was first introduced, some critics believed that it would be too difficult to use, even for experienced clinicians. Some recent studies address the training and experience needed to assess patients for impairments in personality functioning with the LPFS.

Twenty-two untrained and clinically inexperienced undergraduate psychology students made DSM-5 LPFS ratings on videotaped Operationalized Psychodynamic Diagnosis (OPD) interviews of 10 female patients at a university in Germany (Zimmermann et al. 2014). The median time students had spent reading about PDs in general was 4 hours; students had spent about a median of 1 hour reading about the OPD interview and 0 hours reading about the LPFS. They had no previous experience in clinical assessment. The reliability of individual raters' LPFS ratings was an acceptable 0.51 (ICC [2,1]), and the reliability across raters was an extremely high 0.96 (ICC [2,22]). Students' LPFS ratings also were significantly associated with the presence of a PD as measured by a semistructured interview to assess PDs, the number of PD diagnoses, and structural personality impairments as measured by the OPD system, and they were highly congruent with expert ratings on written case vignettes in a second part of the study. Thus, the students' ratings were not only reliable but also valid. Similar results were found in another study of ratings of Structured Interview of Personality Organization interviews by clinically inexperienced undergraduate students in Italy (Preti et al. 2018).

In another study (Morey 2018), 72 individual indicators from the LPFS that describe core impairments in personality functioning at all five levels of severity were rated for an acquaintance by 194 undergraduate college students at a university in the United States; these students had minimal training in personality pathology and no training in the AMPD. Student ratings of LPFS domains (i.e., identity, self-direction, empathy, and intimacy) and total LPFS scores were highly internally consistent. A principal components extraction identified a single component accounting for 40% of the variance in ratings with an eigenvalue eight times larger than the next component, strongly suggesting that the LPFS is unidimensional, as is intended. Students' LPFS scores were positively correlated with traits of neuroticism and negatively correlated with agreeableness and conscientiousness, consistent with meta-analyses of the relationship between PDs and factors from the five-factor model (FFM) of personality. The indicators strongly predicted personality problems in the target acquaintances according to their severity level on the LPFS, with a very large effect size ($d = 2.04$) obtained for personality problems compared with no problems for severity-weighted LPFS scores. An ROC curve analysis found an AUC (area under the curve) of 0.91 for differentiating the presence from the absence of personality problems in the targets, greater than for any of the FFM variables. These findings support the proposition that effective use of the LPFS might not require much clinical experience or training.

In a fourth study (Garcia et al. 2018), 13 advanced clinical psychology doctoral students at another U.S. university, who had minimal familiarity with the AMPD, rated 15 written case vignettes on LPFS domains and total score over 3 successive weeks.

The vignettes also were rated by experts (the authors) for level of impairment in personality functioning. After the students completed their ratings, the five cases for the week were discussed in class. Interrater reliability for the global LPFS rating for single student raters (ICC [2,1]=0.81) and aggregated across raters (ICC [2,13]= 0.96) was excellent. The reliability of domain ratings was also good. The reliability of the identity and self-direction domains was good to excellent from the first session, but the reliability of the empathy and intimacy domains increased with practice over the three sessions. Students' agreement with experts was also strong. The authors concluded that assessing impairment in personality functioning was learnable with moderate didactic instruction and hands-on experience and was "not that difficult" (p. 1).

See Chapter 3, "Articulating a Core Dimension of Personality Pathology," in this volume for more information about the history and development of the LPFS.

Pathological Personality Traits

DSM-5 Section II defines personality traits as "enduring patterns of perceiving, relating to, and thinking about the environment and oneself that are exhibited in a wide range of social and personal contexts" (American Psychiatric Association 2013, p. 647) and states that it is "only when personality traits are inflexible and maladaptive and cause significant functional impairment or subjective distress [that] they constitute personality disorders" (p. 647). For each specific PD, a summary of its particular "pattern" (i.e., defining traits) is provided in the criteria "stem," which is followed by seven to nine specific criteria designed to indicate the pattern. For example, diagnosis of BPD indicates a pattern of "instability of interpersonal relationships, self-image, and affects, and marked impulsivity," with five or more of nine specific criteria that represent manifestations of this pattern required.

Thus, DSM-5 Section II defines PDs in terms of personality traits. However, there are a number of shortcomings of the Section II implementation of maladaptive personality traits for describing PDs that the DSM-5 Section III AMPD sought to rectify. First, Section II does not provide a comprehensive set of maladaptive personality traits for the criteria of PDs. Instead, 79 specific (adult) PD criteria are provided, which together are an amalgam of traits, behaviors, symptoms, and their consequences. Second, for some Section II PDs, there are inconsistencies between the defining trait(s) (i.e., those in the "stem") and the specific criteria by which the trait(s) is to be indicated. For example, STPD is defined by two basic traits: 1) discomfort with, and reduced capacity for, close relationships and 2) cognitive or perceptual distortions and eccentricities of behavior. However, because STPD is then indicated by nine criteria—four of which relate to interpersonal discomfort and five of which relate to cognitive distortions and eccentricity—and any five of these nine criteria are sufficient for a diagnosis, it is possible to meet criteria for STPD with no indicators of one of the two presumed principal traits. For some Section II PDs, criteria indicators do not appear to reflect the disorder's defining trait(s). For example, ASPD is defined as "disregard for and violation of the rights of others," but Criterion 3, "impulsivity or failure to plan ahead," does not necessarily reflect this trait, because impulsivity need not result in the violation of others' rights.

Furthermore, the Section II PD diagnostic criteria provide a very limited set of indicators for each defining trait. In most cases, there are four or five indicators for a defining trait, which are too few for an internally consistent (reliable) assessment (Clark and Watson 1995). The results of four studies of the internal consistency of DSM criteria sets with a combined sample size of 980 showed that no PD had an average alpha coefficient of 0.80; only AVPD and dependent PD had average alphas of 0.70 or greater, indicating less than optimal reliability (Blais et al. 1998; Clark et al. 2009; Morey 1988; Warren and South 2009). Finally, the specific trait indicators of the Section II PDs have limited applicability across gender, age, culture, or life circumstances. For example, Criterion 7 of PPD, "recurrent suspicions, without justification, regarding fidelity of spouse or sexual partner," would not apply to a person who has no partner, effectively limiting the number of criteria available for the diagnosis. Criterion 1 of AVPD, "avoids occupational activities that involve significant interpersonal contact," could not apply to one of the spouses in a single-earner, two-person household or to a retired person.

To address these shortcomings, the DSM-5 P&PD Work Group recommended several changes. First, the DSM-5 Section III AMPD provides a set of 25 maladaptive personality trait facets whose empirically based structure reflects that of the well-established FFM of personality traits (Krueger and Markon 2014). The model is an extension of the FFM of personality that specifically delineates and encompasses the more extreme and maladaptive personality variants necessary to capture the maladaptive personality dispositions of individuals with PDs (Costa and Widiger 2002). The AMPD includes five broad, higher-order personality trait domains—Negative Affectivity, Detachment, Antagonism, Disinhibition, and Psychoticism—each composed of three to six lower-order, more specific trait facets that are representative of the domains (e.g., manipulativeness and callousness are two of the specific facets in the Antagonism domain) (Krueger and Eaton 2010; Krueger et al. 2011a, 2011b, 2012; Wright et al. 2012). Trait domains and facets can be rated by clinicians on 4-point dimensional scales of descriptiveness: 0=very little or not at all descriptive, 1=mildly descriptive, 2=moderately descriptive, and 3=very descriptive. The structural validity of an original 37-trait model was tested in a three-wave community survey (Krueger et al. 2011b, 2012), and the model was subsequently revised to yield the five-domain, 25-trait model on which the DSM-5 Section III diagnostic criteria for PDs are based. The Appendix to this textbook lists the definitions of the five PD trait domains and 25 facets of DSM-5. (Further explanation on how to evaluate and rate traits can be found in Chapter 5, "Manifestations, Assessment, Diagnosis, and Differential Diagnosis," in this volume.) Patient-report and lay informant–report forms of the PID-5, a semistructured interview; the Structured Clinical Interview for the DSM-5 Alternative Model for Personality Disorders Module II: Personality Traits (Skodol et al. 2018); and other trait-based assessment instruments also have been developed to assist in the evaluation of DSM-5 AMPD personality trait domains and facets.

Extensive evidence indicates that the FFM represents a universal structure of personality traits that encompasses both the normal and the abnormal range of traits in both self and observer ratings, as well as across age groups and diverse cultures (McCrae and Costa 1997). For example, Yamagata et al. (2006) found high congruence for the FFM across descriptive, genetic, and environmental factors in three countries (Canada, Germany, and Japan) in a sample of 1,209 monozygotic and 701 dizygotic twin pairs, and De Fruyt et al. (2009) found a universal structure in observer ratings of more than 5,000 adolescents in 24 countries.

The DSM-5 Section III GCPD require that there be one or more pathological personality traits to diagnose PD. This requirement provides continuity with the DSM-IV definition of PD (as maladaptive personality traits) and with DSM-IV PD diagnoses. Then, rather than providing a limited set of indicators for the traits of each PD, the DSM-5 Section III model includes the traits themselves to constitute the B criteria. Using traits as indicators solves the current problem of the lack of correspondence between the defining traits of the PDs and the specific indicators and allows for variation in the expression of traits, depending on an individual's circumstances and personal characteristics (e.g., age).

From a psychometric perspective, personality traits can be assessed reliably. For example, the personality trait domains all had very good test-retest reliability in the DSM-5 academic center field trials, as measured by a 36-item self-report Patient Rated Personality Scale (ICCs ranged from 0.84 for Negative Affectivity to 0.77 for Antagonism and averaged 0.81). Structured interviews for personality traits also show strong psychometric properties: Stepp et al. (2005) reported ICCs greater than 0.90 for all domains and facets of the Structured Interview for the Five-Factor Model (SIFFM) in clinical and nonclinical samples. In a survey of 123 clinicians rating BPD criteria (Section II) and AMPD traits from case vignettes, traits were rated as reliably as criteria (Morey 2019).

The DSM-5 Section III model lists the component traits for six specific PDs (see section "Translation of Six DSM-IV Personality Disorders" later in this chapter). For PD-TS, the clinician is directed simply to note the patient's prominent maladaptive personality traits, whichever they may be. To maximize continuity with the DSM-IV PDs and also to create a tighter connection between the hallmark features of PDs and the criteria required to make a diagnosis, threshold algorithms for diagnoses are provided for the specific DSM-5 Section III PDs. For example, ASPD is defined by four specific trait facets of the higher-order trait domain of Antagonism and three specific trait facets of the higher-order trait domain of Disinhibition. As determined by empirical methods (Morey and Skodol 2013), a total of six of these seven trait facets are required for diagnosis, thus ensuring that there are at least two trait facets from each of the broad domains that constitute the trait set of ASPD (see also the later subsection "Diagnostic Thresholds").

The 25 facet-level PID-5 scales have been shown to be reliable (alphas reported by Krueger et al. [2012] ranged from 0.72 to 0.96 in the normative U.S. population sample, with a median of 0.86). Domain-level scales of the PID-5 are also highly reliable because they consist of empirically based combinations of facet-level scales (range= 0.84–0.96). (The PID-5, available in several versions, can be accessed online at http:/ /www.psychiatry.org/practice/dsm/dsm5/online-assessment-measures.)

Comprehensive Coverage of DSM-IV Personality Disorders

An initial investigation of the link between the DSM-5 trait facets and the DSM-IV PDs was provided by Hopwood et al. (2012). DSM-IV PDs were assessed with the Personality Diagnostic Questionnaire–4 (PDQ-4; Hyler 1994), a 99-item self-report instrument that assesses each of the diagnostic criteria for the 10 DSM-IV PDs. Traits proposed for DSM-5 Section III PD types (Table 4–2), as assessed by the PID-5, explained substantial variance in DSM-IV PDs as assessed by the PDQ-4, and trait indicators for the six PDs were mostly specific for those disorders. Traits and an indicator of general

TABLE 4–2. **Assignment of 25 trait facets to DSM-5 personality disorders**

Trait domains/facets	Personality disorders					
	ASPD	AVPD	BPD	NPD	OCPD	STPD
Negative Affectivity (vs. Emotional Stability)						
Emotional lability			X			
Anxiousness		X	X			
Separation insecurity			X			
Perseveration					X	
Depressivity			X			
Detachment (vs. Extraversion)						
Withdrawal		X				X
Intimacy avoidance		X			X	
Anhedonia		X				
Restricted affectivity					X	X
Suspiciousness						X
Antagonism (vs. Agreeableness)						
Manipulativeness	X					
Deceitfulness	X					
Grandiosity				X		
Attention seeking				X		
Callousness	X					
Hostility	X		X			
Disinhibition (vs. Conscientiousness)						
Irresponsibility	X					
Impulsivity	X		X			
Risk taking	X		X			
Rigid perfectionism (lack of)					X	
Psychoticism (vs. Lucidity)						
Unusual beliefs and experiences						X
Eccentricity						X
Cognitive and perceptual dysregulation						X

Note. Underlining indicates common facets.
ASPD=antisocial personality disorder; AVPD=avoidant personality disorder; BPD=borderline personality disorder; NPD=narcissistic personality disorder; OCPD=obsessive-compulsive personality disorder; STPD=schizotypal personality disorder.

personality pathology severity also provided incremental information about PDs in this study, further supporting the validity of the hybrid personality functioning–trait model.

An empirically structured set of traits helps make the observed comorbidity between PDs comprehensible. Some PDs share traits in common. For example, BPD and AVPD are both characterized by the trait facet anxiousness, which "builds in" a certain degree of overlap or comorbidity. Similarly, BPD and ASPD may be expected to overlap even more frequently because they have three facets in common: hostility, impulsivity, and risk taking. Importantly, defining PDs by an empirically structured set of trait facets also explains overlap between some disorders that do *not* have any facets in common because of the hierarchical structure of personality traits. Specifically, PDs that are characterized by facets from the same domain can be expected to overlap more than those whose facets are from different domains, because trait facets within a domain are more strongly intercorrelated than trait facets across distinct domains. Thus, even though ASPD and NPD share no specific trait facets, they may be expected to co-occur with some frequency because traits in the Antagonism domain characterize both types. Although the DSM-5 formulation does not eliminate the comorbidity built into the DSM-IV system, the observed empirical overlap is now well explained via shared traits within the hierarchical empirical structure of personality trait variation and by the core components of the LPFS (see also Chapter 3, "Articulating a Core Dimension of Personality Pathology," in this volume).

Convergence With the Empirical Structure of Personality

In addition to providing reproductions of DSM-IV PDs, the DSM-5 trait set provides a *synthetic bridge* between DSM-IV PDs and the empirical structure of human personality, thus creating a pathway for moving systematically not only from DSM-IV to DSM-5 but also from DSM-5 to an even better system grounded in data that will be collected using the proposed structured set of trait facets. This synthetic bridge can be seen by examining the joint structure of the DSM-5 facets and established markers of the five major domains of personality variation. That is, an extensive literature shows that personality constructs are organized empirically into five broad domains (Costa and Widiger 2002; Widiger and Simonsen 2005). These domains often are labeled Neuroticism (tense, anxious), Agreeableness (oriented toward getting along with other people), Extraversion (outgoing, friendly), Openness (to unusual and novel experiences), and Conscientiousness (orderly, planful). These domains have been shown to organize both normal- and abnormal-range personality constructs (Markon et al. 2005). This organizational continuity emerges because abnormal- and normal-range variation are continuous with each other, a fact for which there is considerable and compelling evidence, while on the other hand there is *no* compelling evidence that abnormal personality is different in *kind*, as opposed to being different in *degree*, from normal-range personality (Eaton et al. 2011; Haslam et al. 2012).

Recent studies have validated the relationship of the DSM-5 trait model to existing measures of the FFM and its variants. Thomas et al. (2013) conjointly factor analyzed data on 808 participants from a nonpatient sample collected using the PID-5 and the Five Factor Model Rating Form and found a factor structure that reflected the domains of the FFM. Wright et al. (2012) examined the hierarchical structure of DSM-5 traits measured by the PID-5 in 2,461 students. Exploratory factor analysis replicated the five-factor structure initially reported by the work group (Krueger et al. 2011a). The two-, three-, and four-factor solutions bore a close resemblance to existing models of common mental disorders, temperament, and personality pathology. In another student sample in Belgium, the five-factor structure from the U.S. derivation sample was also confirmed, and the joint structure of the DSM-5 pathological traits and general personality traits as measured by the NEO Personality Inventory–3 resembled the major dimensions of the FFM and the Personality Psychopathology Five (PSY-5;

De Fruyt et al. 2013). Anderson et al. (2013) examined the convergence of PID-5 domains and facets and the PSY-5 domains as measured by the Minnesota Multiphasic Personality Inventory–2 Restructured Form. Correspondence between PSY-5 scales and their PID-5 counterpart domains was high, and a joint factor analysis indicated the five-factor structure shared by the two approaches. The five-factor structure of the PID-5 also has been confirmed in Flemish inpatients (Bastiaens et al. 2016) and in Spanish clinical and community populations (Gutiérrez et al. 2017). A recent meta-analysis of 14 independent samples (N=14,743) by Watters and Bagby (2018) showed that the degree of cross-loading of PID-5 facet scales on more than one factor decreased when multiple samples were combined and provided a clearer picture of the five-factor internal structure of the facet scales.

Finally, in the only sample of clinician ratings of patients on the DSM-5 pathological personality trait system, Morey et al. (2013b) found the same five-factor structure as proposed and replicated in the abovementioned studies that used self-report measures and primarily nonpatient samples.

Revision of Additional DSM-IV General Criteria for Personality Disorder for DSM-5 Section III

Relatively minor changes were made to DSM-IV GCPD (now DSM-5 Section II) Criteria B through F for the DSM-5 Section III alternative model. A brief discussion of each of these criteria follows. (Some criteria letters differ between Section II and Section III GCPD, as clarified in the following text.)

GCPD Criterion B

Section II Criterion B states, "The enduring pattern is inflexible and pervasive across a broad range of personal and social situations" (American Psychiatric Association 2013, p. 646). The DSM-5 Section III model includes a revised GCPD Criterion C: "The impairments in personality functioning and the individual's personality trait expression are *relatively* [italics added] inflexible and pervasive across a broad range of personal and social situations" (American Psychiatric Association 2013, p. 761). The key elements of Criteria A and B (i.e., impairments in personality functioning and the individual's personality trait expression) are repeated in this criterion, as well as all subsequent GCPD, to keep the focus on these key elements, which the other GCPD modify or elaborate. The insertion of "relatively" before "inflexible and pervasive" is intended to dispel the mistaken belief that personality characteristics are cast in stone and to convey that PD features are not absolutely and completely unresponsive to any and all environmental circumstances.

GCPD Criterion C

Criterion C in Section II states, "The enduring pattern leads to clinically significant distress or impairment in social, occupational, or other important areas of functioning" (American Psychiatric Association 2013, p. 646). This criterion has been deleted from the DSM-5 Section III model because it is redundant with the proposed Criterion A for impairment in personality functioning, which includes social functioning. Furthermore, the DSM-5 Impairment and Disability Assessment Study Group recommended that DSM-5 criteria should describe signs, symptoms, and manifestations of disorders, and not their consequences, neither internal (i.e., distress) nor external (e.g., occupational).

GCPD Criterion D

Section II Criterion D refers to the longitudinal course of PDs as follows: "The pattern is stable and of long duration, and its onset can be traced back at least to adolescence or early adulthood" (American Psychiatric Association 2013, p. 647). Criterion D in DSM-5 Section III describes this pattern similarly: "The impairments in personality functioning and the individual's personality trait expression are *relatively* [italics added] stable across time, with onsets that can be traced back to at least adolescence or early adulthood" (American Psychiatric Association 2013, p. 761).

The notion of PDs as stable disorders to be distinguished from the more episodic mental disorders, such as mood disorders, has persisted despite a large number of one-time follow-up studies in the DSM-III and DSM-III-R (American Psychiatric Association 1987) eras that showed that fewer than 50% of patients diagnosed with PDs retained these diagnoses over time (Skodol 2008, 2013). The results of three methodologically rigorous, large-scale studies of the naturalistic course of PDs—the CLPS (Gunderson et al. 2000; Skodol et al. 2005c), The McLean Study of Adult Development (MSAD; Zanarini et al. 2005), and The Children in the Community Study (CICS; Cohen et al. 2005), conducted on patient (CLPS and MSAD) and community (CICS) populations—confirm that the longitudinal course of PD psychopathology is much more waxing and waning than stable. In addition, personality traits show clear temperamental antecedents (Shiner 2005), such that by school age, children's personality structure is similar to adults' structure (Shiner 2009; Tackett et al. 2009). As early as age 3 years, personality traits are moderately stable, but their stability increases across the lifespan until at least age 50 (Roberts and DelVecchio 2000). The insertion of "relatively" to modify "stable" in the revised Criterion D reflects this large body of empirical evidence. The redefinition of PDs in terms of personality functioning and pathological traits is expected to increase the stability of PD diagnoses, because both the functional impairments (Skodol et al. 2005b) and the trait manifestations (Hopwood et al. 2013a) of PDs have been found to be more stable than the symptomatic manifestations (McGlashan et al. 2005; Zanarini et al. 2016). A more detailed discussion of the longitudinal course of PDs can be found in Chapter 9, "Longitudinal Course and Outcomes," in this volume.

GCPD Criterion E

Section II Criterion E states, "The enduring pattern is not better explained as a manifestation or consequence of another mental disorder" (American Psychiatric Association 2013, p. 647). The revised criteria adopt the "standard" DSM-5 language for Criterion E: "The impairments in personality functioning and the individual's personality trait expression are not better explained by another mental disorder" (American Psychiatric Association 2013, p. 761).

GCPD Criterion F

Criterion F is meant to rule out substances and other medical conditions as a cause of personality psychopathology: "The enduring pattern is not attributable to the physiological effects of a substance (e.g., a drug of abuse, a medication) or another medical condition (e.g., head trauma)" (American Psychiatric Association 2013, p. 647). The revised criteria again reflect the "standard" DSM-5 language for this criterion: "The impairments in personality functioning and the individual's personality trait expression are not solely attributable to the physiological effects of a substance or another medical condition (e.g., severe head trauma)" (American Psychiatric Association 2013, p. 761). Mental disorders in DSM-5 are considered medical conditions.

GCPD Criterion G

Criterion G has been added to the DSM-5 Section III model for the GCPD and the individual PDs. It states, "The impairments in personality functioning and the individual's personality trait expression are not better understood as normal for an individual's developmental stage or sociocultural environment" (American Psychiatric Association 2013, p. 761). In Section II, GCPD Criterion A includes the stipulation that the "enduring pattern" must deviate "markedly from the expectations of the individual's culture." In the DSM-5 AMPD, this concept is incorporated into a separate criterion, and developmental considerations are added. This change is consistent with the intention of DSM-5 to be widely applicable in different cultures and developmental age groups.

Translation of Six DSM-IV Personality Disorders

Criteria for individual PDs in DSM-IV were amalgams of traits, cognitions about self and others, behaviors, emotions, signs, symptoms, and interpersonal consequences of maladaptive personality functioning. Many of the individual criteria for the DSM-IV PDs reflected disturbances in sense of self and interpersonal functioning. Also, DSM-IV acknowledged the importance of personality traits in its description of a PD when it said, "Only when personality traits are inflexible and maladaptive and cause significant functional impairment or subjective distress do they constitute Personality Disorders" (American Psychiatric Association 1994, p. 630). Most of the criterion "stems" or lead-ins to the specific PD manifestations in DSM-IV relied heavily on self and interpersonal or trait language. For example, the criteria for NPD began with "A pervasive pattern of grandiosity (in fantasy or behavior), need for admiration, and lack of empathy" (American Psychiatric Association 1994, p. 661), and the criteria for AVPD began with "A pervasive pattern of social inhibition, feelings of inadequacy, and hypersensitivity to negative evaluation" (American Psychiatric Association 1994, p. 664). Many criteria for individual disorders varied from those that were directly trait-based (e.g., ASPD's "deceitfulness," "impulsivity," "irritability and aggressiveness," "reckless disregard for safety," and "irresponsibility") (American Psychiatric Association 1994, p. 650) to those that were more specific manifestations of traits (e.g., STPD's "ideas of reference," "odd beliefs or magical thinking," "unusual perceptual experiences," and "odd thinking and speech" [American Psychiatric Association 1994, p. 645], which are all manifestations of various facets of the broad trait domain of Psychoticism).

One result of the extreme variation in the ways PDs were characterized was their low convergent validity when operationalized in different measures. In an early study, the average kappa across specific PDs between an unstructured clinical interview and the Personality Disorder Questionnaire—Revised (Hyler and Rieder 1987) was an abysmal 0.08 (Hyler et al. 1989). A study comparing the LEAD (Longitudinal Evaluation using All Data; Spitzer 1983) standard with two different structured assessments yielded an average kappa of 0.25 for *any PD*—that is, simply whether individuals did or did not have a PD (Pilkonis et al. 1991). Importantly, these are not isolated examples. Meta-analytic convergence between structured interviews and between structured interviews and personality questionnaires, respectively, yielded kappas of 0.27 for specific PDs and 0.29 for any PD (Clark et al. 1997).

The P&PD Work Group was charged by the DSM-5 Task Force with developing a standard approach to diagnostic criteria sets that would be consistent with core personality functioning and dimensional trait constructs. Therefore, revised diagnostic criteria are included in DSM-5 Section III for six specific PDs: ASPD, AVPD, BPD, NPD, OCPD, and STPD. Each PD is translated into typical impairments in personality functioning (Criterion A) and particular sets of pathological personality traits (Criterion B). The other DSM-IV (and DSM-5 Section II) PDs (paranoid, schizoid, histrionic, and dependent), DSM-IV Appendix B PDs (depressive, passive-aggressive), and the residual category of PDNOS are diagnosed by the DSM-5 Section III model with PD-TS (Skodol 2012), which is represented by moderate or greater impairment in personality functioning, combined with specification by pathological personality traits based on individuals' most prominent descriptive trait features.

Specific Personality Disorders

The PDs with the most extensive empirical evidence of validity and clinical utility are BPD, ASPD, and STPD (Blashfield and Intoccia 2000; Morey and Stagner 2012). In contrast, very few empirical studies have focused explicitly on paranoid, schizoid, or histrionic PD. The rationales for retaining 6 of the 10 DSM-IV PDs (Skodol et al. 2011a) in DSM-5 Section III were based on their prevalence (and its consistency) in community and clinical populations, associated functional impairment, treatment and prognostic significance, and (when information was available) neurobiological and genetic studies. Moreover, the DSM-IV PDs for which the P&PD Work Group elected not to provide full descriptions in DSM-5 were characterized by the relative simplicity of their trait composition, such that they are easily represented. A study published shortly before DSM-5 in a very large outpatient population reported that 84% of PD diagnoses fell into one of the six specific PDs included in DSM-5 Section III (Zimmerman et al. 2012).

In both epidemiological (Torgersen 2009) and clinical (Stuart et al. 1998; Zimmerman et al. 2005) samples, AVPD and OCPD are consistently among the most common PDs. BPD has a moderate prevalence in community studies, but it is one of the most common PDs in clinical settings. STPD has a relatively low prevalence in both populations but is highly impairing. ASPD is less common but has a considerable individual and collective effect on society and related relevance in forensic settings. NPD is one of the less common PDs, but constructs of narcissism have utility in treatment planning.

All DSM-IV PDs have moderate heritability (Coolidge et al. 2001; Kendler et al. 2006; Reichborn-Kjennerud et al. 2007; Torgersen et al. 2000, 2008); however, estimates are inconsistent across samples. Behavioral genetics evidence supports at least five of the six PD types retained for DSM-5 (the exception being NPD). STPD has been found to have the strongest loadings on genetic and environmental risk factors among DSM-IV Cluster A PDs (Kendler et al. 2006); ASPD and BPD have a second genetic and non-shared environmental factor over and above the genetic factor influencing all Cluster B disorders (Torgersen et al. 2008); and of the Cluster C PDs, AVPD has been found to be more heritable than dependent PD, and OCPD has disorder-specific genetic influence not found for the other two PDs (Reichborn-Kjennerud et al. 2007). Significantly, Section II STPD, ASPD, BPD, and AVPD—all retained in the alternative model—have been shown to have 100% genetic overlap with the five DSM-5 Section III personality trait domains, and OCPD (also retained) had 43% of genetic variance shared (Reichborn-Kjennerud et al. 2017). The retained PD types also have been associated with increased rates of various types of abuse and neglect in both prospective (e.g., Johnson et al. 1999; Widom 1989) and retrospective (e.g., Battle et al. 2004; Zanarini et al. 2002b) studies. The retained PDs are associated with high and persistent degrees of functional impairment (Skodol et al. 2002, 2005a, 2005b), and BPD is associated with an increased risk for suicidal behavior (Oldham 2006). The retained specific PDs also are associated with poorer outcomes of a range of mood, anxiety, and substance use disorders (Ansell et al. 2011; Fenton et al. 2012; Grilo et al. 2005, 2010; Hasin et al. 2011; Skodol et al. 2011b).

Criteria Assignment

Initially, assignment of the specific A criteria to the six individual PD types was made by inspection of the related DSM-IV criteria involving self and interpersonal functioning, by consideration of the definitions of the proposed core components of personality functioning, and by clinical judgment; the proposed criteria were then examined in a survey of 337 clinician ratings of patients, hereafter referred to as "the Morey survey." Item-total correlations for the 24 A criteria (four for each of the six PDs) with the entire DSM-5 PD criterion set ranged from 0.70 (ASPD empathy) to 0.25 (OCPD empathy), with an overall mean of 0.48. The item-total correlation range was from 0.64 (ASPD) to 0.38 (OCPD). Self functioning (identity, self-direction) criteria had a mean item-total correlation across the six PDs of 0.45, and interpersonal functioning (empathy, intimacy) criteria had a mean correlation of 0.51 (Morey and Skodol 2013).

Saulsman and Page (2004) conducted a meta-analysis of 15 independent samples on relationships between the DSM-IV PDs and the broad, higher-order trait domains of the FFM as measured by the self-report NEO-PI-R (Costa and McCrae 1992). Samuel and Widiger (2008) conducted a non-overlapping meta-analysis of 18 independent samples, first replicating Saulsman and Page's (2004) domain-level findings and then further examining relationships between the DSM-IV PDs and the more specific, lower-order trait facets of the FFM. In addition to the NEO-PI-R, Samuel and Widiger examined studies that used either the SIFFM (Trull et al. 1998) or the FFM Rating Form (Mullins-Sweatt et al. 2006). The results of the two domain-level meta-analyses showed a high degree of similarity, indicating the robustness of the relations. The results of the FFM facet-level meta-analysis were used for the preliminary assignment of pathological personality traits to the B criteria for PDs, as represented in DSM-5 Section III.

These assignments then were examined by Hopwood et al. (2012) and by Morey et al. (2016). In the Morey survey, each of the 25 traits from the pathological trait model proposed for DSM-5, as rated by clinicians, was correlated to the criterion count for DSM-IV PDs, also rated by the clinicians, to examine the fidelity of the rendering of DSM-IV criteria by trait terms. For ASPD, each of the seven assigned traits had higher correlations with DSM-IV criteria for ASPD than any of the other 18 traits (range 0.49 for hostility to 0.73 for irresponsibility; mean=0.65). The same was true for the six traits assigned to STPD. For OCPD, both of the assigned traits had the highest correlations, and two additional traits with significant correlations consistent with rational-theoretical considerations were added; for AVPD, three of the four assigned traits had the highest correlations; and for BPD, five of seven had the highest correlations. Using Cohen's metric, half the correlations indicated a large effect size, 47% a medium effect size, and only one a small effect size; in all cases, the correlations were statistically significant ($P<0.01$). For NPD, grandiosity had the highest correlation (0.77), but several other traits including callousness, deceitfulness, and manipulativeness had higher correlations than attention seeking (0.54). These results paralleled the findings for NPD in the Hopwood et al. (2012) study. However, adding these traits to NPD increased overlap with ASPD considerably, so rather than being added to the NPD criterion set, they are mentioned as common "trait specifiers" for NPD, to modify the diagnosis and capture the concept of "malignant narcissism." After comparing the results from the Morey survey and the Hopwood et al. study, a change was made to the assigned traits of only one PD: intimacy avoidance and restricted affectivity were added to OCPD.

The new criteria for BPD were rated with moderately good reliability in the DSM-5 field trials (pooled interclass kappa=0.54), despite a monothetic B criterion set used at the time requiring seven of seven traits for a diagnosis (Regier et al. 2013). Subsequent analyses of the field trial data suggested that a polythetic rule for the B criterion set requiring four or five or more of the trait facets would improve reliability and increase correspondence with the DSM-IV diagnosis. It is important to recognize that the DSM-5 Section III model provides a scientifically based framework (of impairment in personality functioning and maladaptive personality traits) in which DSM-IV PD concepts can be faithfully represented, meaning that validated aspects of disorders such as BPD (e.g., Gunderson et al. 2018) will have continuity under the new system. As a demonstration, in the Morey survey comparing patients on all DSM-IV and DSM-5 specific PD criteria and dimensions, the correlations between rated criterion counts of DSM-IV and DSM-5 diagnostic concepts from the 337 patients were as follows: BPD, 0.80; ASPD, 0.80; AVPD, 0.77; NPD, 0.74; STPD, 0.63; and OCPD, 0.57 (Morey and Skodol 2013). In most instances, these values are comparable to the established joint interview reliabilities of these diagnoses under DSM-IV, suggesting that *the agreement between DSM-IV and DSM-5 Section III PD diagnoses is likely to be as high as the agreement between two diagnosticians on DSM-IV (and now DSM-5 Section II) diagnoses.* However, an important difference is that in DSM-5, a coherent framework for representing the potential underlying endophenotypic structure of the PDs is provided, in contrast to the mixed collection of signs, symptoms, traits, and behaviors that make up the DSM-5 Section II diagnostic criteria.

Many studies now confirm that the DSM-5 pathological trait model provides very good coverage of Section II PD criteria, with the possible exception of OCPD (e.g., Bach et al. 2017; Few et al. 2013; Rojas and Widiger 2017; Watters et al. 2019). In a sample of 142 psychiatric outpatients who completed the PID-5 and were interviewed with the SCID-II, Bach et al. (2017) found that, overall, Section II PDs included in the

AMPD were most strongly associated with the Section III personality trait facets representing the B criteria for those PDs. In the Few et al. study (2013), 109 patients were interviewed with a semistructured interview for DSM-IV PDs for the presence of Section III traits and impairments in personality functioning and completed the PID-5. Again, both clinician-rated and self-report personality traits accounted for substantial variance in DSM-IV PD constructs, indicating good overall coverage (but comparatively weaker for OCPD, AVPD, and NPD). Rojas and Widiger (2017) found good coverage overall and for the individual B criteria for the six PDs retained in the AMPD in 425 community adults, all of whom had received mental health treatment, with a few of the criteria for Section II OCPD perhaps needing improved coverage by the Section III trait model. Finally, Watters et al. (2019) examined 25 independent data sets using diverse samples and methods that include measurement of AMPD traits and at least one Section II PD in a meta-analysis designed to empirically develop trait criterion profiles for the six Section III PDs. The results indicated general support for the traits making up the B criteria for the PDs, with OCPD being the exception. The assigned traits did not clearly discriminate between the PDs (although they were relatively distinct), because several of the disorders have assigned traits in common (see Table 4–2). Although important for continuity in clinical practice and research, it should be remembered that congruence between the DSM-5 trait model and the Section II PDs should not be taken as the "gold standard" for evaluating the validity of the trait model because of multiple problems in the conceptualization and articulation of personality pathology according to traditional DSM categorical PDs.

Diagnostic Thresholds

Three scoring rules were compared for the A criteria for each PD using the data from the Morey survey: one or more each from self and from interpersonal functioning, any single A criterion, and any two A criteria. Maximizing sensitivity and specificity for the corresponding DSM-IV PDs were used as the outcomes. Sensitivity values are of particular importance relative to specificity for the A criteria, because all DSM-5 PDs are presumed to have core impairments in personality functioning, and further specificity will likely result from pathological traits (B criteria). Over all six PDs, any two A criteria resulted in the best combination of strong sensitivities and adequate specificities (Morey and Skodol 2013).

Originally, all specified PD traits were required for the diagnosis of a given PD. As mentioned in the previous subsection, these monothetic scoring rules were tested in the DSM-5 field trials. Although monothetic scoring reduces heterogeneity, it also reduces prevalence and reliability, so polythetic decision rules were investigated in the Morey survey. As an example, based on the DSM-5 field trial result that requiring either four or five of seven traits for BPD equally increased the test-retest reliability of the diagnosis, a threshold of any four B criteria was compared with any five using the Morey survey data. A threshold of any four criteria, compared with any five criteria, was associated with a higher kappa of agreement with a DSM-IV diagnosis (0.64 vs. 0.57), a prevalence more closely approximating the DSM-IV prevalence of 40.2% (40.1% vs. 28.7%), better discrimination from four of the five other DSM-5 Section III PDs, and a stronger correlation to functioning (–0.30 vs. –0.25). Requiring only four criteria, however, means that a patient could be diagnosed with BPD with only the four criteria listed under the Negative Affectivity domain and, therefore, without any evidence of Disinhibition or Antagonism. Therefore, "any four criteria" was compared with an algorithm requiring four criteria and also requiring that one criterion of the four be from either the Disinhibition domain (i.e., impulsivity or risk taking) or the Antagonism domain (hostility). This algorithm produced an equivalent kappa to the "any four" rule with DSM-IV BPD of 0.64, little change in prevalence (38.9%), and slightly more overlap with other PDs but a slightly stronger relationship to functioning (–0.32). Thus, the final algorithm requires four or more Criterion B traits, one of which must be a trait from either the Disinhibition or the Antagonism domain (Morey and Skodol 2013).

A similar iterative process was followed for selecting the diagnostic thresholds for the B criteria for the other five specified PDs included in the DSM-5 AMPD. Balancing consideration of agreement with DSM-IV diagnosis (kappa) and prevalence, minimizing overlap with other PDs (i.e., discriminant validity), and maximizing the correlation to the composite of psychosocial functioning (social, occupational, leisure) in the Morey survey, the decision rules for the B criteria were set as listed in Table 4–3.

Elimination of Childhood Conduct Disorder as a Requirement for Antisocial Personality Disorder

In previous DSM editions, ASPD could be diagnosed only if childhood conduct disorder (CCD), with onset before age 15 years, was also present in the developmental history of the patient. In the DSM-5 AMPD, ASPD can be diagnosed in the absence of CCD. This significant change was made for several reasons.

First, the ASPD diagnosis in previous editions of DSM involved retrospective recall and/or review of records to establish that the CCD requirement was met. Retrospective recall has well-known shortcomings: not all patients are accurate reporters of their own history (Moffitt et al. 2010), and historical records with sufficient information content and detail to establish or rule out a CCD diagnosis are not always available for adult patients or may be inaccessible to the clinician for legal reasons (e.g., juvenile criminal records are often inaccessible). Thus, the ASPD diagnosis in the AMPD is based solely on contemporary assessment data pertaining to a person's personality, consistent with all other PDs.

Second, the requirement of CCD for the diagnosis of ASPD implies that adult antisocial behavior (AAB) can present only in persons who met criteria for CCD. This is not empirically accurate. AAB can also present in the absence of CCD. Also, more than 50% of children with CCD do not go on to develop ASPD (Zoccolillo et al. 1992). For example, Silberg et al. (2007) studied CCD and AAB in a sample of male twins and reported a correlation of 0.46 between CCD and AAB, indicating both continuity and discontinuity in the development of antisocial behavior that is not recognized by the CCD requirement for ASPD. Moreover, AAB was associated with novel genetic effects that were not overlapping with genetic effects on CCD, indicating etiological distinctiveness between antisocial behavior syndromes occurring in different developmental periods. By removing the CCD requirement from ASPD, both conduct disorder and ASPD can be diagnosed as appropriate, recognizing the fact that people can and do change in their antisocial propensities over the life course. Children with CCD are also at risk for developing other externalizing and internalizing mental disorders,

TABLE 4–3.   B criteria (trait domains/facets) diagnostic threshold algorithms for six DSM-5 AMPD personality disorder types

Personality disorder	Trait domains (facet *N*s)	Proposed algorithm
Antisocial	Antagonism (4) Disinhibition (3)	6 or more of 7 trait facets
Avoidant	Detachment (3) Negative Affectivity (1)	3 or more of 4 trait facets, and 1 must be anxiousness
Borderline	Negative Affectivity (4) Disinhibition (2) Antagonism (1)	4 or more of 7 trait facets, and 1 must be impulsivity, risk taking, or hostility
Narcissistic	Antagonism (2)	Both trait facets
Obsessive-compulsive	Conscientiousness (1) Negative Affectivity (1) Detachment (2)	3 or more of 4 trait facets, and 1 must be rigid perfectionism
Schizotypal	Psychoticism (3) Detachment (3)	4 or more of 6 trait facets

not only ASPD (e.g., Kim-Cohen et al. 2003). Moreover, other childhood disorders, in addition to CCD, increase the risk for ASPD (e.g., Kasen et al. 2001).

Third, AAB (ASPD in the AMPD) has been studied in both clinical and epidemiological samples and has been found to be both prevalent and consequential. Goldstein and Grant (2011) provided an extensive review of literature on the validity of AAB versus ASPD, focusing on both psychiatric and medical correlates of these syndromes, and concluded as follows: "Findings concerning the similarities between AAB and ASPD indicate the clinical and public health importance of AAB, calling into question the requirement under DSM criteria of CCD for the diagnosis of clinically serious antisociality in adults" (p. 52). They noted also that the prevalence of AAB is greater than the prevalence of ASPD, in spite of both syndromes having similar validity evidence. By removing the CCD requirement from ASPD, the alternative DSM-5 model ASPD recognizes the substantial social costs of antisocial behavior in adulthood that is not necessarily accompanied by antisocial behavior in a developmentally earlier period. (A detailed discussion of antisocial personality and behavior can be found in Chapter 22, "Antisocial Personality Disorder and Other Antisocial Behavior," in this volume.)

Redefinition of PDNOS as PD-TS

DSM-IV stated that PDNOS

> is a category provided for two situations: 1) the individual's personality pattern meets the general criteria for a Personality Disorder and traits of several different Personality Disorders are present, but the criteria for any specific Personality Disorder are not met; or 2) the individual's personality pattern meets the general criteria for a Personality Disorder, but the individual is considered to have a Personality Disorder that is not included in the Classification (e.g., passive-aggressive personality disorder). (American Psychiatric Association 1994, p. 629)

The DSM-5 AMPD includes the more useful category PD-TS to replace PDNOS.

This new diagnosis in the AMPD allows clinicians to turn the residual PDNOS category into a clinically more useful one by selecting from the set of maladaptive traits those that are most characteristic of an individual and assigning an appropriate specific level of impairment in personality functioning. This can be done in both the instances described in DSM-IV (and Section II)—that is, 1) when an individual meets the GCPD but not the specific criteria for one of the specifically named disorders and 2) when an individual has a PD not included in DSM-5, whether it is a disorder from the DSM-IV appendix (i.e., depressive, passive-aggressive) or one that was rendered as a specific disorder in DSM-IV but is not specifically included in the AMPD (i.e., paranoid, schizoid, histrionic, dependent). For example, an individual meeting all the criteria for DSM-IV-TR depressive PD might be characterized by depressivity (e.g., "is pessimistic"), anxiousness (e.g., "is brooding and given to worry"), anhedonia (e.g., "usual mood is dominated by dejection, gloominess, cheerlessness, joylessness, unhappiness"), and hostility (e.g., "is negativistic, critical, and judgmental toward others") (American Psychiatric Association 1994, p. 733).

PD-TS also can be used as the diagnosis when patients have such extensive personality pathology that they meet criteria for several of the specific PDs, with or without additional traits. In such a case, it may be clinically more useful to state, for example, that the individual has extreme and extensive Negative Affectivity, Detachment, and Disinhibition, with manipulativeness and eccentricity, than to list the several diagnoses met (e.g., STPD, BPD, and AVPD plus manipulativeness), because it provides a more precise picture of the individual's specific pattern of trait psychopathology.

Use of Level of Personality Functioning and Pathological Traits as Specifiers

DSM-IV lacked a PD-specific severity specifier. In that iteration of DSM, neither the general severity specifiers nor the Axis V GAF Scale had sufficient specificity for personality psychopathology to be useful in measuring its severity. The LPFS, therefore, functions as a PD-specific severity measure in the alternative DSM-5 Section III model.

Both the severity level of personality functioning and the trait specifiers may be used to record additional personality features that may be present in a PD but are not required for the diagnosis. For example, although moderate or greater impairment in personality functioning is required for the diagnosis of BPD (Criterion A), the severity of impairment in personality functioning can vary between patients and thus can also be specified, if it is more severe and/or if it improves over time. In addition, traits of Psychoticism (e.g., cognitive and perceptual dysregulation) are not diagnostic criteria for BPD but can be specified if present. The provision of 25 pathological personality traits permits more systematic use of personality information to inform clinical case formulation and treatment planning than was possible with DSM-IV or is possible with DSM-5 Section III PDs.

Traits to Augment the Description of Personality Disorders

DSM-IV states that when an individual's disorder meets criteria for more than one PD, both should be diagnosed. This is true in DSM-5 Section III PDs as well; however, in addition, if an individual's disorder meets criteria for a specific PD and has several prominent personality traits besides those needed to diagnose a specific PD, the additional traits may be listed to provide valuable personality information for use in treatment planning.

Traits of Clinical Significance in Patients Who Do Not Have a Personality Disorder

DSM-IV also states that specific maladaptive personality traits that do not meet the threshold for a PD may be listed. This is unchanged in DSM-5 Section III, except for the important difference that DSM-5 Section III provides a set of 25 specific trait facets for clinicians to use in describing the personality difficulties of their patients and in treatment planning. Given that personality has been shown to be an important modifier of a wide range of clinical phenomena and a source of dysfunction (e.g., Lahey 2009; Ozer and Benet-Martinez 2006; Roberts et al. 2007), and is associated with economic costs exceeding those of many mental disorders themselves (Cuijpers et al. 2010), a dimensional trait model will strengthen DSM-5 Section III–based assessments in general.

Clinical Utility of a Hybrid Model of Personality Disorder

In addition to the independent utility of measures of personality functioning and of pathological personality traits in identifying and describing personality pathology and in planning and predicting the outcome of treatment, several recent studies support a model of personality psychopathology that specifically combines ratings of disorder and trait constructs. Each has been shown to add incremental value to the other in predicting important antecedent (e.g., family history, history of child abuse), concurrent (e.g., functional impairment, medication use), and predictive (e.g., functioning, hospitalization, suicide attempts) variables (Hopwood and Zanarini 2010; Morey and Zanarini 2000; Morey et al. 2007, 2012).

Morey and Zanarini (2000) found that FFM personality domains captured substantial variance in the diagnosis of BPD with respect to its differentiation from nonborderline PDs, but also that residual variance not explained by the FFM was related significantly to important clinical correlates of BPD, such as childhood abuse history, family history of mood and substance use disorders, concurrent (especially impulsive) symptoms, and 2- and 4-year outcomes. In the CLPS, dimensional representations of DSM-IV PD diagnoses (i.e., criterion counts) predicted concurrent functional impairment, but their predictive power diminished over time (Morey et al. 2007). By contrast, the FFM (assessed with the NEO-PI-R) provided less information about current behavior and functioning but was more stable over time and more predictive of future outcomes. The model used in the Schedule for Nonadaptive and Adaptive Personality (SNAP; Clark 1993) and its second edition (SNAP-2; Clark et al. 2009) performed the best, both at baseline and prospectively, because it combines the strengths of a pathological disorder diagnosis and more normal-range personality traits by assessing personality traits across the normal-to-abnormal spectrum and by including clinically important trait dimensions (e.g., self-harm, dependency) that are not included in measures of normal-range personality. In fact, a model combining FFM and DSM-IV PD constructs performed much like the SNAP model. The results indicated that models of personality pathology that incorporate stable trait dispositions and dynamic, maladaptive manifestations are most clinically informative.

Hopwood and Zanarini (2010) found that FFM extraversion and agreeableness were incrementally predictive (over a BPD diagnosis) of psychosocial functioning over a 10-year period and that borderline cognitive and impulse action features had incremental effects over FFM traits. They concluded that both BPD symptoms and personality traits are important long-term predictors of clinical functioning and supported the integration of traits and disorder in DSM-5. Morey et al. (2012) extended their earlier findings comparing the FFM, SNAP, and DSM-IV PDs in a 10-year follow-up of CLPS patients. Baseline data were used to predict long-term outcomes, including functioning, Axis I psychopathology, and medication use. Each model was significantly valid, predicting a host of important clinical outcomes. Overall, approaches that integrate normative traits and personality pathology proved to be most predictive: the SNAP generally showed the largest validity coefficients overall, and the DSM-IV PD syndromes and FFM traits tended to provide substantial incremental information relative to one another (Morey et al. 2012). The results again indicated that DSM-5 PD assessment ideally would involve an integration of characteristic PD features and personality traits, to maximize clinical utility. Such a hybrid model is presented in DSM-5 Section III.

Perceived Clinical Utility

In the DSM-5 field trials, clinicians were asked to rate the usefulness of tested diagnostic criteria for all disorders. In both the academic centers and the routine clinical practice field trials (Kraemer et al. 2010), the Section III PD model was rated as "moderately," "very," or "extremely" useful by more than 80% of clinicians. In the academic center field trial, the Section III model was rated as "very" or "extremely" useful compared with DSM-IV by more clinicians than for all other disorders except somatic symptom disorders and feeding and eating disorders. In the routine clinical practice trial, the Section III model was rated as "very" or "extremely" useful compared with DSM-IV by more clinicians than for all other disorders except neurocognitive disorders and substance use and addictive disorders. The Morey survey asked clinicians to rate the perceived utility of the proposed DSM-5 rendering of personality pathology compared with DSM-IV. Questions addressed ease of use and usefulness for communication, description, and treatment planning. Although the clinicians were much more familiar with DSM-IV PDs, they rated all DSM-5 components to be generally "as useful" or "more useful" than DSM-IV for clinical description and treatment planning (Morey et al. 2014).

Relationships to Clinical Judgments

The Morey survey investigated the relationships of DSM-IV PDs and DSM-5 PDs and their components to important clinical validators including psychosocial functioning; risk for self-harm, violence, and criminality; optimal level of treatment intensity; and prognosis (Morey and Benson 2016; Morey et al. 2013a). DSM-5 components together and individually (personality functioning level and traits) had appreciably stronger unadjusted and corrected correlations with these concurrent validators than DSM-IV disorders in 11 of 12 comparisons. The only exceptions were for level of personality functioning and the composite risk prediction, the latter of which was more associated with DSM-IV PDs.

The incremental validity of the DSM-IV and DSM-5 PD systems—that is, the associations between each of the two PD systems and the four validators while controlling for the effects of the other—also was examined. The partial multiple correlations (and corresponding PRESS [predicted residual sums of squares]–corrected [for different numbers of variables] correlations) show that DSM-5 PD renderings significantly added to DSM-IV in predicting all four clinical judgments, while DSM-IV did not provide any validity information above and beyond that provided by DSM-5. Thus, *virtually all valid variance in DSM-IV PD diagnoses was captured by DSM-5, but the converse was not true.* The DSM-5 formulation accounted for significant elements of functioning, risk, treatment needs, and prognosis that were not captured by DSM-IV.

Conclusion and Future Directions

A new alternative model of PD psychopathology is included in DSM-5 Section III, based on dimensional assessments of impairment in personality (self and interpersonal) functioning and of pathological personality traits. Each of these aspects of personality pathology has an extensive empirical basis. Six DSM-IV PDs were translated into consistent criteria sets defined by typical impairments in personality functioning and specific pathological personality traits for DSM-5 Section III. The PDs selected to be represented as specific PDs are those with the greatest research bases and clinical utility. Assignments of revised criteria were based on careful consideration of continuity with DSM-IV, literature reviews, and empirical data. Diagnostic thresholds were set for the first time for all of the PD diagnoses using rational, empirical methods. The AMPD represents DSM-IV (and DSM-5 Section II) PDs with high fidelity, thereby reducing concerns about potentially disruptive effects of the changes on clinical practice or research. The new hybrid model is expected to increase the clinical utility of personality assessment over the 10-category DSM-IV/ DSM-5 Section II PD classification, based on previous research. Data comparing the DSM-IV classification and the DSM-5 AMPD indicate that the revised formulations are viewed by clinicians as equally or more useful than DSM-IV and have considerably greater ability to predict important clinical correlates, including functioning, risks, treatment needs, and prognosis.

More research in diverse settings and populations is obviously desired. First et al. (2002) outlined ideal steps for validating a new model for the PDs in *A Research Agenda for DSM-V*. Specifically, they suggested that alternatives should 1) better account for existing behavioral, neurobiological, genetic, and epidemiological data and adequately represent all clinically important aspects of a PD; 2) be more reliable, specific, and clinically informative; 3) more effectively guide treatment decisions; 4) have adequate levels of temporal stability in clinical settings; 5) relate to motivational and cognitive systems of the brain; 6) provide a better understanding of the interactions between temperaments and environment that result in PD; and 7) explicate the mechanisms by which maladaptive and adaptive personality traits affect physical disease and health. Although previous research on which the Section III alternative model is based has yielded suggestive findings in this regard, only extensive research can address them with certainty.

At the beginning of the deliberations of the DSM-5 work groups, a "paradigm shift" was deemed necessary for DSM-5 because of the shortcomings of the "neo-Kraepelinian model" of mental disorders. The P&PD Work Group persisted in the pursuit of a hybrid dimensional-categorical model for PDs, for which the PD field was eager (Bernstein et al. 2007; Clark 2007; Widiger and Trull 2007) and which the DSM-5 research agenda embraced. Recently, 361 PD experts were asked to rank order their preferences for categorical, dimensional, or mixed-hybrid approaches to PD diagnosis such as the mixed-hybrid approach incorporated in the AMPD (Morey and Hopwood 2019). Respondents preferred a mixed-hybrid approach over a purely dimensional approach and had a clear preference against a categorical model, echoing the findings of Bernstein et al. (2007) published 12 years earlier.

A set of criteria for change was proposed for DSM-5 to be applied across all categories, which focused on traditional measures of validity (antecedent, concurrent, and predictive) to support making changes. It is ironic that the motivation for DSM-5 was that existing categories of mental disorders could not be validated using traditional (e.g., Robins and Guze 1970) criteria, but new options for these disorders seem intended to meet these standards. Furthermore, different validators (e.g., familiality vs. consistent longitudinal course) are known to support different definitions of disorder, and which one is prioritized depends on the specific purpose of the diagnosis (e.g., to study heritability vs. to predict prognosis).

The guidelines for change in DSM-5 stated that the magnitude of a suggested change should be supported by a proportional amount and quality of evidence. In the PD field, the problems with the existing 10-category system for diagnosing PDs were deemed so severe that a reduced threshold for change seemed warranted. Furthermore, the relationship between empirical literature and clinical utility is not entirely clear. Should the recommended changes in the classification reflect and promote progress on understanding pathophysiology and etiology, or should they assist clinicians in doing their essential tasks? When these goals are in conflict, on what basis, by what process, and by whom should decisions be made (Skodol 2011)?

In addition, clinical utility should not be limited to user friendliness, feasibility, and clinician acceptability of diagnostic approaches; rather, the usefulness of such approaches for communication between clinicians or between clinicians and patients or their ability to guide treatment decisions or estimates of prognosis should be considered (First et al. 2004). According to strict definitions of validity (e.g., Kendell and Jablensky 2003), few psychiatric diagnoses can be said to be valid, because few "zones of rarity" (p. 4) in the manifestations of disorders have been found, and few disorders have been identified to have specific mechanisms of pathophysiology or etiology. According to Kendell and Jablensky (2003), however, a diagnosis possesses utility

> if it provides nontrivial information about prognosis and likely treatment outcomes, and/or testable propositions about biological and social correlates....Diagnostic categories provide invaluable information about the likelihood of future recovery, relapse, deterioration, and social handicap; they guide decisions about treatment; and they provide a wealth of information about similar patients encountered in clinical populations or community surveys throughout the world. (p. 9)

Therefore, in addition to the structural, genetic, and neurobiological validity of personality pathology, many of the clinicians and researchers on the P&PD Work Group believed that attention should be paid to the clinical purposes for which diagnostic assessments are used.

In tandem with the development of the DSM-5 Section III alternative model, a new model for the classification and diagnosis of PDs has been proposed for ICD-11 (Tyrer et al. 2019). This model has significant similarities to the DSM-5 AMPD because it incorporates a dimensional severity rating for personality pathology based, in part, on self and interpersonal constructs and five broad trait domains for describing personality pathology that overlap with the DSM-5 AMPD trait domains. Significant differences also exist between the two systems, however; in the ICD-11 proposal, impairment in psychosocial functioning is included in its severity measure, trait domains are rated categorically rather than as dimensions, and it has no PD types, with the exception of a "borderline" categorical specifier consisting of DSM-IV criteria for BPD (Bach and First 2018). How the international mental health community, which has enthusiastically generated much of the research on the DSM-5 alternative model (e.g., Zimmermann et al. 2019), will react to the ICD-11 model in comparison with the AMPD is unknown at this time. Furthermore, a new model for the classification and diagnosis of psychopathology, including personality psychopathology, that eschews diagnostic categories completely—the Hierarchical Taxonomy of Psychopathology (HiTOP)—is generating considerable interest worldwide (Conway et al. 2019; Kotov et al. 2017; Krueger et al. 2018; Ruggero et al. 2019). This empirically based taxonomy groups psychopathology into higher-order spectra that correspond, for the most part, to the personality trait domains of the AMPD and treats personality trait facets and other symptoms of psychopathology as lower-order indicators. Whether the HiTOP model can expand its support beyond the boundaries of academic psychology and into general mental health care also remains to be seen.

DSM-5, as a whole, is intended to be a "living document," with the potential for partial revision in an ongoing process, as research advances in a particular area warrant (Regier et al. 2009). Thus, the edition published in 2013 technically should have been called DSM-5.0, with future revisions called 5.1, 5.2, and so on. Whether the notion of a continuing process of revision will be acceptable and can be implemented by the American Psychiatric Association, or will be too disruptive to practice and research, is also a matter for the future.

References

Ackerman SJ, Hilsenroth MJ, Clemence AJ, et al: The effects of social cognition and object representation on psychotherapy continuation. Bull Menninger Clin 64:386–408, 2000

American Psychiatric Association: Diagnostic and Statistical Manual of Mental Disorders, 3rd Edition. Washington, DC, American Psychiatric Association, 1980

American Psychiatric Association: Diagnostic and Statistical Manual of Mental Disorders, 3rd Edition, Revised. Washington, DC, American Psychiatric Association, 1987

American Psychiatric Association: Diagnostic and Statistical Manual of Mental Disorders, 4th Edition. Washington, DC, American Psychiatric Association, 1994

American Psychiatric Association: Diagnostic and Statistical Manual of Mental Disorders, 5th Edition. Arlington, VA, American Psychiatric Association, 2013

Anderson JL, Sellborn M, Bagby RM, et al: On the convergence between PSY-5 domains and PID-5 domains and facets: implications for assessment of DSM-5 personality traits. Assessment 20:286–294, 2013

Ansell EB, Pinto A, Edelen MO, et al: The association of personality disorders with the prospective 7-year course of anxiety disorders. Psychol Med 41:1019–1028, 2011

Bach B, First MB: Application of the ICD-11 classification of personality disorders. BMC Psychiatry 18:351, 2018

Bach B, Hutsebaut J: Level of Personality Functioning—Brief Form 2.0: utility in capturing personality problems in psychiatric outpatients and incarcerated addicts. J Pers Assess 100:660–670, 2018

Bach B, Anderson J, Simonsen E: Continuity between interview-rated personality disorders and self-reported DSM-5 traits in a Danish psychiatric sample. Personal Disord 8:261–267, 2017

Balsis S, Lowmaster S, Cooper LD, et al: Personality disorder diagnostic thresholds correspond to different levels of latent pathology. J Pers Disord 25:115–127, 2011

Bastiaens T, Claes L, Smits D, et al: The construct validity of the Dutch Personality Inventory for DSM-5 Personality Disorders (PID-5) in a clinical sample. Assessment 23:42–51, 2016

Bateman A, Fonagy P: Eight-year follow-up of patients treated for borderline personality disorder: mentalization-based treatment versus treatment as usual. Am J Psychiatry 165:631–638, 2008

Battle CL, Shea MT, Johnson DM, et al: Childhood maltreatment associated with adult personality disorders: findings from the Collaborative Longitudinal Personality Disorders Study. J Pers Disord 18:193–211, 2004

Bender DS: An ecumenical approach to conceptualizing and studying the core of personality psychopathology; a commentary on Hopwood et al. J Pers Disord 27:311–319, 2013

Bender DS: The p-factor and what it means to be human: commentary on Criterion A of the AMPD in HiTOP. J Pers Assess 101:356–359, 2019

Bender DS, Farber BA, Geller JD: Cluster B personality traits and attachment. J Am Acad Psychoanal 29:551–563, 1997

Bender DS, Morey LC, Skodol AE: Toward a model for assessing level of personality functioning in DSM-5, part I: a review of theory and methods. J Pers Assess 93:332–346, 2011

Benjamin LS: Dimensional, categorical, or hybrid analyses of personality: a response to Widiger's proposal. Psychol Inquiry 4:91–132, 1993

Berghuis H, Kamphuis JH, Verheul R: Core features of personality disorder: differentiating general personality dysfunction from personality traits. J Pers Disord 26:704–716, 2012

Bernstein DP, Iscan C, Maser J, et al: Opinions of personality disorder experts regarding the DSM-IV personality disorders classification system. J Pers Disord 21:536–551, 2007

Blais MA, Benedict KB, Norman DK: Establishing the psychometric properties of the DSM-III-R personality disorders: implications for DSM-V. J Clin Psychol 54:795–802, 1998

Blashfield RK: Variants of categorical and dimensional models. Psychol Inquiry 4:95–98, 1993

Blashfield RK, Intoccia V: Growth of the literature on the topic of personality disorders. Am J Psychiatry 157:472–473, 2000

Clark LA: Schedule for Nonadaptive and Adaptive Personality. Minneapolis, University of Minnesota Press, 1993

Clark LA: Assessment and diagnosis of personality disorder: perennial issues and an emerging reconceptualization. Annu Rev Psychol 58:227–257, 2007

Clark LA, Watson DB: Constructing validity: basic issues in objective scale development. Psychol Assess 7:309–319, 1995

Clark LA, Livesley WJ, Morey L: Personality disorder assessment: the challenge of construct validity. J Pers Disord 11:205–231, 1997

Clark LA, Simms LJ, Wu KD, et al: Schedule for Nonadaptive and Adaptive Personality, 2nd Edition (SNAP-2). Minneapolis, University of Minnesota Press, 2009

Cohen P, Crawford TN, Johnson JG, et al: The Children in the Community Study of developmental course of personality disorder. J Pers Disord 19:466–486, 2005

Conway CC, Forbes MK, Forbush KT, et al: A hierarchical taxonomy of psychopathology can transform mental health research. Perspect Psychol Sci 14:419–436, 2019

Coolidge FL, Thede LL, Jang KL: Heritability of personality disorders in childhood: a preliminary investigation. J Pers Disord 15:33–40, 2001

Costa PT Jr, McCrae RR: NEO PI-R Professional Manual: Revised NEO Personality Inventory and NEO Five-Factor Inventory. Odessa, FL, Personality Assessment Resources, 1992

Costa PT Jr, Widiger TA (eds): Personality Disorders and the Five-Factor Model of Personality, 2nd Edition. Washington, DC, American Psychological Association, 2002

Crawford MJ, Koldobsky N, Mulder R, et al: Classifying personality disorder according to severity. J Pers Disord 25:321–330, 2011

Cuijpers P, Smit F, Pennix BW, et al: Economic costs of neuroticism. Arch Gen Psychiatry 67:1086–1093, 2010

DeFife JA, Goldberg M, Westen D: Dimensional assessment of self and interpersonal functioning in adolescents: implications for DSM-5's general definition of personality disorder. J Pers Disord 29:248–260, 2015

De Fruyt F, De Bolle M, McCrae RR, et al: Assessing the universal structure of personality in early adolescence: the NEO-PI-R and NEO-PI-3 in 24 cultures. Assessment 16:301–311, 2009

De Fruyt F, De Clercq B, De Bolle M, et al: General and maladaptive traits in a five-factor framework for DSM-5 in a university student sample. Assessment 20:295–307, 2013

Diguer L, Pelletier S, Hebert E, et al: Personality organizations, psychiatric severity, and self and object representations. Psychoanal Psychol 21:259–275, 2004

Dimaggio G, Nicolo A, Fiore D, et al: States of minds in narcissistic personality disorder: three psychotherapies analyzed using the grid of problematic states. Psychother Res 18:466–480, 2008

Donaldson ZR, Young LJ: Oxytocin, vasopressin, and the neurogenetics of sociality. Science 322:900–904, 2008

Donegan NH, Sanislow CA, Blumberg HP, et al: Amygdala hyperreactivity in borderline personality disorder: implications for emotional dysregulation. Biol Psychiatry 54:1284–1293, 2003

Eaton NR, Krueger RF, South SC, et al: Contrasting prototypes and dimensions in the classification of personality pathology: evidence that dimensions, but not prototypes, are robust. Psychol Med 41:1151–1163, 2011

Eikenaes E, Hummelen B, Abrahamsen G, et al: Personality functioning in patients with avoidant personality disorder and social phobia. J Pers Disord 27:746–763, 2013

Fair DA, Cohen AL, Dosenbach NUF, et al: The maturing architecture of the brain's default network. Proc Natl Acad Sci USA 105:4028–4032, 2008

Feenstra DJ, Hutsebaut J, Verheul R, et al: Severity Indices of Personality Problems (SIPP-118) in adolescents: reliability and validity. Psychol Assess 23:646–655, 2011

Fenton MC, Keyes K, Geier T, et al: Psychiatric comorbidity and the persistence of drug use disorders in the United States. Addiction 107:599–609, 2012

Few LR, Miller JD, Rothbaum AO, et al: Examination of the Section III DSM-5 diagnostic system for personality disorders in an outpatient clinical sample. J Abnorm Psychol 122:1057–1069, 2013

First MB, Bell CC, Cuthbert B, et al: Personality disorders and relational disorders: a research agenda for addressing crucial gaps in DSM, in A Research Agenda for DSM-V. Edited by Kupfer, DJ, First MB, Regier DA. Washington, DC, American Psychiatric Association, 2002, pp 123–199

First MB, Pincus H, Levine J, et al: Clinical utility as a criterion for revising psychiatric diagnoses. Am J Psychiatry 161:946–954, 2004

Fonagy P, Leigh T, Steele M, et al: The relation of attachment status, psychiatric classification, and response to psychotherapy. J Consult Clin Psychol 64:22–31, 1996

Frances A: The DSM-III personality disorders section: a commentary. Am J Psychiatry 137:1050–1054, 1980

Frances A: Categorical and dimensional systems of personality diagnosis: a comparison. Compr Psychiatry 23:516–527, 1982

Frances A, Clarkin JF, Gilmore M, et al: Reliability of criteria for borderline personality disorder: a comparison of DSM-III and the diagnostic interview for borderline patients. Am J Psychiatry 141:1080–1084, 1984

Frances A, Pincus HA, Widiger TA, et al: DSM-IV: work in progress. Am J Psychiatry 147:1439–1448, 1990

Frances A, First MB, Widiger TA, et al: An A to Z guide to DSM-IV conundrums. J Abnorm Psychol 100:407–412, 1991

Garcia DJ, Skadberg RM, Schmidt M, et al: It's not that difficult: an interrater reliability study of the DSM-5 Section III Alternative Model for Personality Disorders. J Pers Assess 100:612–620, 2018

Goldstein RB, Grant BF: Burden of syndromal antisocial behavior in adulthood, in Antisocial Behavior: Causes, Correlations, and Treatments. Edited by Clarke RM. Hauppauge, NY, Nova Science Publishers, 2011, pp 1–74

Grant BF, Stinson FS, Dawson DA, et al: Co-occurrence of DSM-IV personality disorders in the United States: results from the National Epidemiologic Survey on Alcohol and Related Conditions. Compr Psychiatry 46:1–5, 2005

Grilo CM, Becker DF, Anez LM, et al: Diagnostic efficiency of DSM-IV criteria for borderline personality disorder: an evaluation in Hispanic men and women with substance use disorders. J Consult Clin Psychol 72:126–131, 2004

Grilo CM, Sanislow CA, Shea MT, et al: Two-year prospective naturalistic study of remission from major depressive disorder as a function of personality disorder comorbidity. J Consult Clin Psychol 73:78–85, 2005

Grilo CM, Sanislow CA, Skodol AE, et al: Longitudinal diagnostic efficiency of DSM-IV criteria for borderline personality disorder: a 2-year prospective study. Can J Psychiatry 52:357–362, 2007

Grilo CM, Stout RL, Markowitz JC, et al: Personality disorders predict relapse after remission from an episode of major depressive disorder: a 6-year prospective study. J Clin Psychiatry 71:1629–1635, 2010

Gunderson JG: Introduction to Section IV: Personality Disorders, in DSM-IV Sourcebook, Vol 2. Edited by Widiger TA, Frances AJ, Pincus HA, et al. Washington, DC, American Psychiatric Association, 1996, pp 647–664

Gunderson JG, Kolb JE, Austin V: The diagnostic interview for borderline patients. Am J Psychiatry 138:896–903, 1981

Gunderson JG, Shea MT, Skodol AE, et al: The Collaborative Longitudinal Personality Disorders Study: development, aims, design, and sample characteristics. J Pers Disord 14:300–315, 2000

Gunderson JG, Stout RL, McGlashan TH, et al: Ten-year course of borderline personality disorder: psychopathology and function from the Collaborative Longitudinal Personality Disorders Study. Arch Gen Psychiatry 68:827–837, 2011

Gunderson JG, Herpertz SC, Skodol AE, et al. Borderline personality disorder. Nat Rev Dis Primers 4:18029, 2018

Gutiérrez F, Aluja A, Peri JM, et al: Psychometric properties of the Spanish PID-5 in a clinical and a community sample. Assessment 24:326–336, 2017

Harpaz-Rotem I, Blatt SJ: A pathway to therapeutic change: changes in self-representation in the treatment of adolescents and young adults. Psychiatry 72:32–49, 2009

Hasin D, Fenton MC, Skodol A, et al: Relationship of personality disorders to the three-year course of alcohol, cannabis, and nicotine disorders. Arch Gen Psychiatry 68:1158–1167, 2011

Haslam N, Holland E, Kuppens P: Categories versus dimensions in personality and psychopathology: a quantitative review of taxometric research. Psychol Med 42:903–920, 2012

Hentschel AG, Livesley WJ: The General Assessment of Personality Disorder (GAPD): factor structure, incremental validity of self-pathology, and relations to DSM-IV personality disorders. J Pers Assess 95:479–485, 2013

Herpertz SC, Bertsch K: The social-cognitive basis of personality disorders. Curr Opin Psychiatry 27:73–77, 2014

Herpertz SC, Bertsch K: A new perspective on the pathophysiology of borderline personality disorder: a model of the role of oxytocin. Am J Psychiatry 172:840–851, 2015

Hopwood CJ, Zanarini MC: Borderline personality traits and disorder: predicting prospective patient functioning. J Consult Clin Psychol 78:585–589, 2010

Hopwood CJ, Malone JC, Ansell EB, et al: Personality assessment in DSM-V: empirical support for rating severity, style, and traits. J Pers Disord 25:305–320, 2011

Hopwood CJ, Thomas KM, Markon KE, et al: DSM-5 personality traits and DSM-IV personality disorders. J Abnorm Psychol 121:424–432, 2012

Hopwood CJ, Morey LC, Donnellan MB, et al: Ten-year rank-order stability of personality traits and disorders in a clinical sample. J Pers 81:335–344, 2013a

Hopwood CJ, Wright AG, Ansell EB, et al: The interpersonal core of personality pathology. J Pers Disord 27:270–295, 2013b

Hopwood CJ, Good EW, Morey LC: Validity of the DSM-5 Levels of Personality Functioning Scale—Self Report. J Pers Assess 100:650–659, 2018

Hyler SE: Personality Diagnostic Questionnaire–4 (PDQ-4). New York, New York State Psychiatric Institute, 1994

Hyler SE, Rieder RO: PDQ-R: Personality Diagnostic Questionnaire—Revised. New York, New York State Psychiatric Institute, 1987

Hyler SE, Rieder RO, Williams JB, et al: A comparison of clinical and self-report diagnoses of DSM-III personality disorders in 552 patients. Compr Psychiatry 30:170–178, 1989

Hyman SE: The diagnosis of mental disorders: the problem of reification. Annu Rev Clin Psychol 6:155–179, 2010

Johansen M, Karterud S, Pedersen G, et al: An investigation of the prototype validity of the borderline DSM-IV construct. Acta Psychiatr Scand 109:289–298, 2004

Johnson JG, Cohen P, Brown J, et al: Childhood maltreatment increases risk for personality disorders during early adulthood. Arch Gen Psychiatry 56:600–606, 1999

Jovev M, Jackson HJ: Early maladaptive schemas in personality disordered individuals. J Pers Disord 18:467–478, 2004

Kasen S, Cohen P, Skodol AE, et al: Childhood depression and adult personality disorder: alternative pathways of continuity. Arch Gen Psychiatry 58:231–236, 2001

Kendell R, Jablensky A: Distinguishing between the validity and utility of psychiatric diagnoses. Am J Psychiatry 160:4–12, 2003

Kendler KS, Czajkowski N, Tambs K, et al: Dimensional representation of DSM-IV Cluster A personality disorders in a population-based sample of Norwegian twins: a multivariate study. Psychol Med 36:1583–1591, 2006

Kim-Cohen J, Caspi A, Moffitt TE, et al: Prior juvenile diagnoses in adults with mental disorder: developmental follow-back of a prospective-longitudinal cohort. Arch Gen Psychiatry 60:709–717, 2003

Kotov R, Krueger RF, Watson D, et al: The Hierarchical Taxonomy of Psychopathology (HiTOP): a dimensional alternative to traditional nosologies. J Abnorm Psychol 126:454–477, 2017

Kraemer HC, Kupfer DJ, Narrow WE, et al: Moving toward DSM-5: the field trials. Am J Psychiatry 167:1058–1060, 2010

Krueger RF, Eaton NR: Personality traits and the classification of mental disorders: towards a more complete integration in DSM-5 and an empirical model of psychopathology. Personal Disord 1:97–118, 2010

Krueger RF, Markon KE: The role of the DSM-5 trait model in moving toward a quantitative and empirically based approach to classifying personality and psychopathology. Annu Rev Clin Psychol 10:477–501, 2014

Krueger RF, Skodol AE, Livesley WJ, et al: Synthesizing dimensional and categorical approaches to personality disorders: refining the research agenda for DSM-V Axis II. Int J Methods Psychiatr Res 16 (suppl 1):S65–S73, 2007

Krueger RF, Eaton NR, Clark LA, et al: Deriving an empirical structure for personality pathology for DSM-5. J Pers Disord 25:170–191, 2011a

Krueger RF, Eaton NR, Derringer J, et al: Personality in DSM-5: helping delineate personality disorder content and framing the meta-structure. J Pers Assess 93:325–331, 2011b

Krueger RF, Derringer J, Markon KE, et al: Initial construction of a maladaptive personality trait model and inventory for DSM-5. Psychol Med 42:1879–1890, 2012

Krueger RF, Kotov R, Watson D, et al: Progress in achieving quantitative classification of psychopathology. World Psychiatry 17:282–293, 2018

Kupfer DJ, First MB, Regier DA (eds): A Research Agenda for DSM-V. Washington, DC, American Psychiatric Association, 2002

Lahey BB: Public health significance of neuroticism. Am Psychol 64:241–256, 2009

Levy KN, Meehan KB, Kelly KM, et al: Change in attachment patterns and reflective function in a randomized control trial of transference-focused psychotherapy for borderline personality disorder. J Consult Clin Psychol 74:1027–1040, 2006

Luyten P, Blatt SJ: Integrating theory-driven and empirically derived models of personality development and psychopathology: a proposal for DSM V. Clin Psychol Rev 31:52–68, 2011

Luyten P, Blatt SJ: Interpersonal relatedness and self-definition in normal and disrupted personality development: retrospect and prospect. Am Psychol 68:172–183, 2013

Markon K, Krueger RF, Watson D: Delineating the structure of normal and abnormal personality: an integrative hierarchical approach. J Pers Soc Psychol 88:139–157, 2005

McCrae RR, Costa PT Jr: Personality trait structure as a human universal. Am Psychol 52:509–516, 1997

McGlashan TH, Grilo CM, Sanislow CA, et al: Two-year prevalence and stability of individual DSM-IV criteria for schizotypal, borderline, avoidant and obsessive-compulsive personality disorders: toward a hybrid model of Axis II disorders. Am J Psychiatry 162:883–889, 2005

Moffitt TE, Caspi A, Taylor A, et al: How common are common mental disorders? Evidence that lifetime prevalence rates are doubled by prospective versus retrospective assessment. Psychol Med 40:899–909, 2010

Morey LC: Personality disorders under DSM-III and DSM-III-R: an examination of convergence, coverage, and internal consistency. Am J Psychiatry 145:573–577, 1988

Morey LC: Personality pathology as pathological narcissism, in Personality Disorders (WPA Series: Evidence and Experience in Psychiatry, Vol 8). Edited by Maj M, Akiskal HS, Mezzich JE, Okasha A. Chichester, West Sussex, England, Wiley, 2005, pp 328–331

Morey LC: Development and initial evaluation of a self-report form of the DSM-5 Level of Personality Functioning Scale. Psychol Assess 29:1302–1308, 2017

Morey LC: Application of the DSM-5 Level of Personality Functioning Scale by lay raters. J Pers Disord 32:709–720, 2018

Morey LC: Interdiagnostician reliability of the DSM-5 Section II and Section III alternative model criteria for borderline personality disorder. J Pers Disord 33:721–S18, 2019

Morey LC, Benson KT: Relating DSM-5 Section II and Section III personality diagnostic classification systems to treatment planning. Compr Psychiatry 68:48–55, 2016

Morey LC, Hopwood CJ: Expert preferences for categorical, dimensional, and mixed/hybrid approaches to personality disorder diagnosis. J Pers Disord Jan 16, 2019 (Epub ahead of print)

Morey LC, Skodol AE: Convergence between DSM-IV and DSM-5 diagnostic models for personality disorder: evaluation of strategies for establishing diagnostic thresholds. J Psychiatr Pract 19:179–193, 2013

Morey LC, Stagner BH: Narcissistic pathology as core personality dysfunction: comparing DSM-IV and the DSM-5 proposal for narcissistic personality disorder. J Clin Psychol 68:908–921, 2012

Morey LC, Zanarini MC: Borderline personality: traits and disorder. J Abnorm Psychol 109:733–737, 2000

Morey LC, Hopwood CJ, Gunderson JG, et al: Comparison of alternative models for personality disorders. Psychol Med 37:983–994, 2007

Morey LC, Berghuis H, Bender DS, et al: Toward a model for assessing level of personality functioning in DSM-5, part II: empirical articulation of a core dimension of personality pathology. J Pers Assess 93:347–353, 2011

Morey LC, Hopwood CJ, Markowitz JC, et al: Comparison of alternative models for personality disorders, II: 6-, 8- and 10-year follow-up. Psychol Med 42:1705–1713, 2012

Morey LC, Bender DS, Skodol AE: Validating the proposed DSM-5 severity indicator for personality disorder. J Nerv Ment Dis 201:729–735, 2013a

Morey LC, Krueger RF, Skodol AE: The hierarchical structure of clinician ratings of proposed DSM-5 pathological personality traits. J Abnorm Psychol 122:836–841, 2013b

Morey LC, Skodol AE, Oldham JM: Clinician judgments of clinical utility: a comparison of DSM-IV-TR personality disorders and the alternative model for DSM-5 personality disorders. J Abnorm Psychol 123:398–405, 2014

Morey LC, Benson KT, Skodol AE: Relating DSM-5 Section III personality traits to Section II personality disorder diagnoses. Psychol Med 46:647–655, 2016

Mulay AL, Cain NM, Waugh MH, et al: Personality constructs and paradigms in the Alternative DSM-5 Model of Personality Disorder. J Pers Assess 100:593–602, 2018

Mullins-Sweatt SN, Jamerson JE, Samuel DB, et al: Psychometric properties of an abbreviated instrument of the five-factor nodel. Assessment 13:119–137, 2006

Narrow WE, Clarke DE, Kuromoto SJ, et al: DSM-5 field trials in the United States and Canada, part III: development and reliability testing of a cross-cutting symptom assessment for DSM-5. Am J Psychiatry 170:71–82, 2013

Northoff G: Is the self a higher-order or fundamental function of the brain? The "basis model of self-specificity" and its encoding by the brain's spontaneous activity. Cogn Neurosci 7:203–222, 2016

Northoff G, Heinzel A, de Greck M, et al: Self-referential processing in our brain—a meta-analysis of imaging studies on the self. Neuroimage 31:440–457, 2006

Oldham JM: Borderline personality disorder and suicidality. Am J Psychiatry 163:20–26, 2006

Oldham JM, Skodol AE, Kellman HD, et al: Diagnosis of DSM-III-R personality disorders by two structured interviews: patterns of comorbidity. Am J Psychiatry 149:213–220, 1992

Ozer DJ, Benet-Martinez V: Personality and the prediction of consequential outcomes. Annu Rev Psychol 57:401–421, 2006

Parker G, Both L, Olley A, et al: Defining personality disordered functioning. J Pers Disord 16:503–522, 2002

Peters EJ, Hilsenroth MJ, Eudell-Simmons EM, et al: Reliability and validity of the Social Cognition and Object Relations Scale in clinical use. Psychotherapy Res 16:617–626, 2006

Pilkonis PA, Heape CL, Ruddy J, et al: Validity in the diagnosis of personality disorders: the use of the LEAD standard. Psychol Assess 148:997–1008, 1991

Pincus AL: Some comments on nomology, diagnostic process, and narcissistic personality disorder in the DSM-5 proposal for personality and personality disorders. Personal Disord 2:41–53, 2011

Pincus HA, Frances A, Davis WW, et al: DSM-IV and new diagnostic categories: holding the line on proliferation. Am J Psychiatry 149:112–117, 1992

Piper WE, Ogrodniczuk JS, Joyce AS: Quality of object relations as a moderator of the relationship between pattern of alliance and outcome in short-term individual psychotherapy. J Pers Assess 83:345–356, 2004

Preston SD, Bechara A, Damascio H, et al: The neural substrates of cognitive empathy. Soc Neurosci 2:254–275, 2007

Preti E, Di Pierro R, Costantini G, et al: Using the Structured Interview of Personality Organization for DSM-5 Level of Personality Functioning rating performed by inexperienced raters. J Pers Assess 100:621–629, 2018

Pulay AJ, Dawson DA, Ruan WJ, et al: The relationship of impairment to personality disorder severity among individuals with specific Axis I disorders: results from the National Epidemiologic Survey on Alcohol and Related Conditions. J Pers Disord 22:405–417, 2008

Qin P, Northoff G: How is our self related to midline regions and the default-mode network? Neuroimage 57:1221–1233, 2011

Regier DA, Narrow WE, Kuhl EA, et al: The conceptual development of DSM-V. Am J Psychiatry 166:645–650, 2009

Regier DA, Narrow WE, Clarke DE, et al: DSM-5 field trials in the United States and Canada, part II: test-retest reliability of selected categorical diagnoses. Am J Psychiatry 170:59–70, 2013

Reichborn-Kjennerud T, Czajkowki N, Neale MC, et al: Genetic and environmental influences on dimensional representations of DSM-IV Cluster C personality disorders: a population-based multivariate twin study. Psychol Med 37:645–653, 2007

Reichborn-Kjennerud T, Krueger RF, Ystrom E, et al: Do DSM-5 Section II personality disorders and Section III personality trait domains reflect the same genetic and environmental risk factors? Psychol Med 47:2205–2215, 2017

Ro E, Clark LA: Psychosocial functioning in the context of diagnosis: assessment and theoretical issues. Psychol Assess 21:313–324, 2009

Roberts BW, DelVecchio WF: The rank-order consistency of personality traits from childhood to old age: a quantitative review of longitudinal studies. Psychol Bull 126:3–25, 2000

Roberts BW, Kuncel NR, Shiner R, et al: The power of personality: the comparative validity of personality traits, socioeconomic status, and cognitive ability for predicting important life outcomes. Perspect Psychol Sci 2:313–345, 2007

Robins E, Guze SB: Establishment of diagnostic validity in psychiatric illness: its application to schizophrenia. Am J Psychiatry 126:983–987, 1970

Rojas SL, Widiger TA: Coverage of the DSM-IV-TR/DSM-5 Section II personality disorders with the DSM-5 dimensional trait model. J Pers Disord 31:462–482, 2017

Rounsaville BJ, Alarcon RD, Andrews G, et al: Basic nomenclature issues for DSM-V, in A Research Agenda for DSM-V. Edited by Kupfer DJ, First MB, Regier DA. Washington, DC, American Psychiatric Association, 2002, pp 1–29

Ruggero C, Kotov R, Hopwood CJ, et al: Integrating the Hierarchical Taxonomy of Psychopathology (HiTOP) into clinical practice. J Consult Clin Psychol 87:1069–1084, 2019

Salvatore G, Nicolo G, Dimaggio G: Impoverished dialogical relationship patterns in paranoid personality disorder. Am J Psychother 59:247–265, 2005

Samuel DB, Widiger TA: A meta-analytic review of the relationship between the five-factor model and DSM-IV-TR personality disorders: a facet level analysis. Clin Psychol Rev 28:1326–1342, 2008

Sanislow CA, Pine DS, Quinn KJ, et al: Developing constructs for psychopathology research: research domain criteria. J Abnorm Psychol 119:631–639, 2010

Saulsman LM, Page AC: The five-factor model and personality disorder empirical literature: a meta-analytic review. Clin Psychol Rev 23:1055–1085, 2004

Scalabrini A, Mucci C, Northoff G: Is our self related to personality? A neuropsychodynamic model. Front Hum Neurosci 12:346, 2018

Shiner RL: A developmental perspective on personality disorders: lessons from research on normal personality development in childhood and adolescence. J Pers Disord 19:202–210, 2005

Shiner RL: The development of personality disorders: perspectives from normal personality development in childhood and adolescence. Dev Psychopathol 21:715–734, 2009

Silberg JL, Rutter M, Tracy K, et al: Etiological heterogeneity in the development of antisocial behavior. Psychol Med 37:1193–1202, 2007

Skodol AE: Longitudinal course and outcome of personality disorders. Psychiatr Clin North Am 31:495–503, 2008

Skodol AE: Scientific issues in the revision of personality disorders for DSM-5. Personal Ment Health 5:97–111, 2011

Skodol AE: Personality disorders in DSM-5. Annu Rev Clin Psychol 8:317–344, 2012

Skodol AE: Borderline, schizotypal, avoidant, obsessive-compulsive, and other personality disorders, in Life Course Epidemiology of Mental Disorders. Edited by Koenen K, Rudenstine S, Susser E, et al. New York, Oxford University Press, 2013, pp 174–181

Skodol AE, Gunderson JG, McGlashan TH, et al: Functional impairment in patients with schizotypal, borderline, avoidant, or obsessive-compulsive personality disorder. Am J Psychiatry 159:276–283, 2002

Skodol AE, Oldham JM, Bender DS, et al: Dimensional representations of DSM-IV personality disorders: relationships to functional impairment. Am J Psychiatry 162:1919–1925, 2005a

Skodol AE, Pagano ME, Bender DS, et al: Stability of functional impairment in patients with schizotypal, borderline, avoidant, or obsessive-compulsive personality disorder over two years. Psychol Med 35:443–451, 2005b

Skodol AE, Shea MT, McGlashan TH, et al: The Collaborative Longitudinal Personality Disorders Study (CLPS): overview and implications. J Pers Disord 19:487–504, 2005c

Skodol AE, Bender DS, Morey LC, et al: Personality disorder types proposed for DSM-5. J Pers Disord 25:136–169, 2011a

Skodol AE, Grilo CM, Keyes K, et al: Relationship of personality disorders to the course of major depressive disorder in a nationally representative sample. Am J Psychiatry 168:257–264, 2011b

Skodol AE, Bender DS, Oldham JM: An alternative model for personality disorders: DSM-5 Section III and beyond, in The American Psychiatric Publishing Textbook of Personality Disorders, 2nd Edition. Edited by Oldham JM, Skodol AE, Bender DS. Arlington, VA, American Psychiatric Publishing, 2014, pp 511–544

Skodol AE, First MF, Bender DS, Oldham JM: Structured Clinical Interview for the DSM-5 Alternative Model for Personality Disorders (SCID-5-AMPD) Module II. Washington, DC, American Psychiatric Association Publishing, 2018

Spitzer RL: Psychiatric diagnosis: are clinicians still necessary? Compr Psychiatry 24:399–411, 1983

Stanley B, Siever LJ: The interpersonal dimension of borderline personality disorder: toward a neuropeptide model. Am J Psychiatry 167:24–39, 2010

Stepp SD, Trull TJ, Burr RM, et al: Incremental validity of the Structured Interview for the Five-Factor Model of Personality (SIFFM). Eur J Pers 19:343–357, 2005

Stuart J, Westen D, Lohr N, et al: Object relations in borderlines, major depressives, and normals: analysis of Rorschach human figure responses. J Pers Assess 55:296–318, 1990

Stuart S, Pfohl B, Battaglia M, et al: The co-occurrence of DSM-III-R personality disorders. J Pers Disord 12:302–315, 1998

Tackett JL, Balsis S, Oltmanns TF, et al: A unifying perspective on personality pathology across the life span: developmental considerations for the fifth edition of the Diagnostic and Statistical Manual of Mental Disorders. Dev Psychopathol 21:687–713, 2009

Thomas KM, Yalch MM, Krueger RF, et al: The convergent structure of DSM-5 personality trait facets and five-factor model trait domains. Assessment 20:308–311, 2013

Torgersen S: Prevalence, sociodemographics, and functional impairment, in Essentials of Personality Disorders. Edited by Oldham JM, Skodol AE, Bender DS. Washington, DC, American Psychiatric Publishing, 2009, pp 83–102

Torgersen S, Lygren S, Oien PA, et al: A twin study of personality disorders. Compr Psychiatry 41:416–425, 2000

Torgersen S, Czajkowski N, Jacobson K, et al: Dimensional representations of DSM-IV Cluster B personality disorders in a population-based sample of Norwegian twins: a multivariate study. Psychol Med 38:1617–1625, 2008

Trull TJ, Widiger TA, Useda JD, et al: A structured interview for the assessment of the five-factor model of personality. Psychol Assess 10:229–240, 1998

Tyrer P: The problem of severity in the classification of personality disorders. J Pers Disord 19:309–314, 2005

Tyrer P, Crawford M, Mulder R, et al: The rationale for the reclassification of personality disorder in the 11th revision of the International Classification of Diseases (ICD-11). Personal Ment Health 5:246–259, 2011

Tyrer P, Reed GM, Crawford MJ: Classification, assessment, prevalence, and effect of personality disorder. Lancet 385:717–726, 2015

Tyrer P, Mulder R, Kim YR, et al: The development of the ICD-11 classification of personality disorders: an amalgam of science, pragmatism, and politics. Annu Rev Clin Psychol 15:481–502, 2019

Verheul R, Widiger TA: A meta-analysis of the prevalence and usage of the personality disorder not otherwise specified (PDNOS) diagnosis. J Pers Disord 18:309–319, 2004

Verheul R, Andrea H, Berghout CC, et al: Severity Indices of Personality Problems (SIPP-118): development, factor structure, reliability and validity. Psychol Assess 20:23–34, 2008

Vermote R, Lowyck B, Luyten P, et al: Process and outcome in psychodynamic hospitalization-based treatment for patients with a personality disorder. J Nerv Ment Dis 198:110–115, 2010

Wagner AW, Linehan MM: Facial expression recognition ability among women with borderline personality disorder: implications for emotion regulation? J Pers Disord 13:329–344, 1999

Wakefield JC: The perils of dimensionalization: challenges in distinguishing negative traits from personality disorders. Psychiatr Clin North Am 31:379–393, 2008

Warren JI, South SC: A symptom level examination of the relationship between Cluster B personality disorders and patterns of criminality and violence in women. Int J Law Psychiatry 32:10–17, 2009

Watters CA, Bagby RM: A meta-analysis of the five-factor internal structure of the Personality Inventory for DSM-5. Psychol Assess 30:1255–1260, 2018

Watters CA, Bagby RM, Sellbom M: Meta-analysis to derive an empirically based set of personality facet criteria for the alternative DSM-5 model for personality disorders. Personal Disord 10:97–104, 2019

Waugh MH, Hopwood CJ, Krueger RF, et al: Psychological assessment with the DSM-5 Alternative Model for Personality Disorders: tradition and innovation. Prof Psychol Res Pr 48:79–89, 2017

Weekers LC, Hutsebaut J, Kampuis JH: The Level of Personality Functioning Scale—Brief Form 2.0: update of a brief instrument for assessing level of personality functioning. Personal Ment Health 13:3–14, 2019

Westen D, Ludolph P, Lerner H, et al: Object relations in borderline adolescents. J Am Acad Child Adolesc Psychiatry 29:338–348, 1990

Widiger A, Simonsen E: Alternative dimensional models of personality disorder: finding a common ground. J Pers Disord 19:110–130, 2005

Widiger TA, Trull TJ: Plate tectonics in the classification of personality disorder: shifting to a dimensional model. Am Psychol 62:71–83, 2007

Widiger TA, Frances AJ, Pincus HA, et al: Toward an empirical classification for the DSM-IV. J Abnorm Psychol 100:280–288, 1991

Widiger TA, Frances AJ, Pincus HA, et al (eds): DSM-IV Sourcebook, Vol 2. Washington, DC, American Psychiatric Association, 1996

Widom CS: The cycle of violence. Science 244:160–166, 1989

Williams TF, Scalco MD, Simms LJ: The construct validity of general and specific dimensions of personality pathology. Psychol Med 48:834–848, 2018

Wright AG, Thomas KM, Hopwood CJ, et al: The hierarchical structure of DSM-5 pathological personality traits. J Abnorm Psychol 121:951–957, 2012

Wright AG, Hopwood CJ, Skodol AE, et al: Longitudinal validation of general and specific structural features of personality pathology. J Abnorm Psychol 125:1120–1134, 2016

Yamagata S, Suzuki A, Ando J, et al: Is the genetic structure of human personality universal? A cross-cultural twin study from North America, Europe, and Asia. J Pers Soc Psychol 90:987–998, 2006

Zanarini MC, Frankenburg FR, Vujanovic AA: Inter-rater and test-retest reliability of the Revised Diagnostic Interview for Borderlines. J Pers Disord 16:270–276, 2002a

Zanarini MC, Yong L, Frankenburg FR, et al: Severity of reported childhood sexual abuse and its relationship to severity of borderline personality psychopathology and psychosocial impairment among borderline inpatients. J Nerv Ment Dis 190:381–387, 2002b

Zanarini MC, Vujanovic AA, Parachini EA, et al: Zanarini Rating Scale for Borderline Personality Disorder (ZAN-BPD): a continuous measure of DSM-IV borderline psychopathology. J Pers Disord 17:233–242, 2003

Zanarini MC, Frankenburg FR, Hennen J, et al: The McLean Study of Adult Development (MSAD): overview and implications of the first six years of prospective follow-up. J Pers Disord 19:505–523, 2005

Zanarini MC, Frankenburg FR, Reich DB, et al: Attainment and stability of sustained symptomatic remission and recovery among patients with borderline personality disorder and Axis II comparison subjects: a 16-year prospective follow-up study. Am J Psychiatry 169:476–483, 2012

Zanarini MC, Frankenburg FR, Reich DB, et al: Fluidity of the subsyndromal phenomenology of borderline personality disorder over 16 years of prospective follow-up. Am J Psychiatry 173:688–694, 2016

Zimmerman M, Rothchild L, Chelminski I: The prevalence of DSM-IV personality disorders in psychiatric outpatients. Am J Psychiatry 162:1911–1918, 2005

Zimmerman M, Chelminski I, Young D, et al: Which DSM-IV personality disorders are most strongly associated with indices of psychosocial morbidity in psychiatric outpatients? Compr Psychiatry 53:940–945, 2012

Zimmermann J, Benecke C, Bender DS, et al: Assessing DSM-5 level of personality function from videotaped clinical interviews: a pilot study with untrained and clinically inexperienced students. J Pers Assess 96:397–409, 2014

Zimmermann J, Kerber A, Rek K, et al: A brief but comprehensive review of research on the Alternative DSM-5 Model for Personality Disorders. Curr Psychiatry Rep 21:92, 2019

Zoccolillo M, Pickles A, Quinton D, et al: The outcome of conduct disorder: implications for defining adult personality disorder and conduct disorder. Psychol Med 22:971–986, 1992

CHAPTER 5

Manifestations, Assessment, Diagnosis, and Differential Diagnosis

Andrew E. Skodol, M.D.

In DSM-5 Section II, "Diagnostic Criteria and Codes" (American Psychiatric Association 2013), personality disorders (PDs) are defined by general criteria identical to those in DSM-IV (American Psychiatric Association 1994), despite the virtual absence of theoretical or empirical justifications for key aspects of these criteria. According to DSM-5 Section II, PDs are enduring patterns of inner experience and behavior that are inflexible and pervasive and cause clinically significant distress or impairment in social, occupational, or other areas of functioning. The patterns deviate markedly from the expectations of an individual's culture and are said to be manifested in two or more of the following areas: cognition, affectivity, interpersonal functioning, and impulse control. These features are not specific to PDs, however, and may characterize other chronic mental disorders, thereby contributing to problems in differential diagnosis. An alternative set of general criteria was proposed for DSM-5 (see Chapter 4, "The Alternative DSM-5 Model for Personality Disorders" in this volume) and can be found in Section III, "Emerging Measures and Models," of the manual.

PDs are associated with significant difficulties in self-appraisal and self-regulation, as well as with impaired interpersonal relationships. Thus, the alternative criteria focus on impairments in aspects of what is called *personality functioning*, which has been shown to be at the core of personality psychopathology according to multiple personality theories and research traditions (Bender et al. 2011; Livesley and Jang 2000; Luyten and Blatt 2013; Waugh et al. 2017). Impairments in personality functioning have been empirically demonstrated to discriminate PDs from other types of psychopathology (Morey et al. 2011), thereby facilitating differential diagnosis. In addition, for a PD diagnosis, the Section III general criteria require the presence of *pathological personality traits*, a term that describes the myriad variations in personality features that characterize PDs.

Because the Section II classification of PDs remains the "official" classification for clinical use, I provide guidance in this chapter on assessing personality psychopathology and diagnosing PDs using Section II concepts. The process of diagnosing PDs and distinguishing them from other mental disorders may be more difficult with DSM-5, which has discontinued the multiaxial recording system of DSM-IV (American Psychiatric Association 1994). Because of the many documented problems with the DSM-IV, and now DSM-5 Section II, categorical approach to personality pathology (see Chapter 4 in this volume), I also outline in this chapter the diagnostic process embodied by the Section III alternative hybrid dimensional-categorical PD model.

DSM-5 Section II includes criteria for the diagnosis of 10 specific PDs, arranged into three clusters based on descriptive similarities. Cluster A is commonly referred to as the "odd or eccentric" cluster and includes paranoid, schizoid, and schizotypal PDs. Cluster B, the "dramatic, emotional, or erratic" cluster, includes antisocial, borderline, histrionic, and narcissistic PDs. Cluster C, the "anxious and fearful" cluster, includes avoidant, dependent, and obsessive-compulsive PDs. DSM-5 Section II also provides the residual categories of other specified PD and unspecified PD. The former category is to be used when the general criteria for a PD are met and features of several different types of PD are present but the criteria for a specific PD are not met (i.e., "mixed" PD features) or the patient has a PD not included in the official classification (e.g., self-defeating or depressive PD). The latter category is used when the general criteria for a PD are met but there is no further specification of the PD's characteristics (e.g., when insufficient information is available to make a more specific diagnosis).

DSM-5 Section III provides diagnostic criteria for those 6 of the 10 Section II categories—antisocial, avoidant, borderline, narcissistic, obsessive-compulsive, and schizotypal—that were judged to have the most empirical evidence of validity and/or clinical utility (Skodol et al. 2011a). The other four Section II PDs and all other presentations that meet the Section III general criteria for a PD are diagnosed in the alternative model as personality disorder—trait specified (PD-TS) (Table 5–1). The clinician notes the specific level of impairment in personality functioning and the specific pathological personality traits that describe the patient (see section "Defining Features of Personality Disorders" below). Thus, in all cases for which a PD is diagnosed using the Section III model, important descriptive information about personality functioning and pathological personality traits is recorded for treatment planning and prognosis.

This chapter considers the manifestations, assessment, diagnosis, and differential diagnosis of PDs. Included are descriptions of the clinical characteristics of the 10 DSM-5 PDs according to both Section II and Section III criteria. (In the case of the four Section II PDs represented by PD-TS in Section III, the descriptions are based on typical impairments in personality functioning and characteristic pathological personality traits—see Table 5–1.) Also included are approaches to clinical interviewing, along with discussions of problems in assessing a patient with a suspected PD, such as state versus trait discrimination, trait versus disorder distinctions, and the effects of gender, culture, and age. Despite limitations in the traditional categorical DSM approach to personality psychopathology, PDs diagnosed by this system have been shown since the 1980s to have considerable clinical utility in predicting functional impairment over and above that associated with other comorbid mental disorders, chronicity of other co-occurring mental disorders, extensive and intensive utilization of treatment resources, and, in many cases, adverse psychosocial outcomes (Skodol

TABLE 5–1. **Crosswalk of DSM-5 Section II personality disorders to Section III personality disorders and Criterion B pathological personality traits**

DSM-5 Section II personality disorder	DSM-5 Section III personality disorder (Criterion B decision rules)	Pathological personality traits (domains)
Paranoid	PD-TS[a]	Suspiciousness (DET) Hostility (ANT)
Schizoid	PD-TS	Withdrawal (DET) Intimacy avoidance (DET) Anhedonia (DET) Restricted affectivity (DET)
Schizotypal	Schizotypal (4 or more)	Cognitive and perceptual dysregulation (PSY) Unusual beliefs and experiences (PSY) Eccentricity (PSY) Restricted affectivity (DET) Withdrawal (DET) Suspiciousness (DET)
Antisocial	Antisocial (6 or more)	Manipulativeness (ANT) Callousness (ANT) Deceitfulness (ANT) Hostility (ANT) Risk taking (DIS) Impulsivity (DIS) Irresponsibility (DIS)
Borderline	Borderline (4 or more; at least one of following traits is required: impulsivity, risk taking, hostility)	Emotional lability (NA) Anxiousness (NA) Separation insecurity (NA) Depressivity (NA) Impulsivity (DIS) Risk taking (DIS) Hostility (ANT)
Histrionic	PD-TS	Emotional lability (NA) Attention seeking (ANT) Manipulativeness (ANT)
Narcissistic	Narcissistic (both traits required)	Grandiosity (ANT) Attention seeking (ANT)
Avoidant	Avoidant (3 or more; anxiousness trait is required)	Anxiousness (NA) Withdrawal (DET) Anhedonia (DET) Intimacy avoidance (DET)

TABLE 5–1.   **Crosswalk of DSM-5 Section II personality disorders to Section III personality disorders and Criterion B pathological personality traits (continued)**

DSM-5 Section II personality disorder	DSM-5 Section III personality disorder (Criterion B decision rules)	Pathological personality traits (domains)
Dependent	PD-TS	Submissiveness (NA) Anxiousness (NA) Separation insecurity (NA)
Obsessive-compulsive	Obsessive-compulsive (3 or more; rigid perfectionism trait is required)	Rigid perfectionism (C) Perseveration (NA) Intimacy avoidance (DET) Restricted affectivity (DET)

Note.   ANT=Antagonism; C=Conscientiousness (opposite pole of DIS); DET=Detachment; DIS=Disinhibition; NA=Negative Affectivity; PD-TS=personality disorder—trait specified; PSY=Psychoticism.
ªWhen a patient's level of impairment in personality functioning is moderate or greater, but the pattern of impairments or pathological personality traits do not correspond to one of the specific Section III personality disorders, a diagnosis of PD-TS is made.

2018). Thus, the recognition and accurate diagnosis of personality psychopathology should be an important clinical priority.

Defining Features of Personality Disorders

DSM-5 PDs are defined differently in Section II and Section III. Each section has a set of general criteria defining what is meant by a PD and individual criteria sets for each specific diagnosis. When a diagnosis is being made, it is useful to consider how the specific manifestations of each PD align with the general definitions according to each model.

Patterns of Inner Experience and Behavior Versus Personality Functioning and Personality Traits

The general diagnostic criteria for a PD in DSM-5 Section II indicate that a pattern of inner experience and behavior is manifested by characteristic patterns of 1) cognition (i.e., ways of perceiving and interpreting self, other people, and events); 2) affectivity (i.e., the range, intensity, lability, and appropriateness of emotional response); 3) interpersonal functioning; and 4) impulse control. Persons with PDs are expected to have manifestations in at least two of these areas. In contrast, Section III general criteria focus on impairment in personality functioning and the presence of pathological personality traits. Personality functioning consists of sense of self (identity and self-direction) and interpersonal relatedness (empathy and intimacy), capturing aspects of all four Section II areas. The Section III pathological trait domains of Negative Affectivity and Disinhibition (see subsection "Criterion B: Pathological Personality Traits" below) elaborate on two of the Section II areas. Although the general criteria of the two models overlap, the Section III general criteria have been shown empirically to be associated specifically with PDs (Morey et al. 2011, 2013a), whereas the Section II general criteria have not.

DSM-5 Section III Alternative Model for Personality Disorders

The general criteria for a PD according to DSM-5 Section III (Skodol et al. 2015) require two initial determinations: 1) an assessment of the level of impairment in personality functioning, which is needed for Criterion A, and 2) an evaluation of pathological personality traits, which is required for Criterion B. The impairments in personality functioning and personality trait expression are relatively inflexible and pervasive across a broad range of personal and social situations (Criterion C); relatively stable across time, with onsets that can be traced back to at least adolescence or early adulthood (Criterion D); not better explained by another mental disorder (Criterion E); not attributable to a substance or another medical condition (Criterion F); and not better understood as normal for an individual's developmental stage or sociocultural environment (Criterion G). All Section III PDs described by criterion sets and PD-TS meet these general criteria, by definition. (The appendix to this textbook includes the complete wording of these general criteria.) Figure 5-1 illustrates a stepwise approach to assessment according to the Alternative DSM-5 Model for Personality Disorders (AMPD) general criteria for personality disorder.

Criterion A: Level of Personality Functioning

Disturbances in *self* and *interpersonal* functioning constitute the core of personality psychopathology (Bender et al. 2011). In the alternative Section III diagnostic model, they are evaluated on a continuum, using the Level of Personality Functioning Scale (LPFS). The LPFS assesses capacities that lie at the heart of personality and adaptive functioning. Self functioning involves identity and self-direction; interpersonal functioning involves empathy and intimacy.

- *Identity* is defined as the experience of oneself as unique, with clear boundaries between self and others; stability of self-esteem and accuracy of self-appraisal; and the capacity for, and the ability to regulate, a range of emotional experience.
- *Self-direction* is the pursuit of coherent and meaningful short-term and life goals; the utilization of constructive and prosocial internal standards of behavior; and the ability to self-reflect productively.
- *Empathy* is the comprehension and appreciation of others' experiences and motivations; tolerance of differing perspectives; and an understanding of the effects of one's own behavior on others.
- *Intimacy* reflects the depth and duration of connection with others; a desire and capacity for closeness; and a mutuality of regard reflected in interpersonal behavior.

The LPFS utilizes each of these elements to differentiate five levels of impairment, ranging from *little or no impairment* (i.e., healthy, adaptive functioning; Level 0) to *some* (Level 1), *moderate* (Level 2), *severe* (Level 3), and *extreme* (Level 4) impairment.

Impairment in personality functioning predicts the presence of a PD, and the severity of impairment predicts whether an individual has more than one PD or one of

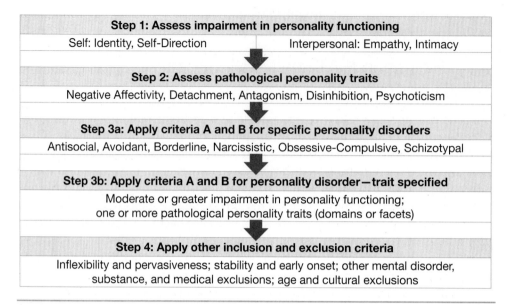

Step 1: Assess impairment in personality functioning	
Self: Identity, Self-Direction	Interpersonal: Empathy, Intimacy

Step 2: Assess pathological personality traits
Negative Affectivity, Detachment, Antagonism, Disinhibition, Psychoticism

Step 3a: Apply criteria A and B for specific personality disorders
Antisocial, Avoidant, Borderline, Narcissistic, Obsessive-Compulsive, Schizotypal

Step 3b: Apply criteria A and B for personality disorder—trait specified
Moderate or greater impairment in personality functioning; one or more pathological personality traits (domains or facets)

Step 4: Apply other inclusion and exclusion criteria
Inflexibility and pervasiveness; stability and early onset; other mental disorder, substance, and medical exclusions; age and cultural exclusions

FIGURE 5–1.   Stepwise approach to assessment according to the alternative model general criteria for personality disorder.

Source.   Reprinted from Skodol AE, Morey LC, Bender DS, et al.: "The Alternative DSM-5 Model for Personality Disorders: a clinical application." *American Journal of Psychiatry* 172:606–613, 2015. Copyright © 2015, American Psychiatric Association. Used with permission.

the more typically severe PDs (Morey et al. 2011). A moderate level of impairment in personality functioning is required for the diagnosis of a PD based on empirical evidence that a moderate level of impairment maximizes the ability of clinicians to accurately and efficiently identify PD pathology (Morey et al. 2013a).

To use the LPFS, the clinician selects the level that most closely captures the individual's *current overall* level of impairment in personality functioning. The rating not only is necessary for the diagnosis of a PD (moderate impairment or greater) but also can be used to specify the severity of impairment present for an individual with any PD at a given point in time. The LPFS may also be used as a global indicator of personality functioning without specification of a PD diagnosis, in the event that personality impairment is subthreshold for a disorder diagnosis, or as a severity change measure during or following treatment. Interrater and test-retest reliability of ratings on the LPFS full scale and on the four domains of personality functioning have been shown to be very good to excellent using a semi-structured interview developed for the LPFS, the Structured Clinical Interview for the DSM-5 Alternative Model for Personality Disorders (SCID-5-AMPD) Module I (Buer Christensen et al. 2018). Reliable ratings have also been achieved, however, even by raters with little clinical experience and training (Garcia et al. 2018; Zimmermann et al. 2014). The full LPFS can be found in the appendix to this textbook.

Criterion B: Pathological Personality Traits

Pathological personality traits in DSM-5 Section III are organized into five broad trait domains: Negative Affectivity, Detachment, Antagonism, Disinhibition, and Psychoticism. Within these five broad domains are 25 specific *trait facets* that have been developed, initially from a review of existing trait models and then through iterative research on samples of persons who sought mental health services (Krueger et al. 2011a, 2011b, 2012). The full trait taxonomy can be found in the appendix to this textbook. Definitions of all personality domains and facets are provided in DSM-5 (American Psychiatric Association 2013, pp. 779–781) and in the appendix. For example, the domain of Negative Affectivity is defined as "frequent and intense experiences of high levels of a wide range of negative emotions (e.g., anxiety, depression, guilt/shame, worry, anger), and their behavioral (e.g., self-harm) and interpersonal (e.g., dependency) manifestations" (p. 779). The trait facet of emotional lability, a component of Negative Affectivity, is defined as "instability of emotional experiences and mood; emotions that are easily aroused, intense, and/or out of proportion to events and circumstances" (p. 779). The B criteria for the specific PDs comprise subsets of the 25 trait facets, based on meta-analytic reviews (Samuel and Widiger 2008; Saulsman and Page 2004) and empirical data on the relationships of the traits to DSM-IV PD diagnoses (Hopwood et al. 2012; Morey et al. 2016). Diagnostic thresholds for the specific PDs in the AMPD were derived to maximize correspondence to DSM-IV PDs, to minimize overlap with other PDs, and to maximize relationships of the PDs to functional impairment (Morey and Skodol 2013).

A *personality trait* is a tendency to feel, perceive, behave, and think in relatively consistent ways across time and across situations in which the trait may be manifested. The clinical utility of the Section III multidimensional personality trait model lies in its ability to focus attention on multiple areas of personality variation in each individual patient. Rather than attention being focused on the identification of one optimal diagnostic label, clinical application of the Section III personality trait model involves reviewing all five broad personality domains. This approach to personality assessment is similar to the well-known review of systems in clinical medicine.

Clinical use of the Section III personality trait model begins with an initial review of all five broad domains of personality. This systematic review may be facilitated by the use of formal psychometric instruments designed to measure specific domains and facets of personality. For example, the personality trait model is operationalized in the Personality Inventory for DSM-5 (PID-5; Krueger et al. 2012). The PID-5 can be completed in its self-report form by patients and in its informant-report form (Markon et al. 2013) by those who know the patient well (e.g., a spouse). In addition, Module II of the SCID-5-AMPD (Skodol et al. 2018) is devoted to the assessment of alternative model personality traits. A detailed clinical assessment might involve collection of data from both patients and informants on all 25 facets of the personality trait model. If this is not possible, because of time or other constraints, assessment focused at the five-domain level is an acceptable clinical option when only a general portrait of a patient's personality is needed. However, the more that personality-based problems are the primary focus of treatment, the more important it will be to assess individuals' trait facets as well as domains (Skodol et al. 2013).

Manifestations of Personality Psychopathology

Cognitive Features

PDs affect the ways individuals think about themselves and about their relationships with other people. Most of the DSM-5 Section II diagnostic criteria for paranoid PD

(PPD) reflect a disturbance in cognition characterized by pervasive distrust and suspiciousness of others. Persons with PPD suspect that others are exploiting, harming, or deceiving them; doubt the loyalty or trustworthiness of others; read hidden, demeaning, or threatening meanings into benign remarks or events; and perceive attacks on their character or reputation. PPD would be diagnosed as PD-TS in the alternative DSM-5 model for PDs (see Table 5–1). The level of impairment in personality functioning typically would be severe or extreme, in part because of serious distortions in sense of self, and relevant pathological personality traits would include suspiciousness and possibly hostility.

Among the major symptoms of Section II schizotypal PD (STPD) are characteristic cognitive and perceptual distortions, such as ideas of reference; odd beliefs and magical thinking (e.g., superstitiousness, belief in clairvoyance or telepathy); bodily illusions; and suspiciousness and paranoia similar to those observed in persons with PPD. STPD is a specific PD in the alternative DSM-5 model. It is characterized by extreme impairments in personality functioning, such as confused boundaries between self and others, and by four or more of six pathological personality traits, which include cognitive and perceptual dysregulation, unusual beliefs and experiences, and suspiciousness—all cognitive manifestations.

Persons with Section II borderline PD (BPD) may also experience transient paranoid ideation when under stress, but the characteristic cognitive manifestations of individuals with BPD are dramatic shifts in their views toward people with whom they are intensely emotionally involved. These shifts emanate from disturbances in mental representations of self and others (Bender and Skodol 2007) and result in the individual's overidealizing others at one point and then devaluating them at another point, when the individual feels disappointed, neglected, or uncared for. This phenomenon is commonly referred to as "splitting." BPD is also a specific PD in Section III, with severe impairments in personality functioning, including a markedly impoverished, poorly developed, or unstable self-image.

Persons with DSM-5 Section II narcissistic PD (NPD) exhibit a grandiose sense of self; have fantasies of unlimited success, power, brilliance, beauty, or ideal love; and believe themselves to be special or unique. DSM-5 Section III criteria for NPD reflect evolved conceptualizations of pathological narcissism in which exaggerated self-appraisal may be either inflated or deflated or vacillating between extremes, and grandiosity may be either overt or covert (Skodol et al. 2014a).

In the area of personal identity, persons with antisocial PD (ASPD), also a specific PD in Section III, exhibit notable egocentrism bordering on grandiosity (although the egocentrism may be masked by relative immunity to stress) and a concomitant sense of entitlement and invulnerability. Self-esteem is disproportionately high, leading to selfishness and overt or covert disregard for legal, moral, or cultural restrictions, because goals are based on "instant gratification."

Persons with avoidant PD (AVPD) have excessively negative opinions of themselves. They see themselves as inept, unappealing, and inferior, and they constantly perceive that they are being criticized or rejected. AVPD is a specific PD in the DSM-5 AMPD. Specific impairments in personality functioning are generally at a moderate level, characterized in part by low self-esteem associated with self-appraisal as socially inept, personally unappealing, or inferior.

Persons with Section II dependent PD (DPD) also lack self-confidence and believe that they are unable to make decisions or to take care of themselves. These individuals are characterized by moderate impairment in personality functioning according to the Section III model because of identities that are dependent on the presence of reassuring others.

Persons with obsessive-compulsive PD (OCPD) are perfectionistic and rigid in their thinking and are often preoccupied with details, rules, lists, and order. Their personality functioning is also at a moderate level of impairment, in part because of a sense of self that is derived predominantly from work or productivity.

Affective Features

Some persons with PDs are emotionally constricted, whereas others are excessively emotional. Among the emotionally constricted individuals are those with schizoid PD, who experience little pleasure in life, appear indifferent to praise or criticism, and are generally emotionally cold, detached, and unexpressive. Persons with STPD also often have constricted or inappropriate affect, although they can exhibit anxiety in relation to their paranoid fears. Persons with OCPD have considerable difficulty expressing loving feelings toward others, and when they do express affection, they do so in a highly controlled or stilted manner. Restricted affectivity is a trait in the Section III B criteria for both STPD and OCPD. Schizoid PD is diagnosed as PD-TS in the AMPD. The relevant pathological personality traits would include anhedonia and restricted affectivity, from the Detachment trait domain.

Among the most emotionally expressive persons with PDs are those with borderline and histrionic PDs. Persons with BPD are emotionally labile and react very strongly, particularly in interpersonal contexts, with a variety of intensely dysphoric emotions, such as depression, anxiety, or irritability. They are also prone to inappropriate, intense outbursts of anger and are often preoccupied with fears of being abandoned by those they are attached to and reliant upon. Emotional lability, depressivity, and hostility are three Criterion B personality traits in the alternative model rendition of BPD. Persons with histrionic PD often display rapidly shifting emotions that seem to be dramatic and exaggerated but are shallow in comparison to the intense emotional expression seen in BPD. Emotional lability would be a relevant trait for such patients, who are diagnosed with PD-TS according to Section III. Persons with ASPD characteristically have problems with irritability and aggressive feelings toward others, as expressed in the context of threat or intimidation. Hostility is one of the trait criteria for ASPD in Section III. Persons with AVPD are dominated by anxiety in social situations; those with DPD are preoccupied by anxiety over the prospects of separation from caregivers and the need to be independent. Anxiousness also characterizes AVPD in the Section III criteria and would be a relevant trait for the PD-TS representation of DPD.

Interpersonal Features

Interpersonal problems are probably most obviously identifiable in PDs (Gunderson 2007; Hill et al. 2008; Hopwood et al. 2013a). Other mental disorders are characterized by prominent cognitive or affective features or by problems with impulse control. All PDs, however, have interpersonal manifestations coupled with problems in sense of self, as captured by the Section III LPFS and the A criteria for the six specific PDs and PD-TS. Each of the six disorders includes characteristic problems with empathy and intimacy.

Persons with ASPD deceive and intimidate others for personal gain. Substantially lacking in empathy, they have no concern for the feelings of others and lack remorse if they hurt someone. In the area of intimacy, they are incapable of having mutually intimate relationships, because they are exploitative or controlling of others. Pathological personality traits include manipulativeness, callousness, deceitfulness, and irresponsibility. Persons with histrionic and narcissistic PDs need to be the center of attention and require excessive admiration. Intimate relationships are generally shallow, and people are sought out predominantly in the service of bolstering self-esteem. Empathic concerns center on issues that have direct implications for the person with the PD. Both disorders would be characterized by the trait of attention seeking according to the Section III AMPD. In addition, histrionic PD might also be characterized by the trait of manipulativeness.

Persons with OCPD have difficulty appreciating others' perspectives and instead need to control others and have them submit to their ways of doing things. Intimacy is circumscribed by stubbornness and rigidity, and a preference for engaging in tasks rather than pursuing close relationships. Traits of rigid perfectionism and intimacy avoidance adversely affect the interpersonal relationships of individuals with OCPD.

The interpersonal relationships of persons with AVPD and DPD are impoverished as a result of fear and submissiveness. Individuals with AVPD are inhibited in interpersonal relationships because they are afraid of being shamed or ridiculed. Empathy is impaired because of a distorted sense of others' appraisal and acute rejection sensitivity. Intimacy avoidance and withdrawal are Criterion B personality traits for Section III AVPD. Individuals with DPD will not disagree with important others for fear of losing their support or approval and will actually do things that are unpleasant, demeaning, or self-defeating to receive nurturance from others. Because of the self-sacrificing approach to relationships, real intimacy and empathy are elusive. Submissiveness and separation insecurity would be relevant Section III AMPD personality trait facets.

The empathy of persons with BPD is biased toward the negative tendencies and vulnerabilities of others. Intimate relationships are extremely challenging, with a pattern of these individuals becoming "deeply" involved and dependent only to turn manipulative and demanding when their needs are not met. They have interpersonal relationships that are unstable and conflicted, and they alternate between overinvolvement with others and withdrawal. Separation insecurity is a relevant Section III Criterion B trait.

The degree of detachment associated with persons with paranoid, schizoid, and schizotypal PDs serves as a pronounced impediment to empathy and intimacy in interpersonal relations. Individuals with schizoid PD manifest an apparent lack of need for closeness with others; those with PPD do not trust others enough to become deeply involved; and those with STPD have few friends or confidants, in part from a lack of trust and in part as a result of poor communication and inadequate relatedness. Section III traits of suspiciousness, withdrawal, and intimacy avoidance lead to social isolation.

Problems With Impulse Control

Problems with impulse control can also be viewed as extremes on a continuum. PDs characterized by a lack of impulse control include ASPD and BPD. Disorders involving problems with overcontrol include AVPD, DPD, and OCPD. ASPD is a prototype of a PD characterized by impulsivity. Persons with ASPD break laws, exploit others, fail to plan ahead, get into fights, ignore commitments and obligations, and exhibit generally reckless behaviors without regard for consequences, such as speeding, driving while intoxicated, having impulsive sex, or abusing drugs. Persons with BPD also show many problems with impulse control, including impulsive spending, indiscriminate sex, substance abuse, reckless driving, and binge eating. In addition, individuals with BPD experience recurrent suicidal thoughts and impulses. Suicide attempts and self-injurious behavior, such as cutting or burning, are common. Section III personality traits that predispose to these behaviors include impulsivity and risk taking from the Disinhibition trait domain and are among the B criteria for both ASPD and BPD. Finally, persons with BPD have problems with anger management, have frequent temper outbursts, and at times may even engage in physical fights. Hostility is a trait in the criteria for both ASPD and BPD.

In contrast to individuals with disinhibited behavior, persons with AVPD are excessively inhibited, especially in relation to people, and are reluctant to take risks or to undertake new activities. Persons with DPD cannot even make basic decisions and do not take initiative to start things. Persons with OCPD are overly conscientious and scrupulous about morality, ethics, and values; they cannot bring themselves to throw away even worthless objects and can be miserly. They are characterized by rigid perfectionism, which is the opposite of the traits characterizing the domain of Disinhibition.

The DSM-5 Section II PD clusters, specific PD types, and their principal defining clinical features are summarized in Table 5–2 and contrasted with central features of the DSM-5 Section III AMPD.

Pervasiveness and Inflexibility

For a PD to be present, the disturbances have to be manifested frequently through a wide range of behaviors, feelings, and perceptions and in many different contexts. In DSM-5 Section II, attempts are made to stress the pervasiveness of the behaviors caused by PDs. Added to the basic definition of each PD and serving as the "stem" to which individual features apply is the phrase "present in a variety of contexts." For example, the diagnostic features of PPD in DSM-5 Section II, preceding the specific criteria, begin as follows: "A pervasive distrust and suspiciousness of others such that their motives are interpreted as malevolent, beginning by early adulthood and present in a variety of contexts, as indicated by four (or more) of the following" (American Psychiatric Association 2013, p. 649). Similarly, for DPD, the criteria are preceded by this description: "A pervasive and excessive need to be taken care of that leads to submissive and clinging behavior and fears of separation, beginning by early adulthood and present in a variety of contexts, as indicated by five (or more) of the following" (American Psychiatric Association 2013, p. 675). The manifestations of Section III personality traits are pervasive by definition, in that they are general tendencies or predispositions to think, feel, and behave in particular patterned ways.

TABLE 5–2.   Defining features of DSM-5 Section II and Section III personality disorders

Personality disorder	Section II features	Section III features
Section II Cluster A	**Odd or eccentric**	
Paranoid	Pervasive distrust and suspiciousness of others such that their motives are interpreted as malevolent	See Table 5–1.
Schizoid	Pervasive pattern of detachment from social relationships and a restricted range of expression of emotions in interpersonal settings	See Table 5–1.
Schizotypal	Pervasive pattern of social and interpersonal deficits marked by acute discomfort with, and reduced capacity for, close relationships as well as by cognitive or perceptual distortions and eccentricities of behavior	Typical features are impairments in the capacity for social and close relationships, and eccentricities in cognition, perception, and behavior that are associated with distorted self-image and incoherent personal goals and accompanied by suspiciousness and restricted emotional expression.
Section II Cluster B	**Dramatic, emotional, or erratic**	
Antisocial	Pervasive pattern of disregard for and violation of the rights of others, occurring since age 15 years; current age at least 18 years	Typical features are a failure to conform to lawful and ethical behavior, and an egocentric, callous lack of concern for others, accompanied by deceitfulness, irresponsibility, manipulativeness, and/or risk taking.
Borderline	Pervasive pattern of instability of interpersonal relationships, self-image, and affects, and marked impulsivity	Typical features are instability of self-image, personal goals, interpersonal relationships, and affects, accompanied by impulsivity, risk taking, and/or hostility.
Histrionic	Pervasive pattern of excessive emotionality and attention seeking	See Table 5–1.
Narcissistic	Pervasive pattern of grandiosity (in fantasy or behavior), need for admiration, and lack of empathy	Typical features are variable and vulnerable self-esteem, with attempts at regulation through attention and approval seeking, and either overt or covert grandiosity.

TABLE 5–2.   Defining features of DSM-5 Section II and Section III personality disorders (*continued*)

Personality disorder	Section II features	Section III features
Section II Cluster C	**Anxious or fearful**	
Avoidant	Pervasive pattern of social inhibition, feelings of inadequacy, and hypersensitivity to negative evaluation	Typical features are avoidance of social situations and inhibition in interpersonal relationships related to feelings of ineptitude and inadequacy, anxious preoccupation with negative evaluation and rejection, and fears of ridicule or embarrassment.
Dependent	Pervasive and excessive need to be taken care of that leads to submissive and clinging behavior and fears of separation	See Table 5–1.
Obsessive-compulsive	Pervasive pattern of preoccupation with orderliness, perfectionism, and mental and interpersonal control, at the expense of flexibility, openness, and efficiency	Typical features are difficulties in establishing and sustaining close relationships, associated with rigid perfectionism, inflexibility, and restricted emotional expression.

Source.   Adapted from the *Diagnostic and Statistical Manual of Mental Disorders,*5th Edition. Arlington, VA, American Psychiatric Association, 2013. Used with permission. Copyright © 2013 American Psychiatric Association.

Inflexibility is a feature that helps to distinguish personality traits or styles and PDs. Inflexibility is indicated by a narrow repertoire of responses that are repeated even when the situation calls for an alternative behavior or in the face of clear evidence that a behavior is inappropriate or not working. For example, a person with OCPD rigidly adheres to rules and organization even in recreation and loses enjoyment as a consequence. A person with AVPD is so fearful of being scrutinized or criticized, even in group situations in which he or she could hardly be the focus of such attention, that life becomes painfully lonely.

Onset and Clinical Course

Personality and PDs have traditionally been assumed to reflect stable descriptions of a person, at least after a certain age. Thus, the patterns of inner experience and behaviors described earlier are called "enduring." PD is also described as "of long duration," with an onset that "can be traced back at least to adolescence or early adulthood" (American Psychiatric Association 2013, pp. 646–647). These concepts persist as integral to the definition of PD despite a large body of empirical evidence that suggests that PD psychopathology is not as stable as the DSM definition would indicate. Longitudinal studies indicate that PDs, as defined by DSM-IV (and DSM-5 Section II) criteria, tend to improve over time, at least from the point of view of their overt clinical signs and symptoms (Gunderson et al. 2011; Johnson et al. 2000; Lenzenweger et al. 2004; Zanarini et al. 2012). These traditional PD criteria sets, however, consist of combinations of pathological personality traits and symptomatic behaviors (McGlashan et al. 2005; Zanarini et al. 2007). Some behaviors, such as self-mutilating behavior (a manifestation of one of the criteria for BPD), may be evidenced much less frequently than traits such as "views self as socially inept, personally unappealing, or inferior to others" (one of the criteria for AVPD). How stable individual manifestations of PDs actually are and what the stable components of PDs are have become areas of active empirical research. It may be that personality psychopathology waxes and wanes (Temes and Zanarini 2018) depending on the circumstances of a person's life (see Chapter 9, "Longitudinal Course and Outcomes," in this volume). Personality traits (Hopwood et al. 2013a) may be more stable than PDs themselves. In DSM-5 Section III, the course of impairments in personality functioning and pathological traits is described, in the criteria, as "relatively" stable to allow for some fluctuation in their manifestations.

Although the onset of PDs has traditionally been considered to be in childhood or adolescence, later onsets can be observed (e.g., Skodol et al. 2007), including onsets in late life (Oltmanns and Balsis 2011). Personality disorder features have been linked to suicidal ideation, poor physical health, and cognitive decline in later life (Cruitt and Oltmanns 2018).

Recently, early recognition of personality pathology in children and adolescents has been encouraged, with an eye toward early intervention and prevention (see Chapter 10, "Early Identification and Prevention of Personality Pathology: An AMPD-Informed Model of Clinical Staging," in this volume). Thus, traditional notions of the course and impact of personality pathology over the life course are changing.

Impairment in Functioning

All PDs are maladaptive and are accompanied by functional problems in school or at work, in social relationships, or at leisure (Skodol 2018). The requirement for impairment in psychosocial functioning is codified in DSM-5 Section II in its Criterion C of the general diagnostic criteria for a PD: "the enduring pattern [of 'inner experience and behavior'—i.e., personality] leads to clinically significant distress or impairment in social, occupational, or other important areas of functioning" (American Psychiatric Association 2013, p. 646).

A number of studies have compared patients with PDs with patients with no PD or with DSM-IV Axis I disorders and have found that patients with PDs were more likely to be functionally impaired (Skodol et al. 2019). Specifically, they are more likely to be separated, divorced, or never married and to have had more unemployment, frequent job changes, or periods of disability. Fewer studies have examined quality of functioning, but in those that have, poorer social functioning or interpersonal relationships and poorer work functioning or occupational achievement and satisfaction have been found among patients with PDs than among patients with other disorders. When patients with different PDs were compared with one another on levels of functional impairment, those with severe PDs, such as STPD and BPD, were found to have significantly more impairment at work, in social relationships, and at leisure than patients with less severe PDs, such as OCPD, or with an impairing other mental disorder, such as major depressive disorder without PD. Patients with AVPD had intermediate levels of impairment. Even the less impaired patients with PDs (e.g., those with OCPD), however, had moderate to severe impairment in at least one area of functioning (or a Global Assessment of Functioning rating of 60 or less) (Skodol et al. 2002). The finding that significant impairment may be in only one area suggests that persons with PDs differ not only in the degree of associated functional impairment but also in the breadth of impairment across functional domains.

Another important aspect of the impairment in functioning in persons with PDs is that it tends to be persistent even beyond apparent improvement in the PD psychopathology itself (Gunderson et al. 2011; Seivewright et al. 2004; Skodol et al. 2005). The persistence of impairment is understandable if one considers that PD psychopathology has usually been long-standing and, therefore, has disrupted a person's work and social development over a period of time (Roberts et al. 2003). The residua, or "scars," of PD pathology take time to heal or be overcome. With time (and treatment), however, improvements in functioning can occur (Zanarini et al. 2010, 2012).

DSM-5 Section III pathological personality traits have been found to incrementally predict impairment in psychosocial functioning over normal-range personality traits, personality disorder criteria counts, and other psychiatric symptoms (Simms and Calabrese 2016). General personality disorder features reflecting disorder severity, however, have been found to be more strongly related longitudinally to impairment in psychosocial functioning than specific features reflecting personality style (Wright et al. 2016).

DSM-5 Section III criteria for PDs do not include a requirement for impairment in psychosocial functioning. This change is in keeping with some other disorders in DSM-5, for which attempts have been made to separate the manifestations of a disorder (i.e., signs, symptoms, traits) from their consequences (i.e., impact on occupational, social, and leisure functioning). Furthermore, Section III PDs all include specific impairments in *personality functioning* at a moderate level or greater. This change is consistent with the distinction between mental *functions* that lead to symptoms (e.g., emotional regulation, reward dependence, reality testing) and the *disabilities* that accompany disturbances in these functions (Sartorius 2009).

Approaches to Clinical Interviewing

Interviewing a patient to assess for a possible PD presents certain challenges that are somewhat unique. Thus, the interviewer is likely to need to rely on a variety of techniques for gathering information to arrive at a clinical diagnosis, including observation and interaction with the patient, direct questioning of the patient, and interviewing of informants.

Observation and Interaction

One problem in evaluating a patient for a PD arises from the fact that many people are not able to view their own personality objectively (Zimmerman 1994). Because personality is, by definition, the way a person sees, relates to, and thinks about himself or herself and the environment, a person's assessment of his or her own personality must be colored by it. The expression of other psychopathology may also be colored by personality style—for example, symptoms of depression are exaggerated by the histrionic personality or minimized by the compulsive personality—but the symptoms of most mental disorders are usually more clearly alien to the patient and more easily identified as problematic. People often learn about their own problem behaviors and their maladaptive patterns of interaction with others through the reactions or observations of other people in their environment.

Traditionally, clinicians have not conducted the same kind of interview in assessing patients suspected of having a personality disturbance as they do with persons suspected of having, for example, a mood or an anxiety disorder. Rather than directly questioning these patients about characteristics of their personality, the clinician, assuming that the patients cannot accurately describe these traits, looks for patterns in the way patients describe themselves, their social relations, and their work functioning. These three areas usually give the clearest picture of personality traits or style in general and of problems in personality functioning specifically. Clinicians have also relied heavily on their observations of how patients interact with them during an evaluation interview or in treatment as manifestations of their patients' personalities (Westen 1997).

These approaches have the advantage of circumventing the potential lack of objectivity patients might have about their personalities, but they also create problems. The clinician usually comes away with a global impression of the patient's personality but frequently is not aware of many of that patient's specific personality characteristics because the clinician has not made a systematic assessment of the manifestations of the wide range of PDs (Blashfield and Herkov 1996; Morey and Benson 2016; Morey and Ochoa 1989; Zimmerman and Mattia 1999). In routine clinical practice, clinicians have tended to use the nonspecific diagnosis of PD not otherwise specified when they believed that a patient's presentation met the general criteria for a PD, because they often did not have enough information to make a specific diagnosis (Verheul and Widiger 2004). Alternatively, clinicians will diagnose PDs hierarchically: once a patient is seen as having one (usually severe) PD, such as BPD, the clinician will not assess whether traits of other PDs are also present (Herkov and Blashfield 1995).

Reliance on the clinician-patient interaction for personality diagnosis runs the risk of generalizing a mode of interpersonal relating that may be limited to a particular situation or context—that is, to the evaluation itself. Although the clinician-patient interaction can be a useful and objective observation, caution should be used in interpreting its significance, and the clinician must attempt to integrate this information into a broader overall picture of a patient's personality functioning.

Direct Questioning

In psychiatric research, a portion of the poor reliability of PD diagnosis has been assumed to be due to the variance in information resulting from unsystematic assessment of personality traits. Therefore, efforts have been made to develop various structured methods for assessing PDs (McDermut and Zimmerman 2008) comparable to those that have been successful in reducing information variance in assessing other mental disorders (Kobak et al. 2008). These methods cover both Section II and Section III approaches to personality psychopathology and include 1) self-report measures such as the Personality Diagnostic Questionnaire–4 (Hyler 1994), the Millon Clinical Multiaxial Inventory–III (Millon et al. 2009), the Minnesota Multiphasic Personality Inventory–2 (Butcher et al. 2001), the aforementioned PID-5 (Krueger et al. 2012), and the new Level of Personality Functioning Scale—Self Report (Morey 2017) and 2) clinical interviews such as the Structured Interview for DSM-IV Personality (Pfohl et al. 1997), the International Personality Disorder Examination (Loranger 1999), the Structured Clinical Interview for DSM-IV Axis II Personality Disorders (First et al. 1997), the Diagnostic Interview for DSM-IV Personality Disorders (Zanarini et al. 1996), the Personality Disorder Interview–IV (Widiger et al. 1995), and the SCID-5-AMPD (First et al. 2018).

The interviews have been based on the general premise that the patient can be asked specific questions that will indicate the presence or absence of each of the criteria of each of the PD types. The self-report instruments are generally considered to require a follow-up interview because of a very high rate of apparently false-positive responses, but data from studies comparing self-report measures with clinical interviews suggest that the former are more helpful in identifying personality disturbances (Hyler et al. 1990). Thus, the clinician can keep in mind that patients do not necessarily deny negative personality attributes. In fact, the evidence suggests that patients may even overreport traits that clinicians might not think are very important, and that patients can, if asked, consistently describe a wide range of personality traits to multiple interviewers. A self-report inventory might be an efficient way to help focus a clinical interview on a narrower range of PD psychopathology. A semistructured interview is useful clinically when the results of an assessment might be subject to close scrutiny, such as in child custody, disability, or forensic evaluations. Both self-report questionnaires and semistructured interview PD diagnoses have been shown to have incremental validity in predicting psychosocial functioning prospectively after 5 years over diagnoses assigned by a treating clinician (Samuel et al. 2013).

Interviewing Informants

Frequently, an individual with a PD consults a mental health professional for evaluation or treatment because another person has found his or her behavior problematic. This person may be a boss, spouse, boyfriend or girlfriend, teacher, parent, or representative of a social agency. Indeed, some people with PDs do not even recognize the problematic aspects of their manner of relating or perceiving except as it has a negative effect on someone with whom they interact.

Because of these "blind spots" that people with PDs may have, the use of a third-party informant in the evaluation can be useful. In some treatment settings, such as a private individual psychotherapy practice, it may be considered counterproductive or contraindicated to include a third party, but in many inpatient and outpatient settings, at least during the evaluation process, it may be appropriate and desirable to see some person close to the patient to corroborate both the patient's report and one's own clinical impressions.

Of course, there is no reason to assume that the informant is free of bias or not coloring a report about the patient with his or her own personality style. In fact, the correspondence between patient self-assessments of PD psychopathology and informant assessments has generally been found to be modest at best (Klonsky et al. 2002). Agreement on pathological personality traits, temperament, and interpersonal problems appears to be somewhat better than on DSM PDs. Informants usually report more personality psychopathology than patients. Agreement on PDs between patient self-assessments and informant assessments is highest for Cluster B disorders (excluding NPD), lower for Clusters A and C, and lowest for traits related to narcissism and entitlement, as might be expected. Therefore, the clinician must make a judgment about the objectivity of the informant and use this as a part, but not a sufficient part, of the overall data on which to base a PD diagnosis. Which source—the patient or the informant—provides information that is more useful for clinical purposes, such as choosing a treatment or predicting outcome (see, e.g., Klein 2003), has yet to be determined definitively.

Problems in Clinical Interviewing

Pervasiveness

The pervasiveness of personality disturbance can be difficult to determine. When a clinician inquires whether a person "often" has a particular experience, a patient will frequently reply "sometimes," which then has to be judged for clinical significance. What constitutes a necessary frequency for a particular trait or behavior and in how many different contexts or with how many different people the trait or behavior needs to be expressed has not been well worked out. Clinicians are forced to rely on their own judgment, keeping in mind also that maladaptivity and inflexibility are hallmarks of pathological traits.

For the clinician interviewing a patient with a possible PD, data about the many areas of functioning, the interpersonal relationships with people interacting in different social roles with the patient, and the nature of the patient-clinician relationship should be integrated into a comprehensive assessment of pervasiveness. Too often, clinicians place disproportionate importance on a patient's functioning at a particular job or with a particular boss or significant other person. Therefore, it is very important to ask patients to describe their relationships and functioning across several different areas of life.

State Versus Trait

An issue that cuts across all PD diagnoses and presents practical problems in differential diagnosis is the distinction between clinical state and personality trait. Personality is presumed to be a relatively enduring aspect of a person, yet assessment of personality ordinarily takes place cross-sectionally—that is, over a brief interval in time. Thus, the clinician is challenged to separate out long-term dispositions of the patient from other, more immediate or situationally determined characteristics. This task is made more complicated by the fact that the patient often comes for evaluation when there is some particularly acute problem, which may be a social or job-related crisis or the onset of another mental disorder. In either case, the situation in which the patient is being evaluated is frequently a state that is not completely characteristic of the patient's life over the longer run.

Assessing an Enduring Pattern

DSM-5 Section II indicates that PDs are of long duration and are not "better explained as a manifestation or consequence of another mental disorder" (American Psychiatric Association 2013, p. 647). Making these determinations in practice is not easy. First of all, an accurate assessment requires recognition of current state. An assessment of current state, in turn, includes knowledge of the circumstances that have prompted the person to seek treatment, the consequences in terms of the decision to seek treatment, the current level of stress, and any other psychopathology, if present.

It is not clear from the diagnostic criteria of DSM-5 how long a pattern of personality disturbance needs to be present, or when it should become evident, for a PD to be diagnosed. Earlier iterations of DSM stated that patients were usually 18 years or older when a PD was diagnosed because it can be argued that, up to that age, a personality pattern could neither have been manifest long enough nor have become significantly entrenched to be considered a stable constellation of behavior. DSM-5 states in Section II, however, that some manifestations of PD are usually recognizable by adolescence or earlier and that PDs can be diagnosed in persons younger than 18 years who have manifested symptoms for at least 1 year. Longitudinal research has shown that PD symptoms evident in childhood or early adolescence may not persist into adult life (Johnson et al. 2000). It has also shown that there is continuity between certain disorders of childhood and adolescence and PDs in early adulthood (Kasen et al. 1999, 2001). Thus, a young boy with oppositional defiant or attention-deficit/hyperactivity disorder in childhood may go on to develop conduct disorder as an adolescent, which can progress to full-blown ASPD in adulthood (Bernstein et al. 1996; Lewinsohn et al. 1997; Rey et al. 1995; Zoccolillo et al. 1992). ASPD is the only diagnosis not given before age 18 years; an adolescent exhibiting significant antisocial behavior before age 18 is diagnosed with conduct disorder.

Regarding the course of a PD, DSM-5 states that PDs are relatively stable over time, although certain of them (e.g., ASPD and BPD) may become somewhat attenuated with age, whereas others (e.g., OCPD and STPD) may not or may, in fact, become more pronounced. As mentioned earlier (see the subsection "Onset and Clinical Course") and discussed in greater detail in Chapter 9 of this volume, this degree of stability may not necessarily pertain to all of the features of all DSM-5 PDs equally.

To assess stability retrospectively, the clinician must ask questions about periods of a person's life that are of various degrees of remoteness from the current situation. Retrospective reporting is subject to distortion, however, and the only sure way of demonstrating stability over time, therefore, may be to do prospective follow-up evaluations. Thus, from a practical, clinical point of view, PD diagnoses made cross-sectionally and on the basis of retrospectively collected data might be considered tentative or provisional pending confirmation by longitudinal evaluation. On an inpatient service, a period of intense observation by many professionals from diverse perspectives may suffice to establish a pattern over time. In a typical outpatient setting, in which encounters with the patients are much less frequent, more time may be required. Ideally, features of a PD should be evident over several years, but it is not practical to wait inordinate amounts of time before coming to a diagnostic conclusion. Interestingly, even PDs that improve with time are associated with adverse outcomes of a variety of other comorbid mental disorders (Ansell et al. 2011; Grilo et al. 2005).

Assessing the Effect of a Comorbid Disorder

The presence of another comorbid mental disorder can complicate the diagnosis of a PD in several ways (Zimmerman 1994). Another mental disorder may cause changes in a person's behavior or attitudes that can appear to be signs of a PD. Depression, for example, may cause a person to seem excessively dependent, avoidant, or self-defeating. Cyclothymic or bipolar II disorder may lead to periods of grandiosity, impulsivity, poor judgment, and depression that might be confused with manifestations of NPD or BPD.

The clinician must be aware of the other psychopathology and assess it within the context of an individual's personality. The clinician can attempt this by asking about aspects of personality functioning at times when the patient is not experiencing other mental disorder symptoms. This approach is particularly feasible when the other disorder is of recent onset and short duration or, if more chronic, the course of the disorder has been characterized by relatively clear-cut episodes with complete remission and symptom-free periods of long duration. When the other disorder is chronic and unremitting, that psychopathology and personality functioning blend together to an extent that can make differentiating between them seem artificial. Nonetheless, research has shown that PDs diagnosed in the presence of another mental disorder, specifically major depressive disorder, have a clinical course and outcomes very similar to those of PDs diagnosed in the absence of major depressive disorder (Morey et al. 2010).

Another example of the ways in which other mental disorders and PDs interact to obscure differential diagnosis is the case of apparent personality psychopathology that in fact is the prodrome of another mental disorder. Distinguishing Cluster A PDs, such as paranoid, schizoid, and schizotypal, from the early signs of disorders in the schizophrenia spectrum and other psychotic disorders class can be particularly difficult. When evaluating a patient early in the course of the initial onset of a psychotic disorder, a clinician may be confronted with changes in the person toward increasing suspiciousness, social withdrawal, eccentricity, or reduced functioning. Because the diagnosis of psychotic disorders, including schizophrenia, requires that the patient have an episode of active psychosis with delusions, hallucinations, or disorganized speech, it is not possible to diagnose this prodrome as a psychotic disorder. In fact, until the full-blown disorder is present, the clinician cannot be certain if it is, indeed, a prodrome.

If a change in behavior is of recent onset, then it may not meet the stability criteria for a PD. In such cases, the clinician is forced to diagnose another specified or unspecified mental disorder. If, however, the pattern of suspiciousness or social withdrawal with or without eccentricities has been well established, it may legitimately be a PD and be diagnosed as such.

If the clinician follows such a patient over time and the patient develops a full-fledged psychotic disorder, the personality disturbance is no longer adequate for a complete diagnosis because no PD includes persistent, frankly psychotic symptoms. This fairly obvious point is frequently overlooked in practice. All of the PDs that have counterpart psychotic disorders have milder or "attenuated" symptoms in which reality testing is, at least in part, intact. For instance, a patient with PPD may have referential ideas but not frank delusions of reference, and a patient with STPD may have illusions but not hallucinations. A possible exception is BPD, in which brief psychotic experiences (lasting minutes to an hour or two at most) are included in the Section II diagnostic criteria. In all cases, however, when the patient becomes psychotic for even a day or two, an additional psychotic disorder diagnosis is necessary.

For the patient with a diagnosis of STPD, the occurrence of a 1-month-long psychotic episode (active-phase symptoms) almost certainly means the disturbance will meet the criteria for schizophrenia, with the symptoms of STPD "counting" as prodromal symptoms toward the 6-month continuous duration requirement. Under these circumstances, the diagnosis of schizophrenia, with its pervasive effects on cognition, perception, functional ability, and so on, is sufficient, and a diagnosis of STPD is redundant. When the patient becomes nonpsychotic again, he or she would be considered to have "residual schizophrenia" instead of STPD.

Personality Traits Versus Personality Disorders

Another difficult distinction is between personality traits or styles and PDs. All patients—all people for that matter—can be described in terms of distinctive patterns of personality, but all do not necessarily warrant a diagnosis of PD. Overdiagnosing is particularly common among inexperienced evaluators. The important features that distinguish pathological personality traits from normal traits are their inflexibility and maladaptiveness.

DSM-5 acknowledges that it is important to describe personality style as well as to diagnose PDs. Therefore, instructions are included to list personality traits even when a PD is absent, or to include them as modifiers of one or more diagnosed PDs (e.g., BPD with histrionic features). In practice, however, this option has been seldom used, even though in addition to the approximately half of clinic patients whose presentation meets criteria for a PD, another one-third may warrant information descriptive of their personality styles. This issue is likely to become exacerbated by the elimination of Axis II in DSM-5, although the comprehensive pathological trait model in Section III gives the clinician more guidance about potentially relevant traits and explicitly states that they are intended to be used whether a person has a PD or not.

The following case example describes a patient with a mental disorder whose ongoing treatment was very much affected by personality traits, none of which met the criteria for a specific PD.

Case Example

Sara, a 25-year-old single female receptionist, was referred for outpatient therapy following hospitalization for her first manic episode. The patient had attended college for 1 year but dropped out in order to "go into advertising." Over the next 5 years, she had held a series of receptionist, secretarial, and sales jobs, each of which she quit because she wasn't "getting ahead in the world." Sara lived alone on the north side of Chicago in an apartment that her parents had furnished for her. She ate all of her meals, however, at her mother's house and claimed not even to have a box of crackers in her cupboard. Between her jobs, her parents paid her rent.

Sara's "career" problems stemmed from the fact that although she felt quite ordinary and without talent for the most part, she had fantasies of a career as a movie star or high fashion model. She took acting classes and singing lessons, but she had never had even a small role in a play or show. What she desired was not so much the careers themselves as the glamour associated with them. Although she wanted to move in the circles of the "beautiful people," she was certain that she had nothing to offer them. Sara sometimes referred to herself as nothing but a shell and scorned herself because of it. She was unable to picture herself working her way up along any realistic career line, feeling both that it would take too long and that she would probably fail.

Sara had had three close relationships with men that were characterized by an intense interdependency that initially was agreeable to both parties. She craved affection and attention and fell deeply in love with these men. However, she eventually became overtly self-centered, demanding, and manipulative, and the man would break off the relationship. After breaking up, she would almost immediately start claiming that the particular man was "going nowhere," was not for her, and would not be missed. Between these relationships, Sara often had periods in which she engaged in a succession of one-night stands, having sex with half a dozen partners in a month. Alternatively, she would frequent rock clubs and bars—"in-spots" as she called them—merely on the chance of meeting someone who would introduce her to the glamorous world she dreamed of.

Sara had no female friends other than her sister. She could see little use for such friendships. She preferred spending her time shopping for stylish clothes or watching television alone at home. She liked to dress fashionably and seductively, but often felt that she was too fat or that her hair was the wrong color. She had trouble controlling her weight and would periodically go on eating binges for a few days that might result in a 10-pound weight gain. She read popular novels but had very few other interests. She admitted she was bored much of the time but also asserted that cultural or athletic pursuits were a waste of time.

Sara was referred for outpatient follow-up without a PD diagnosis. In fact, her long-term functioning failed to meet DSM-5 criteria for any specific type of PD. On the other hand, her presentation almost met the criteria for several PDs, especially BPD: the patient showed signs of impulsivity (overeating, sexual promiscuity), intense interpersonal relationships (manipulativeness, overidealization/devaluation), identity disturbance, and chronic feelings of emptiness. She did not, however, display intense anger, intolerance of being alone, physically self-damaging behavior, stress-related paranoia or dissociation, or affective instability independent of her mood disorder. Similarly, Sara had symptoms of histrionic PD: she was inappropriately sexually seductive and used her physical appearance to draw attention to herself, but she was not emotionally overdramatic. She had shallow expression of emotions and was uncomfortable when she was not the center of attention, but was not overly suggestible. Sara also had some features of narcissistic, avoidant, and dependent PDs. A DSM-5 Section II diagnosis of other specified PD (mixed features) could be made.

In terms of the DSM-5 alternative model of PDs, Sara might be best described as having PD-TS. Her level of impairment in personality functioning would be "severe," with impairment in identity, self-direction, empathy, and intimacy. She has a poor sense of autonomy and agency and experiences the lack of a true identity and emptiness. She vacillates between overidentification with and dependence on others and overemphasis on independence. She has fragile, incoherent self-esteem that includes both self-denigration and self-aggrandizement. She has difficulty establishing and achieving her goals in life. She is unaware of the effects of her own actions on others. Her relationships with others are based on her needs, with little mutuality, as others are in her life primarily to satisfy her fantasies and desires. Pathological personality traits that describe her include attention seeking, manipulativeness, and grandiosity from the Antagonism domain, impulsivity and risk-taking from the Disinhibition domain, and submissiveness from the Negative Affectivity domain. The attention paid to personality functioning and traits in her evaluation conveys a vivid picture of Sara's complicated personality pathology, which would be the focus of her subsequent therapy.

Effects of Gender, Culture, and Age

Gender

Although definitive estimates about the sex ratio of PDs cannot be made because ideal epidemiological studies do not exist, some PDs are believed to be more common in clinical settings among men and others among women. PDs listed in Section II of DSM-5 as occurring in clinical settings more often among men are paranoid, schizoid, schizotypal, antisocial, narcissistic, and obsessive-compulsive PDs. Those occurring more often in women are borderline, histrionic, and dependent PDs. Avoidant PD is said to be equally common in men and women. Apparently elevated sex ratios that do not reflect true prevalence rates can be the result of sampling or diagnostic biases in clinical settings (Widiger 1998). True differences may be due to biological factors such as hormones, social factors such as child-rearing practices, and their interactions (Morey et al. 2005).

Culture

Apparent manifestations of PDs must be considered in the context of a patient's cultural reference group and the degree to which behaviors such as diffidence, passivity, emotionality, emphasis on work and productivity, and unusual beliefs and rituals are culturally sanctioned. Only when such behaviors are clearly in excess or discordant with the standards of a person's cultural milieu would the diagnosis of a PD be considered. Certain sociocultural contexts may lend themselves to eliciting and reinforcing behaviors that might be mistaken for PD psychopathology. Members of minority groups, immigrants, or refugees, for example, might appear overly guarded or mistrustful, avoidant, or hostile in response to experiences of discrimination, language barriers, or problems in acculturation (Alarcon 2005).

Age

Although PDs usually are not diagnosed prior to age 18 years, certain thoughts, feelings, and behaviors suggestive of personality psychopathology may be apparent in childhood. For example, dependency, social anxiety and hypersensitivity, disruptive behavior, or identity problems may be developmentally expected. Follow-up studies of children have shown decreases in such behaviors over time (Johnson et al. 2000), although children with elevated rates of PD-type signs and symptoms do appear to be at higher risk for personality and other mental disorders in young adulthood (Johnson et al. 1999; Kasen et al. 1999). Thus, some childhood problems may not turn out to be transitory, and PD may be viewed developmentally as a failure to mature out of certain age-appropriate or phase-specific feelings or behaviors. A developmental perspective on PDs is presented more fully in Chapter 7, "Development, Attachment, and Childhood Experiences: A Mentalization Perspective," in this volume. Early identification of personality pathology is a subject of Chapter 10, "Early Identification and Prevention of Personality Pathology: An AMPD-Informed Model of Clinical Staging."

Until recently, little was known about the nature and importance of personality and PDs in later life. Anecdotal clinical information was abundant, but systematic data were sparse. Many important issues persist concerning the prevalence of PDs in later life and their manifestations, development and course, and impact on aspects of living (Oltmanns and Balsis 2011). Personality pathology may not be accurately diagnosed in older populations if the clinician employs the same criteria that are used in younger ones. Modifications have to be made to account for changes in life circumstances, such as the loss of a spouse or friends, retirement from work, or physical infirmity, that make some criteria not applicable. Some early-onset PDs (e.g., BPD and ASPD) may improve with advancing age, whereas others (e.g., NPD and OCPD) may get worse. PDs may actually have an onset in later life. The long-term consequences of pathological versus adaptive personalities for health, longevity, marital and other social relationships, and the experience of important late-life events are currently under study (see, e.g., Oldham and Skodol 2013). Specific personality traits or types may represent risk factors for the development of depression, dementia, or other psychiatric syndromes in later life. In contrast, other traits or types serve as protective factors against the development of these conditions, or could even enhance healthy aging. The Section III personality functioning and personality trait model enhances the clinician's ability to assess and track important personality characteristics throughout the lifespan.

Differential Diagnosis

In this section, the focus is on differential diagnosis of PDs as defined by the DSM-5 Section III alternative model. The guidelines for the differential diagnosis of Section II PDs remain unchanged from DSM-IV and can be found in DSM-5. Differential diagnosis of PDs is facilitated by consideration of pathological trait domains, because these broad propensities toward particular ways of thinking, feeling, and behaving underlie certain PDs and other mental disorders (Kotov et al. 2017; Krueger and Eaton 2010; Krueger et al. 2007) with which they are commonly comorbid.

At the broadest level, PDs and other mental disorders can be divided into externalizing and internalizing disorders (Krueger et al. 2011b). *Externalizing disorders* are characterized primarily by Disinhibition, that is, an "orientation toward immediate gratification, leading to impulsive behavior driven by current thoughts, feelings, and external stimuli, without regard for past learning or consideration of future consequences" (American Psychiatric Association 2013, p. 780). Externalizing disorders are also characterized by Antagonism, that is, "behaviors that put the individual at odds with other people, including an exaggerated sense of self-importance and a concomitant expectation of special treatment, as well as a callous antipathy toward others, encompassing both an unawareness of others' needs and feelings and a readiness to use others in the service of self-enhancement" (American Psychiatric Association 2013, p. 780). Disruptive behavior disorders (e.g., conduct disorder), substance-related and addictive disorders, and ASPD are representative of the externalizing "meta-cluster" of disorders.

Internalizing disorders are characterized by Negative Affectivity, that is, "frequent and intense experiences of high levels of a wide range of negative emotions (e.g., anxiety, depression, guilt/shame, worry, anger) and their behavioral (e.g., self-harm) and interpersonal (e.g., dependency) manifestations" (American Psychiatric Association 2013, p. 779). An internalizing meta-cluster of disorders would include depressive disorders, anxiety disorders characterized by distress (e.g., generalized anxiety disorder) or fear (e.g., phobic disorders), and PDs such as AVPD. At least one PD—that is, BPD—appears to straddle both externalizing and internalizing spectra (Eaton et al. 2011). A third meta-cluster of disorders is characterized by Psychoticism; that is, they include "a wide range of culturally incongruent odd, eccentric, or unusual behaviors and cognitions, including both process (e.g., perception, dissociation) and content (e.g., beliefs)" (American Psychiatric Association 2013, p. 781). In this cluster would be found schizophrenia spectrum and other psychotic disorders, bipolar disorder, and STPD (Keyes et al. 2013).

Other DSM-5 trait domains are related more strongly to the principal domains within these large spectra. Detachment is correlated more strongly with Negative Affectivity than with Disinhibition (Morey et al. 2013b). Detachment has also been shown to correlate with Psychoticism. Individual PDs in the AMPD are characterized by different combinations of underlying trait domains: ASPD is a combination of Antagonism and Disinhibition; BPD is a combination of Negative Affectivity, Antagonism, and Disinhibition; AVPD is a combination of Negative Affectivity and Detachment; STPD is a combination of Psychoticism and Detachment; and OCPD is a combination of Compulsivity (the opposite of Disinhibition), Negative Affectivity, and Detachment. Of the specific PDs in Section III, only NPD is characterized by a single trait domain (Antagonism). Thus, thinking about differential diagnosis in terms of underlying dispositions—with shared pathophysiologies (e.g., Iacono et al. 2002) and etiologies (e.g., Kendler et al. 2011)—helps the clinician to include all the disorders that should be under consideration and also to discern the critical differences between them, in order to arrive at the most accurate and appropriate diagnosis.

In general, the major issues for differential diagnosis of PDs are 1) distinguishing PDs from other PDs with similar features, 2) distinguishing personality pathology from the psychopathology of other mental disorders, and 3) distinguishing personality pathology warranting a PD diagnosis from personality pathology that arises from the use of a substance of abuse or from a co-occurring other medical condition. PDs can be distinguished from one another on the basis of their characteristic impairments in personality functioning, described by Criterion A for each specific disorder, or on the basis of their characteristic patterns of pathological personality traits, described by Criterion B. PDs can be distinguished from other mental disorders on the basis of the presence of impairments in personality functioning at the moderate level or greater for the diagnosis of a PD. Applying the single-item LPFS as a first step in differential diagnosis can discriminate the presence of a PD with very good accuracy (i.e., sensitivity and specificity) (Morey et al. 2013a). In many cases, PDs and other mental disorders co-occur, based on shared trait vulnerabilities or predispositions, and in such cases both types of disorders should be diagnosed, because it has been shown that PDs worsen the course (i.e., longer time to remission, shorter time to relapse, more time in episodes) of disorders such as major depressive disorder, anxiety disorders, and substance use disorders (Ansell et al. 2011; Fenton et al. 2012; Grilo et al. 2005; Hasin et al. 2011; Skodol et al. 2011b, 2014b) and require special treatment. Comorbidity among other mental disorders and PDs has been shown to increase the risk for negative prognoses with respect to adult attainments and functioning (Crawford et al. 2008).

Substance- or medication-induced personality change is distinguished from PD primarily on the basis of the relationship in time of the personality disturbance to the exposure to the substance or medication. If there is a close historical association between the onset of the personality change and the exposure to substances (also corroborated when possible by physical examination or laboratory tests), then the personality pathology is probably due to the substance or medication. There is no diagnosis for substance/medication-induced PD in DSM-5, however, so a clinician would use the diagnosis of an "other substance–induced disorder" (specifying the substance, if possible). If the PD preceded involvement with substances or persists for a considerable time after the cessation of substance use, it most likely represents an independent disorder. Again, a substance use disorder can co-occur with a PD because of underlying traits of impulsivity or risk taking. In that case, both disorders should be diagnosed. Similarly, evidence from history, physical examination, and laboratory tests, coupled with a temporal sequence suggesting the primacy of another medical condition, distinguishes personality change due to another medical condition (Section II) from a PD.

Externalizing Personality Pathology

Antagonism and Disinhibition

Personality disorders.   BPD has some trait features in common with ASPD (e.g., similarities in the domains of Antagonism [hostility trait] and Disinhibition [impulsivity and risk-taking traits]), but individuals with BPD show more Negative Affectivity (e.g., emotional lability, separation insecurity), whereas individuals with ASPD show a broader range of traits of Antagonism (e.g., callousness, manipulativeness) associated with imposing on and/or controlling others. Impulsivity in BPD is more often oriented toward self than toward others (i.e., self-harmful or suicidal behaviors). Suicide attempts and overall psychological distress are also higher in BPD.

Individuals with NPD and those with ASPD are both self-centered and lacking in empathy. Individuals with ASPD, however, are more manipulative, deceitful, callous, hostile, irresponsible, and impulsive than individuals with NPD. Those with NPD do use others to enhance self-esteem needs and for personal gain, but they are not as openly exploitative of others as are individuals with ASPD, and they are more likely to use charm or seduction than coercion or intimidation to get what they want from others. If other traits from the Antagonism domain are present, such as manipulativeness, deceitfulness, or callousness, they can be added to the NPD diagnosis as "specifiers," which indicate a particularly severe form of NPD often referred to as "malignant narcissism."

NPD is characterized by self-appraisal that may be inflated or deflated, or that may vacillate between extremes. Individuals with BPD also have unstable self-images. Both disorders are characterized by problems with empathy. The absence of impulsivity, risk taking, separation insecurity, and fears of abandonment in NPD helps to distinguish between the disorders. In addition, individuals with NPD tend to be disdainful and dismissive of others, especially when the others are not meeting the needs of the individuals with NPD, whereas individuals with BPD can be both disdainful and very interpersonally needy.

The entitlement and superiority seen in individuals with NPD may be confused with the rigid perfectionism (at the opposite pole from the Disinhibition domain) of OCPD, which leads the individual to believe that there is only one right way to do things. Both disorders are also characterized by personal standards that may be unreasonably high. Individuals with either PD also have problems with empathy: their ability to recognize, understand, or identify with the feelings and needs of others is impaired, and relationships can be largely superficial. Individuals with NPD, however, rely on positive reactions from others for self-definition and self-esteem regulation and seek the attention of others, in contrast to individuals with OCPD, whose sense of self is derived predominantly from work or productivity, often at the expense of interpersonal relationships.

Individuals with NPD may also profess a commitment to perfection and believe that others cannot do things as well, but these individuals are preoccupied with striving for perfection as a means of shoring up a fragile self-image, whereas those with OCPD are concerned about receiving punishment or criticism for inadequate achievement. Individuals with AVPD are usually self-critical but lack the behavioral and cognitive rigidity that characterizes those with OCPD.

Other mental disorders. Impulsivity, irresponsibility, risk-taking behaviors (including law breaking), hostility, and self-centeredness can be seen in manic or hypomanic episodes of bipolar I or II disorder, but, compared with individuals with externalizing PDs, individuals with bipolar disorders frequently do not demonstrate callousness or manipulativeness and are more likely to exhibit behavioral disorganization of psychotic proportions. Agitated or anxious patients with major depressive disorder may present with an impulsive act (e.g., a suicide attempt) but also have morbid self-destructive tendencies of mood disturbances.

Posttraumatic stress disorder may be manifested by impulsive behaviors, antagonism/hostility, incapacity for intimacy, or unreliability, and a history of early traumatic experiences also seen in externalizing PDs. However, posttraumatic stress disorder has other well-defined clinical features (e.g., reexperiencing and intrusion symptoms, specific avoidance behaviors) that are not diagnostic of PDs.

Attention-deficit/hyperactivity disorder (ADHD), typically first detected in childhood or early adolescence, has also been described in adulthood. Characterized mostly by distractibility, motor restlessness, and cognitive performance deficits, ADHD does not include prominent antagonistic features such as callousness, deceitfulness, manipulativeness, or hostility. Conduct disorder, particularly in its adult version, must be distinguished from ASPD on the basis of an absence in the former of the severe manifestations (secondary to impulsivity, violence proneness, etc.) and serious consequences (e.g., behavioral, legal, ethical) seen in the latter.

The grandiosity that is frequently manifested in individuals with NPD may suggest a manic or hypomanic episode. The absence of other manic or hypomanic symptoms, such as decreased need for sleep, pressured speech, flight of ideas, and psychomotor agitation, helps to distinguish NPD from bipolar I or bipolar II disorder.

Despite the similarity in names, obsessive-compulsive disorder is usually easily distinguished from OCPD by the presence of true obsessions and compulsions in the former. When criteria for both personality and obsessive-compulsive spectrum disorders are met, both diagnoses should be recorded.

Substance use and other medical conditions.   When externalizing behavior in an adult is associated with a substance use disorder, the diagnosis of ASPD (according to DSM-5 Section II) is not made unless signs of such behavior were also present in childhood (i.e., conduct disorder) and have continued into adulthood. The onset of ASPD typically precedes, for example, that of alcohol dependence by several years. When substance use and antisocial behavior both began in childhood and continued into adulthood, both disorders should be diagnosed if the criteria for both are met, even though some antisocial behaviors may be a consequence of the substance use disorder (e.g., illegal drug selling, theft to obtain money for drugs). In adults, particularly older adults, the appearance or significant, unexpected worsening of antisocial behaviors (or isolated traits of them) should be the subject of a careful diagnostic assessment to rule out other medical conditions as triggering factors. Common conditions include brain tumors or other occult malignancies, sequelae of head injuries, degenerative neurological diseases, or late-life metabolic disturbances (e.g., affecting the liver, thyroid, parathyroid, pancreas, or hypothalamic-pituitary-adrenal axis).

Internalizing Personality Pathology

Negative Affectivity

Personality disorders.   NPD and BPD may both be characterized by angry reactions to minor stimuli and fluctuations in self-image, but the lack of self-destructiveness, impulsivity, and separation insecurity in NPD distinguishes this disorder from BPD. AVPD and OCPD both are characterized by high Negative Affectivity, although different trait facets are required for the diagnosis. In OCPD the core Negative Affectivity feature is perseveration—persistence at tasks long after the behavior has ceased to be functional or effective—whereas in AVPD the core Negative Affectivity feature is anxiousness, with particular apprehension in social situations and fears of embarrassment.

Other mental disorders. BPD often co-occurs with major depressive disorder or other disorders of anxiety or mood, and multiple disorders should be diagnosed when present. However, because the cross-sectional presentation of BPD can resemble an episode of a depressive, bipolar, or anxiety disorder, the clinician should use caution in giving multiple diagnoses based only on a cross-sectional presentation.

The most important differential diagnosis for AVPD is social anxiety disorder (social phobia), and the two disorders are highly comorbid. There are no discernible qualitative differences between the two disorders with regard to demographic features (including age at onset), social skills deficits, cognitive features, physiological reactions, and comorbid depression, although the clinical picture of individuals with AVPD typically is more severe and is associated with a broader pattern of avoidance, including of positive emotions and novel situations. Importantly, in AVPD, the anxiousness from hypersensitivity to social evaluation is associated with core impairment in identity, specifically the belief that the self is inferior. Thus, an important distinction between the disorders is how social anxiety, which they have in common, relates to the self-concept. Although avoidant behavior also characterizes agoraphobia, in AVPD the focus is on social evaluation, whereas in agoraphobia it is on the difficulty of escape or the lack of help in the event of incapacitation.

Detachment/Thought Disorder

Detachment and Psychoticism

Personality disorders. Regarding Detachment traits, AVPD and STPD share (social) withdrawal, but STPD is further characterized by restricted affectivity (constricted emotional experience and expression), whereas AVPD is further characterized by anhedonia (deficits in the capacity to feel pleasure or take interest in things) and intimacy avoidance (avoidance of interpersonal attachments, especially romantic relationships). Also, in AVPD, withdrawal is driven by a fear of rejection and reluctance to enter into situations or relationships that may ultimately lead to rejection, whereas in STPD, Detachment is more pervasive, not easily reversed even when there are guarantees of acceptance, and characterized by extreme difficulty in negotiating the affective/cognitive complexities of interpersonal relationships. Finally, individuals with AVPD lack the traits of Psychoticism (e.g., cognitive and perceptual dysregulation, eccentricity, unusual beliefs and experiences) that characterize individuals with STPD.

Individuals with BPD may display psychotic-like symptoms, but such symptoms are more intense and transient, and more related to affective shifts, than the chronic, pervasive suspiciousness or typically less dramatic cognitive distortions in individuals with STPD. BPD, however, may be comorbid with STPD.

Some individuals traditionally diagnosed with AVPD may actually be better characterized as having covert/vulnerable narcissistic personality characteristics. Social withdrawal is a common factor among both individuals with AVPD and those with the covert presentation of NPD. However, whereas individuals with AVPD are afraid of not being liked or accepted, those with covert narcissistic tendencies crave admiration to bolster their fragile self-esteem and secretly or unconsciously feel entitled to it.

Other mental disorders. STPD is distinct from psychotic schizophrenia spectrum disorders, including schizophrenia itself, as well as other psychotic disorders such as delusional disorder or mood disorder with psychotic features, because individuals with STPD do not have overt persistent psychotic symptoms (i.e., delusions and hallucinations). Although psychotic symptoms may occur in the context of a discrete psychotic disorder in the course of STPD, this is unusual because STPD must have been present before the onset of the psychotic symptoms and must persist even when the psychotic symptoms are in remission. If STPD features are observed for more than 6 months in an individual who later develops overt psychosis (i.e., delusions, hallucinations, or disorganized speech) of 1 month or longer and severe functional impairments required for a schizophrenia diagnosis, the schizotypal features would be considered a "premorbid" or prodromal state of schizophrenia rather than STPD. Individuals with STPD may exhibit restricted affect and have the associated depression or dysphoria of mood disorders, but may not complain of any psychotic-like symptoms. In such individuals, STPD may be present but overlooked.

In children or adolescents, features of STPD may be difficult to discriminate from those of developmental disorders in the autism spectrum because both may be characterized by social isolation, eccentricity, and peculiarities of language and behavior. Individuals with autism spectrum disorder, however, often exhibit stereotyped behaviors and interests that are not typical for STPD and social and nonverbal communication deficits and lack of emotional reciprocity that may be more prominent than in STPD.

Personality Disorder—Trait Specified

Personality Disorder—Trait Specified Versus Pathological Personality Traits

One major differential diagnostic issue with PD-TS is the determination of whether a diagnosis of PD is warranted, or whether one simply should note the individual's relevant pathological personality features. The DSM-5 personality trait model can be used to record personality features regardless of whether they are manifestations of a PD diagnosis. Therefore, the evidence for Criterion A (disturbances in self and interpersonal functioning) should be carefully assessed to determine whether a diagnosis of PD is warranted; the LPFS is provided to assist in this determination.

Personality Disorder—Trait Specified Versus a Specific Personality Disorder

A second important differential diagnostic issue with PD-TS is the determination of whether a diagnosis of one of the six specific PD types or of PD-TS should be made. This determination is based on the clinician's judgment of the degree to which the patient's 1) self and interpersonal disturbance (Criterion A) and 2) personality trait configuration (Criterion B) match the characterization of a specific PD. If an individual's specific personality disturbance and trait configuration match those of a specific PD well, that PD diagnosis should be made. If, however, there are notable discrepancies between the individual's specific personality disturbance and trait configuration and those of a specific PD, including the presence of additional prominent personality traits, then a PD-TS diagnosis should be made. For example, if an individual's personality functioning disturbance matches that of the AVPD well and the individual's trait profile is characterized by the traits making up AVPD Criterion B (i.e., anxiousness, withdrawal, anhedonia, and intimacy avoidance), but the individual's personality also is characterized by other traits, it must be determined whether the most prominent features of the individual's personality are those of the AVPD or whether the additional personality features are also clinically relevant. In the former case, the diagnosis would be AVPD with additional features specified (e.g., with depressivity), whereas in the latter case, the more appropriate diagnosis would be PD-TS, with specification of all prominent traits (e.g., with depressivity, submissiveness, anxiousness, withdrawal, intimacy avoidance). PD-TS should be diagnosed if an individual's presentation meets the general criteria for PD but lacks one or more of the personality trait facets required for a diagnosis of a specific PD (e.g., subthreshold or other specified PD).

Comorbid Specific Personality Disorders Versus Personality Disorder—Trait Specified

A third important differential diagnostic issue with PD-TS is the determination of whether a diagnosis of two or more of the six specific PDs or of PD-TS should be made. This determination also is based on clinician judgment of the degree to which the individual's self and interpersonal disturbance (Criterion A) and personality trait configuration (Criterion B) match the characterization of multiple specific PDs. If an individual's specific personality disturbance and trait configuration match those of multiple specific PDs, the specific PD diagnoses should be made. If, however, there are notable discrepancies between the individual's specific personality disturbance and trait configuration and those of the multiple specific PDs being considered, then a PD-TS diagnosis should be made.

Other Mental Disorders

With regard to differential diagnosis of other conditions that may resemble PD-TS (e.g., major depressive disorder vs. PD-TS with Criterion B characterized by prominent depressivity and anhedonia), the major consideration is whether Criterion A features (disturbances in self and interpersonal functioning) are present or absent. In general, any and all personality trait features pertinent to the clinical presentation should be recorded, together with any major diagnoses for which the individual meets criteria. Personality change (e.g., increased Negative Affectivity) also can be an early sign of onset of dementia (Low et al. 2013), so consideration of whether the individual's personality trait expression is due solely to another medical condition is important.

Conclusion

The accurate diagnosis of PD presents many hurdles for the clinician. The assessment process is fraught with challenges, and learning how to recognize the psychopathology of personality and its relationship with other disorders requires care and diligence. The importance of personality pathology for the overall functioning of the individual patient and for his or her prognosis, however, cannot be overstated.

In this chapter, two DSM-5 models of personality pathology—the Section II categorical approach carried over from DSM-IV and the new Section III hybrid dimensional-categorical AMPD—are reviewed from the perspectives of manifestations, assessment, diagnosis, and differential diagnosis. Although clinicians may continue to use the criteria of Section II for official purposes, they are encouraged to study and use the Section III model, which presents a coherent conceptual basis for all personality psychopathology, an efficient and effective approach to assessment, and a more empirically based formulation of PD criteria than Section II.

References

Alarcon RD: Cross-cultural issues, in The American Psychiatric Publishing Textbook of Personality Disorders. Edited by Oldham JM, Skodol AE, Bender DS. Washington, DC, American Psychiatric Publishing, 2005, pp 561–578

American Psychiatric Association: Diagnostic and Statistical Manual of Mental Disorders, 4th Edition. Washington, DC, American Psychiatric Association, 1994

American Psychiatric Association: Diagnostic and Statistical Manual of Mental Disorders, 5th Edition. Arlington, VA, American Psychiatric Association, 2013

Ansell EB, Pinto A, Edelen MO, et al: The association of personality disorders with the prospective 7-year course of anxiety disorders. Psychol Med 41:1019–1028, 2011

Bender DS, Skodol AE: Borderline personality as a self-other representational disturbance. J Pers Disord 21:500–517, 2007

Bender DS, Morey LC, Skodol AE: Toward a model for assessing level of personality functioning in DSM-5, part I: a review of theory and methods. J Pers Assess 93:332–346, 2011

Bernstein DP, Cohen P, Skodol AE, et al: Childhood antecedents of adolescent personality disorders. Am J Psychiatry 153:907–913, 1996

Blashfield RK, Herkov MJ: Investigating clinician adherence to diagnosis by criteria: a replication of Morey and Ochoa (1989). J Pers Disord 10:219–228, 1996

Buer Christensen T, Papp MCS, Arnesen M, et al: Interrater reliability of the Structured Clinical Interview for the DSM-5 Alternative Model for Personality Disorders, Module I: Level of Personality Functioning Scale. J Pers Assess 100:630–641, 2018

Butcher JN, Graham JR, Ben-Porath YS, et al: Minnesota Multiphasic Personality Inventory-2: Manual for Administration and Scoring, Revised Edition. Minneapolis, University of Minnesota Press, 2001

Crawford TN, Cohen P, First MB, et al: Comorbid Axis I and Axis II disorders in early adolescence: outcomes 20 years later. Arch Gen Psychiatry 65:641–648, 2008

Cruitt PJ, Oltmanns TE: Age-related outcomes associated with personality pathology in later life. Curr Opin Psychol 21:89–93, 2018

Eaton NR, Krueger RF, Keyes KM, et al: Borderline personality disorder comorbidity: relationship to the internalizing-externalizing structure of common mental disorders. Psychol Med 41:1041–1050, 2011

Fenton MC, Keyes K, Geier T, et al: Psychiatric comorbidity and the persistence of drug use disorders in the United States. Addiction 107:599–609, 2012

First M, Gibbon M, Spitzer RL, et al: User's Guide for the Structured Clinical Interview for DSM-IV Axis II Personality Disorders. Washington, DC, American Psychiatric Press, 1997

First MB, Skodol AE, Bender DS, et al: User's Guide for the Structured Clinical Interview for the DSM-5 Alternative Model for Personality Disorders (SCID-5-AMPD). Arlington, VA, American Psychiatric Association Publishing, 2018

Garcia DJ, Skadberg RM, Schmidt M, et al: It's not that difficult: an interrater reliability study of the DSM-5 Section III Alternative Model for Personality Disorders. J Pers Assess 100:612–620, 2018

Grilo CM, Sanislow CA, Shea MT, et al: Two-year prospective naturalistic study of remission from major depressive disorder as a function of personality disorder comorbidity. J Consult Clin Psychol 73:78–85, 2005

Gunderson JG: Disturbed relationships as phenotype for borderline personality disorder. Am J Psychiatry 164:1637–1640, 2007

Gunderson JG, Stout RL, McGlashan TH, et al: Ten-year course of borderline personality disorder: psychopathology and function from the Collaborative Longitudinal Personality Disorders Study. Arch Gen Psychiatry 68:827–837, 2011

Hasin D, Fenton MC, Skodol A, et al: Relationship of personality disorders to the three-year course of alcohol, cannabis, and nicotine disorders. Arch Gen Psychiatry 68:1158–1167, 2011

Herkov MJ, Blashfield RK: Clinicians' diagnoses of personality disorder: evidence of a hierarchical structure. J Pers Assess 65:313–321, 1995

Hill J, Pilkonis P, Morse J, et al: Social domain dysfunction and disorganization in borderline personality disorder. Psychol Med 38:135–146, 2008

Hopwood CJ, Thomas KM, Markon KE, et al: DSM-5 personality traits and DSM-IV personality disorders. J Abnorm Psychol 121:424–432, 2012

Hopwood CJ, Morey LC, Donnnellan MB, et al: Ten year rank-order stability of personality traits and disorders in a clinical sample. J Pers 81:335–344, 2013a

Hopwood CJ, Wright AG, Ansell EB, et al: The interpersonal core of personality pathology. J Pers Disord 27:270–295, 2013b

Hyler SE: Personality Diagnostic Questionnaire–4. New York, New York State Psychiatric Institute, 1994

Hyler SE, Skodol AE, Kellman D, et al: Validity of the Personality Diagnostic Questionnaire: comparison with two structured interviews. Am J Psychiatry 147:1043–1048, 1990

Iacono WG, Carlson SR, Malone SM, et al: P3 event-related potential amplitude and the risk for disinhibitory disorders in adolescent boys. Arch Gen Psychiatry 59:750–757, 2002

Johnson JG, Cohen P, Skodol AE, et al: Personality disorders in adolescence and risk of major mental disorders and suicidality during adulthood. Arch Gen Psychiatry 56:805–811, 1999

Johnson JG, Cohen P, Kasen S, et al: Age-related change in personality disorder trait levels between early adolescence and adulthood: a community-based longitudinal investigation. Acta Psychiatr Scand 102:265–275, 2000

Kasen S, Cohen P, Skodol AE, et al: Influence of child and adolescent psychiatric disorders on young adult personality disorder. Am J Psychiatry 156:1529–1535, 1999

Kasen S, Cohen P, Skodol AE, et al: Childhood depression and adult personality disorder: alternative pathways of continuity. Arch Gen Psychiatry 58:231–236, 2001

Kendler KS, Aggen SH, Knudsen GP, et al: The structure of genetic and environmental risk factors for syndromal and subsyndromal common DSM-IV Axis I and all Axis II disorders. Am J Psychiatry 168:29–39, 2011

Keyes KM, Eaton NR, Krueger RF, et al: Thought disorder in the meta-structure of psychopathology. Psychol Med 43:1673–1683, 2013

Klein DN: Patients' versus informants' reports of personality disorders in predicting 7½-year outcome in outpatients with depressive disorders. Psychol Assess 15:216–222, 2003

Klonsky ED, Oltmanns TF, Turkheimer E: Informant-reports of personality disorder: relation to self-reports and future directions. Clin Psychol Sci Pract 9:300–311, 2002

Kobak KA, Skodol AE, Bender DS: Diagnostic measures for adults, in Handbook of Psychiatric Measures, 2nd Edition. Edited by Rush AJ, First MB, Blacker D. Washington, DC, American Psychiatric Publishing, 2008, pp 35–60

Kotov R, Krueger RF, Watson D, et al: The Hierarchical Taxonomy of Psychopathology (HiTOP): a dimensional alternative to traditional nosologies. J Abnorm Psychol 126:454–477, 2017

Krueger RF, Eaton NR: Personality traits and the classification of mental disorders: towards a more complete integration in DSM-5 and an empirical model of psychopathology. Personal Disord 1:97–118, 2010

Krueger RF, Markon KE, Patrick CJ, et al: Linking antisocial behavior, substance use, and personality: an integrative quantitative model of the adult externalizing spectrum. J Abnorm Psychol 116:645–666, 2007

Krueger RF, Eaton NR, Clark LA, et al: Deriving an empirical structure for personality pathology for DSM-5. J Pers Disord 25:170–191, 2011a

Krueger RF, Eaton NR, Derringer J, et al: Personality in DSM-5: helping delineate personality disorder content and framing the meta-structure. J Pers Assess 93:325–331, 2011b

Krueger RF, Derringer J, Markon KE, et al: Initial construction of a maladaptive personality trait model and inventory for DSM-5. Psychol Med 42:1879–1890, 2012

Lenzenweger MF, Johnson MD, Willett JB: Individual growth curve analysis illuminates stability and change in personality disorder features: the longitudinal study of personality disorders. Arch Gen Psychiatry 61:1015–1024, 2004

Lewinsohn PM, Rohde P, Seeley JR, et al: Axis II psychopathology as a function of Axis I disorder in childhood and adolescence. J Am Acad Child Adolesc Psychiatry 36:1752–1759, 1997

Livesley WJ, Jang KL: Toward an empirically based classification of personality disorder. J Pers Disord 14:137–151, 2000

Loranger AW: International Personality Disorder Examination (IPDE): DSM-IV and ICD-10 Modules. Odessa, FL, Psychological Assessment Resources, 1999

Low L-F, Harrison F, Lackersteen SM: Does personality affect risk for dementia? A systematic review and meta-analysis. Am J Geriatr Psychiatry 21:713–728, 2013

Luyten P, Blatt SJ: Interpersonal relatedness and self-definition in normal and disrupted personality development: retrospect and prospect. Am Psychol 68:172–183, 2013

Markon KE, Quilty LC, Bagby RM, et al: The development and psychometric properties of an informant-report form of the Personality Inventory for DSM-5 (PID-5). Assessment 20:370–383, 2013

McDermut W, Zimmerman M: Personality disorders, personality traits, and defense mechanisms, in Handbook of Psychiatric Measures, 2nd Edition. Edited by Rush AJ, First MB, Blacker D. Washington, DC, American Psychiatric Publishing, 2008, pp 687–729

McGlashan TH, Grilo CM, Sanislow CA, et al: Two-year prevalence and stability of individual DSM-IV criteria for schizotypal, borderline, avoidant and obsessive-compulsive personality disorders: toward a hybrid model of Axis II disorders. Am J Psychiatry 162:883–889, 2005

Millon T, David R, Millon C, et al: Millon Clinical Multiaxial Inventory, 3rd Edition. San Antonio, TX, Pearson, 2009

Morey LC: Development and initial evaluation of a self-report form of the DSM-5 Level of Personality Functioning Scale. Psychol Assess 29:1302–1308, 2017

Morey LC, Benson KT: An investigation of adherence to diagnostic criteria, revisited: clinical diagnosis of the DSM-IV/DSM-5 Section II personality disorders. J Pers Disord 30:130–144, 2016

Morey LC, Ochoa ES: An investigation of adherence to diagnostic criteria. J Pers Disord 3:180–192, 1989

Morey LC, Skodol AE: Convergence between DSM-IV-TR and DSM-5 diagnostic models for personality disorder: evaluation of strategies for establishing diagnostic thresholds. J Psychiatr Pract 19:179–193, 2013

Morey LC, Alexander GM, Boggs C: Gender, in The American Psychiatric Publishing Textbook of Personality Disorders. Edited by Oldham JM, Skodol AE, Bender DS. Washington, DC, American Psychiatric Publishing, 2005, pp 541–559

Morey LC, Shea MT, Markowitz JC, et al: State effects of major depression on the assessment of personality and personality disorder. Am J Psychiatry 167:528–535, 2010

Morey LC, Berghuis H, Bender DS, et al: Toward a model for assessing level of personality functioning in DSM-5, Part II: empirical articulation of a core dimension of personality pathology. J Pers Assess 93:347–353, 2011

Morey LC, Bender DS, Skodol AE: Validating the proposed DSM-5 severity indicator for personality disorder. J Nerv Ment Dis 201:729–735, 2013a

Morey LC, Krueger RF, Skodol AE: The hierarchical structure of clinician ratings of proposed DSM-5 pathological personality traits. J Abnorm Psychol 122:836–841, 2013b

Morey LC, Benson KT, Skodol AE: Relating DSM-5 Section III personality traits to Section II personality disorder diagnoses. Psychol Med 46:647–655, 2016

Oldham JM, Skodol AE: Personality and personality disorders, and the passage of time. Am J Geriatr Psychiatry 21:709–712, 2013

Oltmanns TF, Balsis S: Personality disorders in later life: questions about the measurement, course, and impact of disorders. Annu Rev Clin Psychol 7:321–349, 2011

Pfohl B, Blum N, Zimmerman M: Structured Interview for DSM-IV Personality (SIDP-IV). Washington, DC, American Psychiatric Press, 1997

Rey JM, Morris-Yates A, Singh M, et al: Continuities between psychiatric disorders in adolescents and personality disorders in young adults. Am J Psychiatry 152:895–900, 1995

Roberts BW, Caspi A, Moffitt TE: Work experiences and personality development in young adulthood. J Pers Soc Psychol 84:582–593, 2003

Samuel DB, Widiger TA: A meta-analytic review of the relationship between the five-factor model and DSM-IV-TR personality disorders: a facet level analysis. Clin Psychol Rev 28:1326–1342, 2008

Samuel DB, Sanislow CA, Hopwood CJ, et al: Convergent and incremental validity of clinician, self-report, and diagnostic interview assessment methods for personality disorders over 5 years. J Consult Clin Psychol 81:650–659, 2013

Sartorius N: Disability and mental illness are different entities and should be assessed separately (abstract). World Psychiatry 8(2):86, June 2009

Saulsman LM, Page AC: The five-factor model and personality disorder empirical literature: a meta-analytic review. Clin Psychol Rev 23:1055–1085, 2004

Seivewright H, Tyrer P, Johnson T: Persistent social dysfunction in anxious and depressed patients with personality disorder. Acta Psychiatr Scand 109:104–109, 2004

Simms LJ, Calabrese WR: Incremental validity of the DSM-5 Section III personality traits with respect to psychosocial impairment. J Pers Disord 30:95–111, 2016

Skodol AE: Impact of personality pathology on psychosocial functioning. Curr Opin Psychol 21:33–38, 2018

Skodol AE, Gunderson JG, McGlashan TH, et al: Functional impairment in patients with schizotypal, borderline, avoidant, or obsessive-compulsive personality disorder. Am J Psychiatry 159:276–283, 2002

Skodol AE, Pagano MP, Bender DS, et al: Stability of functional impairment in patients with schizotypal, borderline, avoidant, or obsessive-compulsive personality disorder over two years. Psychol Med 35:443–451, 2005

Skodol AE, Johnson JG, Cohen P, et al: Personality disorder and impaired functioning from adolescence to adulthood. Br J Psychiatry 190:415–420, 2007

Skodol AE, Bender DS, Morey LC, et al: Personality disorder types proposed for DSM-5. J Pers Disord 25:136–169, 2011a

Skodol AE, Grilo CM, Keyes K, et al: Relationship of personality disorders to the course of major depressive disorder in a nationally representative sample. Am J Psychiatry 168:257–264, 2011b

Skodol AE, Krueger RK, Bender DS, et al: Personality disorders in DSM-5 Section III. Focus 11(2):187–288, 2013

Skodol AE, Bender DS, Morey LC: Narcissistic personality disorder in DSM-5. Personal Disord 5:422–427, 2014a

Skodol AE, Geier T, Grant BF, et al: Personality disorders and the persistence of anxiety disorders in a nationally representative sample. Depress Anxiety 31:721–728, 2014b

Skodol AE, Morey LC, Bender DS, et al: The Alternative DSM-5 Model for Personality Disorders: a clinical application. Am J Psychiatry 172:606–613, 2015

Skodol AE, First MB, Bender DS, et al: Module II Structured Clinical Interview for Personality Traits, in Structured Clinical Interview for the DSM-5 Alternative Model for Personality Disorders (SCID-AMPD). Arlington, VA, American Psychiatric Association Publishing, 2018

Skodol AE, Bender DS, Oldham JM: Personality pathology and personality disorders, in The American Psychiatric Association Publishing Textbook of Psychiatry, 7th Edition. Edited by Roberts LW. Washington, DC, American Psychiatric Association Publishing, 2019, pp 711–747

Temes CM, Zanarini MC: The longitudinal course of borderline personality disorder. Psychiatr Clin North Am 41:685–694, 2018

Verheul R, Widiger TA: A meta-analysis of the prevalence and usage of the personality disorder not otherwise specified (PDNOS) diagnosis. J Pers Disord 18:309–319, 2004

Waugh MH, Hopwood CJ, Krueger RF, et al. Psychological assessment with the DSM-5 Alternative Model for Personality Disorders: tradition and innovation. Prof Psychol Res Pr 48:79–89, 2017

Westen D: Divergences between clinical and research methods for assessing personality disorders: implications for research and the evolution of Axis II. Am J Psychiatry 154:895–903, 1997

Widiger TA: Sex biases in the diagnosis of personality disorders. J Pers Disord 12:95–118, 1998

Widiger TA, Mangine S, Corbitt EM, et al: Personality Disorder Interview–IV: A Semistructured Interview for the Assessment of Personality Disorders. Odessa, FL, Psychological Assessment Resources, 1995

Wright AC, Hopwood CJ, Skodol AE, et al: Longitudinal validation of general and specific structural features of personality pathology. J Abnorm Psychol 125:1120–1134, 2016

Zanarini MC, Frankenburg FR, Sickel AE, et al: Diagnostic Interview for DSM-IV Personality Disorders (DIPD-IV). Belmont, MA, Laboratory for the Study of Adult Development, McLean Hospital, and Department of Psychiatry, Harvard Medical School, 1996

Zanarini MC, Frankenburg FR, Reich DB, et al: The subsyndromal phenomenology of borderline personality disorder: a 10-year follow-up study. Am J Psychiatry 164:929–935, 2007

Zanarini MC, Frankenburg FR, Reich DB, et al: Time to attainment of recovery from borderline personality disorder and stability of recovery: a 10-year prospective follow-up study. Am J Psychiatry 167:663–667, 2010

Zanarini MC, Frankenburg FR, Reich DB, et al: Attainment and stability of sustained symptomatic remission and recovery among patients with borderline personality disorder and Axis II comparison subjects: a 16-year prospective follow-up study. Am J Psychiatry 169:476–483, 2012

Zimmerman M: Diagnosing personality disorders: a review of issues and research methods. Arch Gen Psychiatry 51:225–245, 1994

Zimmerman M, Mattia JI: Differences between clinical and research practices in diagnosing borderline personality disorder. Am J Psychiatry 156:1570–1574, 1999

Zimmermann J, Benecke C, Bender DS, et al: Assessing DSM-5 level of personality functioning from videotaped clinical interviews: a pilot study with untrained and clinically inexperienced students. J Pers Assess 96:397–409, 2014

Zoccolillo M, Pickles A, Quinton D, et al: The outcome of conduct disorder: implications for defining adult personality disorder and conduct disorder. Psychol Med 22:971–986, 1992

PART II

Risk Factors, Etiology, and Impact

CHAPTER 6

Prevalence, Sociodemographics, and Functional Impairment

Svenn Torgersen, Ph.D.

From clinical work, therapists get an impression of which personality disorders (PDs) are more common and which are rarer. However, people with some types of PDs may be more likely to seek treatment and obtain treatment compared with people with other types of PDs. Consequently, to find out how prevalent different PDs are in the general population, one needs data about representative samples of the general population. Epidemiological research provides exactly that type of information.

Clinical work also gives therapists ideas about relationships between socioeconomic and sociodemographic factors and PDs. However, in clinical settings, therapists meet only those from an unfavorable environment who have developed a PD. Clinicians do not meet those from an unfavorable environment who have *not* developed a disorder. Furthermore, the combination of a specific PD and specific sociodemographic features may increase the likelihood that a particular person will seek treatment. These complexities mean that only population (epidemiological) studies can demonstrate the "true" relationship between PDs and socioeconomic and sociodemographic variables, or any other variables such as traumas, disastrous events, upbringing, or partner relationships.

Prevalence

A number of studies have been performed to estimate the prevalence of DSM PDs in samples more or less representative of the general population. Table 6–1 presents the results of these studies. Many samples were relatively small. One study consisted of control groups in family studies (Maier et al. 1992), one was a study of relatives of pa-

TABLE 6–1. Prevalence of personality disorders in different epidemiological studies

PD	Zimmerman and Coryell 1989	Maier et al. 1992	Moldin et al. 1994	Klein et al. 1995	Lenzenweger et al. 1997	Torgersen et al. 2001	Samuels et al. 2002
Number	797	452	303	229	258	2000	742
System	DSM-III	DSM-III-R	DSM-III-R	DSM-III-R	DSM-III-R	DSM-III-R	DSM-IV
Method	SIDP	SCID-II	PDE	PDE	PDE	SIDP-R	IPDE
Place	Iowa	Mainz, Germany	New York	New York	New York	Oslo, Norway	Baltimore, Maryland
PPD	0.9	1.8	0.0	1.8	0.4	2.2	0.7
SPD	0.9	0.4	0.0	0.9	0.4	1.6	0.7
STPD	2.9	0.4	0.7	0.0	0.9	0.6	1.8
ASPD	3.3	0.2	2.6	2.6	0.8	0.6	4.5
BPD	1.7	1.1	2.0	1.8	0.0	0.7	1.2
HPD	3.0	1.3	0.3	1.8	1.9	1.9	0.4
NPD	0.0	0.0	0.0	4.4	1.2	0.8	0.1
AVPD	1.3	1.1	0.7	5.7	0.4	5.0	1.4
DPD	1.8	1.6	1.0	0.4	0.4	1.5	0.3
OCPD	2.0	2.2	0.7	2.6	0.0	1.9	1.2
PAPD	3.3	1.8	1.7	1.8	0.0	1.6	
SDPD					0.0	0.8	
SAPD					0.0	0.2	
DEPD					0.0		
Cl A						3.9	3.0
Cl B						3.0	5.8
Cl C						9.2	2.7
Total PD	14.3	10.0	7.3	14.8	3.9	13.1	10.0

TABLE 6–1. Prevalence of personality disorders in different epidemiological studies *(continued)*

	Coid et al. 2006	Lenzenweger et al. 2007	Johnson et al. 2008	Lindal and Stefansson 2009	Barnow et al. 2010	Gerhardt et al. 2011	Range	Median; mean
Number	656	214	568	420	745	110		
System	DSM-IV	DSM-IV	DSM-IV	DSM-IV	DSM-IV	DSM-IV		
Method	SCID-II	IPDE	SCID-II	DIP-Q	SCID-II	SCID-II		
Place	UK	United States	New York	Reykjavik, Iceland	Me.-Vor.	Heidelberg		
PPD	0.7	2.3	2.4	4.8	3.2	2.7	0.0–4.8	1.8; 1.7
SPD	0.8	4.9	1.3	3.1	0.8	0.0	0.0–4.9	0.8; 1.3
STPD	0.1	3.3	0.9	4.5	0.1	0.0	0.0–4.5	0.7; 1.3
ASPD	0.6	1.0	2.2	1.4	0.8	0.0	0.0–4.5	1.0; 1.8
BPD	0.7	1.6	2.2	4.5	2.3	3.6	0.0–4.5	1.7; 1.6
HPD	0.0	0.0	1.5	0.7	0.7	0.0	0.0–3.0	0.7; 1.2
NPD	0.0	0.0	1.1	1.2	0.7	0.9	0.0–4.4	0.7; 0.8
AVPD	0.8	5.2	3.7	5.2	2.3	4.5	0.0–5.2	2.3; 2.7
DPD	0.1	0.6	1.4	1.7	1.3	0.0	0.1–1.8	1.0; 1.0
OCPD	1.9	2.4	1.5	7.1	6.3	4.5	0.0–7.1	2.0; 2.5
PAPD			1.7			0.9	0.0–3.3	2.1; 1.7
SDPD							0.0–0.8	0.4
SAPD							0.0–0.2	0.1
DEPD			1.5				1.5	1.5
Cl A	1.6	6.2			3.8	2.7	1.6–6.2	3.4; 3.5
Cl B	0.5	2.3			3.9	4.5	0.5–5.8	3.5; 3.3
Cl C	2.6	6.8			8.6	9.1	2.6–9.2	7.7; 6.5
Total PD	4.4	11.9	13.3	11.1	12.8	15.5	3.9–15.5	11.9; 11.0

Note. ASPD=antisocial personality disorder; AVPD=avoidant personality disorder; BPD=borderline personality disorder; Cl A=Cluster A; Cl B=Cluster B; Cl C=Cluster C; DEPD=depressive personality disorder; DPD=dependent personality disorder; HPD=histrionic personality disorder; NPD=narcissistic personality disorder; OCPD=obsessive-compulsive personality disorder; PAPD=passive-aggressive personality disorder; PD=personality disorder; PPD=paranoid personality disorder; SAPD=sadistic personality disorder; SDPD=self-defeating personality disorder; SPD=schizoid personality disorder; STPD=schizotypal personality disorder. DIP-Q=DSM-IV and ICD-10 Personality Questionnaire; IPDE=International Personality Disorder Examination; PDE=Personality Disorder Examination; SCID-II=Structured Clinical Interview for DSM-IV Axis II Personality Disorders; SIDP=Structured Interview for DSM-III-R Personality; SIDP-R=Structured Interview for DSM-III-R Personality—Revised.

tients with mood disorders and schizophrenia (Zimmerman and Coryell 1989), and another was a study of subjects with nonspecific chronic back pain (Gerhardt et al. 2011). One consisted of young participants (Johnson et al. 2008), and another focused on a sample in which half the subjects were young children of the other half (Barnow et al. 2010). Many studies were from nearly the same place: New York City or upstate New York (Johnson et al. 2008; Klein et al. 1995; Lenzenweger et al. 1997; Moldin et al. 1994). Most were from urban areas (Gerhardt et al. 2011; Johnson et al. 2008; Klein et al. 1995; Lenzenweger et al. 1997; Lindal and Stefansson 2009; Maier et al. 1992; Moldin et al. 1994; Samuels et al. 2002; Torgersen et al. 2001). Semistructured or structured interviews were used in most studies, except that of Lindal and Stefansson (2009), who used a questionnaire, the DSM-IV and ICD-10 Personality Questionnaire (DIP-Q). One study (Zimmerman and Coryell 1989) was based on DSM-III (American Psychiatric Association 1980), others (Klein et al. 1995; Lenzenweger et al. 1997; Maier et al. 1992; Moldin et al. 1994; Torgersen et al. 2001) were based on DSM-III-R (American Psychiatric Association 1987), and some (Barnow et al. 2010; Coid et al. 2006; Gerhardt et al. 2011; Johnson et al. 2008; Lenzenweger et al. 2007; Lindal and Stefansson 2009; Samuels et al. 2002) were based on DSM-IV (American Psychiatric Association 1994). Some researchers used the Structured Interview for DSM-III-R Personality Disorders (SIDP; Torgersen et al. 2001; Zimmerman and Coryell 1989), some used the Structured Clinical Interview for DSM-IV Axis II Personality Disorders (SCID-II; Barnow et al. 2010; Coid et al. 2006; Gerhardt et al. 2011; Johnson et al. 2008; Maier et al. 1992), and others used versions of the Personality Disorder Examination (PDE; Klein et al. 1995; Lenzenweger et al. 1997, 2007; Moldin et al. 1994; Samuels et al. 2002). Most studies were from the United States (Klein et al. 1995; Lenzenweger et al. 1997, 2007; Moldin et al. 1994; Samuels et al. 2002; Zimmerman and Coryell 1989), although some were from northwestern Europe (Barnow et al. 2010; Coid et al. 2006; Gerhardt et al. 2011; Lindal and Stefansson 2009; Maier et al. 1992; Torgersen et al. 2001). Surprisingly, the prevalence for any PD was very similar in these different studies: 10 of 13 studies reported the prevalence for any PD between 10% and 15%. On average, the prevalence was 11% or 12%, depending on whether the mean or the median was used in the calculations.

Table 6–1 also shows prevalence information about the DSM PD clusters. In five of the six studies that reported such data, Cluster C (anxious/fearful) disorders are reported to be the most frequent. The prevalence rates of Cluster A (odd/eccentric) and Cluster B (dramatic/emotional) disorders average around 3.5% each, and the prevalence of Cluster C disorders averages around 7.0%.

As to the specific PDs, the variation in prevalence across studies is relatively higher. This is not surprising because the percentages are lower, and hence the relative standard errors are larger. However, the rank orders of the specific PDs are not so different from study to study. For obsessive-compulsive and avoidant PDs, the rank is between first and third for the majority of the studies. Borderline PD is between third and fifth, dependent PD between fifth and seventh, schizoid PD between sixth and eighth, and narcissistic PD consistently least or next to least frequent. Paranoid PD is also relatively stable between ranks second and fifth, whereas the ranks of schizotypal, antisocial, and histrionic PDs are spread over the whole range.

An analysis of the correlations between the prevalence of the specific PDs in different studies and the averages, excluding the study investigated, was performed for purposes of this chapter. Six of the 13 studies showed a correlation of 0.57 or higher with the average over all the other studies. All studies with a high correlation with the average were published in 2001 or later (Torgersen et al. 2001 [$r=0.57$]; Coid et al. 2006 [$r=0.77$]; Johnson et al. 2008 [$r=0.68$]; Lindal and Stefansson 2009 [$r=0.70$]; Barnow et al. 2010 [$r=0.62$]; Gerhardt et al. 2011 [$r=.82$]). The intraclass correlation over all 13 studies was 0.75.

On average, the prevalence of specific PDs is around 1%–1.5%. Avoidant and obsessive-compulsive PDs are the most frequent PDs, each affecting around 2.5% of the population. Paranoid, borderline, antisocial, and passive-aggressive PDs (the latter from the DSM-IV appendix) affect around 1.5% each. Schizoid, dependent, schizotypal, and histrionic PDs each affect about 1.0% of the population. The prevalence of narcissistic PD is often below 1%. The few studies of the other PDs from either the DSM-III-R or DSM-IV appendix showed very low prevalence rates for self-defeating and sadistic PDs and a high frequency for depressive PD. Although there is no definitive empirical work justifying retaining any of the provisional PDs in DSM-5 (American Psychiatric Association 2013), individuals who exhibit tendencies such as these can now be characterized with respect to personality functioning and pathological traits in the alternative DSM-5 PD model in Section III, "Emerging Measures and Models." I include data on the prevalence of these provisional PDs for those clinicians and researchers who retain an interest in them.

There are no obvious differences in prevalence of a PD depending on whether DSM-III, DSM-III-R, or DSM-IV is used or what kind of instrument is applied. However, the number of studies in each category is too low to draw any conclusions. Comparison of studies from the United States and northwestern Europe indicates that obsessive-compulsive and paranoid PDs, and possibly avoidant, schizoid, and dependent PDs, are more common in Europe, whereas antisocial and schizotypal PDs, and possibly histrionic and narcissistic PDs, are more common in the United States. It may be the case, therefore, that an affectively inhibited, skeptical, and withdrawn personality style is more common in northwest Europe, whereas an affectively expressive, impulsive, flamboyant, and possibly eccentric style is more likely in America.

In a recent meta-analysis, Volkert et al. (2018) included 9 studies (originally 10, but one was put aside because of a large deviation from the other studies). DSM-III and DSM-III-R were excluded from the analysis, but studies applying questionnaires, studies that did not look at all PDs, and a study of ICD-10 PDs were included, and as a result there was almost no overlap with the studies in Table 6–1. Surprisingly, the authors found exactly the same 11.0 as in Table 6–1 (much lower if only the "expert rating" in six studies was included). An analysis of the correlations between the average prevalence of the specific PDs in Table 6–1 and the average prevalence in the meta-analysis gave a Pearson correlation of 0.51 and an intraclass correlation of 0.62. There thus seems to be some consensus in the literature regarding the prevalence of PDs.

Huang et al. (2009) investigated the prevalence of PDs in areas including the United States, Africa, Asia, and Western Europe. They used a short questionnaire and multiple imputation to estimate the prevalence in different countries. The Western European sample can be disregarded because it included only married couples and had an extremely low prevalence. The average prevalence for any PD among all regions/countries examined was estimated to be as low as 6.1, far lower than in the studies in Table 6–1. The average prevalence of Cluster A PDs was 3.6, but the prevalence of 1.5 for Cluster B and 2.7 for Cluster C is less than half of what was found in other studies with more thorough methodologies. The authors discussed this difference and proposed that the reason for the difference was the instrument and the multiple imputation procedure. What is interesting, however, is the similarity between countries. All (except for Western Europe) show the highest prevalence for Cluster A, followed by Cluster C and then Cluster B. Five of the seven studies show a prevalence between 6.1 and 7.9, including samples from America, Africa, and Asia. Therefore, the study suggests that the prevalence of PDs might show the same pattern all over the world, not excluding differences within the regions.

Lifetime Prevalence

Lifetime prevalence for disorders is necessarily higher than point prevalence. If the percentage of a population with a given disorder is measured during the past 2 weeks, 1 month, 1 year, 2 years, or 5 years, the percentage will be lower than if the population is followed throughout the whole lifespan. This obvious fact has long been established for many mental disorders, and the same will hold true for PDs, provided that the disorders are not present at an early age and do not remain chronic throughout life. Indeed, empirical research shows that many treated individuals are free of their PDs after a relatively short time (Grilo et al. 2004; Shea et al. 2002; Skodol et al. 2005a; Zanarini et al. 2006). The same is true in the general population (Johnson et al. 2008; Lenzenweger 1999). At the same time, the 2- to 5-year point prevalence rates do not diminish much with age, as discussed in the following paragraphs. The implication is that new cases have to debut in the population to replace those that disappear, even if a few reappear (Durbin and Klein 2006; Ferro et al. 1998; Zanarini et al. 2006).

A direct indication of the difference between point prevalence and lifetime prevalence of PDs is found in a study of adolescents in New York followed from age 14 to age 32 years (Johnson et al. 2008) (Table 6–2). Although the mean point prevalence of PDs over the four observation points—ages 14, 16, 22, and 33 years—was 13.4%, the cumulative prevalence over the four time points was 28.2%. The same relationship was observed for the specific PDs. The ratio between the cumulative prevalence and the average prevalence at a specific time was around 3.

In the National Epidemiologic Survey on Alcohol and Related Conditions (NESARC), interviewers tried to obtain a lifetime assessment of PD prevalence instead of a 2- to 5-year assessment (Grant et al. 2004, 2008, 2012; Pulay et al. 2009; Stinson et al. 2008) (Table 6–2). When the prevalence of individual PDs is compared with the average for PDs in all published epidemiological studies, the lifetime prevalence (as far as the respondents can remember) is around three times as high. The implications are that the average lifetime prevalence of a specific PD will be at least 3%–4%, and the lifetime prevalence of any PD will be at least around 30% but probably much higher. Thus, according to the present criteria for PDs as defined in DSM-5 Section II, "Diagnostic Criteria and Codes," a large percentage of people at some point in their lives will qualify for having a PD. The rest of the time, they may be only slightly below the level of a clinical disorder or perhaps far below the level for a shorter or longer time of their lifespan. The reason for this clinical course is the semicontinuous nature of PDs. An individual's personality dysfunction is not stable. Events and life situations can bring the dysfunction up to the threshold for a PD during at least one period in life. The

TABLE 6–2. Difference between point prevalence and lifetime prevalence for personality disorders

Disorder	Mean, all studies, point prevalence	Grant et al. 2004, 2008, 2012; Pulay et al. 2009; Stinson et al. 2008		Johnson et al. 2008			Average ratio
		Lifetime	Ratio: lifetime/point prevalence	Mean over 4 waves, ages 14–32 years	Cumulative over 4 waves, ages 14–32 years	Ratio: point prevalence/cumulative	
PPD	1.7	4.4	2.6	2.1	7.0	3.3	3.1
SPD	1.3	3.1	2.4	1.1	3.9	3.6	3.1
STPD	1.3	3.9	3.0	1.2	4.0	3.3	3.5
ASPD	1.8	3.6	2.0	2.2[a]	(3.2)[a]	(1.6)[a]	(1.8)[a]
BPD	1.6	5.9	3.7	1.5	5.5	3.7	4.0
HPD	1.2	1.8	1.5	1.5	4.6	3.1	2.3
NPD	0.8	6.2	7.8	2.2	6.3	2.9	5.4
AVPD	2.7	2.4	0.9	2.4	8.1	3.4	2.2
DPD	1.0	0.5	0.5	0.8	3.2	4.0	2.3
OCPD	2.5	7.8	3.1	0.7	3.0	4.3	4.1
PAPD				1.9	5.6	2.9	
DEPD				0.8	3.0	3.8	
Average	1.6	4.0	2.8	1.5	4.8	3.2	3.1
Any PD				13.4	28.2	2.1	

Note. ASPD=antisocial personality disorder; AVPD=avoidant personality disorder; BPD=borderline personality disorder; DEPD=depressive personality disorder; DPD=dependent personality disorder; HPD=histrionic personality disorder; NPD=narcissistic personality disorder; OCPD=obsessive-compulsive personality disorder; PAPD=passive-aggressive personality disorder; PD=personality disorder; PPD=paranoid personality disorder; SPD=schizoid personality disorder; STPD=schizotypal personality disorder.

[a]Waves at ages 14 and 16 years do not include ASPD.

dysfunction often decreases back toward the mean in the population, and although it does not necessarily reach this mean level, it remains below the level for a PD. Other individuals who previously met too few criteria for a diagnosis will display an increase and rise over the threshold. Many individuals will reach the above-threshold level at least once in their lifetime. This waxing and waning of personality pathology argues for movement away from traditional categorical approaches to classification and diagnosis and toward more dimensional representations.

Prevalence in Clinical Populations

Knowledge about the prevalence of PDs in clinical populations is very important for clinicians and health administrators. Previously, most information available about the prevalence of PDs stemmed from such clinical populations. Today, much more is known about prevalence in the general population. A comparison of clinical and community prevalence rates provides meaningful information about the varying tendency to be treated among individuals with various PDs.

Table 6–3 presents a comparison between the prevalence of PDs in the general population and prevalences in nine clinical populations adapted from the *Oxford Handbook of Personality Disorders* (Torgersen 2012). Epidemiological studies of the general population make it possible to have a direct comparison of individuals who have been treated for psychological problems and those who have not been treated. As shown in Table 6–3, borderline and dependent PDs are much more prevalent in the clinical population than in the general population. Other PDs relatively much more common in clinical populations are narcissistic, histrionic, avoidant, and schizotypal PDs. Passive-aggressive, paranoid, antisocial, and obsessive-compulsive PDs are relatively a little more common in the clinical population, whereas schizoid PD does not seem to be more common in clinical populations than in the general population. Notably, narcissistic, dependent, and histrionic PDs are quite prevalent in clinical populations, although the quality of life is not as low for these individuals (Cramer et al. 2006, 2007) as for those with schizoid and paranoid PDs, which are relatively uncommon in clinical populations, although these individuals suffer a lot. Strongly dependent and extroverted individuals are more likely to seek help and support, whereas skeptical, introverted individuals prefer to be more self-reliant, try to solve problems themselves, and keep away from treatment. Thus, personality, more than psychological suffering, is a strong factor in illness behavior.

In summary, although the prevalence rates of PDs vary strongly from study to study, the number of published studies makes it possible to draw some conclusions. At least in the United States and Europe, the prevalence rates of specific PDs are as high as 1.5% (Table 6–1). The prevalence of "any PD" is 11%–12%. The sum of the percentages for the specific disorders is higher, close to 20%, pointing to the fact that a large number of individuals with one disorder also have one, two, three, or even more additional disorders. Studying only patients provides a distorted impression of the absolute and relative prevalence of PDs, because individuals with dependent and extroverted traits seek treatment much more often, whereas the opposite is the case for skeptical, introverted persons.

TABLE 6–3. Relative risk of attending or having attended psychiatric care for different personality disorders

Disorder	Common population, international (median; mean)	Clinical population, international (median; mean)	Relative risk (median; mean)	Relative rank of risk	Common population, Oslo, Norway				Relative rank of relative risk, combined
					Nontreated	Treated	Relative risk	Relative rank of risk	
PPD	1.8; 1.7	6.3; 9.6	3.5; 5.6	8	2.1	5.8	2.8	6	6
SPD	0.8; 1.3	1.4; 1.9	1.8; 1.5	11	1.4	7.2	5.1	4	8
STPD	0.7; 1.3	6.4; 5.7	9.1; 4.4	6	0.6	1.4	2.3	8	6
ASPD	1.0; 1.8	3.9; 5.9	3.9; 3.3	9	0.6	0.0	<0.2	11	11
BPD	1.7; 1.6	28.5; 28.5	17.8; 17.8	1	0.5	7.2	14.4	1	1
HPD	0.7; 1.2	8.0; 9.7	11.4; 8.1	4	1.8	4.3	2.4	7	5
NPD	0.7; 0.8	5.1; 10.1	7.3; 12.6	3	0.8	2.9	3.6	5	3
AVPD	2.3; 2.7	21.5; 24.6	9.3; 9.1	5	4.3	23.2	5.4	3	3
DPD	1.0; 1.0	13.0; 15.0	13.0; 15.0	10	1.3	8.7	6.7	2	2
OCPD	2.0; 2.5	6.1; 10.5	3.1; 4.2	7	1.9	2.9	1.5	9	10
PAPD	2.1; 1.7	10.1; 9.5	4.8; 5.6		1.6	1.4	0.9	10	9
Cl A	3.4; 3.5	11.2; 10.2	3.3; 2.9	3	3.6	13.0	3.6	2	3
Cl B	3.5; 3.3	32.1; 31.7	9.2; 9.6	1	3.3	8.7	2.6	3	2
Cl C	7.5; 6.5	27.6; 26.9	3.6; 4.1	2	7.0	26.1	3.7	1	1
Any PD	11.9; 11.0	65.6; 64.4	5.5; 5.9		12.5	31.9	2.6		

Note. ASPD=antisocial personality disorder; AVPD=avoidant personality disorder; BPD=borderline personality disorder; Cl A=Cluster A; Cl B=Cluster B; Cl C=Cluster C; DPD=dependent personality disorder; HPD=histrionic personality disorder; NPD=narcissistic personality disorder; OCPD=obsessive-compulsive personality disorder; PAPD=passive-aggressive personality disorder; PD=personality disorder; PPD=paranoid personality disorder; SPD=schizoid personality disorder; STPD=schizotypal personality disorder.
Source. Adapted from Torgersen 2012, p. 193, and Torgersen et al. 2001.

Sociodemographic Correlates

Gender

Gender differences are common among mental disorders. Mood and anxiety disorders are more common among women, and substance-related disorders are more common among men (Kringlen et al. 2001). Women and men also differ with regard to PDs. Zimmerman and Coryell (1989) observed a higher prevalence of any PD among males, as did Jackson and Burgess (2000) for ICD-10 screening when regression analysis was applied. However, differences between genders were very small, and Torgersen et al. (2001) did not observe any differences. As for the PD clusters, Samuels et al. (2002) and Torgersen et al. (2001) reported that Cluster A and Cluster B disorders or traits were more common among men; Coid et al. (2006) found the same for Cluster B only.

Among the specific Cluster A disorders, Torgersen et al. (2001), Ullrich and Coid (2009), and Zimmerman and Coryell (1990) found that schizoid PD or traits were more common among men; Zimmerman and Coryell (1990) also found this true for paranoid traits. Grant et al. (2004), however, observed that women more often had paranoid PD. Although neither Zimmerman and Coryell (1989, 1990) nor Torgersen et al. (2001) observed any gender difference for schizotypal PD, Pulay et al. (2009) found that schizotypal PD was more common among men, and Ullrich and Coid (2009) found it was more common among women.

Among the Cluster B disorders, antisocial PD was much more common among men (Grant et al. 2004; Torgersen et al. 2001; Ullrich and Coid 2009; Zimmerman and Coryell 1989, 1990). Histrionic PD or traits occurred more often among women (Torgersen et al. 2001; Zimmerman and Coryell 1990). Narcissistic PD and traits were found more often among men (Stinson et al. 2008; Torgersen et al. 2001; Ullrich and Coid 2009; Zimmerman and Coryell 1989, 1990). Although there were few statistically significant gender differences for borderline PD or traits, Ullrich and Coid (2009) reported a higher incidence among women.

Among the Cluster C disorders, dependent PD was much more common among women (Grant et al. 2004; Torgersen et al. 2001; Ullrich and Coid 2009; Zimmerman and Coryell 1989, 1990), and obsessive-compulsive PD or traits were found more often among men (Torgersen et al. 2001; Ullrich and Coid 2009; Zimmerman and Coryell 1989, 1990). Zimmerman and Coryell (1989, 1990), Grant et al. (2004), and Ullrich and Coid (2009) reported more avoidant PD and traits among women.

Regarding PDs "provided for further study" in DSM-III-R or DSM-IV, Torgersen et al. (2001), but not Zimmerman and Coryell (1989, 1990), found that men more often had passive-aggressive PD. Torgersen and colleagues also found that women more often presented with self-defeating traits, and men more often presented with sadistic traits.

The most clear-cut results from the studies were that men with PDs tend to be antisocial and narcissistic, and women with PDs tend to be histrionic and dependent. These results are perhaps not surprising. More surprising, however, are the relatively few indications of gender differences for borderline traits, even though borderline features are often considered to be more common in women than in men. In patient samples, borderline PD was not more prevalent among women than among men (Alnæs and Torgersen 1988; Fossati et al. 2003; Golomb et al. 1995). In one study of patients, borderline PD was, in fact, more common among men than among women (Carter et al. 1999). Reports that paranoid and schizotypal PDs do not show any gender bias, that men more often have schizoid and obsessive-compulsive PDs or traits, and that women more often have avoidant and histrionic PDs or traits are more in accord with common opinion.

Age

For an individual younger than age 18 to be diagnosed with a PD, the features must have been present at least 1 year, although this is not true for PDs diagnosed using the Alternative DSM-5 Model for Personality Disorders (AMPD; American Psychiatric Association 2013). At the same time, it is assumed that PDs start early in life and are relatively stable. For some PDs, especially the dramatic types (Cluster B), it is also assumed that they are typical for young people. On the other hand, the older people are, the longer they have had to develop PDs, even though PDs may also disappear. Suicide and fatal accidents also may happen more often among those with PDs than among other individuals. These facts will influence the rate of specific PDs in older age.

Zimmerman and Coryell (1989) observed that individuals with PDs were younger than those without. Jackson and Burgess (2000) found the same age distribution using a short ICD-10 screening instrument, the International Personality Disorder Screener. Torgersen et al. (2001), however, observed the opposite in a study conducted in Norway. This difference can be explained by the higher prevalence of introverted and the lower prevalence of impulsive personality traits in Norway compared with the United States. Introverted PDs are more prevalent among older people, and impulsive PDs are less prevalent.

With regard to the clusters of PDs, Torgersen et al. (2001) found that individuals with Cluster A disorders were older, whereas Samuels et al. (2002), Coid et al. (2006), and Lenzenweger et al. (2007) did not find any age variations for these disorders. For the Cluster B disorders, Samuels et al. (2002), Coid et al. (2006), and Lenzenweger et al. (2007) found a higher prevalence among the younger subjects, whereas Torgersen et al. (2001) found that the Cluster B trait dimensions decreased with age. For the Cluster C disorders, no age trend was reported in any of the studies.

Among the Cluster A disorders, schizoid PD or traits were generally found to be associated with older people (Engels et al. 2003; Torgersen et al. 2001; Ullrich and Coid 2009; Zimmerman and Coryell 1989, 1990), although Grant et al. (2004) found them to be more common in younger people. In contrast, most researchers found schizotypal PD to be more common in younger individuals (Engels et al. 2003; Pulay et al. 2009; Ullrich and Coid 2009; Zimmerman and Coryell 1989, 1990), but Torgersen et al. (2001) found it to be more common in older individuals. Paranoid PD was observed more among younger people in two studies (Grant et al. 2004; Ullrich and Coid 2009).

Many study authors reported that younger people more frequently had Cluster B disorders or traits: borderline (Engels et al. 2003; Grant et al. 2004, 2008; Torgersen et al. 2001; Ullrich and Coid 2009; Zimmerman and Coryell 1989, 1990), antisocial (Grant et al. 2004, 2008; Torgersen et al. 2001; Ullrich and Coid 2009; Zimmerman and Coryell 1989, 1990), histrionic (Grant et al. 2004; Ullrich and Coid 2009; Zimmerman and

Coryell 1990), and narcissistic (Stinson et al. 2008; Ullrich and Coid 2009; Zimmerman and Coryell 1990).

Individuals with obsessive-compulsive PD and traits appear to be older (Engels et al. 2003; Grant et al. 2012; Torgersen et al. 2001; Ullrich and Coid 2009). One study found that individuals with avoidant PD are older (Torgersen et al. 2001), and another reported that they are younger (Ullrich and Coid 2009). One study observed that those with dependent PD are younger (Grant et al. 2004).

Zimmerman and Coryell (1989) found that individuals with passive-aggressive PD are typically of a younger age, and Torgersen et al. (2001) observed that such traits were negatively correlated with age. The latter study also examined self-defeating and sadistic traits and found that sadistic traits were associated with younger age.

To summarize, persons with borderline, antisocial, and possibly schizotypal, histrionic, and narcissistic PDs seem to be younger, whereas those with schizoid and obsessive-compulsive PDs are older. These findings are in accordance with those from a follow-up study by Seivewright et al. (2002) showing a strong developmental trend from Cluster B to Cluster A disorders and a somewhat weaker change to Cluster C disorders. The reason for the age difference may be that people become less impulsive and overtly aggressive as they age. Agreeableness and conscientiousness increase with age (Srivastava et al. 2003). Cluster B disorders are typically negatively correlated with agreeableness and conscientiousness (Saulsman and Page 2004).

Marital Status

Most of the results concerning marital status are from Zimmerman and Coryell (1989). Some of the data from Torgersen et al. (2001) have been calculated for this chapter to be comparable in format to the tables in Zimmerman and Coryell (1989) (Table 6–4).

As illustrated in Table 6–4, subjects with PDs have more often been separated or divorced compared with those without a PD. They are less likely to be currently married (Jackson and Burgess 2000; Zimmerman and Coryell 1989), and they are also more likely to have never been married (Zimmerman and Coryell 1989). If nonmarried persons living with a partner are considered, subjects with PDs more often live alone without a partner than do subjects without a PD in the general population (Torgersen et al. 2001).

However, because the risk of having a PD is related to gender and age, the real effect of other sociodemographic variables such as marital status is difficult to determine. Younger people are less often married, and education is also related to gender and age. The best way to determine the independent effect of individual sociodemographic variables is to apply multivariate methods; however, these methods have been used in very few studies because they need large samples. In the study by Torgersen et al. (2001), such multivariate analyses have been carried out for living alone versus living with a partner.

Individuals with lifetime Cluster A disorders have more often been divorced or separated (Coid et al. 2006; Samuels et al. 2002); those with current Cluster A disorders are more often divorced at the time of the interview, and they have more seldom been married (Samuels et al. 2002) (Table 6–4). Those with Cluster B disorders are also often unmarried and more often live alone (Torgersen et al. 2001), and they have more often

TABLE 6–4. Marital status and personality disorders, calculated from Torgersen et al. 2001

Personality disorder	N	Single (never married) (%)	Married (%)	Separated[a] (%)	Divorced[a] (%)	Widowed (%)	Ever separated[b] (%)	Ever divorced[c] (%)
Paranoid	46	34.8	34.8	6.5	21.7[c]	2.2	15.8	36.7
Schizoid	32	56.3	31.3	0.0	6.3	6.3	20.0	28.6
Schizotypal	12	50.0	33.3	0.0	8.3	8.3	20.0	16.7
Antisocial	12	75.0[d]	8.3[d]	0.0	16.7	0.0	0.0	66.7
Borderline	14	57.1	35.7	7.1	0.0	0.0	20.0	16.7
Histrionic	39	46.2	35.9	0.0	17.9	0.0	0.0	47.6[d]
Narcissistic	17	35.6	52.9	0.0	5.9	5.9	10.0	9.1
Avoidant	102	45.1	36.3	1.0	14.7	2.9	7.5	28.6
Dependent	31	58.1[d]	25.8[d]	3.2	12.9	0.0	11.1	30.8
Obsessive-compulsive	39	41.6	43.6	0.0	10.3	5.1	5.6	21.7
Passive-aggressive	32	35.3	31.3	6.3	9.4	3.1	18.2	31.3
Self-defeating	17	35.3	17.6[d]	0.0	41.2[e]	5.9	25.0	63.6
Sadistic	4	50.0	56.0	0.0	0.0	0.0	0.0	0.0
Cluster A: eccentric	80	45.6	33.8[d]	3.8	15.0	2.5	13.8	34.1
Cluster B: dramatic	62	49.3	35.2	1.4	12.7	1.4	8.3	33.3
Cluster C: fearful	189	45.5	36.5[d]	1.3	14.1	2.6	8.2	28.2
Any personality disorder	269	43.9	36.8[f]	2.2	15.6[d]	1.5	7.9	33.1[f]
No personality disorder	1,784	38.8	46.5	2.4	10.4	1.8	5.1	23.2
Total	2,053	693.0	830.0	43.0	185.0	33.0	43.0	253.0

[a]At the time of interview.
[b]Excluding those who were never married.
[c]Excluding those who were never married and those who are divorced.
[d]χ^2 test, $P<0.05$. [e]χ^2 test, $P<0.001$. [f]χ^2 test, $P<0.01$.

been separated or divorced (Coid et al. 2006). Those with Cluster C disorders are also less often married (Samuels et al. 2002) and more often live alone (Torgersen et al. 2001).

Difficulties arise in comparing the different studies when examining the specific PDs. Marital status does not seem to be as important in the Norwegian study (Torgersen et al. 2001), perhaps because many Norwegians live in stable relationships without being married. When "living together with a partner" from the study of Torgersen et al. (2001) is included as being analogous to marriage, the findings of this study and the study by Zimmerman and Coryell (1989) are more similar. It is important to note that the observations in the study by Torgersen and colleagues were based on logistic and linear regression analysis, taking into account a number of other sociodemographic variables.

Among individuals with Cluster A disorders, those with paranoid PD are more often single (never married) (Grant et al. 2004), divorced (Grant et al. 2004) (Table 6–4), or living alone (Torgersen et al. 2001). Those with schizoid PD are less often separated (Zimmerman and Coryell 1989), more often ever separated/divorced/widowed or never married (Grant et al. 2004), and more often living alone (Torgersen et al. 2001). Those with schizotypal PD have more often been separated (Zimmerman and Coryell 1989) and more often living alone (Torgersen et al. 2001). They are more often separated/divorced/widowed or never married (Pulay et al. 2009), all compared with those without the specific PDs.

Among the Cluster B disorders, persons with histrionic PD have more often been separated or divorced (Zimmerman and Coryell 1989). They are also more often not married at the time of the interview (Zimmerman and Coryell 1989); more often divorced, separated, widowed, or never married (Grant et al. 2004); and more often living alone (Torgersen et al. 2001). Those with antisocial PD also have more often been divorced, separated (Zimmerman and Coryell 1989), or never married (Grant et al. 2004) (Table 6–4); are less often married at the time of the interview; and are more often living alone (Torgersen et al. 2001). Persons with borderline PD also have more often been separated if married, are more often divorced, and are not married at the time of the interview (Zimmerman and Coryell 1989). They are more often never married (Zimmerman and Coryell 1989); are more often living alone (Torgersen et al. 2001); and are more often separated, divorced, or widowed (Grant et al. 2008). Finally, those with narcissistic PD also more often live alone (Torgersen et al. 2001), and they are more often separated, divorced, widowed or never married (Stinson et al. 2008).

Among persons with Cluster C disorders, those with avoidant PD have more often been separated (Zimmerman and Coryell 1989). They are more often separated, divorced, or widowed, and more often have never married (Grant et al. 2004). Those with dependent PD more often have been separated at the time of the interview (Zimmerman and Coryell 1989); have never married (Grant et al. 2004) (Table 6–4); or are separated, divorced, or widowed (Grant et al. 2004). Those with obsessive-compulsive traits are less often married (Torgersen et al. 2001), and females with obsessive-compulsive PD are less often separated, divorced, or widowed at the time of the interview.

Among the proposed PDs, persons with passive-aggressive PD have more often been divorced and are less often married at the time of the interview (Zimmerman and Coryell 1989), and are more likely to live alone (Torgersen et al. 2001). Those with self-defeating PD have more often been divorced (Zimmerman and Coryell 1989), are more often divorced (see Table 6–4) or not married at the time of the interview (Zimmerman and Coryell 1989), and are more likely to live alone (Torgersen et al. 2001).

In summary, persons with PDs, particularly those with self-defeating, borderline, or schizotypal PD, typically live alone. Those with obsessive-compulsive PD may be an exception. Never having been married is often observed among those with antisocial and dependent PDs. The risk of divorce or separation is high among those with paranoid PD. In cultures where it is more common to live together unmarried, a breakup in the relationship is less easy to record. For whatever reason, living without a partner is very common among people with PDs.

Education and Income

Relatively few studies have investigated the relationship between PDs and education and income. Torgersen et al. (2001) observed that people with any PD had less education than those without a PD. The same was observed for those with disorders or traits in any of the clusters (Clusters A, B, or C). Samuels et al. (2002) and Lenzenweger et al. (2007) confirmed that those with Cluster B disorders, but not those with Cluster A or Cluster C disorders, had less education. Coid et al. (2006), however, found lower education among those with Cluster A disorders.

In applying logistic regression analysis and taking into account a number of other sociodemographic variables, Torgersen et al. (2001) observed that paranoid and avoidant PDs and traits and schizoid, schizotypal, antisocial, borderline, dependent, and self-defeating personality traits were related to lower education. Interestingly, individuals with obsessive-compulsive PD or traits had higher education. Only histrionic, narcissistic, and passive-aggressive PDs or traits were unrelated to education. In Wave 1 of the NESARC, Grant et al. (2004) found that lower education was related to all the studied PDs (paranoid, schizoid, antisocial, histrionic, avoidant, and dependent), with the exception of obsessive-compulsive PD, which was related to higher education (as Torgersen et al. [2001] found). In NESARC Wave 2, Grant et al. (2008) found that borderline PD was more common among those with lower education and income. The same was true for low income and schizotypal PD (Pulay et al. 2009) but not narcissistic PD (Stinson et al. 2008).

Coid et al. (2006) found that Cluster A disorders were related to unemployment and lower social class, Cluster B disorders were related to lower social class, and Cluster C disorders were related to being "economically inactive" but not unemployed. Grant et al. (2004) found that lower income was related to all of the studied (NESARC Wave 1) PDs except obsessive-compulsive PD. Lenzenweger et al. (2007) found that only borderline PD was related to unemployment. Samuels et al. (2002) also investigated the relationship between income and PDs but did not find any association. Jackson and Burgess (2000) did not find any relationship between PDs and unemployment. It is important to note that these studies applied multivariate methods, taking into account other sociodemographic variables.

In summary, with a few exceptions, PDs are related to economic problems and lower socioeconomic status. This holds true for all of the Cluster A disorders (paranoid, schizoid, and schizotypal) and for at least two Cluster B disorders (antisocial and borderline). It is not true for narcissistic PD, and the socioeconomic status of those with histrionic PD is equivocal. As for Cluster C disorders, avoidant and dependent

PDs imply poorer socioeconomic status, whereas the opposite is true for obsessive-compulsive PD. Only one study (Torgersen et al. 2001) examined the provisional disorders, and this study suggested lower education for those with self-defeating and sadistic, but not passive-aggressive, PDs.

Urban Location

The study of Torgersen et al. (2001) showed that persons living in the populated center of the city (in this case, Oslo) more often had PDs than those in less populated areas. The same was true for all clusters of PDs and all specific disorders except antisocial, sadistic, avoidant, and dependent PDs. In Wave 1 of the NESARC, Grant et al. (2004) found this to be true for paranoid and avoidant PDs but not for antisocial, histrionic, schizoid, dependent, or obsessive-compulsive PDs. No difference was found for schizotypal (Pulay et al. 2009), borderline (Grant et al. 2008), or narcissistic (Stinson et al. 2008) PDs in Wave 2. The Norwegian and American studies agree that paranoid PD, but not antisocial and dependent PDs, is related to urbanicity. They disagree about schizoid, schizotypal, borderline, histrionic, narcissistic, avoidant, and obsessive-compulsive PDs.

Quality of life is generally lower in the center of the city (Cramer et al. 2004), and there is a higher rate of symptom disorders in the city or in the center of the city (Kringlen et al. 2001; Lewis and Booth 1992, 1994; Marcelis et al. 1998; Sundquist et al. 2004; van Os et al. 2001). One reason may be that the concentrated urban life creates stress, leading to PDs. Another reason may be that individuals with personality problems drift to cities, where they can lead anonymous lives. A third explanation may be that less social control in cities simply makes it easier to express less socially acceptable aspects of one's personality. Historically, it was believed that excessive social control creates mental problems. Perhaps social control hinders the development of accentuated eccentric, narcissistic, and impulsive personality styles.

Quality of Life and Dysfunction

Central to the definition of PDs are the interpersonal problems, reduced well-being, and dysfunction that individuals with PDs experience. In the sample studied by Torgersen et al. (2001), quality of life was assessed by interview and included the following aspects: subjective well-being, self-realization, relation to friends, social support, negative life events, relation to family of origin, and neighborhood quality (published in Cramer et al. 2003, 2006, 2007). All aspects were integrated in a global quality-of-life index.

PDs turned out to be more strongly related to quality of life than were Axis I mental disorders, somatic health, or any other socioeconomic, demographic, or life situation variable (Cramer et al. 2007). Among the specific PDs, avoidant PD was most strongly related to poor quality of life after the researchers controlled for all the aforementioned variables. Next came schizotypal, then paranoid, schizoid, borderline, dependent, and antisocial PDs, followed by narcissistic and self-defeating PDs to a lesser degree. Histrionic, obsessive-compulsive, and passive-aggressive PDs were unrelated to quality of life. It may be surprising that borderline PD was not more strongly related to reduced quality of life; the reason for this is that the disorder is related to a number of other variables that are related to quality of life. Hence, the variables become weaker in a multiple regression analysis.

Cramer et al. (2003) created a dysfunction index by combining quality of life (reversed); the answer to the Structured Interview for DSM-III Personality Disorders—Revised question "Do you feel that the way you usually deal with people and handle situations causes you problems?"; the number of lifetime Axis I diagnoses; and any incidence of seeking treatment with varying degrees of seriousness, from private psychologists and psychiatrists—via outpatient and inpatient clinics—to psychiatric hospitals. The dysfunction index was related to PD, much as the global quality-of-life index was. The only differences found in comparing results derived from the dysfunction index with those from the global quality-of-life index were that those persons with borderline, histrionic, dependent, or self-defeating PD appeared more dysfunctional, and those persons with antisocial PD appeared less dysfunctional. The reason for the differences is mainly that individuals with borderline, histrionic, dependent, and self-defeating PDs are more likely to seek treatment, and those with antisocial PD are less likely to seek treatment.

However, the most important result in the Cramer et al. (2003, 2006, 2007) study was that for both quality of life and dysfunction, there was a perfect linear dose-response relationship to number of criteria fulfilled for all PDs together and to the number of criteria fulfilled for any specific PD. Thus, if a person has one criterion fulfilled for one or another PD, his or her quality of life is lower and dysfunction is higher than among those with no criteria fulfilled. Those with two criteria fulfilled for one or more specific disorders have more problems than those with one, those with three criteria have more problems than those with two, and so on. In other words, when persons with zero criteria on all disorders were grouped together—that is, those with a maximum of one criterion on any specific disorder, those with a maximum of two, and so on—the relationship to global quality of life and dysfunction was perfectly linear (Figures 6–1 and 6–2). This result means that there are no arguments for any specific number of criteria to define a PD if one uses quality of life or dysfunction as validation variables. There is no natural cutoff point. These results are consistent with those of Hopwood et al. (2011), who found that a general dimension of severity of personality pathology based on counts of criteria met was the single strongest determinant of current and prospective (3-year) psychosocial dysfunction. In DSM-5 Section III, the Level of Personality Functioning Scale measures the overall severity of impairment in personality functioning on a continuum and is predictive of the presence of a PD, PD comorbidity, and the presence of a severe PD.

A high level of dysfunction and disability was also observed among individuals with schizotypal PD, followed by borderline and avoidant PDs, in a large-scale multicenter study (Skodol et al. 2002). It was also observed in this study that individuals with obsessive-compulsive PD showed much less disability than individuals with other types of PD, even though they had severe impairment in at least one area of functioning. Applying dimensional representation of PDs gave the same order of dysfunction (Skodol et al. 2005b).

In another study, Ullrich et al. (2007) found that obsessive-compulsive PD was not related to poor functioning—in fact, it was quite the opposite. Also, histrionic PD was positively related to "status and wealth," whereas narcissistic and paranoid PDs were

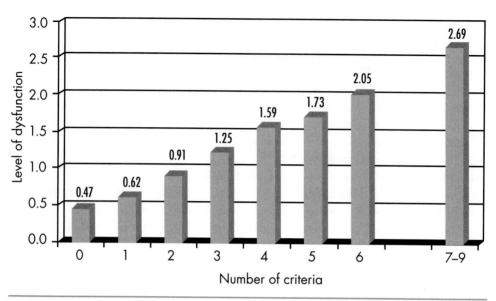

FIGURE 6–1. Relationship between maximum number of criteria fulfilled on any personality disorder and dysfunction.

As explained in the text, the ordinate (dysfunction) is a composite of life quality (reversed), treatment seeking, the number of lifetime Axis I diagnoses, and the notion that one's behavior causes problems. The mean and standard deviation are 1.

unrelated to this index, as well as to "successful intimate relationships." Taken together, individuals with schizoid PD scored poorest on these two indexes, followed by those with antisocial, schizotypal, avoidant, borderline, and dependent PDs.

Zimmerman and Coryell (1989) also found a high frequency of psychosexual dysfunction among persons with avoidant PD. Surprisingly, this dysfunction was infrequent among persons with borderline PD; not surprisingly, it was also infrequent among those with antisocial PD.

Grant et al. (2004) applied a short form of a quality-of-life assessment, the 12-item Short Form Health Survey, Version 2 (SF-12v2; Ware et al. 2002), in NESARC Wave 1 and found that individuals with dependent PD had the poorest quality of life, followed by those with avoidant, paranoid, schizoid, or antisocial PD. There was no reduction in quality of life for those with histrionic PD and a reduction on only one of three scores for those with obsessive-compulsive PD. The mental disability part of the same SF-12v2 was applied in NESARC Wave 2 and showed that individuals with borderline PD displayed a high level of dysfunction, similar to dependent and avoidant PDs in Wave 1 (Grant et al. 2008); those with schizotypal PD were in the middle, similar to paranoid and schizoid PDs in Wave 1 (Pulay et al. 2009); and those with narcissistic PD demonstrated an acceptable functional level, similar to those with antisocial and obsessive-compulsive PDs in Wave 1 (Stinson et al. 2008). Vaughn et al. (2010) looked at the likelihood of receiving public assistance among those with PDs in Wave 1 of NESARC. Public assistance was common among those with paranoid, antisocial, dependent, and avoidant PDs but not for those with histrionic, schizoid, and obsessive-compulsive PDs. Similarly, Knudsen et al. (2012) found that those with borderline, dependent, and schizotypal PDs were most likely to receive disability benefits.

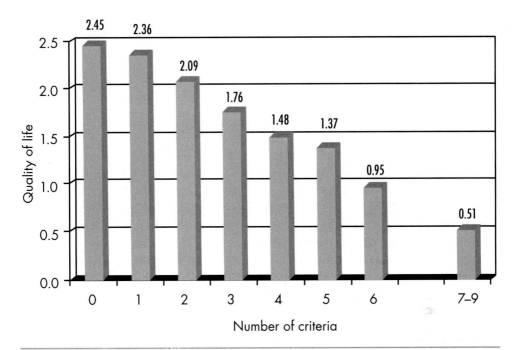

FIGURE 6–2.   Relationship between maximum number of criteria fulfilled on any personality disorder and quality of life.

As explained in text, the ordinate (quality of life) is a composite of subjective well-being, self-realization, social support, negative life events, and relationship with family, friends, and neighbors. The mean is set to 2, and the standard deviation is 1.

Those with avoidant, narcissistic, schizoid, and obsessive-compulsive PDs followed, whereas those with antisocial and histrionic PDs were not more likely to receive disability benefits than people without PDs in the United Kingdom.

Crawford et al. (2005) studied impairment using the Global Assessment of Functioning scale. Subjects with borderline PD had the poorest functioning, followed by those with avoidant, schizotypal, narcissistic, antisocial, paranoid, histrionic, dependent, and schizoid PDs. Only those with obsessive-compulsive PD had no indication of dysfunction.

Skodol (2018) recently reviewed clinical and community-based studies of the relationship between personality pathology and psychosocial functioning, especially referring to the Alternative DSM-5 Model for Personality Disorders (AMPD). Personality disorders have been found to impair social, occupational, leisure, and global functioning more than major depressive disorder. Impairment has been found in clinical and community populations and is independent of co-occurring other mental disorders. Impairment is more stable over time than are PD diagnoses themselves. Personality traits are also impairing and are predictive of outcomes over time, but a hybrid of personality disorder features and normal range personality traits may be the most predictive model. A general, "transdiagnostic," self-other severity factor may be important for understanding the relationship of personality pathology and psychosocial functioning over time. The AMPD may be useful for the study and understanding of psychosocial functioning in individuals with personality pathology.

An older Danish registry study found that individuals who had received a diagnosis of PD were more likely to be a victim of homicide, to die by suicide, and, to a lesser degree, to die by accidents, compared with people with diagnoses of 10 other categories of mental disorders (Hiroeh et al. 2001). Only individuals with drug use, alcoholism, and organic psychoses (psychoses associated with CNS syphilis, epilepsy, or other physical illness) were more vulnerable.

Generally, few recent studies of dysfunction among individuals with PDs have looked at specific PDs. In conclusion, all studies taken together show that reduced quality of life and dysfunction are highest among persons with avoidant PD, followed closely by those with schizotypal and borderline PDs. Those with paranoid, schizoid, dependent, and antisocial PDs follow. There are few studies showing impaired quality of life for persons with histrionic, narcissistic, or obsessive-compulsive PD. The same is true for the quality of life of persons with the provisional passive-aggressive, self-defeating, and sadistic PDs.

There is reason to question, on the basis of quality-of-life and dysfunction studies, whether histrionic and obsessive-compulsive PDs, in spite of their long histories, deserve their status as PDs. Narcissistic PD was not included in ICD-10 (World Health Organization 1992), which some would view as a wise decision. All 10 of the DSM-IV PDs have been retained as specific disorders in DSM-5, although in the AMPD, histrionic, paranoid, schizoid, and dependent PDs may be diagnosed as *personality disorder—trait specified*. On the basis of the studies of dysfunction and quality of life, deemphasizing histrionic PD in the AMPD seems reasonable. Demoting paranoid, schizoid, and dependent PDs as specific PDs in the AMPD while keeping obsessive-compulsive and narcissistic PDs may be questioned according to the research on dysfunction and quality of life. As mentioned previously in the section "Sociodemographic Correlates," there has been insufficient evidence for retaining as full-fledged disorders the DSM-III-R and DSM-IV provisional disorders "provided for further study," but personality traits consistent with those descriptions may be specified by the AMPD. (See also Chapter 4, "The Alternative DSM-5 Model for Personality Disorders," in this volume for a more detailed discussion of the rationale for retaining specific PDs in the alternative model.)

Conclusion

There is a linear reduction in quality of life and a linear increase in dysfunction for each additional PD criterion manifested. Thus, people exist on a continuum from those with no or small personality problems to those with moderate problems and those with severe problems. No natural cutoff point exists. Any definition of how many criteria are required for a PD to be diagnosed is arbitrary. Even so, having a definition is important for communication. However, a change in criteria will immediately change the prevalence estimates of a PD. Consequently, correlations between PDs and other variables are more important than prevalence rates. These correlations appear to be independent of how strictly PDs are defined.

Because of the continuous nature of PDs, their tendency to disappear, and the even distribution of point prevalence over age, then new PDs must necessarily have an onset over the life span, in order to keep those prevalence rates steady. Consequently, the likelihood of having a PD once in the lifetime may be surprisingly high.

Epidemiological research has perhaps changed some stereotypical notions about PDs; for example, borderline PD is not a "female disorder." PDs are more frequent in the general population than we generally believed, especially the introverted PDs. Living without a partner is a risk factor for PDs, but being unmarried is less a risk factor than many would have believed. People living in a partnership without being married function well.

Care must be taken to avoid believing that correlations display one-directional causal relationships. PDs may hinder obtaining higher levels of education and may create socioeconomic difficulties. Problematic personality traits may prevent a person from going into a relationship or may lead to the breaking up of relationships, rather than relationship issues and problems being the cause of problematic personality traits. Poor quality of life may be a consequence just as much as a cause of PDs. Future genetically informative, longitudinal epidemiological studies may disclose the causal pathways and hence increase our understanding of this important group of mental disorders.

References

Alnæs R, Torgersen S: DSM-III symptom disorders (Axis I) and personality disorders (Axis II) in an outpatient population. Acta Psychiatr Scand 78:348–355, 1988

American Psychiatric Association: Diagnostic and Statistical Manual of Mental Disorders, 3rd Edition. Washington, DC, American Psychiatric Association, 1980

American Psychiatric Association: Diagnostic and Statistical Manual of Mental Disorders, 3rd Edition, Revised. Washington, DC, American Psychiatric Association, 1987

American Psychiatric Association: Diagnostic and Statistical Manual of Mental Disorders, 4th Edition. Washington, DC, American Psychiatric Association, 1994

American Psychiatric Association: Diagnostic and Statistical Manual of Mental Disorders, 5th Edition. Arlington, VA, American Psychiatric Association, 2013

Barnow S, Stopsack M, Ulrich I, et al: Prevalence and familiarity of personality disorders in Deutschland: results of the Greifswald family study (in German). Psychother Psychosom Med Psychol 60:334–341, 2010

Carter JD, Joyce PR, Mulder RT, et al: Gender differences in the frequency of personality disorders in depressed outpatients. J Pers Disord 13:67–74, 1999

Coid J, Yang M, Tyrer P, et al: Prevalences and correlates of personality disorder in Great Britain. Br J Psychiatry 188:423–431, 2006

Cramer V, Torgersen S, Kringlen E: Personality disorders, prevalence, sociodemographic correlations, quality of life, dysfunction, and the question of continuity. Persønlichkeitsstørungen Theorie und Therapie 7:189–198, 2003

Cramer V, Torgersen S, Kringlen E: Quality of life in a city: the effect of population density. Soc Indic Res 69:103–116, 2004

Cramer V, Torgersen S, Kringlen E: Personality disorders and quality of life: a population study. Compr Psychiatry 47:178–184, 2006

Cramer V, Torgersen S, Kringlen E: Sociodemographic conditions, subjective somatic health, Axis I disorders and personality disorders in the common population: the relationship to quality of life. J Pers Disord 21:552–567, 2007

Crawford TN, Cohen P, Johnson JG, et al: Self-reported personality disorder in the Children in the Community sample: convergent and prospective validity in late adolescence and adulthood. J Pers Disord 19:30–52, 2005

Durbin EC, Klein DN: Ten-year stability of personality disorders among outpatients with mood disorders. J Abnorm Psychol 115:75–84, 2006

Engels GI, Duijsens IJ, Harrigma R, et al: Personality disorders in the elderly compared to four younger age groups: a cross-sectional study of community residents and mental health patients. J Pers Disord 17:447–459, 2003

Ferro T, Klein DN, Schwartz JE, et al: 30-month stability of personality disorder diagnoses in depressed outpatients. Am J Psychiatry 155:653–659, 1998

Fossati A, Feeney JA, Donati D, et al: Personality disorders and adult attachment dimensions in a mixed psychiatric sample: a multivariate study. J Nerv Ment Dis 191:30–37, 2003

Gerhardt A, Hartmann M, Schuller-Roma B, et al: The prevalence and type of Axis-I and Axis-II mental disorders in subjects with non-specific chronic back pain: results from a population-based study. Pain Med 12:1231–1240, 2011

Golomb M, Fava M, Abraham M, et al: Gender differences in personality disorders. Am J Psychiatry 152:579–582, 1995

Grant BF, Hasin DS, Stinson FR, et al: Prevalence, correlates, and disability of personality disorders in the United States: results from the national epidemiologic survey on alcohol and related conditions. J Clin Psychiatry 65:948–958, 2004

Grant BF, Chou SP, Goldstein RB, et al: Prevalence, correlates, disability and comorbidity of DSM-IV borderline personality disorder: results from the Wave 2 National Epidemiologic Survey on Alcohol and Related Conditions. J Clin Psychiatry 69:533–545, 2008

Grant JE, Mooney ME, Kushner MG: Prevalence, correlates, and comorbidity of DSM-IV obsessive-compulsive personality disorder: results from the National Epidemiologic Survey on Alcohol and Related Conditions. J Psychiatr Res 46:469–475, 2012

Grilo CM, Sanislow CA, Gunderson JG, et al: Two-year stability and change of schizotypal, borderline, avoidant, and obsessive-compulsive personality disorders. J Consult Clin Psychol 72:767–775, 2004

Hiroeh U, Appleby L, Mortensen PB, et al: Death by homicide, suicide, and other unnatural causes in people with mental illness: a population-based study. Lancet 358:2110–2112, 2001

Hopwood CJ, Malone JC, Ansell EB, et al: Personality assessment in DSM-5: empirical support for rating severity, style, and traits. J Pers Disord 25:305–320, 2011

Huang Y, Kotov R, Girolamo G, et al: DSM-IV personality disorders in the WHO World Mental Health Surveys. Br J Psychiatry 195:46–53, 2009

Jackson HP, Burgess PM: Personality disorders in the community: a report from the Australian National Survey of Mental Health and Wellbeing. Soc Psychiatry Psychiatr Epidemiol 35:531–538, 2000

Johnson JG, Cohen P, Kasen S, et al: Cumulative prevalence of personality disorders between adolescence and adulthood. Acta Psychiar Scand 118:410–413, 2008

Klein DN, Riso LP, Donaldson SK, et al: Family study of early onset dysthymia: mood and personality disorders in relatives of outpatients with dysthymia and episodic major depressive and normal controls. Arch Gen Psychiatry 52:487–496, 1995

Knudsen AK, Skogen JC, Harvey, SB, et al: Personality disorders, common mental disorders and receipt of disability benefits: evidence from the British National Survey of Psychiatric morbidity. Psychol Med 42:2631–2640, 2012

Kringlen E, Torgersen S, Cramer V: A Norwegian psychiatric epidemiological study. Am J Psychiatry 158:1091–1098, 2001

Lenzenweger MF: Stability and change in personality disorder features: the Longitudinal Study of Personality Disorders. Arch Gen Psychiatry 56(11):1009–1015, 1999

Lenzenweger MF, Loranger AW, Korfine L, et al: Detecting personality disorders in a nonclinical population: application of a 2-stage procedure for case identification. Arch Gen Psychiatry 54:345–351, 1997

Lenzenweger MF, Lane MC, Loranger AW, et al: DSM-IV personality disorders in the national comorbidity survey replication. Biol Psychiatry 62:553–564, 2007

Lewis G, Booth M: Regional differences in mental health in Great Britain. J Epidemiol Community Health 46:608–611, 1992

Lewis G, Booth M: Are cities bad for your mental health? Psychol Med 24:913–915, 1994

Lindal E, Stefansson JG: The prevalence of personality disorders in the greater-Reykjavik area. Laeknabladid 95:179–184, 2009

Maier W, Lichtermann D, Klingler T, et al: Prevalences of personality disorders (DSM-III-R) in the community. J Pers Disord 6:187–196, 1992

Marcelis M, Navarro-Mateu F, Murray R: Urbanization and psychosis: a study of 1942–1978 birth cohorts in the Netherlands. Psychol Med 28:1197–1203, 1998

Moldin SO, Rice JP, Erlenmeyer-Kimling L, et al: Latent structure of DSM-III-R Axis II psychopathology in a normal sample. J Abnorm Psychol 103:259–266, 1994

Pulay AJ, Stinson FS, Dawson DA, et al: Prevalence, correlates, disability and comorbidity of DSM-IV schizotypal personality disorder: results from the Wave 2 National Epidemiologic Survey on Alcohol and Related Conditions. Prim Care Companion J Clin Psychiatry 11(2):53–67, 2009

Samuels J, Eaton WW, Bienvenu OJ III, et al: Prevalences and correlates of personality disorders in a community sample. Br J Psychiatry 180:536–542, 2002

Saulsman LM, Page AC: The five-factor model and personality disorders empirical literature: a meta-analytic review. Clin Psychol Rev 23:1055–1085, 2004

Seivewright H, Tyrer P, Johnson T: Change in personality status in neurotic disorders. Lancet 359:2253–2254, 2002

Shea MT, Stout R, Gunderson J, et al: Short-term diagnostic stability of schizotypal, borderline, avoidant, and obsessive-compulsive personality disorders. Am J Psychiatry 159:2036–2041, 2002

Skodol AE: Personality pathology and psychosocial functioning. Curr Opin Psychol 21:33–38, 2018

Skodol AE, Gunderson JG, McGlashan TH, et al: Functional impairment in patients with schizotypal, borderline, avoidant, or obsessive-compulsive personality disorder. Am J Psychiatry 159:276–283, 2002

Skodol AE, Gunderson JG, Shea MT, et al: The Collaborative Longitudinal Personality Disorders Study (CLPS): overview and implications. J Pers Disord 19:487–504, 2005a

Skodol AE, Oldham JM, Bender DS, et al: Dimensional representation of DSM-IV personality disorders: relationship to functional impairment. Am J Psychiatry 162:1919-1925, 2005b

Srivastava S, John OP, Gosling SD, et al: Development of personality in early and middle adulthood: set like plaster or persistent change? J Pers Soc Psychol 84:1041–1053, 2003

Stinson FS, Dawson DA, Goldstein RB, et al: Prevalence, correlates, disability, and comorbidity of DSM-IV narcissistic personality disorder: results from the Wave 2 National Epidemiologic Survey on Alcohol and Related Conditions. J Clin Psychiatry 69:1033–1045, 2008

Sundquist K, Frank G, Sundquist J: Urbanisation and incidence of psychosis and depression. Br J Psychiatry 184:293–298, 2004

Torgersen S: Epidemiology, in The Oxford Handbook of Personality Disorders. Edited by Widiger TA. Oxford, UK, Oxford University Press, 2012, pp 186–205

Torgersen S, Kringlen E, Cramer V: The prevalence of personality disorders in a community sample. Arch Gen Psychiatry 58:590–596, 2001

Ullrich S, Coid J: The age distribution of self-reported personality disorder traits in a household population. J Pers Disord 23:187–200, 2009

Ullrich S, Farrington DP, Coid JW: Dimensions of DSM-IV personality disorders and life-success. J Pers Disord 21:657–663, 2007

van Os J, Hanssen M, Bijl RV, et al: Prevalence of psychotic disorder and community level of psychotic symptoms: an urban-rural comparison. Arch Gen Psychiatry 58:663–668, 2001

Vaughn MG, Fu Q, Beaver D, et al: Are personality disorders associated with social welfare burden in the United States? J Pers Disord 24:709–720, 2010

Volkert J, Gablonski T-C, Rabung S: Prevalence of personality disorders in the general adult population in Western countries: systematic review and meta-analysis. Br J Psychiatry 213:709–715, 2018

Ware JE, Kosinski M, Turner-Bowker DM, et al: How to Score Version 2 of the SF-12 Health Survey. Lincoln, RI, Quality Metric, 2002

World Health Organization: The ICD-10 Classification of Mental and Behavioral Disorders: Clinical Description and Diagnostic Guidelines. Geneva, World Health Organization, 1992

Zanarini MC, Frankenburg FR, Hennen J, et al: Prediction of the 10-year course of borderline personality disorder. Am J Psychiatry 163:827–832, 2006

Zimmerman M, Coryell W: DSM-III personality disorder diagnoses in a nonpatient sample: demographic correlates and comorbidity. Arch Gen Psychiatry 46:682–689, 1989

Zimmerman M, Coryell WH: Diagnosing personality disorders in the community: a comparison of self-report and interview measures. Arch Gen Psychiatry 47:527–531, 1990

CHAPTER 7

Development, Attachment, and Childhood Experiences

A Mentalizing Perspective

Peter Fonagy, Ph.D.

Anthony W. Bateman, M.A., FRCPsych

Nicolas Lorenzini, Ph.D.

Patrick Luyten, Ph.D.

Chloe Campbell, Ph.D.

This chapter will set out current developmental thinking around the emergence of personality disorder (PD). We will begin with an account of attachment theory, because this has been the touchstone for many developmental accounts of disorder in recent decades. We will then describe recent developments in research and thinking that suggest a multilevel perspective on the emergence of personality pathology. We will maintain that early attachment interactions are central to the development of the child's ability to regulate affect and stress, to mentalize, and to acquire attentional control and a sense of self-agency (Fonagy et al. 2010). It is in the context of attachment relationships that infants develop a robust capacity for mentalizing—the ability to appreciate others', and one's own, subjective dispositional and motivational states. We will suggest that, in addition, early attachment relationships act as a channel through which social and cultural information is intergenerationally transmitted among human beings (Fonagy and Allison 2014; Fonagy et al. 2017). Finally, we will draw attention to the influence of broader environmental and sociocultural factors, as well as biological factors, in the development of PD.

Attachment Theory

Attachment theory (Bowlby 1969) describes how individuals manage their most intimate relationships with their "attachment figures": their parents, children, and romantic partners. Attachment, at an evolutionary level, is an adaptation for survival—it is the mechanism by which babies elicit essential care needed for survival. As more is understood about the interface of brain development and early psychosocial experience, however, it becomes clear that the evolutionary role of the attachment relationship goes far beyond giving physical protection to the human infant (Feldman 2017).

Beginning at birth, the infant's interactions with his or her primary caregivers will form a characteristic pattern that will shape personality development and affect close relationships in later life, as well as expectations of social acceptance and attitudes toward rejection. When the attachment figure responds appropriately to an infant who is undergoing a stressful experience by providing stability and safety, the infant is reassured, confident, and able to explore the surroundings. Through the consistent experience of this reassuring interaction, the child is able to build mental models of self and of others (internal working models), which can often endure across life.

Attachment has traditionally been measured through assessments of characteristic patterns of relating. The most influential protocol for observing individual differences in infants' attachment security has been the Strange Situation (Ainsworth et al. 1978), during which an infant is briefly separated from his or her caregiver and left with a stranger in an unfamiliar setting. Three distinct attachment patterns have been identified in the behavior of infants up to 2 years old: secure (approximately 63% of children tested in nonclinical populations), anxious/resistant or ambivalent (16%), and avoidant (21%). The corresponding attachment styles in adults are secure/autonomous (58% of the nonclinical population), anxious/preoccupied (19%), and avoidant/dismissing (23%) (Bakermans-Kranenburg and van IJzendoorn 2009). The Adult Attachment Interview (AAI; George et al. 1984; Hesse 2016), which is based on reported attachment narratives of the subject's childhood, is the measure used to classify adults' attachment styles. A fourth pattern was later identified and labeled as unresolved/disorganized for adults and disoriented/disorganized for infants (Levy et al. 2011).

During the Strange Situation procedure, a securely attached infant curiously investigates his or her new surroundings in the primary caregiver's presence, appears anxious in the stranger's presence, is distressed by the caregiver's brief absence, rapidly seeks contact with the caregiver when the caregiver returns, and is easily reassured enough to resume exploration and investigation. Analogously, an adult categorized as secure/autonomous during the AAI coherently integrates attachment memories into a meaningful narrative and shows an appreciation for attachment relationships.

An avoidant infant appears less anxious at separation, may not seek contact with the caregiver on his or her return, and may not seem to prefer the caregiver over the stranger. In adults, avoidant/dismissing AAI narratives will seem incoherent; these adults will struggle to recall specific memories in support of general arguments and will idealize or devalue their early relationships (Hesse 2016). These behaviors are the result of a deactivation of the attachment system. The individual will characteristically appear inhibited when it comes to seeking proximity, seem determined to manage stress alone, and tend to adopt noninterpersonal strategies for regulating negative emotions and handling moments of vulnerability.

An anxious/resistant infant shows less interest in exploration and play in the new environment, becomes highly distressed by the separation, and struggles to settle after being reunited with the caregiver. Correspondingly, an anxious/preoccupied adult's AAI narratives will also lack coherence and will express confusion, anger, or fear in relation to early attachment figures. This strategy, entailing the hyperactivation of proximity-seeking and protection-seeking behaviors, is an adaptation to hypersensitivity toward signs of possible rejection or abandonment and to an intensification of undesirable emotions during these moments.

A disoriented/disorganized infant will show undirected or bizarre behavior (e.g., freezing, clapping the hands, or head banging) or may try to escape the situation. An unresolved/disorganized adult's AAI narratives about bereavements or childhood traumas will contain semantic and/or syntactic confusions. This corresponds to the breakdown of strategies to cope with stress, which leads to emotion dysregulation.

Attachment styles are assumed to be associated with enduring strategies for dealing with emotions and social contact. For example, the increased sense of agency in the secure child allows him or her to move toward the ownership of inner experience and toward an understanding of self and others as intentional beings whose behavior is organized by mental states, thoughts, feelings, beliefs, and desires. Consistent with this, longitudinal research has demonstrated that children with a history of secure attachment are independently rated as more resilient, self-reliant, socially oriented (Sroufe 1983; Waters et al. 1979), and empathic to distress (Kestenbaum et al. 1989), and as having deeper relationships and higher self-esteem (Groh et al. 2017; Sroufe et al. 1990). Securely attached individuals trust their attachment figures and do not exaggerate environmental threat; as a result, they can respond proportionately to challenges (Fonagy and Allison 2014; Fonagy et al. 2017; Nolte et al. 2011).

Avoidant/dismissing individuals may have a higher tolerance for experiencing negative emotions, whereas anxious/preoccupied individuals, who tend to be wary following a history of inconsistent support from caregivers, are likely to have a lower threshold for perceiving environmental threat and, therefore, stress. This is likely to contribute to frequent activation of the attachment system, with the concomitant distress and anger such activation can cause being likely to manifest as compulsive care-seeking and overdependency. Unresolved/disorganized individuals—the adult analog of disoriented/disorganized infants—frequently have parents who are themselves unresolved regarding their own losses or abuse experiences.

It should be noted that although there is some evidence of an association between insecure attachment styles—particularly disorganized attachment—and risk of mental health disorder, the association is "relatively weak and probabilistic" (Fearon 2017, p. 31). Insecure attachment styles are not regarded as disorders; they seem to represent understandable adaptations to a given environment and may range from highly adaptive to maladaptive (Belsky et al. 2010; Ein-Dor et al. 2010; Fearon 2017). The two categories of disorder related to attachment—reactive attachment disorder and disinhibited social engagement disorder (American Psychiatric Association 2013)—are different entities and are normally associated with extreme environments such as institutional care (Fearon 2017).

Attachment theory and research have certainly radically extended our understanding of the impact of early relational experiences on children's social and emotional development, and have resulted in a wide body of cross-sectional and longitudinal work indicating the role of sensitive caregiving in the development of secure or insecure attachment styles. This association has been well replicated, but its effect is not large. As one of the foremost attachment researchers has written: "while sensitivity of parenting may be thought of as the most important immediate determinant of attachment security, a host of broader contextual factors also appear to be consistently associated with security and insecurity, including parental depression, social support, marital quality and poverty" (Fearon 2017, p. 31). The approach to the emergence of PD described in this chapter involves a developmental model that integrates the multilayered influences on developmental psychopathology through an emphasis on human sensitivity and responsiveness to cues about the social environment and that environment's richness in collaboration, support, and trust. In the next section, we will review a number of challenges to traditional attachment theory.

Challenges to Attachment Theory

Developmental research increasingly points to the complex, multifactorial nature of human developmental processes, particularly in the field of attachment. Recent research suggests, for example, that evocative person–environment correlations—that is, features of the child that evoke certain responses in the caregivers and in the wider social environment—may contest an environmentalist interpretation of associations between parental behaviors and child outcomes, and offer a primarily genetic account of family influence on development (Klahr and Burt 2014). Such research presents a major challenge for traditional attachment theory, which assumes that the attachment style of the caregivers plays a major role in determining the developmental trajectory of the child (Fraley 2002). Meta-analyses have regularly indicated that contextual factors, such as risk status (e.g., family conflict, parental separation, minority ethnic status, male sex), decrease the correspondence between parents' attachment classifications and those of their children (Verhage et al. 2018).

Overall, developmental research presents four challenges to attachment theory. First, the relationship between childhood attachment status and developmental outcome is weaker than might be expected from some assumptions within traditional attachment theory (Fearon et al. 2010; Groh et al. 2012; Madigan et al. 2013). Second, meta-analyses have suggested that attachment is only moderately stable across development, a finding that contrasts with key assumptions of attachment approaches (Fraley 2002; Pinquart et al. 2013). Although attachment is somewhat more stable in adolescence and adulthood than in childhood (Fraley and Roberts 2005; Jones et al. 2018), meta-analyses have revealed that risk status is typically associated with lower attachment stability (e.g., Verhage et al. 2018). These findings make sense if attachment is seen as an interpersonal strategy to optimize adaptation to a given environment. The stability of attachment therefore seems to be largely a function of the stability of the environment—as has been evidenced by studies in which the dynamic structural relationships among psychological factors, in this case, attachment, environmental factors, and constant factors over time, were modeled on the basis of existing longitudinal studies of attachment (Fraley and Roberts 2005). Third, a meta-analysis (Verhage et al. 2016) found that parental sensitivity, which is regarded as key in the intergenerational transmission of attachment, explained only a small proportion of the variance (effect sizes $r = 0.31$ for secure-autonomous attachment and 0.21 for unresolved attachment) in the association between parent and infant attachment. Parental reflective functioning similarly accounts for only a small proportion of the variance in the intergenerational transmission of attachment (Zeegers et al. 2017). Fourth, while there is clear evidence that infant attachment status is largely governed by the environment, the picture is less clear for older adolescence and adulthood (see Oliveira and Fearon 2019). There is increasing evidence that genes may play an important role in shaping developmental trajectories associated with attachment beyond infancy (Fearon et al. 2014). As Oliveira and Fearon (2019) pointed out, the role of genes may also be less direct and may reflect genetically determined differences in susceptibility to environmental influence (Belsky and Pluess 2013). We return to this in the section below on attachment, mentalizing, and epistemic trust, where we explain in more detail how these challenges have played a major role in changing our view on the role of attachment and PD.

Attachment History and Personality Disorder

Many leading authorities in PD research have linked enduring and persistent dysfunctional adaptation (i.e., personality pathology) to attachment theory and research (Agrawal et al. 2004; Cohen 2008; Gunderson 1996; Levy 2005; Oldham 2009; Steele and Siever 2010; Westen et al. 2006). The endorsement of attachment theory by these authors is understandable and appropriate given a number of characteristics of this theory: 1) its biological basis and universal applicability; 2) its capacity to link early childhood to later patterns of enduring adaptation; 3) its description of patterns of interpersonal relating that are analogous to dispositional characteristics of individuals with PD; 4) its epistemological commitment to an empirical approach alongside an interest in a psychodynamic perspective on development and function; and 5) its helpful framework for focusing psychotherapeutic interventions.

The characteristics, behaviors, and symptoms associated with insecurely attached adults are often manifested by individuals with a PD (Adshead and Sarkar 2012; Lorenzini and Fonagy 2013). Studies of attachment patterns in people with PDs, particularly those in DSM-5 Cluster B (Bender et al. 2001), indicate that such individuals show higher rates of insecure attachment than the general population. Individuals who are diagnosed with borderline PD (BPD) and avoidant PD rarely fall into the secure attachment category (Baryshnikov et al. 2017; Eikenaes et al. 2016; Westen et al. 2006). High levels of preoccupied attachment (reflecting attachment hyperactivating strategies) and disorganized/unresolved patterns of attachment (reflecting the use of both attachment hyperactivating and deactivating strategies) have been found in BPD patients (for a review, see Fonagy and Luyten 2016). Studies have found that 50%–80% of patients with BPD show either or both of those two attachment styles (Agrawal et al. 2004; Barone et al. 2011); this makes sense in light of both the approach-avoidance social dynamics and sensitivity to rejection (preoccupied dimension) and the cognitive-linguistic slippage (incoherent/disorganized dimension) that are evident in patients with BPD.

However, because of the overlap in phenomenology between BPD and patterns of preoccupied and disorganized attachment, these studies are not particularly compelling. Prospective studies showing very high rates of trauma (including complex trauma) in individuals with BPD provide more convincing evidence for hypothesized associations between disruptions in the development of the attachment behavioral system and BPD. One review of 39 prospective studies (covering 24 unique samples) found that exposure to different types of trauma, including emotional abuse, neglect, and physical and sexual abuse, was associated with increased risk of BPD (Stepp et al. 2016). This review also provides support for more recent formulations emphasizing the broader socioecological context in the etiology of BPD, as it found that BPD patients are typically exposed to a broader adverse context characterized by parental psychopathology, lower socioeconomic status, and/or violence.

Although the prevalence of trauma in BPD is often as high as 90% and patients with BPD typically report higher levels of trauma than patients with other PDs (Fonagy and Luyten 2016), genetic factors, including gene-environment correlations and interactions, may also play an important role in the etiology of BPD. BPD has an estimated heritability of 40%–50% (Distel et al. 2008). A study of over 5,000 twins and almost 1,300 siblings found that the unique environmental variance explaining BPD features increased in a linear fashion with the number of traumatic life events to which an individual had been exposed (from 54% with no events to 64% with six events) (Distel et al. 2011). In a nationally representative birth cohort of more than 1,100 families with twins in the United Kingdom, maltreatment was highly associated with BPD symptoms, but only in those with a family history of psychopathology as an index of genetic vulnerability (Belsky et al. 2012). In families with no history of psychopathology, maltreatment was reported by only 7% of individuals with BPD, compared with almost 50% of those with a family history of psychopathology. Hence, consistent with our recent theoretical formulations, vulnerability to BPD is best considered within a multifactorial and socioecological framework (Luyten et al. 2020b).

We suggest that if traumatic events provoke the activation of the attachment system, then individuals who respond to these experiences by inhibiting mentalizing and emotional regulation are less likely to resolve these events and more likely to show personality pathology later in life (Bateman and Fonagy 2019), because the inhibition of mentalizing entails the closure of epistemic channels that are essential for learning from the environment. Even if the environment is benign (nontraumatizing) later in life, the individual's long-standing mentalizing problems will make it difficult for them to learn from new experiences and adapt accordingly (Fonagy and Allison 2014; Fonagy et al. 2015, 2017; Landrum et al. 2015).

Most research assessing the relationship between attachment and PDs does not control for comorbidity, which could result in diffuse patterns of association. For example, in the case of BPD, different symptom disorder comorbidities are associated with different attachment styles: BPD with comorbid anxiety or mood disorders tends to be associated with preoccupied attachment, whereas BPD with comorbid substance or alcohol abuse tends toward a dismissing style (Barone et al. 2011; Westen et al. 2006).

The research limitations examined above accentuate the value of current efforts toward dimensional rather than categorical diagnostic systems (American Psychiatric Association 2013; Cartwright-Hatton et al. 2011; Hopwood et al. 2018; Krueger et al. 2018; Oltmanns and Widiger 2018; Widiger et al. 2011) and toward person-centered rather than symptom-centered ways of addressing mental disorders (Hagan et al. 2016; O'Donnell et al. 2017). Such ways of understanding and conceptualizing psychopathology (particularly PDs) are necessarily longitudinal because only a developmental perspective can offer insight into the processes underlying symptomatic manifestations and allow the therapist to assess a particular patient's risks and strengths, account for high rates of comorbidity, tailor interventions, and maintain a fruitful therapeutic relationship. Following the same line, recent advances in the understanding of comorbidity in general, and in PDs in particular, suggest that the almost ubiquitous presence of comorbidities in mental ill health reflect the presence of a single general psychopathology factor (Caspi and Moffitt 2018; Caspi et al. 2014; Lahey et al. 2017; Sharp et al. 2015). The so-called p factor seems to us to correspond conceptually most closely to a general lack of resilience, which could perhaps be traced back in development to impairments in the capacity to appraise stressful social experiences (Kalisch et al. 2015a, 2015b) due to the incomplete development of mentalizing capacities (Bateman et al. 2018; Borelli et al. 2018; Duval et al. 2018). As we will suggest below, based on a general model of social communication (Sperber et al. 2010), the vulnerability created by dysfunctional social cognition may limit an individual's capacity to learn about the social world from others and to recognize when other individuals or groups are trustworthy as a source of such knowledge (Fonagy et al. 2015; van Harmelen et al. 2017).

The complexity of the evidence reviewed in this section suggests that although early attachment is a significant factor, it is unlikely to constitute the final common pathway in the development of PDs. In the next section, we will develop a social-communicative position on the development of personality pathology. We will suggest that attachment styles are themselves one part of social communication about the most effective way to function in the prevailing culture, which is promoted by the familial context. The instinct for communication should thus be understood as another important element in the pathway between early attachment and other psychosocial experience and PDs.

Communication, Natural Pedagogy, and Epistemic Trust

Communication is considered to be the instinct driving the transmission of knowledge and culture, which gives human beings unique evolutionary advantages. If we were to consider culture as any learned behavior, then human communication would not be distinct from that of other animals—some of which show highly evolved capacities for, for example, cognitive mapping, object characterization, and creative problem solving. Shared social skills, including the recognition of third-party social relationships and the prediction of future behavior, are also characteristic of some primates (Tomasello and Call 1997). However, critically, according to Tomasello (2014), while some primate species have shown the ability to learn some form of human-like communication, some key elements of human communication are missing, namely, "all of those aspects of human grammar that conceptually structure constructions for others and their knowledge, expectations, and perspective" (p. 105). In other words, what makes human communication and learning unique is that they are fundamentally socially constituted and do not consist of purely instrumental signals that function to achieve a desired goal. In humans, learned behaviors are understood as being underpinned by intention. The key feature of human cultural learning is the understanding that others act for internal reasons and, like oneself, have a perspective on the world that may be understood and shared.

These socio-evolutionary findings are relevant for our understanding of the emergence of PD. A child must learn a great deal about the culture in which he or she lives in the first years of life. In order to survive in a given cultural context, the child must rapidly develop knowledge of the properties and uses of tools and symbols that integrate both procedural and semantic information, which must then be generalized—that is, the information must not be restricted to the particular context in which the child has learned it (Gergely and Jacob 2012). Because much cultural information cannot simply be deductively learned, the learner is dependent on the reliability and trustworthiness of those who are communicating that information (Wilson and Sperber 2012). However, in order to assess the reliability of the communicator, the learner must at the same time remain vigilant about the truthfulness of information he or she is receiving. Without this *epistemic vigilance* (Sperber et al. 2010), the learner runs the risk of being misinformed. Taking in knowledge based on authority requires the communication to have certain characteristic features that will lift the natural barrier of epistemic vigilance, encouraging the learner to incorporate the knowledge as something that is known by everyone belonging to his or her group (Gergely and Jacob 2012). These features have been termed *ostensive cues* (Russell 1940; Sperber and Wilson 1995). They form part of the human repertoire of teaching behaviors subsumed under the theory of *natural pedagogy* (Csibra and Gergely 2009). These behaviors are used by an individual (communicator) to alert the addressee (learner) that the individual intends to communicate, and they act as a cue for the reduction of epistemic vigilance in the learner. Human infants display a (species-specific) sensitivity to ostensive cues (Csibra and Gergely 2006, 2009, 2011). They attend preferentially to signals such as eye contact, turn-taking contingent reactivity, and the use of a special vocal tone by the communicator, all of which appear to trigger a special mode of learning in the infant.

By using ostensive cues, the communicator explicitly recognizes the listener (whether a child or adult) as a person with intentionality. When the listener is given special attention in this way, he or she adopts an attitude of *epistemic trust* and is ready to receive personally relevant knowledge about the social world that can be generalized beyond that specific instance. In this way, he or she acquires knowledge about how to manage in the social world more widely.

Csibra and Gergely (2009) summarized several developmental experiments that give powerful support to the theory of natural pedagogy. In one of these experiments, 6-month-olds were shown to follow an adult's gaze shift to an object only if the gaze shift had been preceded by either eye contact with the infant or infant-directed speech (Senju and Csibra 2008). Shared attention with an agent is triggered by the infant experiencing the agent's interest in the infant. The interest triggers the infant's expectation that there may be something relevant for the infant to learn, and facilitates epistemic trust in the agent.

Perhaps the most persuasive understanding about how mentalizing develops is given in an account that centers on collaboration as the essential species-specific attribute of humans (Tomasello 2018). Human sociality is explained by the capacity humans have to share the mental states of others. Tomasello (2018) pointed out that the key to this capacity is being able to coordinate different perspectives and to appreciate the distinction between the subjective (i.e., one's own view) and the objective (i.e., physical reality) and coordinate these with knowledge of another's mental state. We would suggest, as did Tomasello, that a joining of minds is the crucial ingredient of mentalizing. Joint attention defines a common object at the same time as acknowledging that different people have different perspectives on that object. Identifying the potential for difference is the first and necessary step toward the alignment of these perspectives, which is the critical underpinning for human collaboration. Tomasello (2014) identified this process as the creation of a dual-level structure of shared intentionality, which encompasses both a shared focus on something and individual perspectives on the same thing (Tomasello 2016).

If we assume that increasing cooperation was the motivator of selective advantage, it is not surprising that humans developed a skill that immeasurably advanced the capacity for social coordination and communication. Building on joint attention (Liszkowski et al. 2004), humans evolved the capacity for sharing minds—for joining together in a moment of combined attention an awareness of internal states in the self and the other. The feeling of "we-ness" associated with this joint intentionality may be underpinned by—and certainly generates the potential for—social collaboration. In the "we-mode" of social cognition (Gallotti and Frith 2013), the individual has the experience of being part of a set of thoughts and feelings that extend beyond his or her own. This sharing of minds in a collective mode of cognition has been recognized by many writers, including developmentalists (e.g., Tronick 2008), psychoanalysts of most classical schools (e.g., Winnicott 1956), and, increasingly, neuroscientists (e.g., Gallotti and Frith 2013).

Attachment, Mentalizing, and Epistemic Trust

Learning about culturally transmitted and relevant knowledge first occurs in the context of early caregiving relationships. We suggest that secure attachment is created by a system that is capable of generating a sense of safety (as Bowlby [1969] defined) alongside epistemic trust. Secure attachment is not a necessary condition for generating epistemic trust, but it may often be sufficient to do so. In early childhood especially, determinants of secure attachment may be efficient indicators of trustworthiness, identifying an adult's investment in and capacity to equip the child with the most useful cultural know-how.

The biological predisposition of the caregiver to respond contingently to the infant's automatic expressive displays creates the foundation for the infant to acquire further knowledge from that caregiver. During what have been termed "marked mirroring interactions," the caregiver signals their expression of the infant's mental state, that is, gives referential displays through ostensive cueing, to indicate the generalizability of knowledge and to instruct the infant about the infant's own subjective experience (Fonagy et al. 2002, 2007; Gergely and Watson 1996). Marking by the caregiver as part of good-enough mirroring serves as an ostensive cue to the infant that the concurrent mirroring of affect signals by the caregiver is both relevant and generalizable.

In this sense, demonstration of parental sensitivity, which is regarded as key for the transmission of attachment security in infancy, as described earlier in this chapter, may have other functions too. There is good evidence from cross-sectional and longitudinal research that secure attachment is associated with higher levels of mentalizing in childhood. Studies (systematically reviewed in Luyten et al. 2020a) suggest that secure attachment in children fosters both the cognitive components of mentalizing—including joint attention, perspective-taking, and theory of mind—and the affective components, such as emotion processing, empathy, and the use of mental-state language (e.g., Becker Razuri et al. 2017; Claussen et al. 2002; Kobak et al. 2017; Kokkinos et al. 2016; McQuaid et al. 2008; Meins et al. 2008; Troyer and Greitemeyer 2018; Zaccagnino et al. 2015).

The propensity of parents to treat their infant as a psychological agent is similarly known to be conducive to the development of secure attachment in the infant. Zeegers et al.'s (2017) meta-analysis identified 20 effect sizes (total number of participants = 974) examining the impact of parental mentalizing on attachment security and reported a pooled correlation of $r=0.30$ between parental mentalizing and infant attachment. Parental sensitivity and mentalizing together explained 12% of the variance in attachment security. However, sensitivity measured in terms of behaviors did not account for the association between mentalizing and attachment. Similarly, the relationship between sensitivity and attachment remained significant after parental mentalizing was controlled for ($r=0.19$). Thus, sensitivity (observed behaviorally) and parental mentalizing (assessed primarily through verbal reports) appeared to be relatively independent influences on attachment, although a small proportion of the impact of parental mentalizing seemed to be mediated by behavioral sensitivity ($r=0.07$). These observations suggest that there may be two parallel ways in which infants and children establish a sense of joining or being with their caregiver: one physical (indicated by behavioral connectivity) and the other cognitive-affective (driven by verbal indications of mutual understanding).

Studies have also suggested that higher levels of parental mentalizing foster mentalizing in children (e.g., Meins et al. 2002) and adolescents (e.g., Rosso and Airaldi 2016; Rosso et al. 2015). Although associations between parental mentalizing and infant attachment are typically small (with effect sizes, defined in terms of Cohen's d, of 0.20), the association between parental and infant mentalizing is stronger, with medium to large effect sizes (Cohen's $d=0.50$–0.80). Rosso and Airaldi (2016) reported a particularly strong association between mothers' ability to mentalize negative and mixed-ambivalent mental states and the corresponding ability in their adolescent children ($r\approx0.40$–0.50). Findings such as these suggest that caregivers' capacity to reflect on difficult and affect-charged mental states may be particularly important in the context of the intergenerational transmission of mentalizing.

Studies on mentalizing and adversity have provided some of the strongest evidence for the association between caregivers' mentalizing capacities and the development of child mentalizing. Early adversity and complex trauma (i.e., early negative life experiences involving neglect and/or abuse, typically within an attachment/caregiving context) have the potential to severely impair mentalizing, with impairments evident as strongly biased mentalizing, hypersensitivity to the mental states of others, defensive inhibition of mentalizing, or a combination of these features (for reviews, see Borelli et al. 2019; Luyten and Fonagy 2019). There is also increasing evidence that high levels of parental reflective functioning, particularly with regard to the parents' own traumatic experiences rather than generic reflective functioning (Ensink et al. 2017), may be an important buffer in the relationship between early adversity and child outcomes (reviewed by Borelli et al. 2019). For instance, higher trauma-related reflective functioning in parents with a history of being sexually abused and/or neglected in childhood was found to be associated with a lower risk of infant attachment disorganization (Berthelot et al. 2015) and a substantially lower risk of exposure to childhood sexual abuse in their own infants (Borelli et al. 2019).

For infants in highly insecure attachment contexts, this pattern associated with the integrated functioning of the attachment and mentalizing systems may never fully develop. Insecure attachment experiences typically lead to increased vulnerability to stress, expressed in impairments in hypothalamic-pituitary-adrenal axis and reward system functioning, and in the synchronous functioning of the mentalizing and reward systems more generally (Feldman 2017). For individuals with this developmental background, interpersonal relationships are not rewarding and may even be highly aversive. For these individuals, it may be the case that attachment figures were not available, leading to them adopting a dismissive pattern of relating to others, or attachment figures were only intermittently available, leading to the use of hyperactivating attachment strategies to try to obtain love, care, and support, but with an underlying belief that others will not be available to provide these. As a consequence, a pattern of either compulsive autonomy, characterized by downplaying attachment relationships and hyporesponsivity to distress, or excessive seeking of love and care, combined with hyperresponsivity to distress (particularly associated with rejection), arises (Luyten and Fonagy 2015). These ideas may be particularly relevant to our understanding of patterns of relating associated with social isolation and lack of interest in social relationships or, conversely, excessive suspiciousness, which are traditionally linked with PDs from a trait perspective, or from a level of personality functioning perspective, in impairments in self and interpersonal functioning (American Psychiatric Association 2013).

Implications for Personality Disorder

The theory of natural pedagogy explains how knowledge acquisition is smoother for secure infants: it gives a theoretical and analytical underpinning to an understanding of the development of mentalizing and the growth of an agentive sense of self. We suggest that it might also provide a powerful developmental explanation for how key social and interpersonal difficulties of PD might emerge. It is important to understand that the relevance of early attachment experiences is precisely that of facilitating mentalizing to allow understanding of and adaptation to the social world. The role of attachment is by no means unique in the development of PD, but, as we have described in the earlier sections of this chapter, it is one (albeit important) element in a complex chain of causation that ultimately manifests as the rigidity of thought and belief that characterizes PD.

Given that secure attachment may provide a powerful basis for an attitude of confidence in one's own experience and beliefs, children with insecure and disorganized attachment tend to mistrust information from their own experience just as much as information offered by others. These children are then left with an insoluble dilemma about whose information they can trust, which, in our view, lays the groundwork for a potentially interminable search: seeking others to confirm or deny one's own under-standing but then finding it impossible to trust information from others once it has been received. For individuals in this situation, the primary avenue for modifying sta-ble beliefs about the world is closed off. This, in addition to already well-established findings concerning the impact of trauma on the developing stress and emotion reg-ulation systems and socioemotional development more generally, may account for the enduring educational difficulties observed in children who have experienced trauma (Elklit et al. 2018), as well as generic problems in learning from experience (Hanson et al. 2017).

Considering these ideas, early adversity is understood as undermining or even de-stroying the capacity for (epistemic) trust (Allen 2013). Compared with nonclinical controls, individuals with BPD judge faces as being less trustworthy and approach-able, in line with these individuals' experiences of childhood trauma (Nicol et al. 2013). Maltreatment at a formative stage of development may be the most common reason for mistrust. Among individuals with PDs, rates of childhood trauma are high, with 73% reporting abuse (of which 34% is sexual abuse) and 82% reporting neglect (Ball and Links 2009). Specifically, BPD patients are four times as likely as clinically normal controls to have experienced early trauma (Johnson et al. 1999), in particular emotional abuse, neglect, and lack of emotional support (Gratz et al. 2008; Huang et al. 2012; Machizawa-Summers 2007; Specht et al. 2009).

We have thus far in this section, and in the earlier iterations of our thinking on epis-temic trust (Fonagy et al. 2015), largely conceptualized the adversity that is associated with disruptions in epistemic trust in terms of attachment difficulties. More recently, we have come to think of this adversity more broadly, in terms of potentially cumula-tive and interactive combinations of factors that may include attachment (but not nec-essarily), genetic propensity (possibly, in the case of BPD, expressed as a tendency to hypermentalize in adolescence), and the epistemic isolation that may arise from living in a consistently nonmentalizing social environment—examples of which may involve the experience and expectation of violence, discrimination, and persistent hostility or denigration. These experiences are all are at odds with the recognition of psychological agency, which we described earlier in this chapter as being so significant in supporting the development of the capacity to mentalize and stimulating epistemic trust.

In sum, we consider PD as an expression of difficulties in social communication. The apparent rigidity that is characteristic of PD (which has led clinicians to associate it with personality—an enduring psychological structure) may result from the inca-pacity to exercise epistemic trust and thus to learn from social experiences that would enable adaptation to different interpersonal contexts. For these individuals, the regu-lar process for modifying stable beliefs about the world, and about oneself in relation to others, is unavailable.

Rigidity, resulting from unmodifiable epistemic vigilance, is apparent not only in the day-to-day life and relationships of a person with a PD; it is also shown in the clin-ical context. Therapists might reasonably expect patients with PD to modify their be-havior on the basis of information they have received—and that they have apparently understood—during therapy; however, in the absence of epistemic trust, the capacity to change is also absent. Interventions made (information offered) by the therapist are not used by the patient to update his or her social understanding, given that the patient has lost the capacity for learning. From the therapist's standpoint, these patients are interpersonally inaccessible. Patients cannot change because they cannot accept that the information they receive is from a trustworthy source, and therefore it is not experienced as relevant to them and usefully generalizable to other social contexts. It is received episodically and can be remembered as something that happened as part of the process of autobiographical recall, but it is not incorporated into the procedural and semantic systems that govern the individual's behavior in social situations.

Epistemic mistrust is not a lack of interest. On the contrary, we may anticipate what can be thought of as epistemic hunger (an urgent need to seek validation of one's own experience) to be combined with mistrust if an individual experiences uncertainty in relation to personal experience. From the patient's perspective, the situation is associated with an unbearable sense of isolation generated by epistemic mistrust. Therapists' inability to communicate with patients causes frustration and a tendency on the part of the therapist to blame the patient for the failure to communicate: the therapist feels that the patient is just not listening. However, it may be more productive for therapists to think that these patients find it hard to trust the truth and relevance of what they hear. Hence, the apparent rigidity that seems to be characteristic of patients with PD can be thought of not as primarily residing within the person with PD but as describing the relationships the individual with PD has with others, including the therapist.

Nevertheless, there is evidence that various types of psychotherapy can achieve positive changes in people with PD (Bateman and Fonagy 2000; Bateman et al. 2015; Budge et al. 2013; Kliem et al. 2010; Leichsenring and Leibing 2003; Leichsenring et al. 2011; Muran et al. 2005; Winston et al. 1994). (See Chapters 12 through 16 in Part III, "Treatment," of this volume for information on psychotherapies that are effective for individuals with PDs.) If different therapeutic models are effective, it is legitimate to ask whether these therapies work for the reasons their developers suggested. The argument has raged for many years of whether the so-called Dodo Bird Verdict on the effectiveness of psychological therapies could not be most parsimoniously accounted for by a limited number of nonspecific factors that are both common to all therapies and necessary for bringing about change (Budd and Hughes 2009; Mansell 2011): the centrality of the therapeutic relationship (including the establishment of a strong working alliance [see Chapter 11, "Therapeutic Alliance," in this volume], the therapist's attitude of caring, and the agreement between patient and therapist on treatment roles); a clear and credible treatment frame that promotes a sense in the patient that the therapeutic environment is safe and structured, and has clear principles for addressing dimensions of personality pathology; and an intervention that increases the patient's sense of competence, agentiveness, and self-efficacy.

It is noteworthy that the paradigmatic common factor—the therapeutic relationship—has key components that include the therapist's capacity for understanding, the patient feeling supported and cared about, and the establishment of a commonly adopted set of treatment goals, as well as an idea that the alliance is based on a high-quality working relationship. It appears that the therapist's capacity to create a secure attachment relationship with the patient is central to the effectiveness of treatments for PDs, and the mechanism through which this secure relationship is established is the mentalizing capacity of the therapist. It has been demonstrated that the therapeutic process of identifying, acknowledging, and sequencing emotional experiences correlates highly with the reduction of BPD symptoms in patients (Goldman and Gregory 2010). The subjective experience of having another person (the therapist) who has the patient's mind in mind, and the rekindling of the patient's capacity to interpret behavior as being motivated by mental states (both in themselves and in others), bring about therapeutic change.

We propose that change in psychological interventions is the outcome of particular forms of social learning derived from the patient's environment, and that effective treatments are in essence a form of social relearning fostered by changes in what we have conceptualized as three communication systems (Fonagy et al. 2019).

The first communication system, the lowering of epistemic vigilance, refers to the fact that all effective psychological treatments convey a particular model of mind to the patient that feels meaningful and relevant. This often involves the therapist using specific ostensive cues that (ideally) will activate social learning in the patient. The channel for learning is opened to the extent that patients recognize benign intentions and feel recognized as an agent. Their epistemic vigilance lessens, and the corresponding growth of epistemic trust creates the potential for the patient to learn and change. Mutual mentalizing plays a key role in this process: the therapist needs to tailor his or her intervention to the specific patient in a way that demonstrates the therapist's ability to see the patient's problems from the patient's perspective, and the patient needs to be able to recognize this (i.e., there needs to be joint intentionality).

The second communication system, the enabling mechanisms of social learning, is activated by the patient's increase in epistemic trust achieved in the first communication system. Reactivation of the patient's capacity to mentalize is fostered by the background of trust and the patient's experience of therapy; ideally, the patient adopts the mentalizing stance modeled by the therapist. The (re)emergence of mentalizing further facilitates epistemic trust. Hence, while we continue to believe that mentalizing is a common factor in most psychological interventions, we now argue that the aim of therapy is not to increase mentalizing in itself. Rather, increased mentalizing increases epistemic trust and opens up the potential for the patient to learn new skills, acquire self-knowledge, and restructure their internal working models. This new learning enables a virtuous cycle marked by salutogenesis—that is, the capacity to benefit from further positive social influences, both in therapy and in the wider interpersonal world outside treatment.

The third and final communication system consists of reengaging with the social world. Being mentalized by another person (the therapist) frees the patient from his or her state of temporary or chronic social isolation, and (re)activates the capacity to learn in the context of relationships outside therapy. This view implies that it is not just the facts and techniques taught in treatment that are important, but also—and perhaps primarily—that when the patients' capacity for social learning is activated, they may seek new experiences, and the reconstruing of their existing relationships is likely to improve adaptation. The patient is thus enabled to use his or her environment in a different way.

This brings us to a major limitation of most psychotherapies. What happens with clinical interventions with patients whose wider social environment does not support mentalizing? Epistemic trust is helpful only if the social world can be relied upon not to abuse openness, and if it is reliable and worthy of trust. The consolidation of therapeutic gains—and indeed any meaningful improvement in quality of life for the patient—is contingent on the patient's social environment tolerating and supporting the changes in the patient brought about by therapy. It is naive almost to the point of dereliction to assume that the practice of psychotherapy and its potential effectiveness can be isolated from the wider social climate in which it is taking place. An implication of this is that psychological interventions may need to intervene at the level of the social environment—for example, a young person's school environment or an adult's housing situation—when possible or appropriate.

Conclusion

Throughout this chapter we have drawn attention to the way developmental psychology can enrich our understanding of the process of therapy. We have relied heavily on the insights of George Gergely and colleagues, who recognized the evolutionary significance of natural pedagogy, a remarkable aspect of human biological makeup that enables individuals to teach and learn cultural information efficiently, established in the context of the earliest relationships via a mechanism that is made use of throughout life. This mechanism governs individual learning as well as the accumulation of collective understanding, and it motivates the epistemic trust that, we believe, underpins the evolution of culture. While humans are by no means the only species to acquire skills that are then transmitted to the next generation, no other species comes close in terms of the complexity of information that humans are able to learn and impart to sustain individual socialization into a community and to enable that community to have ideas that uniquely define it. For that kind of learning, humans had to go beyond discovery by observation or discovery by trial and error, and evolved a particular mode of knowledge acquisition through receptiveness to deliberate instruction. This mode of learning enables humans to transmit beliefs and expectations based on communal experience. It was for these complex understandings that a special communication process was required, perhaps evolving out of the attachment system, through sensitive responding, to become a way of identifying trustworthy sources of information by a feeling of interpersonal recognition generating the experience of epistemic trust. This mechanism ultimately enables individuals to acquire knowledge about themselves, others, and the wider world. It was probably also a selective advantage for openness to learning from experience to be powerfully moderated by the quality of the relationship between communicator/teacher and child/learner. Negative experiences with a communicator should reinforce natural epistemic vigilance and perhaps create hypervigilance, closing off the possibility of social learning.

The importance of developing epistemic trust in therapy is that it makes it possible for the patient to engage productively in the therapeutic process and to benefit from the process, in terms of learning new ways of being and new ways of understanding other people and themselves. However, this is not the main benefit of developing trust. We assume that enabling patients to be more trusting in relationships *beyond* therapy will help to increase their capacity for social learning more generally.

How does improved mentalizing enhance epistemic trust to enable social learning? There are a number of components that highlight how mentalizing interfaces with epistemic trust, which makes the systematic addressing of mentalizing in therapy so important.

1. The patient needs a minimum capacity for mentalizing to be able to create a narrative that is coherent enough for anyone to be able to discern and respond to it in a manner that could create a sense of joining with the patient.
2. As pointed out above, the process of generating epistemic trust is reciprocal, and epistemic trust must also be created in the therapist by the patient so that the patient's narrative is trusted; for this to happen, the patient must acquire some capacity to mentalize.
3. Further progress in mentalizing is needed for the patient to be able to perceive the therapist's representation of the patient and interpret it accurately.
4. Mentalizing is required for the image of the patient created by the therapist, and the self-image on which it is based, to match. The general aim of enhancing mentalizing will serve the purpose of making the entire process of social learning possible.

Mentalizing is a key part of the therapeutic process because it enhances the ability to learn. It is a generic way of establishing epistemic trust, so that individuals can begin to learn from experience and achieve change in their understanding of the social relationships of which they are a part, and of their own behavior and actions. Having the experience of one's subjectivity being understood is the necessary key to open the individual up to learning—which then has the potential to change the individual's perception of their social world. Teaching people to mentalize better is not psychotherapy; it is a key to accessing a biologically determined method of modifying lasting structures of knowledge about the world. As such, it is part of the process that underpins the transmission of knowledge from generation to generation. It enables individuals to garner knowledge that is relevant to them and to use it across contexts independent of the specific context in which learning took place (i.e., to generalize knowledge acquired in therapy to the world outside the consulting room). The experience of feeling thought about in therapy—that is, of being mentalized by the therapist—makes patients feel safe enough to think about themselves in relation to their social world.

The therapist's ability to see the world from the patient's standpoint opens up the patient's mind by establishing epistemic trust and creating a collaboration. The patient becomes able to trust the social world as a learning environment. This means that perhaps it is not what therapists teach patients in therapy that matters; perhaps the (re-)kindling of the evolutionarily determined capacity for learning from social situations is what generates the most change.

References

Adshead G, Sarkar J: The nature of personality disorder. Adv Psychiatr Treat 18:162–172, 2012

Agrawal HR, Gunderson J, Holmes BM, et al: Attachment studies with borderline patients: a review. Harv Rev Psychiatry 12:94–104, 2004

Ainsworth MDS, Blehar MC, Waters E, et al: Patterns of Attachment: A Psychological Study of the Strange Situation. Hillsdale, NJ, Erlbaum, 1978

Allen JG: Mentalizing in the Development and Treatment of Attachment Trauma. London, Karnac Books, 2013

American Psychiatric Association: Diagnostic and Statistical Manual of Mental Disorders, 5th Edition. Arlington, VA, American Psychiatric Association, 2013

Bakermans-Kranenburg MJ, van IJzendoorn MH: The first 10,000 Adult Attachment Interviews: distributions of adult attachment representations in clinical and non-clinical groups. Attach Hum Dev 11:223–263, 2009

Ball JS, Links PS: Borderline personality disorder and childhood trauma: evidence for a causal relationship. Curr Psychiatry Rep 11:63–68, 2009

Barone L, Fossati A, Guiducci V: Attachment mental states and inferred pathways of development in borderline personality disorder: a study using the Adult Attachment Interview. Attach Hum Dev 13:451–469, 2011

Baryshnikov I, Joffe G, Koivisto M, et al: Relationships between self-reported childhood traumatic experiences, attachment style, neuroticism and features of borderline personality disorders in patients with mood disorders. J Affect Disord 210:82–89, 2017

Bateman AW, Fonagy P: Effectiveness of psychotherapeutic treatment of personality disorder. Br J Psychiatry 177:138–143, 2000

Bateman A, Fonagy P (eds): Handbook of Mentalizing in Mental Health Practice. Washington, DC, American Psychiatric Association Publishing, 2019

Bateman AW, Gunderson J, Mulder R: Treatment of personality disorder. Lancet 385:735–743, 2015

Bateman A, Campbell C, Luyten P, et al: A mentalization-based approach to common factors in the treatment of borderline personality disorder. Curr Opin Psychol 21:44–49, 2018

Becker Razuri E, Hiles Howard AR, Purvis KB, et al: Mental state language development: the longitudinal roles of attachment and maternal language. Infant Ment Health J 38:329–342, 2017

Belsky DW, Caspi A, Arseneault L, et al: Etiological features of borderline personality related characteristics in a birth cohort of 12-year-old children. Dev Psychopathol 24:251–265, 2012

Belsky J, Pluess M: Beyond risk, resilience, and dysregulation: phenotypic plasticity and human development. Dev Psychopathol 25:1243–1261, 2013

Belsky J, Houts RM, Fearon RM: Infant attachment security and the timing of puberty: testing an evolutionary hypothesis. Psychol Sci 21:1195–1201, 2010

Bender DS, Dolan RT, Skodol AE, et al: Treatment utilization by patients with personality disorders. Am J Psychiatry 158:295–302, 2001

Berthelot N, Ensink K, Bernazzani O, et al: Intergenerational transmission of attachment in abused and neglected mothers: the role of trauma-specific reflective functioning. Infant Ment Health J 36:200–212, 2015

Borelli JL, Ensink K, Hong K, et al: School-aged children with higher reflective functioning exhibit lower cardiovascular reactivity. Front Med 5:196, 2018

Borelli JL, Cohen C, Pettit C, et al: Maternal and child sexual abuse history: an intergenerational exploration of children's adjustment and maternal trauma-reflective functioning. Front Psychol 10:1062, 2019

Bowlby J: Attachment and Loss, Vol 1: Attachment. London: Hogarth Press/Institute of Psycho-Analysis, 1969

Budd R, Hughes I: The Dodo Bird Verdict—controversial, inevitable and important: a commentary on 30 years of meta-analyses. Clin Psychol Psychother 16:510–522, 2009

Budge SL, Moore JT, Del Re AC, et al: The effectiveness of evidence-based treatments for personality disorders when comparing treatment-as-usual and bona fide treatments. Clin Psychol Rev 33:1057–1066, 2013

Cartwright-Hatton S, McNally D, Field AP, et al: A new parenting-based group intervention for young anxious children: results of a randomized controlled trial. J Am Acad Child Adolesc Psychiatry 50:242–251.e6, 2011

Caspi A, Moffitt TE: All for one and one for all: mental disorders in one dimension. Am J Psychiatry 175:831–844, 2018

Caspi A, Houts RM, Belsky DW, et al: The p factor: one general psychopathology factor in the structure of psychiatric disorders? Clin Psychol Sci 2:119–137, 2014

Claussen AH, Mundy PC, Mallik SA, et al: Joint attention and disorganized attachment status in infants at risk. Dev Psychopathol 14:279–291, 2002

Cohen P: Child development and personality disorder. Psychiatr Clin North Am 31:477–493, 2008

Csibra G, Gergely G: Social learning and social cognition: the case for pedagogy, in Processes of Change in Brain and Cognitive Development (Attention and Performance Series, Vol XXI). Edited by Johnson MH, Munakata Y. Oxford, UK, Oxford University Press, 2006, pp 249–274

Csibra G, Gergely G: Natural pedagogy. Trends Cogn Sci 13:148–153, 2009

Csibra G, Gergely G: Natural pedagogy as evolutionary adaptation. Philos Trans R Soc Lond B Biol Sci 366:1149–1157, 2011

Distel MA, Trull TJ, Derom CA, et al: Heritability of borderline personality disorder features is similar across three countries. Psychol Med 38:1219–1229, 2008

Distel MA, Middeldorp CM, Trull TJ, et al: Life events and borderline personality features: the influence of gene-environment interaction and gene-environment correlation. Psychol Med 41:849–860, 2011

Duval J, Ensink K, Normandin L, et al: Measuring reflective functioning in adolescents: relations to personality disorders and psychological difficulties. Adolesc Psychiatry 8:5–20, 2018

Eikenaes I, Pedersen G, Wilberg T: Attachment styles in patients with avoidant personality disorder compared with social phobia. Psychol Psychother 89:245–260, 2016

Ein-Dor T, Mikulincer M, Doron G, et al: The attachment paradox: how can so many of us (the insecure ones) have no adaptive advantages? Perspect Psychol Sci 5:123–141, 2010

Elklit A, Michelsen L, Murphy S: Childhood maltreatment and school problems: a Danish national study. Scandinavian Journal of Educational Research 62:150-159, 2018

Ensink K, Begin M, Normandin L, et al: Parental reflective functioning as a moderator of child internalizing difficulties in the context of child sexual abuse. Psychiatry Res 257:361–366, 2017

Fearon P: Attachment theory: research and application to practice and policy, in Transforming Infant Wellbeing: Research, Policy and Practice for the First 1001 Critical Days. Edited by Leach P. Abingdon, UK, Routledge, 2017, pp 28–36

Fearon RP, Bakermans-Kranenburg MJ, van Ijzendoorn MH, et al: The significance of insecure attachment and disorganization in the development of children's externalizing behavior: a meta-analytic study. Child Dev 81:435–456, 2010

Fearon P, Shmueli-Goetz Y, Viding E, et al: Genetic and environmental influences on adolescent attachment. J Child Psychol Psychiatry 55:1033–1041, 2014

Feldman R: The neurobiology of human attachments. Trends Cogn Sci 21:80–99, 2017

Fonagy P, Allison E: The role of mentalizing and epistemic trust in the therapeutic relationship. Psychotherapy 51:372–380, 2014

Fonagy P, Luyten P: A multilevel perspective on the development of borderline personality disorder, in Developmental Psychopathology, Vol 3: Maladaptation and Psychopathology. Edited by Cicchetti D. New York, Wiley, 2016, pp 726–792

Fonagy P, Gergely G, Jurist E, et al: Affect Regulation, Mentalization, and the Development of the Self. New York, Other Press, 2002

Fonagy P, Gergely G, Target M: The parent–infant dyad and the construction of the subjective self. J Child Psychol Psychiatry 48:288–328, 2007

Fonagy P, Luyten P, Bateman A, et al: Attachment and personality pathology, in Psychodynamic Psychotherapy for Personality Disorders: A Clinical Handbook. Edited by Clarkin JF, Fonagy P, Gabbard GO. Washington, DC, American Psychiatric Publishing, 2010, pp 37–88

Fonagy P, Luyten P, Allison E: Epistemic petrification and the restoration of epistemic trust: a new conceptualization of borderline personality disorder and its psychosocial treatment. J Pers Disord 29:575–609, 2015

Fonagy P, Luyten P, Allison E, et al: What we have changed our minds about: Part 2. Borderline personality disorder, epistemic trust and the developmental significance of social communication. Borderline Personal Disord Emot Dysregul 4:9, 2017

Fonagy P, Allison E, Campbell C: Mentalizing, resilience, and epistemic trust, in Handbook of Mentalizing in Mental Health Practice. Edited by Bateman A, Fonagy P. Washington, DC, American Psychiatric Association Publishing, 2019, pp 63–77

Fraley RC: Attachment stability from infancy to adulthood: meta-analysis and dynamic modeling of developmental mechanisms. Pers Soc Psychol Rev 6:123–151, 2002

Fraley RC, Roberts BW: Patterns of continuity: a dynamic model for conceptualizing the stability of individual differences in psychological constructs across the life course. Psychol Rev 112:60–74, 2005

Gallotti M, Frith CD: Social cognition in the we-mode. Trends Cogn Sci 17:160–165, 2013

George C, Kaplan N, Main M: Adult Attachment Interview. Berkeley, Department of Psychology, University of California at Berkeley, 1984

Gergely G, Jacob P: Reasoning about instrumental and communicative agency in human infancy, in Rational Constructivism in Cognitive Development (Advances in Child Development and Behavior Series, Vol 43). Edited by Benson JB, Xu F, Kushnir T. Waltham, MA, Academic Press, 2012, pp 59–94

Gergely G, Watson JS: The social biofeedback theory of parental affect-mirroring: the development of emotional self-awareness and self-control in infancy. Int J Psychoanal 77:1181–1212, 1996

Goldman GA, Gregory RJ: Relationships between techniques and outcomes for borderline personality disorder. Am J Psychother 64:359–371, 2010

Gratz KL, Tull MT, Baruch DE, et al: Factors associated with co-occurring borderline personality disorder among inner-city substance users: the roles of childhood maltreatment, negative affect intensity/reactivity, and emotion dysregulation. Compr Psychiatry 49:603–615, 2008

Groh AM, Roisman GI, van Ijzendoorn MH, et al: The significance of insecure and disorganized attachment for children's internalizing symptoms: a meta-analytic study. Child Dev 83:591–610, 2012

Groh AM, Fearon RMP, van IJzendoorn MH, et al: Attachment in the early life course: meta-analytic evidence for its role in socioemotional development. Child Dev Perspect 11:70–76, 2017

Gunderson JG: The borderline patient's intolerance of aloneness: insecure attachments and therapist availability. Am J Psychiatry 153:752–758, 1996

Hagan MJ, Sulik MJ, Lieberman AF: Traumatic life events and psychopathology in a high risk, ethnically diverse sample of young children: a person-centered approach. J Abnorm Child Psychol 44:833–844, 2016

Hanson JL, van den Bos W, Roeber BJ, et al: Early adversity and learning: implications for typical and atypical behavioral development. J Child Psychol Psychiatry 58:770–778, 2017

Hesse E: The Adult Attachment Interview: protocol, method of analysis, and selected empirical studies: 1985-2015, in Handbook of Attachment. Edited by Cassidy J, Shaver PR. New York, Guilford, 2016, pp 553–597

Hopwood CJ, Kotov R, Krueger RF, et al: The time has come for dimensional personality disorder diagnosis. Personal Ment Health 12:82–86, 2018

Huang J, Yang Y, Wu J, et al: Childhood abuse in Chinese patients with borderline personality disorder. J Pers Disord 26:238–254, 2012

Johnson JG, Cohen P, Brown J, et al: Childhood maltreatment increases risk for personality disorders during early adulthood. Arch Gen Psychiatry 56:600–606, 1999

Jones JD, Fraley RC, Ehrlich KB, et al: Stability of attachment style in adolescence: an empirical test of alternative developmental processes. Child Dev 89:871–880, 2018

Kalisch R, Muller MB, Tüscher O: Advancing empirical resilience research. Behav Brain Sci 38:e128, 2015a

Kalisch R, Muller MB, Tüscher O: A conceptual framework for the neurobiological study of resilience. Behav Brain Sci 38:e92, 2015b

Kestenbaum R, Farber E, Sroufe LA: Individual differences in empathy among preschoolers' concurrent and predictive validity, in Empathy and Related Emotional Responses: New Directions for Child Development. Edited by Eisenberg N. San Francisco, Jossey-Bass, 1989, pp 51–56

Klahr AM, Burt SA: Elucidating the etiology of individual differences in parenting: a meta-analysis of behavioral genetic research. Psychol Bull 140:544–586, 2014

Kliem S, Kroger C, Kosfelder J: Dialectical behavior therapy for borderline personality disorder: a meta-analysis using mixed-effects modeling. J Consult Clin Psychol 78:936–951, 2010

Kobak R, Zajac K, Abbott C, et al: Atypical dimensions of caregiver–adolescent interaction in an economically disadvantaged sample. Dev Psychopathol 29:405–416, 2017

Kokkinos CM, Kakarani S, Kolovou D: Relationships among shyness, social competence, peer relations, and theory of mind among pre-adolescents. Soc Psychol Educ 19:117–133, 2016

Krueger RF, Kotov R, Watson D, et al: Progress in achieving quantitative classification of psychopathology. World Psychiatry 17:282–293, 2018

Lahey BB, Krueger RF, Rathouz PJ, et al: Validity and utility of the general factor of psychopathology. World Psychiatry 16:142–144, 2017

Landrum AR, Eaves BS Jr, Shafto P: Learning to trust and trusting to learn: a theoretical framework. Trends Cogn Sci 19:109–111, 2015

Leichsenring F, Leibing E: The effectiveness of psychodynamic therapy and cognitive behavior therapy in the treatment of personality disorders: a meta-analysis. Am J Psychiatry 160:1223–1232, 2003

Leichsenring F, Leibing E, Kruse J, et al: Borderline personality disorder. Lancet 377:74–84, 2011

Levy KN: The implications of attachment theory and research for understanding borderline personality disorder. Dev Psychopathol 17:959–986, 2005

Levy KN, Ellison WD, Scott LN, et al: Attachment style. J Clin Psychol 67:193–203, 2011

Liszkowski U, Carpenter M, Henning A, et al: Twelve-month-olds point to share attention and interest. Dev Sci 7:297–307, 2004

Lorenzini N, Fonagy P: Attachment and personality disorders: a short review. FOCUS 11:155–166, 2013

Luyten P, Fonagy P: The neurobiology of mentalizing. Personal Disord 6:366–379, 2015

Luyten P, Fonagy P: Mentalizing and trauma, in Handbook of Mentalizing in Mental Health Practice. Edited by Bateman A, Fonagy P. Washington, DC, American Psychiatric Association Publishing, 2019, pp 79–99

Luyten P, Campbell C, Allison E, et al: The mentalizing approach to psychopathology: state of the art and future directions. Annu Rev Clin Psychol 16:297–325, 2020a

Luyten P, Campbell C, Fonagy P: Borderline personality disorder, complex trauma, and problems with self and identity: a social-communicative approach. J Pers 88:88–105, 2020b

Machizawa-Summers S: Childhood trauma and parental bonding among Japanese female patients with borderline personality disorder. Int J Psychol 42:265–273, 2007

Madigan S, Atkinson L, Laurin K, et al: Attachment and internalizing behavior in early childhood: a meta-analysis. Dev Psychol 49:672–689, 2013

Mansell W: Core processes of psychopathology and recovery: "Does the Dodo bird effect have wings?" Clin Psychol Rev 31:189–192, 2011

McQuaid N, Bigelow AE, McLaughlin J, et al: Maternal mental state language and preschool children's attachment security: relation to children's mental state language and expressions of emotional understanding. Soc Dev 17:61–83, 2008

Meins E, Fernyhough C, Wainwright R, et al: Maternal mind-mindedness and attachment security as predictors of theory of mind understanding. Child Dev 73:1715–1726, 2002

Meins E, Harris-Waller J, Lloyd A: Understanding alexithymia: associations with peer attachment style and mind-mindedness. Pers Individ Dif 45:146–152, 2008

Muran JC, Safran JD, Samstag LW, et al: Evaluating an alliance-focused treatment for personality disorders. Psychotherapy 42:532–545, 2005

Nicol K, Pope M, Sprengelmeyer R, et al: Social judgement in borderline personality disorder. PLoS One 8:e73440, 2013

Nolte T, Guiney J, Fonagy P, et al: Interpersonal stress regulation and the development of anxiety disorders: an attachment-based developmental framework. Front Behav Neurosci 5:55, 2011

O'Donnell ML, Schaefer I, Varker T, et al: A systematic review of person-centered approaches to investigating patterns of trauma exposure. Clin Psychol Rev 57:208–225, 2017

Oldham JM: Borderline personality disorder comes of age. Am J Psychiatry 166:509–511, 2009

Oliveira P, Fearon P: The biological bases of attachment. Adopt Foster 43:274–293, 2019

Oltmanns JR, Widiger TA: A self-report measure for the ICD-11 dimensional trait model proposal: the personality inventory for ICD-11. Psychol Assess 30:154–169, 2018

Pinquart M, Feussner C, Ahnert L: Meta-analytic evidence for stability in attachments from infancy to early adulthood. Attach Hum Dev 15:189–218, 2013

Rosso AM, Airaldi C: Intergenerational transmission of reflective functioning. Front Psychol 7:1903, 2016

Rosso AM, Viterbori P, Scopesi AM: Are maternal reflective functioning and attachment security associated with preadolescent mentalization? Front Psychol 6:1134, 2015

Russell B: An Inquiry into Meaning and Truth. London, Allen & Unwin, 1940

Senju A, Csibra G: Gaze following in human infants depends on communicative signals. Curr Biol 18:668–671, 2008

Sharp C, Wright AG, Fowler JC, et al: The structure of personality pathology: both general ("g") and specific ("s") factors? J Abnorm Psychol 124:387–398, 2015

Specht MW, Chapman A, Cellucci T: Schemas and borderline personality disorder symptoms in incarcerated women. J Behav Ther Exp Psychiatry 40:256–264, 2009

Sperber D, Wilson D: Relevance: Communication and Cognition, 2nd Edition. Malden, MA, Blackwell, 1995

Sperber D, Clement F, Heintz C, et al: Epistemic vigilance. Mind and Language 25:359–393, 2010

Sroufe LA: Infant-caregiver attachment and patterns of adaptation in preschool: the roots of maladaption and competence, in Development and Policy Concerning Children With Special Needs (Minnesota Symposium in Child Psychology, Vol 16). Edited by Perimutter M. Hillsdale, NJ, Erlbaum, 1983, pp 41–81

Sroufe LA, Egeland B, Kreutzer T: The fate of early experience following developmental change: longitudinal approaches to individual adaptation in childhood. Child Dev 61:1363–1373, 1990

Steele H, Siever L: An attachment perspective on borderline personality disorder: advances in gene-environment considerations. Curr Psychiatry Rep 12:61–67, 2010

Stepp SD, Lazarus SA, Byrd AL: A systematic review of risk factors prospectively associated with borderline personality disorder: taking stock and moving forward. Personal Disord 7:316–323, 2016

Tomasello M: A Natural History of Human Thinking. Cambridge, MA, Harvard University Press, 2014

Tomasello M: A Natural History of Human Morality. Cambridge, MA, Harvard University Press, 2016

Tomasello M: How children come to understand false beliefs: a shared intentionality account. Proc Natl Acad Sci USA 115:8491–8498, 2018

Tomasello M, Call J: Primate Cognition. Oxford, UK, Oxford University Press, 1997

Tronick EZ: Emotional connections and dyadic consciousness in infant-mother and patient-therapist interactions: commentary on paper by Frank M. Lachmann. Psychoanal Dial 11:187–194, 2008

Troyer D, Greitemeyer T: The impact of attachment orientations on empathy in adults: considering the mediating role of emotion regulation strategies and negative affectivity. Pers Individ Dif 122:198–205, 2018

van Harmelen A-L, Kievit RA, Ioannidis K, et al: Adolescent friendships predict later resilient functioning across psychosocial domains in a healthy community cohort. Psychol Med 47:2312–2322, 2017

Verhage ML, Schuengel C, Madigan S, et al: Narrowing the transmission gap: a synthesis of three decades of research on intergenerational transmission of attachment. Psychol Bull 142:337–366, 2016

Verhage ML, Fearon RMP, Schuengel C, et al: Examining ecological constraints on the intergenerational transmission of attachment via individual participant data meta-analysis. Child Dev 89:2023–2037, 2018

Waters E, Wippman J, Sroufe LA: Attachment, positive affect, and competence in the peer group: two studies in construct validation. Child Dev 50:821–829, 1979

Westen D, Nakash O, Thomas C, et al: Clinical assessment of attachment patterns and personality disorder in adolescents and adults. J Consult Clin Psychol 74:1065–1085, 2006

Widiger TA, Huprich S, Clarkin J: Proposals for DSM-5: introduction to special section of Journal of Personality Disorders. J Pers Disord 25:135, 2011

Wilson D, Sperber D: Meaning and Relevance. Cambridge, UK, Cambridge University Press, 2012

Winnicott DW: Mirror role of mother and family in child development, in Playing and Reality. London, Tavistock, 1956, pp 111–118

Winston A, Laikin M, Pollack J, et al: Short-term psychotherapy of personality disorders. Am J Psychiatry 151:190–194, 1994

Zaccagnino M, Cussino M, Preziosa A, et al: Attachment representation in institutionalized children: a preliminary study using the Child Attachment Interview. Clin Psychol Psychother 22:165–175, 2015

Zeegers MAJ, Colonnesi C, Stams GJM, et al: Mind matters: a meta-analysis on parental mentalization and sensitivity as predictors of infant-parent attachment. Psychol Bull 143:1245–1272, 2017

CHAPTER 8

Genetics and Neurobiology

Sharely Fred Torres, M.D.

M. Mercedes Perez-Rodriguez, M.D., Ph.D.

Antonia S. New, M.D.

Daniel R. Rosell, M.D., Ph.D.

Harold W. Koenigsberg, M.D.

Since 1980, there has been a rapid explosion in knowledge regarding the neurobiology of brain substrates of the severe personality disorders. Once conceived solely in traditional psychodynamic or behavioral terms, these disorders are increasingly understood as emerging from biological susceptibilities shaped by genetic dispositions in concert with environmental insults. These advancements have stimulated the development of interactional models of the personality disorders ultimately leading to new forms of treatment both in the pharmacological and in the psychosocial treatment arenas. They have also opened the door to the identification and development of possible neurobiological predictors to clinical responses to these treatments.

Personality disorders have been traditionally conceptualized in terms of categories that stem from a long-standing clinical tradition. Of the multiple categories included in versions of the American Psychiatric Association's *Diagnostic and Statistical Manual of Mental Disorders*, the categories of schizotypal, borderline, antisocial, and avoidant personality disorders emerge as having the greatest number of studies of external val-

The authors wish to express their gratitude to Larry J. Siever, M.D., who pioneered the study of the neurobiology of the personality disorders and who has made seminal contributions to the conceptualization of these complex disorders. Larry has been a colleague, mentor, and inspiration to us. His contributions have enabled much of the work described in this chapter.

idators. Complementary to this approach is a dimensional approach consonant with a long tradition in academic psychology of defining personality disorders as continuous dimensions of pathology or as emerging from multiple interactive traits. This latter perspective parallels the approach taken by the National Institute of Mental Health for studying psychopathology—namely, the Research Domain Criteria (RDoC). Both the categorical and dimensional systems are acknowledged in Section III of DSM-5 (American Psychiatric Association 2013), in the Alternative DSM-5 Model for Personality Disorders. Major domains or dimensions of psychopathology that we consider in this chapter include affect or emotion regulation, impulse/action modulation, interpersonal/social cognition, and a dimension of anxiety as related to defenses against its emergence.

The goal of our chapter is to summarize the most salient research on the neurobiology of borderline personality disorder, schizotypal personality disorder, antisocial personality disorder, and avoidant personality disorder, by presenting studies that have examined these personality disorders categorically, as well as studies that have focused on specific dimensions of the disorders. These dimensions capture core features of the disorders, representing intermediate phenotypes known as *endophenotypes*. Endophenotypes are heritable and state-independent and thus present at the onset of illness and independent of symptoms (Gottesman and Gould 2003; Leboyer et al. 1998). Organizing the neurobiological research of personality disorders around core endophenotypes is helpful, since it has been postulated that endophenotypes may even be more closely related to the genotype and biological underpinnings of the disorder than the categorically defined disorder itself (Roussos and Siever 2012; Ruocco and Carcone 2016).

Borderline Personality Disorder

Most research on personality disorders has focused on borderline personality disorder (BPD). BPD is a pervasive illness characterized by emotional intensity and instability, identity disturbance, impulsive and self-destructive behaviors, and unstable interpersonal relationships (American Psychiatric Association 2013).

Epidemiological research estimates that the point prevalence of BPD is on average 1%, with reported ranges from 0.5% to 3.9% in the community population and a lifetime prevalence of 5.9% (Ellison et al. 2018; Grant et al. 2008). Furthermore, BPD affects approximately 12% of psychiatric outpatients and 22% of inpatients (Ellison et al. 2018). As with other personality disorders, BPD is highly comorbid with other disorders, especially substance use disorders (Helle et al. 2019) and mood disorders, including major depressive disorder (MDD) and bipolar disorder (Skodol et al. 2002b). Attempts to study BPD in isolation, by eliminating these confounding disorders, has been a challenge and has been construed as a limitation of existing neurobiological research of BPD. However, it has also been argued that comorbidities are at the core of BPD and that excluding comorbid disorders from BPD research would lead to unrepresentative study samples.

We will review the extensive body of research on BPD first by examining studies that focus on the DSM BPD category per se, and then by examining findings relating to candidate endophenotypes relevant to BPD.

Studies of the Borderline Personality Disorder Category

Genetics of Borderline Personality Disorder

There is strong evidence for the heritability of BPD, with estimates from twin studies varying between 40% and 60% (Distel et al. 2008; Kendler et al. 2008; Torgersen 2009; Torgersen et al. 2000, 2012). A recent study of over a million families, including monozygotic and dizygotic twins, reports a heritability of 46% (Skoglund et al. 2019). Despite ample evidence that the disorder is genetically transmitted, the exact candidate genes are not yet known, partly because genome-wide association studies (GWASs) are scant and those published include small sample sizes (Bassir Nia et al. 2018). Nevertheless, there is preliminary evidence for a number of candidate genes underlying dimensions of BPD that will be discussed in further detail below.

Genome-wide association studies (GWASs) have been critical in the identification of risk alleles of many complex disorders. To date, there have only been two GWASs in BPD, one of which focused not on patients with the full BPD diagnosis but on self-reported BPD traits. The GWAS of almost 1,000 subjects with the categorical diagnosis of BPD identified two genes that might be implicated in the pathogenesis of BPD: the dihydropyrimidine dehydrogenase (*DPYD*) and plakophilin-4 (*PKP4*) genes on chromosomes 1 and 2, respectively. Dihydropyrimidine dehydrogenase is the initial and rate-limiting enzyme in pyrimidine metabolism, and plakophilin-4 is involved in cell adhesion and cytoskeleton organization. It is unclear how impairments in these molecular pathways may confer increased susceptibility to developing BPD. This GWAS also found significant overlap of BPD with bipolar disorder, MDD, and schizophrenia (Witt et al. 2017), providing genetic evidence for the high rates of comorbidities in BPD and supporting the notion that genetic findings so far do not appear to be specific to BPD, but rather likely reflect effects on transdiagnostic dimensions shared by these disorders.

In a genome-wide linkage study with 711 twin pairs, chromosome 9 was found to have the highest linkage peak, compared with chromosomes 1, 4, and 18, which were also implicated in the heritability of BPD (Distel et al. 2008). In a later GWAS of subclinical self-reported BPD traits (affect instability, identity problems, negative relations, and self-harm) based on the Personality Assessment Inventory—Borderline Scale, *serinc5*, on chromosome 5, was implicated in the development of BPD traits (Lubke et al. 2014). *serinc5* plays a role in the synthesis of lipids in the nervous system. While these genetic studies suggest preliminary genetic factors that may relate to the development of BPD traits, it is likely that over time these genetic predispositions interact with episodic and situational circumstances that contribute to the heterogeneous presentation of the disorder (Conway et al. 2018).

Epigenetic Findings in Borderline Personality Disorder

Epigenetics focuses on the impact of the environment on molecular alterations of gene expression. Epigenetic mechanisms that impact gene expression include DNA methylation, histone remodeling, and non-coding RNA silencing. Most epigenetic research in BPD has focused on DNA methylation, which typically reduces expression of genes. Three major studies (Dammann et al. 2011; Teschler et al. 2013, 2016) reported an average 1.2 times greater methylation at CpG sites, and thus reduced gene expression, of candidate neuropsychiatric genes in individuals with BPD compared with healthy controls (HCs). These include the serotonin receptor 2A (*HTRA2A*), monoamine oxidase A and B (*MAOA* and *MOAB*), catechol-O-methyltransferase (*SCOMT*), and the proline-rich membrane anchor 1 (*prima1*) genes, all with key functions in major neurotransmitter systems. However, a limitation of these studies is small sample size.

Several other epigenetic studies in BPD have examined the relationship of trauma, or childhood adversity, to methylation (Groleau et al. 2014; Martín-Blanco et al. 2014; Perroud et al. 2011, 2016; Prados et al. 2015; Thaler et al. 2014). Several of these studies have identified an interaction between severity of childhood trauma and methylation of the NR3C1 promoter of the glucocorticoid receptor gene conferring a greater risk for the development of BPD (Dammann et al. 2011; Martín-Blanco et al. 2014).

Finally, there are emerging data suggesting that epigenetic changes in BPD can be altered by psychotherapy. Perroud and colleagues (2013) reported that in individuals with BPD, dialectical behavior therapy (Linehan 1987), an evidenced-based treatment for BPD, can result in methylation changes in the brain-derived neurotrophic factor gene (*BDNF*), which is involved in neurogenesis (Perroud et al. 2013). This provides evidence that epigenetic correlates in BPD may be altered by treatment.

Gene-Environment Interaction in Borderline Personality Disorder

As it is best understood, contributors to the development of BPD include both biological vulnerabilities and exposure to environmental factors such as childhood adversity (Carpenter et al. 2012; Cattane et al. 2017; Sharp and Kim 2015). The previously mentioned genome-wide linkage study that found evidence for the heritability of BPD to be approximately 40% also found that the environment explained 58% variance in BPD twin cohorts across three countries (Distel et al. 2008). These researchers subsequently performed the largest gene x environment study in BPD to date. This later study of more than 5,000 twin pairs showed that while genes may confer an increased risk for BPD, interestingly, they may also increase the likelihood of exposure to traumatic experiences (Distel et al. 2011). A more recent study that recruited a large sample of more than 1,000 twin, adoptive, and biological families from the community found evidence for both genetic and environmental transmission of BPD, further strengthening the notion that both nature and nurture are critical to the etiology of BPD (Fatimah et al. 2020).

Much of the research highlighting the role of gene-environment interactions in BPD has focused on the hypothalamic-pituitary-adrenal (HPA) axis. Compared with HCs, individuals with BPD have been found to have higher urinary levels of the stress hormone cortisol (Lieb et al. 2004; Southwick et al. 2003; Wingenfeld et al. 2007). A study that assessed the impact of early life stress on the HPA axis similarly identified a heightened cortisol response in female BPD patients who experienced childhood abuse (Rinne et al. 2002). Abnormalities in the HPA axis have been replicated in a genetic association study that found two risk alleles of the FK506 binding protein 5 gene (*FKBP5*), which result in inhibition of glucocorticoid receptor activity, to be more represented in patients with BPD (Martín-Blanco et al. 2016). Cortisol elevations may play a role in BPD patients' fast reaction time to emotional stimuli (Carvalho Fernando et al. 2013), contributing to affective instability in BPD. However, these findings are limited by the high rates of comorbid posttraumatic stress disorder (PTSD) in the BPD cohorts and evidence of shared neuropathological pathways in both of these disorders (Amad et al. 2019). Other gene-environment studies have shed light on the serotonin metabolic pathway. One recent study found evidence for polymorphisms of the gene encoding tryptophan hydroxylase I, which is the rate-limiting enzyme in serotonin synthesis, interacting with child abuse to pose a greater risk of developing BPD (Wilson et al. 2012).

Neural Correlates of Borderline Personality Disorder

A growing literature of anatomical and functional neuroimaging studies of BPD has identified structural and functional anomalies in BPD. Several studies have suggested that the volumes of emotional processing brain regions are altered in individuals with BPD. Patients with BPD have decreased cingulate gray matter and hippocampal volume compared with HCs (Brambilla et al. 2004; Denny et al. 2016; Hazlett et al. 2005; Minzenberg et al. 2008; Nunes et al. 2009; Ruocco et al. 2012; Tebartz van Elst et al. 2003). Smaller left orbitofrontal and right anterior cingulate cortex (ACC) size has also been reported in BPD (Minzenberg et al. 2008; Tebartz van Elst et al. 2003). A decreased volume of the orbitofrontal cortex (OFC) and ACC has been identified in BPD as early as adolescence (Brunner et al. 2010), suggesting that BPD may be a neurodevelopmental disorder. Studies have yielded inconsistent findings with respect to amygdala volumes. This may be due to confounding comorbidities in BPD, namely MDD (Minzenberg et al. 2008; New et al. 2007). Despite these possible confounds, most studies report the amygdala of individuals with BPD to be decreased in size compared to healthy individuals (Kimmel et al. 2016; Nunes et al. 2009; O'Neill and Frodl 2012; Ruocco and Carcone 2016;Ruocco et al. 2012). One study highlighted a gender effect, finding decreased ACC volumes only in males (Soloff et al. 2008). Recent studies have also highlighted unique gray matter findings in frontolimbic circuits and the default mode network (DMN) of individuals with BPD (Aguilar-Ortiz et al. 2020; Yang et al. 2016). A recent study reported that compared with HCs, those with BPD had increased volume of the hypothalamus, which, interestingly, was correlated with a history of childhood trauma in BPD patients (Kuhlmann et al. 2013). Some of the variability in the neuroimaging findings may be the result of the heterogeneity of individuals who met the required five or more of nine criteria for BPD in DSM-IV (American Psychiatric Association 1994).

Finally, a puzzling observation has emerged as neurobiological findings are interpreted in the context of behavioral reports of emotion processing in BPD. One early affective startle study in our lab demonstrated that, as expected, BPD patients exhibited showed an exaggerated physiological response to aversive words compared with HCs (Hazlett et al. 2007). However, surprisingly, the BPD subjects rated these negative words to which they were more physiologically sensitive more neutrally than HCs. Thus, there appears to be a disconnect between neurophysiological response and subjective reports by patients with BPD. A subsequent imaging study showed that BPD subjects had a heightened functional MRI (fMRI) blood oxygen level–dependent (BOLD) amygdala response to positive and negative images, yet a more blunted emotional rating, most pronounced with negatives images (Hazlett et al. 2012b). New and colleagues also reported that BPD patients reported greater difficulty in identifying feelings (alexithymia) than both HCs and individuals with avoidant personality disorder (New et al. 2012). Therefore, measurable neural markers, including imaging and physiologic parameters, may provide a more accurate representation of the underlying emotional reactivity in BPD than do self-reports. Subsequent research in our lab has confirmed that individuals with BPD had high rates of alexithymia on a self-report questionnaire, called the Toronto Alexithymia Scale (New et al. 2012). Heartbeat evoked potentials (HEPs), which are an indicator of cortical processing of bodily systems from the cardiovascular system, have been associated with impaired emotional processing in BPD. One study found that compared with HCs, patients with BPD had reduced HEPs, which negatively correlated with emotion dysregulation (Müller et al. 2015). Given ample evidence that patients with BPD have a lack of emotional awareness, treatments for this population might benefit from a focus on enhancing self-referential processing and self-reflection (Choi-Kain et al. 2016, 2017).

Studies of Candidate Endophenotypes in Borderline Personality Disorder

Specific endophenotypes of BPD may be associated with discrete biological mechanisms. There are three well-studied endophenotypes of BPD that we will consider in detail: 1) affective instability (Nica and Links 2009; Trull et al. 2008), 2) impulsive aggression (Links et al. 1999), and 3) interpersonal disturbances (Gunderson 2007). We organize our review by examining genetic, behavioral, and neural concomitants of each dimension in BPD.

Affective Instability in Borderline Personality Disorder

Affective instability of BPD is characterized by rapid shifts in affective state, often in response to psychosocial cues. Affect may shift from baseline to either depression, anger, happiness, or fear rather suddenly. These affective states may last for a few hours but usually not more than a day at a time. In a study that assessed the degree to which affective instability was associated with individual and interpersonal disturbances in BPD, affective instability was found to be strongly associated with many dysfunctional patterns, including chronic emptiness, boredom, and even suicidality (Koenigsberg et al. 2001; Links et al. 2007). While affective instability is seen in many disorders (Bradley et al. 2011; Koenigsberg 2010) and may be a candidate transdiagnostic domain, in BPD it is distinct from the longer-lasting affect states seen in mood disorders, which persist for weeks or longer and are less immediately reactive to social triggers (Perez-Rodriguez et al. 2018).

Genetics of affective instability in BPD. Genetics research has not yet identified candidate genes specific for affective instability in BPD. Candidate genes have been identified for mood instability in other psychiatric disorders. One GWAS in the UK biobank sample provided evidence of several genes playing a role in self-reported mood instability, including genes for the DCC netrin 1 receptor (*DCC*), eukaryotic translation initiation factor 2B subunit beta (*eIF2B2*), placental growth factor (*PGF*), and protein tyrosine phosphatase receptor type D (*PTPRD*); the authors concluded that there likely is a polygenic basis for mood instability (Ward et al. 2017). Alternatively, familial, twin, and adoptive studies have provided preliminary evidence for a common genetic pathway in affective instability, but the exact common pathway is still being explored. A large twin study found that 51% variance among four core domains of BPD (affective instability, identity problems, negative relationships, and self-harm) was explained by a unitary genetic factor. For three of the four BPD dimensions, including affective instability, 50% variance was explained by a unitary latent factor (Distel et al. 2010).

Behavioral manifestations of affective instability in BPD. Affective instability in BPD may be driven by a high sensitivity to emotional stimuli. Specifically, many studies suggest that patients with BPD require less visual information to identify facial emotions (Lynch et al. 2006; Wagner and Linehan 1999), and because of this increased ability to detect subtle changes in facial expression, they may have an exaggerated emotional response even to neutral social situations. Others have suggested that affective instability in BPD is driven by a bias to identifying negative emotions (Meehan et al. 2017). For example, a facial recognition study of more than 100 undergraduates found that more self-reported BPD features related to a decreased accuracy detecting neutral faces, but an increased accuracy detecting negative faces, particularly at low intensity thresholds. A separate study found this bias to negative emotions in BPD to be exacerbated under stress (Deckers et al. 2015).

In addition to heightened sensitivity to the perception of emotional stimuli, evidence suggests a number of other processes may be implicated in affective instability. Imaging findings summarized below suggest that impairments in the capacity to habituate to negative stimuli or in cognitive emotion regulatory processes may play a role. Consistent with this impaired "top down" control theory, a group of researchers found that among college students with BPD traits, self-reported regulation by effortful control influenced how strongly facial emotions were experienced (Meehan et al. 2017). Our work, too, supports a deficit in cognitive control mechanisms as a contributor to affective instability. We found that BPD patients are impaired in their capacity to engage cognitive reappraisal, a frequently used and highly adaptive emotion regulation strategy, to downregulate negative responses to aversive social cues (Koenigsberg et al. 2009). We discuss brain-based evidence addressing these possibilities in the neuroimaging section below.

Neural correlates of affective instability in BPD. A number of studies examining emotion processing in BPD patients provide support for the "bottom up" model of affective instability rooted in observations of hypersensitivity of the amygdala, insula, and other limbic structures in BPD (Bertsch et al. 2018). In an early study, Donegan et al. (2003) reported that relative to HCs, BPD patients showed greater activation of the left amygdala when viewing fearful, sad, happy, and neutral faces. Studies utilizing more complex emotional and social stimuli have also identified increased amygdala and fusiform gyrus activation in individuals with BPD (Herpertz et al. 2001; Koenigsberg et al. 2009). In addition, greater activity has been reported in visual areas and the superior temporal gyrus (STG) in individuals with BPD (Koenigsberg et al. 2009). A meta-analysis integrating 24 studies of BPD reported that during processing of negative emotional stimuli, BPD patients showed hyperactivation of the left amygdala and posterior cingulate cortex, as well as blunted response of the prefrontal cortex (PFC), compared with HCs (Schulze et al. 2016).

In addition to hypersensitivity to emotional stimuli, individuals with BPD demonstrate an impairment in the ability to regulate emotions, a factor that could contribute to affective instability. Two regulatory mechanisms that have been implicated are cognitive reappraisal and habituation. Cognitive reappraisal, which entails a voluntary reconceptualization of a distressing cue in a less disturbing fashion, is one of the most highly adaptive emotion regulatory mechanisms (Gross 1998, 2002). It is accomplished by focusing on the cue as would an objective, uninvolved observer (emotional distancing) or by creating an alternative narrative for the cue that renders it less toxic (situational reappraisal). Emotion habituation is an implicit process in which repeated exposure to adverse stimuli results in reduction of the experienced emotional intensity and subjective distress. Both of these strategies are frequently utilized by healthy individuals to regulate emotions (Buhle et al. 2014; Gross 2015). Studies that have investigated the mechanism of emotion dysregulation in BPD have identified impairments in both these realms.

To examine the hypothesis that affective instability may be associated with poor implementation of emotion regulatory processes, our group compared BPD patients with HCs as they carried out a cognitive reappraisal task during fMRI. BPD patients attempting cognitive reappraisal by emotional distancing were less able to downregulate amygdala activity and engage cortical regions such as the dorsal anterior cingulate and inferior parietal cortex, which are known to play a role in cognitive reappraisal in healthy individuals (Koenigsberg et al. 2009). This finding was extended by Schulze et al. (2011), who showed an impaired ability to downregulate insula activity in BPD patients when engaging in cognitive reappraisal.

Imaging studies have also highlighted impairments in emotional habituation in BPD. While the intensity of an emotional reaction to a stimulus typically decreases as one is repeatedly exposed to that stimulus, there is neuroimaging evidence that BPD patients fail to habituate as healthy subjects do, and may even sensitize to repeated presentations of a negative stimulus (Denny et al. 2018; Hazlett et al. 2012b; Koenigsberg et al. 2014). When reexposed to the same negative images, HCs who habituate show an increase in mid-posterior insula to amygdala functional connectivity, whereas BPD patients do not (Koenigsberg et al. 2014).

Further supporting the link between affective instability and impaired habituation, our group found the degree of affective instability in BPD patients to be correlated with the degree to which they showed low anterior cingulate activity during habituation (Koenigsberg et al. 2014). Impairment in habituation in BPD patients correlates with the degree of experienced childhood adversity (Bilek et al. 2019) and with BDNF genotypes (Perez-Rodriguez et al. 2017), suggesting that there may be genetic and environmental influences underlying this phenomenon.

These neural findings might explain why patients with BPD are clinically observed to become overinvolved emotionally. Thus, given an inability to employ healthy emotion regulation strategies like cognitive reappraisal or emotional habituation, patients with BPD are more susceptible to distressing emotional situations, leading to increased affective instability as vulnerable neural systems interact with real-world stressors.

Several recent imaging studies have examined the impact of treatment on neural processes. In a single-arm trial of 24 female BPD patients, four runs of real-time fMRI neurofeedback of the amygdala over the span of six weeks were found to decrease BPD symptoms and emotion-modulated startle to negative pictures (Zaehringer et al. 2019). Studies of response to dialectical behavior therapy found that patients with BPD showed decreased amygdala activation, and improved self-reported emotion regulation, compared to HCs (Goodman et al. 2014; Schmitt et al. 2016).

Impulsive Aggression in Borderline Personality Disorder

The features of BPD that fall under behavioral dysregulation include impulsivity, impulsive aggression, self-injury, and suicidality (Zanarini et al. 2008). Several of these dimensions map onto the RDoC construct of "frustrative nonreward," in the Negative Valence domain. Although BPD patients frequently engage in self-destructive behaviors, they often report remorseful feelings after they act. For this reason, it has been suggested that low levels of distress tolerance may be an underlying factor of behavioral dysregulation, because it was found to be a stronger predictor of self-injury than daily experiences in BPD, including daily negative affect or urges to hurt oneself (Ammerman et al. 2017).

Genetics of impulsive aggression in BPD.   There is strong evidence for a genetic predisposition to impulsive aggression, although it is not necessarily specific to BPD. One meta-analysis of twin studies estimated the heritability of impulsive aggression to be 44%–72% (Miles and Carey 1997). Studies looking at candidate genes of impulsive aggression have found greatest evidence for the involvement of the monoamine oxidase A (MAO-A), 5-hydroxytryptamine receptor, tryptophan hydroxylase-2, dopamine beta-hydroxylase, and catechol-O-methyltransferase genes. For behavioral dysregulation in BPD specifically, one "risk" haplotype has been identified in the gene coding for tryptophan hydroxylase-2 (*TPH-2*), the rate-limiting enzyme in serotonin synthesis. A study from our lab showed that this risk haplotype is associated with higher rates of impulsive aggression and suicidality in BPD patients (Perez-Rodriguez et al. 2010). Another candidate gene for impulsivity in BPD is the gene for MAO-A, an enzyme involved in degradation of serotonin and norepinephrine. This enzyme is known to play a role in aggression, impulsivity, suicide, and mood lability, which are all features of behavioral dysregulation in BPD. A positron emission tomography (PET) study showed that MAO-A density in the PFC and ACC is increased in BPD patients with severe symptoms and is associated with depressive symptoms and suicidality (Kolla et al. 2016). An earlier study showed that a specific polymorphism resulting in higher activity of the variable number tandem repeat (VNTR) polymorphism in the promoter of *MAOA* is associated with BPD (Ni et al. 2006).

Finally, genetic studies have also highlighted specific alleles associated with dysregulated neurotransmitters in BPD. One study demonstrated that BPD patients have a higher frequency of the rs6318G allele and of the G/G genotype of the serotonin 5-HT_2 receptor gene (*5-HT2C*), which may be associated with aggression and suicidality (Ni et al. 2009). A similar study looked at alleles for dopaminergic genes and, after examining data from 987 BPD cases and 1,110 HCs, this study found a significant association between BPD diagnosis and a single nucleotide polymorphism (SNP) rs12718541 of the dopa decarboxylase gene (*DDC*) (Mobascher et al. 2014). Finally, just as studies have suggested dysfunction of the HPA axis to be involved in the general development of BPD, it has also been suggested that the HPA axis may play a specific role in impulsivity. Carvalho Fernando et al. (2013) found that laboratory-induced increases in cortisol levels were associated with decreased reaction times to emotional stimuli in BPD patients and HCs; this response was attenuated among BPD patients with comorbid PTSD. Thus, it could be that HPA axis abnormalities in BPD confer greater susceptibility to impulsivity through abnormalities in response inhibition of task-irrelevant distracters.

Neural correlates of impulsive aggression in BPD.   In a study of BPD patients and HCs, activation of the amygdala was significantly associated with aggression in males with BPD. In particular, males with greater aggressive tendencies showed increased activity of the left superficial and laterobasal amygdala. While no differences in amygdala volume were noted between BPD patients and HCs, for males with BPD, there was a trend-level association between right amygdala volume and aggression (Mancke et al. 2018a). These findings confirm the role of the amygdala in behavioral dysregulation in BPD. Coupled with findings from another study demonstrating that aggressive males with BPD, but not females, showed preferential activation of the left amygdala, it is possible that male gender may be a mediator of aggression driven by amygdala activity in individuals with BPD (Mancke et al. 2018a, 2018b; Herpertz et al. 2017).

Other brain regions known to play a role in aggression, in part due to brain lesion studies, are the OFC and the anterior cingulate gyrus (ACG). Studies on aggression in BPD have suggested that these regions are also smaller in size. Soloff and colleagues report that compared with HCs, individuals with BPD with suicidal behavior have smaller volume of the orbitofrontal gyrus (Soloff et al. 2012). Reduced prefrontal gray matter volume may also be a correlate of aggression, as demonstrated both in antisocial personality disorder (ASPD) (Raine et al. 2000) and BPD (Coccaro et al. 2011). One reason reduced gray matter volume in these regions may result in aggression in BPD is that the PFC exerts top-down control on the amygdala (Roxo et al. 2011). In impulsively aggressive individuals, a lower volume of the OFC and ACG may result in reduced inhibition of brain regions that drive dysregulated behaviors. During anger provocation, individuals with BPD showed diminished medial OFC input (Pietrini et al. 2000). Another study highlighted an association between reduced gray matter volume in the right ventrolateral PFC and aggression in individuals with BPD who had a history of trauma (Morandotti et al. 2013). Our group has identified disrupted OFC-amygdala coupling in BPD in response to angry faces (New et al. 2007), which has also been demonstrated in intermittent explosive disorder (Coccaro et al. 2007). Consistent with the model of impaired OFC downregulation of amygdala activity in aggression was a study that showed that when females with BPD were asked to imagine self-injurious behavior, they showed reduced activation of the OFC, increased activity of the dorsolateral PFC (DLPFC), and decreased activity in the mid-cingulate compared with HCs (Kraus et al. 2010). Several authors have reported that aggression in BPD is associated with decreased gray matter volume of the hippocampus, a structure that plays a role in the regulation of aggressive behavior (Haller 2013; Sala et al. 2011; Zetzsche et al. 2007). Finally, a study from our group (Perez-Rodriguez et al. 2012) found abnormal striatal activity only in highly aggressive males with BPD, but not in females, during an aggression provocation paradigm.

Diffusion tensor imaging (DTI) has been used to assess the role of white matter integrity in aggression in BPD. In DTI studies, fractional anisotropy (FA) represents directional coherence of the white matter tracts. Several DTI studies have highlighted reduced FA in individuals with BPD compared with HCs (Lischke et al. 2015; Vandekerckhove et al. 2020; Whalley et al. 2015). A study from our lab specifically highlights decreased FA in the temporal lobe of adolescents (New et al. 2013), but not adults, with BPD. One study specifically identified decreased frontal white matter integrity in women who engage in self-injury (Grant et al. 2007), suggesting that deficient white matter coherence may predispose to aggression in BPD. A separate study found de-creased FA of the superior longitudinal fasciculus to be associated with intermittent explosive disorder and general impulsive aggression (Lee et al. 2016). Rüsch and col-leagues (2007) demonstrated increased mean diffusivity of the inferior frontal cortex of angry patients.

In addition to assessing variations in brain size and connectivity, other studies have examined neurotransmitter levels in BPD. Dysfunction of the serotoninergic system has been associated with BPD (Lieb et al. 2004; Ni et al. 2006) and with several features of behavioral dysregulation in this cohort, including higher rates of impul-sivity, aggression, affective lability, and suicide (Audenaert et al. 2006; Bondy et al. 2006; Courtet et al. 2005; Popova 2006; Savitz et al. 2010; Skodol et al. 2002a, 2002b). Studies have highlighted decreased levels of 5-hydroxyindoleacetic acid in the cere-brospinal fluid of suicide attempters (Audenaert et al. 2006; Gardner et al. 1990), and genetics studies have highlighted associations between polymorphisms of serotonin genes and suicidality (Bondy et al. 2006; Courtet et al. 2005). One study that assessed serotonin in BPD found that compared with individuals with other personality disor-ders, individuals with BPD show a blunted prolactin response to fenfluramine, an amphetamine derivative that stimulates the release of serotonin from vesicles. This suggests that individuals with BPD may have a reduced central serotonin response, which has been directly correlated with impulsive aggression (Hansenne et al. 2002). This could be a consequence of reduced 5-HT_{1A} receptor sensitivity in BPD. In fact, aggressive BPD individuals have been found to have decreased serotonergic respon-siveness, as demonstrated by decreased *d,l*-fenfluramine activation of the OFC and ACG, and increased activity in the posterior cingulate, a region involved in facial emotion recognition (New et al. 2002; Siever et al. 1999; Soloff et al. 2000). Further-more, a study in our lab demonstrated normalization of OFC function with the selec-tive serotonin reuptake inhibitor fluoxetine (New et al. 2004). There have, in fact, been several studies demonstrating reduced synthesis of serotonin in men and women with BPD. Distinct regions have been implicated in men and women. In men, there appears to be reduced serotonin synthesis in the medial frontal gyrus, ACG, STG, and corpus striatum, while in women the right ACG and STG show reduced serotonin synthesis (Leyton et al. 2001). Another study demonstrated reduced availability of the 5-HT transporter in the ACG of individuals with personality disorders with impul-sive aggression (Frankle et al. 2005), further strengthening the serotonin dysregula-tion theory of impulsivity in BPD.

Non-suicidal self-injury (NSSI), a common feature of BPD, is a manifestation of self-directed impulsive aggression. The pain associated with the tissue damage in NSSI and the evidence of a dysregulated opioid system in BPD (see subsection "Neu-romolecular and Genetic Correlates of Interpersonal Impairments in BPD" below) call for examination of pain processing in BPD. Several studies have demonstrated that BPD patients have decreased pain sensitivity (Schmahl et al. 2010), with the pain sensitivity further decreasing during emotional states. An imaging study showed that when exposed to comparable subjective levels of thermal pain, compared with HCs, those with BPD show increased activation of the DLPFC, which has been shown to be involved in pain control, and deactivation of the perigenual ACC and right amygdala, which form part of the affective-motivational pain pathway (Schmahl et al. 2006). The DMN, which is involved in self-referential thinking, has also been implicated in pain processing in BPD. During pain processing specifically, BPD patients appear to have decreased attenuation of activity in the posterior DMN, which is correlated with greater symptom severity and dissociation (Krause-Utz and Elzinga 2019). Pain induction has been shown to decrease amygdala activity in BPD patients, but not HCs (Niedtfeld et al. 2010; Reitz et al. 2015), suggesting that in BPD, pain may actually reduce negative emotional states These findings raise the possibility that NSSI, which lowers amygdala activity, may function to lower stress, possibly via the stimulation of endogenous opioids, in BPD patients.

Interpersonal Relationship Disturbances in Borderline Personality Disorder

One of the most striking and unique features of BPD is the pattern of interpersonal disturbances that characterize the disorder. BPD patients experience others and themselves alternately as accepting or rejecting, idealizing or devaluing, loving or hating. These shifts in perception gives rise to intense, turbulent, push-pull interpersonal relationships (Kernberg 1975) that may generate feelings of chronic emptiness, self-identity disturbances, and difficulty sustaining long-term relationships. This impairment has actually been suggested to be the core feature of the disorder (Stanley and Siever 2010) and is known to cause significant morbidity (Brodsky et al. 2006). A study from our lab linked interpersonal and identity disturbances to the more established domains of affective instability and impulsivity (Koenigsberg et al. 2001), further strengthening the importance of this domain in BPD.

Neural correlates of interpersonal impairments in BPD.   The mechanisms of interpersonal and social impairments in BPD are not yet known. They may be related to disruptions in systems of social processing and cognition, or of attachment and emotion regulation (Beeney et al. 2015). Other research suggests interpersonal impairments could be due to a hypersensitivity to stressors (Gunderson and Lyons-Ruth 2008). Just as increased sensitivity to detecting emotion in faces might contribute to affective instability, it could also lead to misinterpretation of social cues and interpersonal impairments in BPD. One study showed that BPD patients demonstrate a greater bias toward detecting angry and fearful faces, and have difficulty accurately labeling the facial emotions they detect (Domes et al. 2009).

It is possible that disruptions in the empathy domain of social cognition could underlie identity disturbances in BPD. Empathy, which broadly refers to the ability to appreciate the feelings of others, has been partitioned into cognitive and emotional empathy. *Cognitive empathy* refers to the capacity to infer the feelings of others, which overlaps with the constructs of "mentalization" and "theory of mind" (Dziobek et al. 2011). *Emotional empathy* refers to the capacity to have feelings appropriate to a social situation. Several studies have demonstrated impairments in both cognitive and emotional empathy in BPD patients. Research has consistently identified cognitive empathy deficits in BPD patients, but there have been inconsistent findings regarding emotional empathy in these individuals. Using an ecologically valid laboratory video task, Dziobek and colleagues demonstrated impaired emotional empathy and cognitive empathy in BPD, which were associated with increased activity in the right superior temporal sulcus (STS) and insula and decreased activity in the left STS, respectively (Dziobek et al. 2011). A more recent imaging study highlighted neural correlates of empathy in BPD. In this study, individuals with BPD were shown pictures of hands exposed to pain after they had first viewed pictures of varied facial expressions. Compared with healthy individuals, individuals with BPD demonstrated differential activation of the insula depending on the preceding facial expression, suggesting that empathy in BPD may be dependent on emotional context (Flasbeck et al. 2019). Another possible mediator of impaired theory of mind in BPD is hyperactivation of the amygdala, as demonstrated by a study that showed that compared with healthy individuals, when asked to deduce the emotions portrayed in facial expressions, patients with BPD showed increased activity of the amygdala (Mier et al. 2013).

Other possible contributors to the interpersonal instability in BPD are rejection sensitivity and frequent efforts to avoid abandonment. These behaviors often lead to clinginess, dependence, and overly controlling tendencies, which are thought to play a role in affective instability and rage (Berenson et al. 2011). Behavioral studies that have sought to elucidate these responses have utilized the CyberBall paradigm (Lazarus et al. 2014; Williams and Jarvis 2006). This virtual ball-tossing game mimics situations of exclusion and inclusion in social groups. CyberBall studies found patients with BPD, compared with HCs, to report a higher frequency of feeling rejected (Domsalla et al. 2014) and simultaneously show strong emotional expressions during exclusion (Renneberg et al. 2012; Staebler et al. 2011). It is possible, then, that in states of rejection, patients with BPD may actually display confusing emotional signals to others, further alienating themselves. A more recent CyberBall imaging study supported these findings: compared with HCs, patients with BPD showed greater activation of the ACC, medial PFC, and right precuneus during social exclusion, all regions involved in facial emotion processing (Wrege et al. 2019).

Another behavioral paradigm of social interaction is the Trust Game, an economic exchange game in which one subject pseudo-invests money with another player, the trustee. The investment is tripled. Throughout the game, the trustee must decide how much money to keep and how much to return to the investor, who must then decide how much to invest in the following round. In a study where BPD patients assumed the role of trustee, they were less able to "coax" investigators to invest at a high rate compared with HCs (King-Casas et al. 2008). After several rounds there was a breakdown in cooperation, which was not seen when the trustee was an HC. Imaging showed that while insula activation in HCs tracked the unfairness of each offer, in BPD subjects insula activation was insensitive to the norm violations represented by low investments. This suggests that BPD patients could not monitor the appropriateness of monetary offers. Such an insensitivity to social norm violations might engender a protective hypervigilance to being slighted in BPD patients.

Neuromolecular and genetic correlates of interpersonal impairments in BPD. Several studies have attempted to find molecular correlates of social behavior in BPD. A neuropeptide that has been implicated in misreading of social cues and attachment difficulties is oxytocin (Stanley et al. 2010). Dysregulation of oxytocin has been shown in BPD and is thought to contribute to the hypersensitivity seen in the disorder (Herpertz and Bertsch 2015). A study found that compared with HCs, women with BPD had lower plasma levels of oxytocin (Bertsch et al. 2013), particularly if they had maladaptive attachment styles (Jobst et al. 2016). After experiencing social exclusion, women with BPD demonstrate even lower oxytocin levels (Jobst et al. 2015), suggesting an association between oxytocin levels in BPD and feelings of rejection. Oxytocin was found to increase affective empathy and approach motivation in BPD patients and HCs (Domes et al. 2019). A similar finding was reported for a different neuropeptide involved in social behavior, arginine vasopressin (AVP). A recent study demonstrated that exposure to early child adversity resulted in impaired social functioning, which was mediated by AVP levels in BPD participants (Brydges et al. 2019). Furthermore, as higher oxytocin levels result in less avoidant behaviors in patients with BPD (Brüne et al. 2013), it is possible that the bias toward detecting anger in facial expressions by BPD patients (Domes et al. 2008) may be moderated by oxytocin. Several genetic studies have identified gene-environment interactions between the oxytocin receptor gene (*OXTR*) variant rs53576 and the experience of childhood trauma in the development of BPD in young adults. Two studies of children from low-income backgrounds, in particular, have suggested that the inheritance of at least one A allele of rs53576 in females, and the inheritance of two homozygous G alleles in males, along with the experience of childhood trauma, is associated with a greater number of BPD traits (Cicchetti et al. 2014; Hammen et al. 2015). Another class of molecules that may underlie interpersonal difficulties in individuals with BPD is opioids (Stanley and Siever 2010). Genetic studies have linked low opioid levels to greater feelings of social rejection and higher rates of depression (Slavich et al. 2014). One model posits that BPD patients have lower opioid levels at baseline, and this could explain feelings of chronic dysphoria and emptiness. Moreover, lower opioid levels could contribute to NSSI as a possible compensatory strategy, since NSSI has been found to transiently increase endogenous opioid levels (Stanley et al. 2010). Supporting this theory are studies demonstrating the effectiveness of naltrexone, an opioid antagonist, in reducing NSSI in BPD (Sonne et al. 1996). A recent PET imaging study that measured opioid activity in individuals with BPD found that at baseline, BPD patients had greater μ-opioid receptor availability in the OFC, caudate, nucleus accumbens, and left amygdala relative to HCs. During sadness induction, BPD patients showed greater reduction in opioid binding, and increased recruitment of endogenous opioid activation in the pregenual anterior cingulate, left OFC, left ventral pallidum, left amygdala, and left temporal cortex. Thus, a deficiency of endogenous opioids could explain the baseline increased opioid receptor availability. However, during sadness, it appears that BPD patients tend to enhance opiate availability more than HCs (Prossin et al. 2010).

Summary: Neurobiology of Borderline Personality Disorder

The last decade has seen a dramatic growth in the body of neurobiological research focused on BPD. This research has drawn on state-of-the-art genetic, neuroimaging, and social game theory methods. Although a definitive neurobiological model of BPD has yet to emerge, this body of research has suggested a number of mechanisms that may contribute to BPD and the transdiagnostic dimensions convergent in this disorder. There is strong evidence for bottom-up hypersensitivity to emotional cues and deficits in both implicit (e.g., impaired habituation) and explicit (e.g., cognitive reappraisal) emotion regulation strategies implemented by prefrontal regions. Associated with these neural correlates is a negative bias in emotional facial recognition that could undermine social interactions. Moreover, the capacity to identify social norm violations has been shown to be blunted in BPD patients. Interestingly, there is a disconnect between the strong physiological reactivity to aversive cues and subjective awareness of aversive states, which manifests in high alexithymia ratings. Additionally, impaired top-down regulation permits release of impulsive aggressive behavior. These features converge to generate turbulent interpersonal relationships, which are associated with significant morbidity. Evidence has also emerged linking early childhood adversity and trauma with anomalies in neural functioning. Although an overarching neurobiological model of BPD remains elusive, a number of the currently available findings have implications for new treatment approaches. These include behavioral treatments designed to enhance use of cognitive emotion regulation strategies or to normalize reactivity to emotional facial cues as well as new pharmacologic interventions directed toward the oxytocin or opioid system.

Schizotypal Personality Disorder

The diagnosis of schizotypal personality disorder (STPD) emerged to describe relatives of patients with schizophrenia (SCZ) who were observed to have similar, yet attenuated, cognitive impairments to those seen in their SCZ relatives. According to DSM-5, individuals with STPD demonstrate a pervasive pattern of odd beliefs and behaviors, including magical thinking and eccentric appearance, as well as marked interpersonal and social deficits, that do not meet criteria for overt psychosis or for a diagnosis of SCZ. These impairments result in significant morbidity in this clinical cohort (McClure et al. 2013). STPD patients report high rates of childhood trauma, which are particularly associated with a greater number of cognitive-perceptual and interpersonal symptoms, along with worse cognitive functioning (Velikonja et al. 2019).

This complex personality disorder that is closely linked to SCZ (ICD-11 has even moved it to the psychosis section) consists of at least three domains—cognitive-perceptual, interpersonal, and oddness/disorganization—that have been associated with a latent vulnerability factor (Fossati et al. 2005). This suggests that while there may be multiple dimensions to the disorder, it is possible that one general neurobiological construct encompasses the pathogenesis of STPD. The cognitive-perceptual dimension is characterized by referential and magical thinking, as well as perceptual disturbances like paranoia and suspiciousness. The interpersonal dimension is characterized primarily by social anxiety and social anhedonia (Barkus and Badcock 2019). Finally, the dimension of oddness/disorganization is characterized by odd speech, thought, appearance, and behavior, as well as constricted affect. Neurobiological research on the first two of these dimensions has highlighted unique biological substrates associated with each of these impairments. We review studies of STPD as a DSM categorical disorder first and then examine the cognitive and interpersonal dimensions below.

Genetics of Schizotypal Personality Disorder

Early evidence for a genetic basis of STPD stemmed from more frequent observations of the disorder in first-degree relatives of patients with SCZ (Kendler et al. 1993). Subsequent research demonstrated that patients with STPD and those with SCZ share common genetic variants (Rosell et al. 2014). However, more recent research summarized below has identified unique genetic variants specific to STPD.

Heritability estimates for STPD range from 20% to 60% (Kendler et al. 2008; Torgersen 1984; Torgersen et al. 2000). Findings from genetic studies that have identified associations between dopamine genetic variants and development of symptoms in STPD provide further evidence for a genetic basis of this disorder. One genetic variant that has been consistently implicated in the pathogenesis of STPD is the enzyme COMT, which is located on chromosome 22. Increased activity of this enzyme, which metabolizes dopamine, has been implicated in the development of psychosis and SCZ (Matthysse and Baldessarini 1972; Poitou et al. 1974). Inheritance of the valine-158 allele results in higher activity of COMT, and thus decreased dopamine levels, compared with the methionine-158 allele. Several studies have demonstrated that the Val-158 allele confers an increased risk for the development of STPD (Avramopoulos et al. 2002; Savitz et al. 2010) and is more represented than the Met allele in this cohort (Roussos et al. 2013). Furthermore, several studies assessing cognitive performance in relation to the COMT genotype found that homozygotes for the Val allele had worse cognitive function than single Val allele carriers (Leung et al. 2007). Further strengthening the association of the COMT Val allele with STPD pathology, it is also possible that the Val allele moderates the effect of childhood trauma on the development of STPD (Savitz et al. 2010). In fact, beyond heritability, the pathogenesis of STPD is more accurately thought to be due to gene-environment interactions (Ericson et al. 2011). In particular, adverse childhood experiences are thought to play an important role in the development of STPD (Kendler et al. 2008). One twin gene-environment study suggested that while there are genetic factors that predispose to schizotypy, unique environmental factors also increase the risk of developing each of the three core dimensions of STPD (Lin et al. 2007). Finally, another allele that has been implicated in the pathogenesis of STPD is the Ser9Gly polymorphism of the dopamine D_3 receptor gene (*DRD3*), which is associated with greater affinity to the dopamine receptor (Roussos et al. 2013). A study from our group found significant associations between the minor alleles of three SNPs within the glycine receptor alpha-1 subunit gene (*GLRA1*) and the disorganized schizotypy dimension, but not the categorical disorder itself (Vora et al. 2018).

Additional genes that have been associated with SCZ may be implicated in STPD. These include polymorphisms of the neuregulin-1 gene (*NRG1*), which have been associated with psychotic disturbances in adolescents (Lin et al. 2005); the Disrupted in Schizophrenia 1 gene (*DISC1*), which has been associated with social anhedonia (Tomppo et al. 2009); the proline dehydrogenase gene (*PRODH*), which has been associated with impairments in working memory and trait anxiety (Roussos et al. 2013; Tomppo et al. 2009); the zinc finger protein gene (*ZNF804A*) involved in neurogenesis, which has been associated with paranoid and suspicious tendencies in STPD (Stefanis et al. 2013); and the p250GAP gene (*ARHGAP32*), associated with N-methyl-D-aspartate receptor function, which has been associated with anxiety in social situations and interpersonal deficits (Ohi et al. 2012). Although not specific to STPD, given the prevalence of social anxiety in this disorder, it is also possible that anxiety genes may confer greater susceptibility to STPD as well. The largest GWAS of anxiety traits was published in 2020, with the genetic data of almost 200,000 individuals. Several significant signals were identified, on chromosomes 3, 6, and 7, that could have implications for genetic vulnerability across many psychiatric disorders (Levey et al. 2020).

Neural Correlates of Schizotypal Personality Disorder

As with SCZ (Levitt et al. 2010), reductions in frontotemporal cortical gray matter volume have been consistently identified in STPD (Asami et al. 2013; Fervaha and Remington 2013; Kawasaki et al. 2004; Takahashi et al. 2009). These have been linked to greater interpersonal and cognitive impairments in this cohort. However, in STPD, frontotemporal reductions appear to be only about 50% reduced compared with SCZ. Furthermore, reductions in STPD spare much of the frontal lobe, including key regions like Brodmann area 10 (Hazlett et al. 2014; Liu et al. 2016), which is implicated in memory recall and executive function. Thus, it appears that frontotemporal volume reductions, and perhaps temporal reductions specifically, since these are shared among individuals with SCZ and STPD, pose a risk for developing a schizophrenia spectrum disorder (Davis et al. 2016; Downhill et al. 2001). A longitudinal metaanalysis suggests that temporal lobe volume reduction could be a static vulnerability that results from shared genetic predisposition as in SCZ; where temporal lobe reductions are greater, there is no evidence of progression of temporal lobe volume reduction over time (Olabi et al. 2011).

Several studies have examined the volume of the temporal lobe regions, including the STG, medial temporal gyrus (MTG), and inferior temporal gyrus (ITG), in STPD. Studies of the STG, which plays a role in deducing the intentions of others, have demonstrated reduced gray matter volume in STPD (Asami et al. 2013; Dickey et al. 2003; Goldstein et al. 2009), including reductions in Heschel's gyrus (Dickey et al. 2002; Takahashi et al. 2006a), which contains the primary auditory cortex, and the planum temporale (Kawasaki et al. 2004), which forms part of Wernicke's language area. Given the function of these regions in language, it is possible that reductions of the STG represent a neural correlate of odd speech, and the oddness/disorganization domain, in STPD (Downhill et al. 2001). Furthermore, a reduction in volume of the STG may explain why individuals with STPD experience social anxiety, as they may be unable to accurately assess actions of others, and worry in social situations where it may not be warranted. While longitudinal studies in SCZ show progressive deterioration of the STG, this does not appear to be the case with STPD (Takahashi and Suzuki 2018; Takahashi et al. 2009, 2010), suggesting that the preservation of STG size may protect against overt psychosis. Finally, volume reductions of the MTG (Asami et al. 2013; Hazlett et al. 2008, 2014) and ITG (Asami et al. 2013; Downhill et al. 2001) have also been documented in STPD.

Similar to temporal lobe findings, gray matter volume of the frontal lobes, particularly of the DLPFC, has been found to be significantly less reduced in STPD compared with SCZ. One study showed that while patients with SCZ and those with STPD both demonstrated gray matter reductions of the inferior frontal, medial temporal, and insula regions, STPD patients showed less reduction of the left orbitofrontal regions compared with SCZ patients (Kawasaki et al. 2004). Another study even found DLPFC volumes in patients with STPD to be larger than those in HCs (Suzuki et al. 2005). It may be that increased prefrontal volume is an additional protective factor in STPD, because it buffers against the development of psychosis (Hazlett et al.

2008; Siever and Davis 2004). In fact, subsequent studies have suggested that size of the DLPFC (Hazlett et al. 2014), or, more generally, frontotemporal coherence (Blain et al. 2020), may be a protective factor in STPD.

Although several imaging studies have assessed cortical atrophy in patients with SCZ (Chen et al. 2015; Crespo-Facorro et al. 2011; Kuperberg et al. 2003; Narr et al. 2005), until recently no study had compared cortical thickness in STPD. In an fMRI study of more than 100 SCZ patients and almost 50 STPD patients, along with HCs, individuals with SCZ were found to have significant cortical thinning of the frontal and temporal regions compared with HCs. Patients with STPD similarly demonstrated reduced cortical thickness of the left fusiform and parahippocampal gyri, right medial superior frontal gyrus, right inferior frontal gyrus, and right medial orbitofrontal cortex as compared with HCs. However, SCZ patients differed from STPD patients in that they had thinner cortices in the left precentral and paracentral gyri (Takayanagi et al. 2020).

Other imaging studies have highlighted disrupted connectivity in the brains of individuals with STPD. Several DTI studies have highlighted reduced FA of the temporal and frontal lobes of patients with SCZ (Goldstein et al. 2019; Kubicki et al. 2007; Tamnes and Agartz 2016). In STPD, similar findings have been demonstrated: compared with HCs, patients with STPD were found to have lower FA in the uncinated fasciculus (Gurrera et al. 2007; Nakamura et al. 2005) and the inferior longitudinal fasciculus (Sun et al. 2016). One study from members of our lab showed that there appears to be a gradient of FA directly correlated with severity of psychosis, because FA was highest in HCs, intermediate in STPD patients, and lowest in SCZ patients, particularly in the left hemisphere (Lener et al. 2015). These findings were replicated in another study from our lab that showed that compared with HCs, subjects with STPD had reduced FA in the left sagittal striatum and superior longitudinal fasciculus, the latter of which was associated with greater severity of disorganization symptoms (Chan et al. 2018). In other studies, abnormalities in white matter integrity have been associated with positive STPD symptoms and interpersonal difficulties (Lener et al. 2015; Nakamura et al. 2005; Sun et al. 2016). Finally, reductions have been identified in projections from the thalamic nuclei to the pulvinar region, which projects to temporal and sensory cortices, in both STPD and SCZ (Di Carlo et al. 2020). However, the mediodorsal nucleus, which projects extensively to the frontal cortex, is reduced in size in SCZ patients, but not in STPD patients (Siever et al. 2002), highlighting yet another unique variant of STPD compared with SCZ.

An additional neurobiological correlate that has been identified in patients with STPD is asymmetry. As with SCZ (Oertel-Knochel et al. 2012), recent studies that have examined frontotemporal lobe asymmetry in STPD have identified asymmetry in STPD specifically, including that of the ACG in females with STPD (Takahashi et al. 2002) and of the parahippocampal gyrus (Dickey et al. 1999). One study of individuals with STPD reported normal asymmetry in the MTG and ITG (Takahashi et al. 2006b), while a recent study in our lab reported reduced right MTG volume asymmetry in STPD. This study also found that compared with HCs, patients with STPD showed an increase of right > left asymmetry in the sagittal stratum (Chan et al. 2018). Another study reported reduced left < right whole and caudal STG asymmetry in STPD patients compared with HCs (Takahashi et al. 2006a), while another reported a trend toward greater left > right asymmetry in STPD (Dickey et al. 1999). Therefore, it is imperative to continue to expand on research of asymmetry in STPD to better understand inconsistencies.

Neural Correlates of Cognitive Dysfunction in Schizotypal Personality Disorder

One hallmark of the pathophysiology of STPD is impaired cognitive function. Individuals with STPD demonstrate deficits in executive function, including working memory, processing speed (McClure et al. 2013; Mitropoulou et al. 2005), and verbal learning and attention (Mitropoulou et al. 2002). Research on neural correlates of executive function has identified physiological anomalies in smooth pursuit eye movements (SPEMs) in STPD, which have been associated with interpersonal difficulties, such as fewer friends and greater discomfort in social relationships (Siever and Davis 2004). This suggests that impairments in cognition may underlie symptoms across many domains, including the interpersonal domain, in STPD. Furthermore, impairments in SPEMs and working memory have been associated with volume reductions in the frontal lobe, and deficits in verbal learning have been associated with temporal lobe abnormalities (Hazlett et al. 2012a). Additionally, impairments in the white matter tracts of temporal and frontal lobes, particularly in the superior longitudinal fasciculus, have been identified in individuals with STPD who have cognitive impairment (Hazlett et al. 2012a). It has also been hypothesized that differentiation between cognitive control networks and social and emotional networks, such as the DMN, may be attenuated in STPDs. This impaired differentiation may limit the ability of cognitive control networks to couple with other attention networks, explaining cognitive deficits (Rosell et al. 2015).

In addition to impaired cognition, within the cognitive-perceptual domain of STPD, deficits in reality testing, characterized by high rates of paranoia and suspiciousness of others' intentions, are characteristic of this disorder. One biological correlate of this impairment may be dysfunction of the dopaminergic system. Just as with SCZ, in STPD, higher dopaminergic activity is thought to play a role in the pathogenesis of perceptual disturbances (Ripoll et al. 2011; Siever and Davis 2004). Evidence for its role stems largely from studies that have reported improvement in psychotic-like experiences in STPD with antipsychotics (Jakobsen et al. 2017; Koenigsberg et al. 2003). Conversely, lower dopaminergic activity has been associated with negative symptoms in STPD (Abi-Dargham et al. 2004; Roussos et al. 2013), suggesting a bivariate relationship of dopamine with positive and negative symptoms in this population. In fact, the first ever SPECT study of iodobenzamide, which binds competitively to D_2 receptors, found that individuals with STPD do not show the same increased release of dopamine noted in SCZ patients with overt psychosis (Abi-Dargham et al. 2004). This suggests that compared to SCZ, cognitive impairments in STPD may be explained by elevated, yet attenuated, dopamine levels.

Further information on neurological correlates of cognitive deficits in STPD has been derived from studies identifying treatments for these impairments. In STPD, cognitive deficits have been noted to improve with amphetamine (Siegel et al. 1996) and catecholaminergic agents (Siever et al. 2002). Additionally, the dopamine agonist pergolide was found to improve working memory, verbal learning, and executive function in STPD (McClure et al. 2010; Williams and Castner 2006). This suggests that lower dopaminergic activity in the prefrontal cortex of STPD may underlie impairments in cognition in SPD. This finding was strengthened by a PET study with a D_1 receptor radioligand that found working memory deficits to be associated with increased D_1 receptor availability in the frontal cortex of individuals with STPD (Abi-Dargham et al. 2002). Finally, the α_2-adrenergic agonist guanfacine (McClure et al. 2007, 2019) has also been found to improve cognitive function in this cohort, suggesting that alternate neurotransmitters may underlie impairments in cognition in STPD.

Neural Correlates of Interpersonal Dysfunction in Schizotypal Personality Disorder

As previously mentioned in the bivariate theory in the previous subsection, dysfunction of the dopaminergic system may underlie negative symptoms in STPD. The specific negative symptoms experienced by this cohort are constricted affect and minimal reactivity to the environment. There is a trend in imaging studies for alterations of dopamine receptors associated with anhedonia, but these symptoms are also thought to be due to the constellation of social and cognitive deficits present in this disorder, associated with dysfunctional dopaminergic tones. Cognitive deficits in theory of mind, specifically, are associated with interpersonal difficulties. Individuals with STPD are thought to have impaired empathic representations of others, leading to difficulties interpersonally, including feelings of detachment, aloofness, and discomfort (Ripoll et al. 2013). In fact, a recent cognitive fMRI study of more than 70 individuals with schizotypy reported higher right posterior superior temporal sulcus (pSTS) activity in response to neutral facial expressions, which was significantly associated with disorganization symptoms. A positive association between right-left pSTS connectivity and disorganization symptoms was specifically revealed. These findings suggest that right pSTS activity may predispose individuals with schizotypy to perceive neutral stimuli as emotionally salient, when in fact they are neutral, and in this way contribute to social cognitive difficulties in STPD (Yan et al. 2020). Finally, impulsive aggression in STPD is most likely explained by biological correlates of impulsivity in other disorders. As with BPD, it is likely that impulsive aggression in STPD could be explained by deficient top-down control of limbic structures, such as the amygdala, or dysfunction of the serotonergic system, as demonstrated by amelioration of aggression in this cohort with serotonergic agents (Coccaro 1998).

Of all the impaired domains in STPD, social anxiety is one that is consistently thought to be at the core of the disorder. In individuals with STPD, social anxiety is unique in that it does not attenuate with familiarity, it is more global and concrete, and it is described as a negative perception of being watched. By contrast, in other personality disorders, such as avoidant, social anxiety appears to be more specific and characterized by fear of what others think, rather than a general paranoia of being observed. Given the unique experience of social anxiety in STPD, research has sought to elucidate neurobiological underpinnings of this phenomenon. One study found a strong correlation between reduced facial affect recognition and schizotypal-like social anxiety in healthy individuals (Abbott and Green 2013). Given that facial affect recognition has been found to be mediated by dopamine levels (Delaveau et al. 2005; Soeiro-de-Souza et al. 2012), future directions of neurobiological research in STPD should seek to elucidate whether social anxiety might be explained by dysfunction of the dopaminergic system as well. In general, because STPD represents an intermediate schizophrenia spectrum phenotype, better understanding of the genetics, pathogenesis, and treatment of this disorder can inform our knowledge of many related psychotic illnesses as well.

Summary: Neurobiology of Schizotypal Personality Disorder

Although STPD is a disorder that is historically rooted in its similarity to SCZ, advancements in neurobiological research have provided ample evidence, and thus been critical, for distinguishing STPD as a separate disorder. Findings from structural imaging studies consistently demonstrate differences in reductions of frontotemporal regions in STPD patients, compared with both SCZ patients and HCs. In particular, differences in reductions of key regions like the DLPFC and STG may underlie symptoms in the oddness/disorganization and interpersonal domains and protect against the development of full-blown psychosis. Similarly, differences in cortical atrophy and connectivity of brain regions in STPD patients, compared with SCZ patients and HCs, may underlie the unique symptoms of this disorder. There is more research needed in the realm of asymmetry to better understand the significance of these findings to date. Finally, although several neurotransmitters have been implicated, dopamine appears to play a critical role in all three domains of STPD, most likely through a bivariate mechanism in which high dopamine levels contribute to perceptual disturbances and low dopamine levels contribute to interpersonal difficulties, including social anxiety. Pharmacological treatments and therapies targeting social cognitive impairments in this cohort are critical to alleviating symptom burden in this population.

Antisocial Personality Disorder

Antisocial personality disorder is a chronic illness that is characterized by a pervasive pattern of disregard for, and violation of, the rights of others. According to DSM-5, in order for criteria for ASPD to be met, individuals must have shown at least three of seven callous-unemotional traits since the age of 15, including 1) failure to conform to social norms, by repeatedly engaging in acts that are grounds for arrest; 2) deceitfulness, demonstrated through repeated lying or conning of others for personal profit; 3) impulsivity or failure to plan ahead; 4) irritability and aggressiveness, resulting in frequent fights and assaults; 5) reckless behavior endangering personal and others' safety; 6) irresponsibility, demonstrated by inability to sustain work or financial obligations; and 7) lack of remorse, characterized by feelings of indifference to having mistreated others. Section III of DSM-5 also highlights trait-specific classifications that encompass personality impairments in ASPD, including disinhibition (or impulsivity) and antagonism. (See Chapter 4, "The Alternative DSM-5 Model for Personality Disorders," in this volume for a more detailed discussion of the impairments in personality functioning and the pathological personality traits that constitute the criteria for ASPD.) Another personality trait that has been consistently highlighted in ASPD is novelty seeking.

The prevalence of this disorder is estimated to be 1%–3% in the general population and 40%–70% in prison populations (Holzer and Vaughn 2017). Thus, better understanding the neurological correlates is imperative given the high rates of the disorder and significant burden to communities and high societal costs.

Genetics of Antisocial Personality Disorder

Many studies support a genetic correlate in the development of ASPD. Twin studies that have focused on the trait of aggression have found substantial evidence for aggression to be heritable (Coccaro et al. 1993, 1997). One twin study in particular found strong support for the genetic influence in ASPD, highlighting two dimensions with significant heritability: aggressive disregard and disinhibition (Kendler et al. 2012). The heritability of ASPD has been estimated to be 40%–50% (Ferguson 2010; Kendler et al. 2008). These findings were strengthened by an adoption study that found strong evidence for a genetic component of ASPD, mediated by ADHD (Cadoret and Stewart 1991). Although inconsistent, evidence from several GWASs further supports genetic underpinnings of ASPD. One GWAS on ASPD did not find evidence for candidate genes in ASPD (Tielbeek et al. 2012). However, a more recent GWAS (Rautiainen et al. 2016) highlighted two polymorphisms in the LINC00951–LRFN2 gene region of chromosome 6, expressed in the frontal cortex, as being associated with ASPD. Several GABA receptor genes have also been associated with both ASPD and alcohol use disorder (Deak et al. 2019), which may also underlie the frequent comorbidity of these disorders. In this GWAS of more than 1,500 individuals, a strong association was reported between the rs11941860 polymorphism of *GABRG1* and antisocial behavior, highlighting the need to study the role of the GABAergic system in relation to ASPD. In general, however, serotonin and dopamine genes probably show the strongest evidence for predisposition to ASPD (Gunter et al. 2010).

Behavioral Correlates of Disinhibition in Antisocial Personality Disorder

One challenge of ASPD research is that this disorder shares significant overlap with psychopathy. Psychopathy is a construct characterized by more pronounced problems in emotional processing that extend beyond lack of remorse. Psychopaths are known to have reduced guilt, empathy, and attachment to others compared with those with ASPD. While individuals with psychopathy are at increased risk for developing antisocial behavior, psychopathy is a distinct concept, and not all psychopaths meet criteria for antisocial personality disorder. In fact, only about 10% of those with antisocial personality disorder meet criteria for psychopathy as well (National Collaborating Centre for Mental Health 2010). An important distinction between individuals with ASPD and individuals with psychopathy is that while psychopaths tend to show instrumental, or planned, aggression, individuals with ASPD show impulsive or reactive aggression, which reflects a lack of impulse control (Dolan and Park 2002). For this reason, research has focused on understanding neurological correlates of disinhibition in this population.

Several studies have attempted to elucidate whether impulsivity in ASPD may be related to cognitive processing deficits. These studies have yielded inconsistent results, with some demonstrating impaired executive function in ASPD and others failing to replicate these results (Crowell et al. 2003; Morgan and Lilienfeld 2000). While a challenge has been teasing apart the relative contributions of ASPD and psychopathy to executive function given the presence of neurocognitive deficits in psychopathy (Blair 2019), one study did report that among individuals with ASPD there was no association between impaired executive function and psychopathy traits (Dolan 2012). This finding suggests that executive impairments in ASPD are distinct from those in psychopathy.

Additional studies on inhibition, or impulse control, in ASPD have utilized the Go/No-Go Task, a computerized inhibitory control challenge. Measuring event-related brain potentials evoked by the Go/No-Go Task, one study found that in healthy individuals, demands of inhibitory control modulated frontal P3 amplitude to negative words (Verona et al. 2012). The group with psychopathy showed blunted processing of negative emotional words, regardless of demands to inhibit, while those with ASPD showed enhanced processing of negative words. Whereas individuals with psychopathy showed decreased response to negative stimuli, those with ASPD showed an enhanced response that interfered with inhibition, possibly underlying distinct aggressive tendencies.

Additional biological research in ASPD has highlighted impairments in decoding facial emotions. Both individuals with ASPD and individuals with psychopathy have been found to less accurately detect facial expressions (Pham and Philippot 2010), although education level appears to be an important moderator. Those with criminal records, regardless of a whether they had a diagnosis of psychopathy, showed similar impairments, highlighting criminality as a possible confounding variable. However, a large meta-analysis did provide further support for impaired social cognition in ASPD (Dolan and Fullam 2004) by highlighting impairments in fear recognition not accounted for by a diagnosis of psychopathy (Marsh and Blair 2008).

Neural Correlates of Antisocial Personality Disorder and Psychopathy

A substantial portion of neuroimaging research in ASPD has focused on neural correlates of impulsive and reactive aggression, to further distinguish impairments in ASPD from those in psychopathy (Blair 2007b; Dolan 2010; Ostrov and Houston 2008). Reactive aggression, present in ASPD, has been conceptualized as a gradated response to threat, so that when escape seems nearly impossible, individuals with ASPD react impulsively with aggression. Structures implicated in the threat system include the amygdala, hypothalamus, and periaqueductal gray, mediated by the medial, orbital, and inferior frontal cortices (Blair 2007a, 2007b, 2010). Findings from studies in BPD patients would suggest that impulsive aggression is associated with heightened activity of the amygdala and reduced frontal regulatory activity. A study in ASPD and psychopathy suggested a different mechanism in each of these disorders. This study found that while individuals with psychopathy demonstrated greater amygdala reactivity than healthy individuals, those with ASPD did not, challenging the notion that aggressive tendencies in ASPD are driven by amygdala activity (Hyde et al. 2014). On the other hand, instrumental, or deliberate, aggression in psychopathy is thought to be mediated by the motor cortex and the caudate. A recent study found that weakened amygdala–ventral medial PFC functional connectivity to fearful but not neutral or angry faces was related to higher psychopathic traits in young adults (Waller et al. 2019), suggesting that an impaired top-down connectivity could underlie aggressive tendencies. These impairments of the amygdala and OFC also lead to difficulty socializing, secondary to a dysfunction in stimulus reinforcement, and poor decision making (Blair 2010). In general, these imaging studies on aggression show consistent impairments of the amygdala and PFC in people with psychopathic traits, but the research for ASPD specifically is limited (Nordstrom et al. 2011; Yang et al. 2009).

More recent studies have provided additional neural evidence distinguishing between ASPD and psychopathy. Individuals with psychopathy have a more efficiently organized dorsal attention network and decreased flow of subcortical structures, such as the amygdala, caudate, and hippocampus, associated with greater callous-unemotional traits (Tillem et al. 2019). By contrast, individuals with ASPD appear to have altered modular organization and impaired neurologic network efficiency (Jiang et al. 2017), which could possibly underlie impulsive, and less planned, aggression. Several PET studies have suggested that disruptions of the serotonergic system, with an emphasis on MAO-A (Kolla and Vinette 2017), an enzyme linked to low mood and suicidality in BPD, may be implicated in feelings of anger and aggression in individuals with ASPD (Kolla and Houle 2019). Alternatively, one of the only known proton magnetic resonance spectroscopy studies to assess glutamine levels in relation to aggression in ASPD found that compared with HCs, individuals with ASPD had significantly elevated levels of glutamine in the left DLPFC and supragenual ACC, two brain regions associated with impulsivity and behavior control. Furthermore, glutamine levels in the DLPFC were found to be positively correlated with aggression in only the ASPD group (Smaragdi et al. 2019).

An imaging study looking at reward processing found evidence for an enlarged striatum in individuals with antisocial traits, suggesting that individuals with ASPD may abnormally process reward, even when it is absent, so that they continue to feel rewarded by stimuli that are otherwise nonrewarding (Glenn and Yang 2012). Another case-control fMRI study of 50 men with ASPD, including 12 with comorbid psychopathy and 20 without any comorbidity, found that compared with individuals without psychopathy, those with comorbid ASPD and psychopathy had increased activation of the posterior cingulate cortex and anterior insula in response to punished errors, and decreased activation of the superior temporal cortex to reward (Gregory et al. 2015), highlighting neural correlates specific to psychopathy. An earlier study from this research team similarly highlighted unique reductions in gray matter volume of the anterior rostral PFC (Brodmann area 10) and temporal cortex (Brodmann area 20/38) in individuals with ASPD and psychopathy compared with those with only ASPD (Gregory et al. 2012). A final neural correlate that has been identified specific to psychopathy is thinning of the cortex (Ly et al. 2012), adding to findings of decreased frontal activity/size conferring greater risk for development of psychopathic traits.

Although imaging research in ASPD is limited (Boccardi et al. 2010; Gregory et al. 2012; Tiihonen et al. 2008), reductions in volume of frontal cortices has been consistently identified in ASPD, even when substance use is controlled for (Dolan 2010; Raine et al. 2000, 2010; Tiihonen et al. 2008). A neuroimaging study on inhibitory control expanded on these findings by highlighting unique activation of frontal brain regions in ASPD during the Go/No-Go Task. Given known frontal lobe dysfunction in

ASPD, it was hypothesized that individuals with ASPD would show attenuated OFC activation. However, compared with HCs, those with ASPD and BPD showed more bilateral, extended activation of medial, superior, and inferior frontal gyri, which could be associated with aggressive and violent traits (Völlm et al. 2004). Furthermore, ASPD is strongly associated with impaired development of the cavum septum pellucidum, suggesting that deficits in limbic development may be a predisposing factor for this disorder (Blair and Zhang 2020; Dolan 2010). The findings of impaired cavum septum pellucidum in ASPD remain even after confounds such as trauma, injuries, and comorbidities have been controlled for, and have also been identified in psychopathy and conduct disorder (Blair and Zhang 2020). Individuals with ASPD have also been found to have longer and thinner corpus callosa (Raine et al. 2003). For example, one study assessing gray matter volume in ASPD and psychopathy reported smaller gray matter volume in the anterior frontal lobe region of Brodmann area 10 in ASPD, which is a region involved with risk taking (Gregory et al. 2012). A recent retrospective structural MRI study of more than 600 individuals with life-course-persistent antisocial behavior expanded these findings. This study found that compared with HCs, individuals with life-course-persistent antisocial behavior had smaller mean surface areas of 282 anatomical areas, and lower cortical thickness of frontal and temporal regions associated with executive function, affect regulation, and motivation (Carlisi et al. 2020). Finally, compared with HCs, individuals with ASPD have also been found to have smaller temporal lobes, whole brain volumes, and cingulate cortex, as well as larger putamen, occipital and parietal lobes, cerebellum, and insula and postcentral gyri (Tiihonen et al. 2008).

Summary: Neurobiology of Antisocial Personality Disorder

Although in recent years there have been advances in neurobiological research of ASPD, compared with other personality disorders, research remains rather limited. One major challenge is the frequent overlap of ASPD and psychopathy. Behavioral research, utilizing tasks like the Go/No-Go Task, have emphasized impaired impulse control as a neural correlate of impulsive aggression in ASPD. Expanding on these findings, neuroimaging research has highlighted impaired frontolimbic (top-down) connections in psychopathy, dysfunction of the reward circuitry, and unique alterations and size of brain structures, associated with aggressive tendencies. In general, genetics research in ASPD is relatively limited (Gunter et al. 2010). Future research in ASPD should examine the role of the serotonergic, dopaminergic, or GABAergic systems in aggression.

Avoidant Personality Disorder

Avoidant personality disorder (AVPD) is estimated to occur in 1%–2% of the population and in about 14.7% of psychiatric outpatients (Torgersen 2009; Zimmerman et al. 2005). It is characterized primarily by three main features: 1) hypersensitivity to negative evaluation, 2) feelings of inadequacy, and 3) social inhibition secondary to a fear of being criticized (Skodol et al. 2002a; Weinbrecht et al. 2016). Despite the prevalence and evident morbidity of this disorder, there is relatively little research in AVPD compared with the other personality disorders discussed in this chapter.

One major challenge to neurobiological research in AVPD is that this disorder has significant overlap with social anxiety disorder (SAD) or general social phobia. In fact, there is some controversy as to whether these disorders constitute separate diagnoses (Herbert et al. 1992; Lampe 2016; Reich 2000) or whether they represent different levels of severity of the same social anxiety disorder. High rates of comorbidity of AVPD and SAD have been documented (Cox et al. 2009; Friborg et al. 2013).

Despite ample similarities between AVPD and SAD, it appears that the experiences of anxiety versus avoidance are distinguishing features between these disorders, with avoidance more prominent in AVPD and anxiety more characteristic of SAD. In fact, AVPD has been conceptualized as arising from high harm avoidance in childhood, or the propensity to withdraw and worry, that stems from the experience of parental neglect (Joyce et al. 2003). This tendency to withdraw could be associated with even greater functional impairments in AVPD compared with SAD, a hypothesis supported by the finding that, compared with patients with SAD, patients with AVPD reported more psychosocial problems and dysfunction related to self-esteem, identity, and relationships (Eikenaes et al. 2013). These results provide further evidence for AVPD as a distinct disorder from SAD.

Genetics of Avoidant Personality Disorder

Research on the genetics of AVPD has been limited. Most of what we know with regard to genetic transmission of this disorder stems from several twin studies that have estimated the heritability of AVPD to be between 25% and 65% (Gjerde et al. 2012; Kendler et al. 2008; Torgersen et al. 2000). Studies assessing the stability of AVPD over time have supported trait rather than state features of the disorder (Shea et al. 2002). Data from the Collaborative Longitudinal Personality Disorders Study, a large multisite prospective study of four personality disorders, found that approximately half of patients with AVPD retained the diagnosis 2 years later (Grilo et al. 2004; Skodol et al. 2005). The traits that appear to be most stable in AVPD are feelings of social ineptitude and of inadequacy of self compared to others (McGlashan et al. 2005).

Behavioral Correlates of Avoidant Personality Disorder

Behavioral research in AVPD has suggested that a heightened sensitivity to detecting negative facial expressions may underlie the interpersonal avoidant patterns noted in AVPD. One facial emotion recognition study found that when asked to identify the emotion of morphed facial expressions, compared with healthy individuals, AVPD patients were less able to correctly identify fearful faces (Rosenthal et al. 2011).

Subsequent studies assessing mentalization in individuals with AVPD found that an impaired ability to accurately interpret other people's internal states was particularly notable for subjects with AVPD compared with individuals with other psychiatric comorbidities (Moroni et al. 2016), including social phobia (Pellecchia et al. 2018). Thus, it could be that a biological correlate distinguishing individuals with AVPD from people with general social phobia is that the former differ in their ability to represent other peoples' thoughts and emotions, which is an impairment strongly associated with social withdrawal (Semerari et al. 2014).

Finally, similar to BPD, one explanation for the avoidance behavior in AVPD could be decreased emotional awareness, or high rates of alexithymia, compared with healthy individuals (Johansen et al. 2013; Nicolò et al. 2011). A review found strong evidence for debilitating degrees of emotional avoidance in AVPD, supporting the notion that avoidance in this population extends beyond social situations. It appears that individuals with AVPD experience significant discomfort with both positive and negative emotions, which could be the primary driver of social isolation (Taylor et al. 2004). A study that measured subjective anxiety and fearful thoughts, as well as using electrocardiographic and respiratory measures, in individuals with AVPD and SAD while they spoke to an audience found that those with AVPD reported the highest rates of subjective anxiety, although their heart rate did not differ from that of healthy individuals (Hofmann et al. 1995).

Neural Correlates of Avoidant Personality Disorder

To date, there have been few functional imaging studies of avoidant personality AVPD. To our knowledge, we have been the only group to publish imaging studies of AVPD. Relative to HCs, individuals with AVPD do not appear to significantly differ in volume of the amygdala, medial PFC, or ACC (Denny et al. 2016). However, right amygdala volume was directly correlated with reported anxiety. Additional results from imaging studies highlight hyperactivation of the amygdala in anticipation of emotion regulation (Denny et al. 2015), and hypoactivation of the dorsal anterior cingulate cortex during habituation (Koenigsberg et al. 2014), in individuals with AVPD. Similar to the previously mentioned study, heightened amygdala activation was found to be associated with increased self-reports of anxiety, although this finding was not replicated in a more recent imaging study of salience network activity in AVPD (Denny et al. 2018). These findings suggest that further research should focus on the role of the amygdala in AVPD.

Summary: Neurobiology of Avoidant Personality Disorder

Neurobiological research of AVPD has been quite limited and faces the challenge of identifying distinct neural correlates that distinguish between AVPD and SAD, or general social phobia. Behavioral studies have identified a bias toward detecting negative emotions and alexithymia as correlates of avoidant behavior in AVPD. Coupled with genetic research, studies suggest that individuals with AVPD may have a heightened stress response. Neuroimaging research addressing AVPD has been limited, and additional work is called for. Pharmacological and psychotherapeutic treatments that are effective for anxiety symptoms are frequently found to improve symptoms in AVPD as well (Herpertz et al. 2007; Ripoll et al. 2011). However, treatments targeting unique neurobiological features of AVPD might be even more effective.

Conclusion and Future Directions

The development of new technologies in neuroimaging, advances in molecular genetics, and the development of specific pharmacodynamic probes have led to exponential growth in neurobiological research of personality disorders, particularly over the last decade. Borderline personality disorder, schizotypal personality disorder, antisocial personality disorder, and avoidant personality disorder have been most extensively studied. There is still much research needed to examine the neurobiological correlates of the other DSM-5 personality disorders. In addition, few studies have applied the same research paradigms to several personality disorders within a single study to permit distinguishing features that are shared among several personality disorders from those specific to individual disorders. Some neurobiological features cut across multiple personality disorder diagnoses and may be better understood as correlates of personality trait disturbances, such as those proposed in Section III of DSM-5. Much remains to be learned about the relationships among the neurobiological features of the personality disorders and their relationship to environmental influences and specific gene-environment interactions. Finally, another important area for further research is the developmental trajectory of the biological features of personality disorders across the lifespan.

References

Abbott GR, Green, MJ: Facial affect recognition and schizotypal personality characteristics. Early Interv Psychiatry 7:58–63, 2013

Abi-Dargham A, Mawlawi O, Lombardo I, et al: Prefrontal dopamine D1 receptors and working memory in schizophrenia. J Neurosci 22:3708–3719, 2002

Abi-Dargham A, Kegeles LS, Zea-Ponce Y, et al: Striatal amphetamine-induced dopamine release in patients with schizotypal personality disorder studied with single photon emission computed tomography and [123I]iodobenzamide. Biol Psychiatry 55:1001–1006, 2004

Aguilar-Ortiz S, Salgado-Pineda P, Vega D, et al: Evidence for default mode network dysfunction in borderline personality disorder. Psychol Med 50:1746–1754, 2020

Amad A, Radua J, Vaiva G, et al: Similarities between borderline personality disorder and post traumatic stress disorder: evidence from resting-state meta-analysis. Neurosci Biobehav 105:52–59, 2019

American Psychiatric Association: Diagnostic and Statistical Manual of Mental Disorders, 4th Edition. Arlington, VA, American Psychiatric Association, 1994

American Psychiatric Association: Diagnostic and Statistical Manual of Mental Disorders, 5th Edition. Arlington, VA, American Psychiatric Association, 2013

Ammerman BA, Olino TM, Coccaro EF, et al: Predicting nonsuicidal self-injury in borderline personality disorder using ecological momentary assessment. J Pers Disord 31:844–855, 2017

Asami T, Whitford TJ, Bouix S, et al: Globally and locally reduced MRI gray matter volumes in neuroleptic-naive men with schizotypal personality disorder: association with negative symptoms. JAMA Psychiatry 70:361–372, 2013

Audenaert K, Peremans K, Goethals I, et al: Functional imaging, serotonin and the suicidal brain. Acta Neurol Belg 106:125–131, 2006

Avramopoulos D, Stefanis NC, Hantoumi I, et al: Higher scores of self-reported schizotypy in healthy young males carrying the COMT high activity allele. Mol Psychiatry 7:706–711, 2002

Barkus E, Badcock JC: A transdiagnostic perspective on social anhedonia. Front Psychiatry 10:216, 2019

Bassir Nia A, Eveleth MC, Gabbay JM, et al: Past, present, and future of genetic research in borderline personality disorder. Curr Opin Psychol 21:60–68, 2018

Beeney JE, Stepp SD, Hallquist MN, et al: Attachment and social cognition in borderline personality disorder: specificity in relation to antisocial and avoidant personality disorders. Personal Disord 6:207–215, 2015

Berenson KR, Downey G, Rafaeli E, et al: The rejection-rage contingency in borderline personality disorder. J Abnorm Psychol 120:681–690, 2011

Bertsch K, Grothe M, Prehn K, et al: Brain volumes differ between diagnostic groups of violent criminal offenders. Eur Arch Psychiatry Clin Neurosci 263:593–606, 2013

Bertsch K, Hillmann K, Herpertz SC: Behavioral and neurobiological correlates of disturbed emotion processing in borderline personality disorder. Psychopathology 51:76–82, 2018

Bilek E, Itz ML, Stößel G, et al: Deficient amygdala habituation to threatening stimuli in borderline personality disorder relates to adverse childhood experiences. Biol Psychiatry 86:930–938, 2019

Blain SD, Grazioplene RG, Ma Y, DeYoung CG: Toward a neural model of the openness-psychoticism dimension: functional connectivity in the default and frontoparietal control networks. Schizophr Bull 46:540–551, 2020

Blair RJR: The amygdala and ventromedial prefrontal cortex in morality and psychopathy. Trends Cogn Sci 11:387–392, 2007a

Blair RJR: Dysfunctions of medial and lateral orbitofrontal cortex in psychopathy. Ann NY Acad Sci 1121:461–479, 2007b

Blair RJR: Neuroimaging of psychopathy and antisocial behavior: a targeted review. Curr Psychiatry Rep 12:76–82, 2010

Blair RJR: Dysfunctional neurocognition in individuals with clinically significant psychopathic traits. Dialogues Clin Neurosci 21:291–299, 2019

Blair RJR, Zhang R: Recent neuroimaging findings with respect to conduct disorder, callous-unemotional traits and psychopathy. Curr Opin Psychiatry 33:45–50, 2020

Boccardi M, Ganzola R, Rossi R, et al: Abnormal hippocampal shape in offenders with psychopathy. Hum Brain Mapp 31:438–447, 2010

Bondy B, Buettner A, Zill P: Genetics of suicide. Mol Psychiatry 11:336–351, 2006

Bradley B, DeFife JA, Guarnaccia C, et al: Emotion dysregulation and negative affect: association with psychiatric symptoms. J Clin Psychiatry 72:685–691, 2011

Brambilla P, Soloff PH, Sala M, et al: Anatomical MRI study of borderline personality disorder patients. Psychiatry Res 131:125–133, 2004

Brodsky BS, Groves SA, Oquendo MA, et al: Interpersonal precipitants and suicide attempts in borderline personality disorder. Suicide Life Threat Behav 36:313–322, 2006

Brüne M, Ebert A, Kolb M, et al: Oxytocin influences avoidant reactions to social threat in adults with borderline personality disorder. Hum Psychopharmacol 28:552–561, 2013

Brunner R, Henze R, Parzer P, et al: Reduced prefrontal and orbitofrontal gray matter in female adolescents with borderline personality disorder: is it disorder specific? NeuroImage 49:114–120, 2010

Brydges NM, Hall J, Best C, et al: Childhood stress impairs social function through AVP-dependent mechanisms. Transl Psychiatry 9:330, Dec 9, 2019

Buhle JT, Silvers JA, Wager TD, et al: Cognitive reappraisal of emotion: a meta-analysis of human neuroimaging studies. Cereb Cortex 24:2981–2990, 2014

Cadoret RJ, Stewart MA: An adoption study of attention deficit/hyperactivity/aggression and their relationship to adult antisocial personality. Compr Psychiatry 32:73–82, 1991

Carlisi CO, Moffitt TE, Knodt AR, et al: Associations between life-course-persistent antisocial behaviour and brain structure in a population-representative longitudinal birth cohort. Lancet Psychiatry 7:245–253, 2020

Carpenter RW, Tomko RL, Trull TJ, et al: Gene-environment studies and borderline personality disorder: a review. Curr Psychiatry Rep 15(1):336, 2012

Carvalho Fernando S, Beblo T, Schlosser N, et al: Acute glucocorticoid effects on response inhibition in borderline personality disorder. Psychoneuroendocrinology 38:2780–2788, 2013

Cattane N, Rossi R, Lanfredi M, et al: Borderline personality disorder and childhood trauma: exploring the affected biological systems and mechanisms. BMC Psychiatry 17(1):221, 2017

Chan CC, Szeszko PR, Wong E, et al: Frontal and temporal cortical volume, white matter tract integrity, and hemispheric asymmetry in schizotypal personality disorder. Schizophr Res 197:226–232, 2018

Chen X, Liang S, Pu W, et al: Reduced cortical thickness in right Heschl's gyrus associated with auditory verbal hallucinations severity in first-episode schizophrenia. BMC Psychiatry 15:152, 2015

Choi-Kain LW, Albert EB, Gunderson JG: Evidence-based treatments for borderline personality disorder: implementation, integration, and stepped care. Harv Rev Psychiatry 24:342–356, 2016

Choi-Kain LW, Finch EF, Masland SR, et al: What works in the treatment of borderline personality disorder. Curr Behav Neurosci Rep 4:21–30, 2017

Cicchetti D, Rogosch FA, Hecht KF, et al: Moderation of maltreatment effects on childhood borderline personality symptoms by gender and oxytocin receptor and FK506 binding protein 5 genes. Dev Psychopathol 26:831–849, 2014

Coccaro EF: Clinical outcome of psychopharmacologic treatment of borderline and schizotypal personality disordered subjects. J Clin Psychiatry 59 (suppl 1):30–35; discussion 36–37, 1998

Coccaro EF, Bergeman CS, McClearn GE: Heritability of irritable impulsiveness: a study of twins reared together and apart. Psychiatry Res 48:229–242, 1993

Coccaro EF, Bergeman CS, Kavoussi RJ, et al: Heritability of aggression and irritability: a twin study of the Buss-Durkee aggression scales in adult male subjects. Biol Psychiatry 41:273–284, 1997

Coccaro EF, McCloskey MS, Fitzgerald DA, et al: Amygdala and orbitofrontal reactivity to social threat in individuals with impulsive aggression. Biol Psychiatry 62:168–178, 2007

Coccaro EF, Sripada CS, Yanowitch RN, et al: Corticolimbic function in impulsive aggressive behavior. Biol Psychiatry 69:1153–1159, 2011

Conway CC, Hopwood CJ, Morey LC, et al: Borderline personality disorder is equally trait-like and state-like over ten years in adult psychiatric patients. J Abnorm Psychol 127:590–601, 2018

Courtet P, Jollant F, Castelnau D, et al: Suicidal behavior: relationship between phenotype and serotonergic genotype. Am J Med Genet C Semin Med Genet 133C:25–33, 2005

Cox BJ, Pagura J, Stein MB, et al: The relationship between generalized social phobia and avoidant personality disorder in a national mental health survey. Depress Anxiety 26:354–362, 2009

Crespo-Facorro B, Roiz-Santiáñez R, Pérez-Iglesias R, et al: Global and regional cortical thinning in first-episode psychosis patients: relationships with clinical and cognitive features. Psychol Med 41:1449–1460, 2011

Crowell TA, Kieffer KM, Kugeares S, et al: Executive and nonexecutive neuropsychological functioning in antisocial personality disorder. Cogn Behav Neurol 16:100–109, 2003

Dammann G, Teschler S, Haag T, et al: Increased DNA methylation of neuropsychiatric genes occurs in borderline personality disorder. Epigenetics 6:1454–1462, 2011

Davis J, Eyre H, Jacka FN, et al: A review of vulnerability and risks for schizophrenia: beyond the two hit hypothesis. Neurosci Biobehav Rev 65:185–194, 2016

Deak JD, Gizer IR, Otto JM, et al: Effects of common and rare chromosome 4 GABAergic gene variation on alcohol use and antisocial behavior. J Stud Alcohol Drugs 80:585–593, 2019

Deckers JWM, Lobbestael J, van Wingen GA, et al: The influence of stress on social cognition in patients with borderline personality disorder. Psychoneuroendocrinology 52:119–129, 2015

Delaveau P, Salgado-Pineda P, Wicker B, et al: Effect of levodopa on healthy volunteers' facial emotion perception: an fMRI study. Clin Neuropharmacol 28:255–261, 2005

Denny BT, Fan J, Liu X, et al: Elevated amygdala activity during reappraisal anticipation predicts anxiety in avoidant personality disorder. J Affect Disord 172:1–7, 2015

Denny BT, Fan J, Liu X, et al: Brain structural anomalies in borderline and avoidant personality disorder patients and their associations with disorder-specific symptoms. J Affect Disord 200:266–274, 2016

Denny BT, Fan J, Fels S, et al: Sensitization of the neural salience network to repeated emotional stimuli following initial habituation in patients with borderline personality disorder. Am J Psychiatry 175:657–664, 2018

Di Carlo P, Pergola G, Antonucci LA, et al: Multivariate patterns of gray matter volume in thalamic nuclei are associated with positive schizotypy in healthy individuals. Psychol Med 50:1501–1509, 2020

Dickey CC, McCarley RW, Voglmaier MM, et al: Schizotypal personality disorder and MRI abnormalities of temporal lobe gray matter. Biol Psychiatry 45:1393–1402, 1999

Dickey CC, McCarley RW, Shenton ME: The brain in schizotypal personality disorder: a review of structural MRI and CT findings. Harv Rev Psychiatry 10:1–15, 2002

Dickey CC, McCarley RW, Voglmaier MM, et al: An MRI study of superior temporal gyrus volume in women with schizotypal personality disorder. Am J Psychiatry 160:2198–2201, 2003

Distel MA, Hottenga J-J, Trull TJ, et al: Chromosome 9: linkage for borderline personality disorder features. Psychiatr Genet 18:302–307, 2008

Distel MA, Willemsen G, Ligthart L, et al: Genetic covariance structure of the four main features of borderline personality disorder. J Pers Disord 24:427–444, 2010

Distel MA, Middeldorp CM, Trull TJ, et al: Life events and borderline personality features: the influence of gene-environment interaction and gene-environment correlation. Psychol Med 41:849–860, 2011

Dolan M: What imaging tells us about violence in anti-social men. Crim Behav Ment Health 20:199–214, 2010

Dolan M: The neuropsychology of prefrontal function in antisocial personality disordered offenders with varying degrees of psychopathy. Psychol Med 42:1715–1725, 2012

Dolan M, Fullam R: Theory of mind and mentalizing ability in antisocial personality disorders with and without psychopathy. Psychol Med 34:1093–1102, 2004

Dolan M, Park I: The neuropsychology of antisocial personality disorder. Psychol Med 32:417–427, 2002

Domes G, Czieschnek D, Weidler F, et al: Recognition of facial affect in borderline personality disorder. J Pers Disord 22:135–147, 2008

Domes G, Schulze L, Herpertz SC: Emotion recognition in borderline personality disorder—a review of the literature. J Pers Disord 23:6–19, 2009

Domes G, Ower N, von Dawans B, et al: Effects of intranasal oxytocin administration on empathy and approach motivation in women with borderline personality disorder: a randomized controlled trial. Transl Psychiatry 9(1):328, 2019

Domsalla M, Koppe G, Niedtfeld I, et al: Cerebral processing of social rejection in patients with borderline personality disorder. Soc Cogn Affect Neurosci 9:1789–1797, 2014

Donegan NH, Sanislow CA, Blumberg HP, et al: Amygdala hyperreactivity in borderline personality disorder: implications for emotional dysregulation. Biol Psychiatry 54:1284–1293, 2003

Downhill JE, Buchsbaum MS, Hazlett EA, et al: Temporal lobe volume determined by magnetic resonance imaging in schizotypal personality disorder and schizophrenia. Schizophr Res 48:187–199, 2001

Dziobek I, Preissler S, Grozdanovic Z, et al: Neuronal correlates of altered empathy and social cognition in borderline personality disorder. NeuroImage 57:539–548, 2011

Eikenaes I, Hummelen B, Abrahamsen G, et al: Personality functioning in patients with avoidant personality disorder and social phobia. J Pers Disord 27:746–763, 2013

Ellison WD, Rosenstein LK, Morgan TA, et al: Community and clinical epidemiology of borderline personality disorder. Psychiatr Clin North Am 41:561–573, 2018

Ericson M, Tuvblad C, Raine A, et al: Heritability and longitudinal stability of schizotypal traits during adolescence. Behav Genet 41:499–511, 2011

Fatimah H, Wiernik BM, Gorey C, et al: Familial factors and the risk of borderline personality pathology: genetic and environmental transmission. Psychol Med 50:1327–1337, 2020

Ferguson CJ: Genetic contributions to antisocial personality and behavior: a meta-analytic review from an evolutionary perspective. J Soc Psychol 150:160–180, 2010

Fervaha G, Remington G: Neuroimaging findings in schizotypal personality disorder: a systematic review. Prog Neuropsychopharmacol Biol Psychiatry 43:96–107, 2013

Flasbeck V, Enzi B, Brüne M: Enhanced processing of painful emotions in patients with border-line personality disorder: a functional magnetic resonance imaging study. Front Psychiatry 10:357, 2019

Fossati A, Citterio A, Grazioli F, et al: Taxonic structure of schizotypal personality disorder: a multiple-instrument, multi-sample study based on mixture models. Psychiatry Res 137:71–85, 2005

Frankle WG, Lombardo I, New AS, et al: Brain serotonin transporter distribution in subjects with impulsive aggressivity: a positron emission study with [11C]McN 5652. Am J Psychiatry 162:915–923, 2005

Friborg O, Martinussen M, Kaiser S, et al: Comorbidity of personality disorders in anxiety disorders: a meta-analysis of 30 years of research. J Affect Disord 145:143–155, 2013

Gardner DL, Lucas PB, Cowdry RW: CSF metabolites in borderline personality disorder compared with normal controls. Biol Psychiatry 28:247–254, 1990

Gjerde LC, Czajkowski N, Røysamb E, et al: The heritability of avoidant and dependent personality disorder assessed by personal interview and questionnaire. Acta Psychiatr Scand 126:448–457, 2012

Glenn AL, Yang Y: The potential role of the striatum in antisocial behavior and psychopathy. Biol Psychiatry 72:817–822, 2012

Goldstein KE, Hazlett EA, New AS, et al: Smaller superior temporal gyrus volume specificity in schizotypal personality disorder. Schizophr Res 112:14–23, 2009

Goldstein KE, Haznedar MM, Alloy LB, et al: Short communication: diffusion tensor anisotropy in the cingulate in borderline and schizotypal personality disorder. Psychiatry Res 279:353–357, 2019

Goodman M, Carpenter D, Tang CY, et al: Dialectical behavior therapy alters emotion regulation and amygdala activity in patients with borderline personality disorder. J Psychiatr Res 57:108–116, 2014

Gottesman II, Gould TD: The endophenotype concept in psychiatry: etymology and strategic intentions. Am J Psychiatry 160:636–645, 2003

Grant BF, Chou SP, Goldstein RB, et al: Prevalence, correlates, disability, and comorbidity of DSM-IV borderline personality disorder: results from the Wave 2 National Epidemiologic Survey on Alcohol and Related Conditions. J Clin Psychiatry 69:533–545, 2008

Grant JE, Correia S, Brennan-Krohn T, et al: Frontal white matter integrity in borderline personality disorder with self-injurious behavior. J Neuropsychiatry Clin Neurosci 19:383–390, 2007

Gregory S, Ffytche D, Simmons A, et al: The antisocial brain: psychopathy matters. Arch Gen Psychiatry 69:962–972, 2012

Gregory S, Blair RJ, Ffytche D, et al: Punishment and psychopathy: a case-control functional MRI investigation of reinforcement learning in violent antisocial personality disordered men. Lancet Psychiatry 2:153–160, 2015

Grilo CM, Sanislow CA, Gunderson JG, et al: Two-year stability and change of schizotypal, borderline, avoidant, and obsessive-compulsive personality disorders. J Consult Clin Psychol 72:767–775, 2004

Groleau P, Joober R, Israel M, et al: Methylation of the dopamine D2 receptor (DRD2) gene promoter in women with a bulimia-spectrum disorder: associations with borderline personality disorder and exposure to childhood abuse. J Psychiatr Res 48:121–127, 2014

Gross JJ: Antecedent- and response-focused emotion regulation: divergent consequences for experience, expression, and physiology. J Pers Soc Psychol 74:224–237, 1998

Gross JJ: Emotion regulation: affective, cognitive, and social consequences. Psychophysiology 39:281–291, 2002

Gross JJ: Emotion regulation: current status and future prospects. Psychol Inq 26:1–26, 2015

Gunderson JG: Disturbed relationships as a phenotype for borderline personality disorder. Am J Psychiatry 164:1637–1640, 2007

Gunderson JG, Lyons-Ruth K: BPD's interpersonal hypersensitivity phenotype: a gene-environment-developmental model. J Pers Disord 22:22–41, 2008

Gunter TD, Vaughn MG, Philibert RA: Behavioral genetics in antisocial spectrum disorders and psychopathy: a review of the recent literature. Behav Sci Law 28:148–173, 2010

Gurrera RJ, Nakamura M, Kubicki M, et al: The uncinate fasciculus and extraversion in schizotypal personality disorder: a diffusion tensor imaging study. Schizophr Res 90:360–362, 2007

Haller J: The neurobiology of abnormal manifestations of aggression—a review of hypothalamic mechanisms in cats, rodents, and humans. Brain Res Bull 93:97–109, 2013

Hammen C, Bower JE, Cole SW: Oxytocin receptor gene variation and differential susceptibility to family environment in predicting youth borderline symptoms. J Pers Disord 29:177–192, 2015

Hansenne M, Pitchot W, Pinto E, et al: 5-HT1A dysfunction in borderline personality disorder. Psychol Med 32:935–941, 2002

Hazlett EA, New AS, Newmark R, et al: Reduced anterior and posterior cingulate gray matter in borderline personality disorder. Biol Psychiatry 58:614–623, 2005

Hazlett EA, Speiser LJ, Goodman M, et al: Exaggerated affect-modulated startle during unpleasant stimuli in borderline personality disorder. Biol Psychiatry 62:250–255, 2007

Hazlett EA, Buchsbaum MS, Haznedar MM, et al: Cortical gray and white matter volume in unmedicated schizotypal and schizophrenia patients. Schizophr Res 101:111–123, 2008

Hazlett EA, Goldstein KE, Kolaitis JC: A review of structural MRI and diffusion tensor imaging in schizotypal personality disorder. Curr Psychiatry Rep 14:70–78, 2012a

Hazlett EA, Zhang J, New AS, et al: Potentiated amygdala response to repeated emotional pictures in borderline personality disorder. Biol Psychiatry 72:448–456, 2012b

Hazlett EA, Lamade RV, Graff FS, et al: Visual-spatial working memory performance and temporal gray matter volume predict schizotypal personality disorder group membership. Schizophr Res 152:350–357, 2014

Helle AC, Watts AL, Trull TJ, Sher KJ: Alcohol use disorder and antisocial and borderline personality disorders. Alcohol Res 40(1):05, 2019

Herbert JD, Hope DA, Bellack AS: Validity of the distinction between generalized social phobia and avoidant personality disorder. J Abnorm Psychol 101:332–339, 1992

Herpertz SC, Bertsch K: A new perspective on the pathophysiology of borderline personality disorder: a model of the role of oxytocin. Am J Psychiatry 172:840–851, 2015

Herpertz SC, Dietrich TM, Wenning B, et al: Evidence of abnormal amygdala functioning in borderline personality disorder: a functional MRI study. Biol Psychiatry 50:292–298, 2001

Herpertz SC, Zanarini M, Schulz CS, et al: World Federation of Societies of Biological Psychiatry (WFSBP) guidelines for biological treatment of personality disorders. World J Biol Psychiatry 8:212–244, 2007

Herpertz SC, Nagy K, Ueltzhöffer K, et al: Brain mechanisms underlying reactive aggression in borderline personality disorder. Sex matters. Biol Psychiatry 82:257–266, 2017

Hofmann SG, Newman MG, Ehlers A, et al: Psychophysiological differences between subgroups of social phobia. J Abnorm Psychol 104:224–231, 1995

Holzer KJ, Vaughn MG: Antisocial personality disorder in older adults: a critical review. J Geriatr Psychiatry Neurol 30:291–302, 2017

Hyde LW, Byrd AL, Votruba-Drzal E, et al: Amygdala reactivity and negative emotionality: divergent correlates of antisocial personality and psychopathy traits in a community sample. J Abnorm Psychol 123:214–224, 2014

Jakobsen KD, Skyum E, Hashemi N, et al: Antipsychotic treatment of schizotypy and schizotypal personality disorder: a systematic review. J Psychopharmacol 31:397–405, 2017

Jiang W, Shi F, Liao J, et al: Disrupted functional connectome in antisocial personality disorder. Brain Imaging Behav 11:1071–1084, 2017

Jobst A, Sabass L, Palagyi A, et al: Effects of social exclusion on emotions and oxytocin and cortisol levels in patients with chronic depression. J Psychiatr Res 60:170–177, 2015

Jobst A, Padberg F, Mauer M-C, et al: Lower oxytocin plasma levels in borderline patients with unresolved attachment representations. Front Hum Neurosci 10:125, 2016

Johansen MS, Normann-Eide E, Normann-Eide T, et al: Emotional dysfunction in avoidant compared to borderline personality disorder: a study of affect consciousness. Scand J Psychol 54:515–521, 2013

Joyce PR, McKenzie JM, Luty SE, et al: Temperament, childhood environment and psychopathology as risk factors for avoidant and borderline personality disorders. Aust N Z J Psychiatry 37:756–764, 2003

Kawasaki Y, Suzuki M, Nohara S, et al: Structural brain differences in patients with schizophrenia and schizotypal disorder demonstrated by voxel-based morphometry. Eur Arch Psychiatry Clin Neurosci 254:406–414, 2004

Kendler KS, McGuire M, Gruenberg AM, et al: The Roscommon Family Study, I: methods, diagnosis of probands, and risk of schizophrenia in relatives. Arch Gen Psychiatry 50:527–540, 1993

Kendler KS, Aggen SH, Czajkowski N, et al: The structure of genetic and environmental risk factors for DSM-IV personality disorders: a multivariate twin study. Arch Gen Psychiatry 65:1438–1446, 2008

Kendler KS, Aggen SH, Patrick CJ: A multivariate twin study of the DSM-IV criteria for antisocial personality disorder. Biol Psychiatry 71:247–253, 2012

Kernberg OF: Borderline Conditions and Pathological Narcissism. New York, Jason Aronson, 1975

Kimmel CL, Alhassoon OM, Wollman SC, et al: Age-related parieto-occipital and other gray matter changes in borderline personality disorder: a meta-analysis of cortical and subcortical structures. Psychiatry Res Neuroimaging 251:15–25, 2016

King-Casas B, Sharp C, Lomax-Bream L, et al: The rupture and repair of cooperation in borderline personality disorder. Science 321:806–810, 2008

Koenigsberg HW: Affective instability: toward an integration of neuroscience and psychological perspectives. J Pers Disord 24:60–82, 2010

Koenigsberg HW, Harvey PD, Mitropoulou V, et al: Are the interpersonal and identity disturbances in the borderline personality disorder criteria linked to the traits of affective instability and impulsivity? J Pers Disord 15:358–370, 2001

Koenigsberg HW, Reynolds D, Goodman M, et al: Risperidone in the treatment of schizotypal personality disorder. J Clin Psychiatry 64:628–634, 2003

Koenigsberg HW, Fan J, Ochsner KN, et al: Neural correlates of the use of psychological distancing to regulate responses to negative social cues: a study of patients with borderline personality disorder. Biol Psychiatry 66:854–863, 2009

Koenigsberg HW, Denny BT, Fan J, et al: The neural correlates of anomalous habituation to negative emotional pictures in borderline and avoidant personality disorder patients. Am J Psychiatry 171:82–90, 2014

Kolla NJ, Houle S: Single-photon emission computed tomography and positron emission tomography studies of antisocial personality disorder and aggression: a targeted review. Curr Psychiatry Rep 21(4):24, 2019

Kolla NJ, Vinette SA: Monoamine oxidase A in antisocial personality disorder and borderline personality disorder. Curr Behav Neurosci Rep 4:41–48, 2017

Kolla NJ, Chiuccariello L, Wilson AA, et al: Elevated monoamine oxidase–A distribution volume in borderline personality disorder is associated with severity across mood symptoms, suicidality, and cognition. Biol Psychiatry 79:117–126, 2016

Kraus A, Valerius G, Seifritz E, et al: Script-driven imagery of self-injurious behavior in patients with borderline personality disorder: a pilot FMRI study. Acta Psychiatr Scand 121:41–51, 2010

Krause-Utz AD, Elzinga BM: Neural mechanisms of dissociation: implication for borderline personality disorder (in German). Tijdschr Psychiatr 61:267–275, 2019

Kubicki M, McCarley R, Westin C-F, et al: A review of diffusion tensor imaging studies in schizophrenia. J Psychiatr Res 41:15–30, 2007

Kuhlmann A, Bertsch K, Schmidinger I, et al: Morphometric differences in central stress-regulating structures between women with and without borderline personality disorder. J Psychiatry Neurosci 38:129–137, 2013

Kuperberg GR, Broome MR, McGuire PK, et al: Regionally localized thinning of the cerebral cortex in schizophrenia. Arch Gen Psychiatry 60:878–888, 2003

Lampe L: Avoidant personality disorder as a social anxiety phenotype: risk factors, associations and treatment. Curr Opin Psychiatry 29:64–69, 2016

Lazarus SA, Cheavens JS, Festa F, et al: Interpersonal functioning in borderline personality disorder: a systematic review of behavioral and laboratory-based assessments. Clin Psychol Rev 34:193–205, 2014

Leboyer M, Bellivier F, Nosten-Bertrand M, et al: Psychiatric genetics: search for phenotypes. Trends Neurosci 21:102–105, 1998

Lee R, Arfanakis K, Evia AM, et al: White matter integrity reductions in intermittent explosive disorder. Neuropsychopharmacology 41:2697–2703, 2016

Lener MS, Wong E, Tang CY, et al: White matter abnormalities in schizophrenia and schizotypal personality disorder. Schizophr Bull 41:300–310, 2015

Leung WW, McClure MM, Siever LJ, et al: Catechol-O-methyltransferase Val158Met genotype in healthy and personality disorder individuals: preliminary results from an examination of cognitive tests hypothetically differentially sensitive to dopamine functions. Neuropsychiatr Dis Treat 3:925–934, 2007

Levey DF, Gelernter J, Polimanti R, et al: Reproducible genetic risk loci for anxiety: results from approximately 200,000 participants in the Million Veteran Program. Am J Psychiatry 177:223–232, 2020

Levitt JJ, Bobrow L, Lucia D, et al: A selective review of volumetric and morphometric imaging in schizophrenia. Curr Top Behav Neurosci 4:243–281, 2010

Leyton M, Okazawa H, Diksic M, et al: Brain regional alpha-[11C]methyl-L-tryptophan trapping in impulsive subjects with borderline personality disorder. Am J Psychiatry 158:775–782, 2001

Lieb K, Zanarini MC, Schmahl C, et al: Borderline personality disorder. Lancet, 364:453–461, 2004

Lin CCH, Su C-H, Kuo P-H, et al: Genetic and environmental influences on schizotypy among adolescents in Taiwan: a multivariate twin/sibling analysis. Behav Genet 37:334–344, 2007

Lin H-F, Liu Y-L, Liu C-M, et al: Neuregulin 1 gene and variations in perceptual aberration of schizotypal personality in adolescents. Psychol Med 35:1589–1598, 2005

Linehan MM: Dialectical behavior therapy for borderline personality disorder: theory and method. Bull Menninger Clin 51:261–276, 1987

Links PS, Heslegrave R, van Reekum R: Impulsivity: core aspect of borderline personality disorder. J Person Disord 13:1–9, 1999

Links PS, Eynan R, Heisel MJ, et al: Affective instability and suicidal ideation and behavior in patients with borderline personality disorder. J Person Disord 21:72–86, 2007

Lischke A, Domin M, Freyberger HJ, et al: Structural alterations in white-matter tracts connecting (para-)limbic and prefrontal brain regions in borderline personality disorder. Psychol Med 45:3171–3180, 2015

Liu K, Zhang T, Zhang Q, et al: Characterization of the fiber connectivity profile of the cerebral cortex in schizotypal personality disorder: a pilot study. Front Psychol 7:809, 2016

Lubke GH, Laurin C, Amin N, et al: Genome-wide analyses of borderline personality features. Mol Psychiatry 19:923–929, 2014

Ly M, Motzkin JC, Philippi CL, et al: Cortical thinning in psychopathy. Am J Psychiatry 169:743–749, 2012

Lynch TR, Rosenthal MZ, Kosson DS, et al: Heightened sensitivity to facial expressions of emotion in borderline personality disorder. Emotion 6:647–655, 2006

Mancke F, Herpertz SC, Hirjak D, et al: Amygdala structure and aggressiveness in borderline personality disorder. Eur Arch Psychiatry Clin Neurosci 268:417–427, 2018a

Mancke F, Schmitt R, Winter D, et al: Assessing the marks of change: how psychotherapy alters the brain structure in women with borderline personality disorder. J Psychiatry Neurosci 43:171–181, 2018b

Marsh AA, Blair RJR: Deficits in facial affect recognition among antisocial populations: a meta-analysis. Neurosci Biobehav Rev 32:454–465, 2008

Martín-Blanco A, Ferrer M, Soler J, et al: Association between methylation of the glucocorticoid receptor gene, childhood maltreatment, and clinical severity in borderline personality disorder. J Psychiatr Res 57:34–40, 2014

Martín-Blanco A, Ferrer M, Soler J, et al: The role of hypothalamus-pituitary-adrenal genes and childhood trauma in borderline personality disorder. Eur Arch Psychiatry Clin Neurosci 266:307–316, 2016

Matthysse S, Baldessarini RJ: S-adenosylmethionine and catechol-O-methyl-transferase in schizophrenia. Am J Psychiatry 128:1310–1312, 1972

McClure MM, Barch DM, Romero MJ, et al: The effects of guanfacine on context processing abnormalities in schizotypal personality disorder. Biol Psychiatry 61:1157–1160, 2007

McClure MM, Harvey PD, Goodman M, et al: Pergolide treatment of cognitive deficits associated with schizotypal personality disorder: continued evidence of the importance of the dopamine system in the schizophrenia spectrum. Neuropsychopharmacology 35:1356–1362, 2010

McClure MM, Harvey PD, Bowie CR, et al: Functional outcomes, functional capacity, and cognitive impairment in schizotypal personality disorder. Schizophr Res 144:146–150, 2013

McClure MM, Graff F, Triebwasser J, et al: Guanfacine augmentation of a combined intervention of computerized cognitive remediation therapy and social skills training for schizotypal personality disorder. Am J Psychiatry 176:307–314, 2019

McGlashan TH, Grilo CM, Sanislow CA, et al: Two-year prevalence and stability of individual DSM-IV criteria for schizotypal, borderline, avoidant, and obsessive-compulsive personality disorders: toward a hybrid model of axis II disorders. Am J Psychiatry 162:883–889, 2005

Meehan KB, De Panfilis C, Cain NM, et al: Facial emotion recognition and borderline personality pathology. Psychiatry Res 255:347–354, 2017

Mier D, Lis S, Esslinger C, et al: Neuronal correlates of social cognition in borderline personality disorder. Soc Cogn Affect Neurosci 8:531–537, 2013

Miles DR, Carey G: Genetic and environmental architecture of human aggression. J Pers Soc Psychol 72:207–217, 1997

Minzenberg MJ, Fan J, New AS, et al: Frontolimbic structural changes in borderline personality disorder. J Psychiatr Res 42:727–733, 2008

Mitropoulou V, Harvey PD, Maldari LA, et al: Neuropsychological performance in schizotypal personality disorder: evidence regarding diagnostic specificity. Biol Psychiatry 52:1175–1182, 2002

Mitropoulou V, Harvey PD, Zegarelli G, et al: Neuropsychological performance in schizotypal personality disorder: importance of working memory. Am J Psychiatry 162:1896–1903, 2005

Mobascher A, Bohus M, Dahmen N, et al: Association between dopa decarboxylase gene variants and borderline personality disorder. Psychiatry Res 219:693–695, 2014

Morandotti N, Dima D, Jogia J, et al: Childhood abuse is associated with structural impairment in the ventrolateral prefrontal cortex and aggressiveness in patients with borderline personality disorder. Psychiatry Res 213:18–23, 2013

Morgan AB, Lilienfeld SO: A meta-analytic review of the relation between antisocial behavior and neuropsychological measures of executive function. Clin Psychol Rev 20:113–136, 2000

Moroni F, Procacci M, Pellecchia G, et al: Mindreading dysfunction in avoidant personality disorder compared with other personality disorders. J Nerv Ment Dis 204:752–757, 2016

Müller LE, Schulz A, Andermann M, et al: Cortical representation of afferent bodily signals in borderline personality disorder: neural correlates and relationship to emotional dysregulation. JAMA Psychiatry 72:1077–1086, 2015

Nakamura M, McCarley RW, Kubicki M, et al: Fronto-temporal disconnectivity in schizotypal personality disorder: a diffusion tensor imaging study. Biol Psychiatry 58:468–478, 2005

Narr KL, Toga AW, Szeszko P, et al: Cortical thinning in cingulate and occipital cortices in first episode schizophrenia. Biol Psychiatry 58:32–40, 2005

National Collaborating Centre for Mental Health: Antisocial Personality Disorder: Treatment, Management and Prevention. National Clinical Practice Guideline No 77. Leicester, UK, British Psychological Society, 2010

New AS, Hazlett EA, Buchsbaum MS, et al: Blunted prefrontal cortical 18fluorodeoxyglucose positron emission tomography response to meta-chlorophenylpiperazine in impulsive aggression. Arch Gen Psychiatry 59:621–629, 2002

New AS, Buchsbaum MS, Hazlett EA, et al: Fluoxetine increases relative metabolic rate in prefrontal cortex in impulsive aggression. Psychopharmacology 176:451–458, 2004

New AS, Hazlett EA, Buchsbaum MS, et al: Amygdala-prefrontal disconnection in borderline personality disorder. Neuropsychopharmacology 32:1629–1640, 2007

New AS, aan het Rot M, Ripoll LH, et al: Empathy and alexithymia in borderline personality disorder: clinical and laboratory measures. J Pers Disord 26:660–675, 2012

New AS, Carpenter DM, Perez-Rodriguez MM, et al: Developmental differences in diffusion tensor imaging parameters in borderline personality disorder. J Psychiatr Res 47:1101–1109, 2013

Ni X, Chan K, Bulgin N, et al: Association between serotonin transporter gene and borderline personality disorder. J Psychiatr Res 40:448–453, 2006

Ni X, Chan D, Chan K, et al: Serotonin genes and gene-gene interactions in borderline personality disorder in a matched case-control study. Prog Neuropsychopharmacol Biol Psychiatry 33:128–133, 2009

Nica EI, Links PS: Affective instability in borderline personality disorder: experience sampling findings. Curr Psychiatry Rep 11:74–81, 2009

Nicolò G, Semerari A, Lysaker PH, et al: Alexithymia in personality disorders: correlations with symptoms and interpersonal functioning. Psychiatry Res 190:37–42, 2011

Niedtfeld I, Schulze L, Kirsch P, et al: Affect regulation and pain in borderline personality disorder: a possible link to the understanding of self-injury. Biol Psychiatry 68:383–391, 2010

Nordstrom BR, Gao Y, Glenn AL, et al: Neurocriminology. Adv Genet 75:255–283, 2011

Nunes PM, Wenzel A, Borges KT, et al: Volumes of the hippocampus and amygdala in patients with borderline personality disorder: a meta-analysis. J Pers Disord 23:333–345, 2009

Oertel-Knochel V, Knochel C, Stablein M, et al: Abnormal functional and structural asymmetry as biomarker for schizophrenia. Curr Top Med Chem 12:2434–2451, 2012

Ohi K, Hashimoto R, Nakazawa T, et al: The p250GAP gene is associated with risk for schizophrenia and schizotypal personality traits. PLoS ONE 7:e35696, 2012

Olabi B, Ellison-Wright I, McIntosh AM, et al: Are there progressive brain changes in schizophrenia? A meta-analysis of structural magnetic resonance imaging studies. Biol Psychiatry 70:88–96, 2011

O'Neill A, Frodl T: Brain structure and function in borderline personality disorder. Brain Struct Funct 217:767–782, 2012

Ostrov JM, Houston RJ: The utility of forms and functions of aggression in emerging adulthood: association with personality disorder symptomatology. J Youth Adolesc 37:1147–1158, 2008

Pellecchia G, Moroni F, Colle L, et al: Avoidant personality disorder and social phobia: does mindreading make the difference? Compr Psychiatry 80:163–169, 2018

Perez-Rodriguez MM, Weinstein S, New AS, et al: Tryptophan-hydroxylase 2 haplotype association with borderline personality disorder and aggression in a sample of patients with personality disorders and healthy controls. J Psychiatr Res 44:1075–1081, 2010

Perez-Rodriguez MM, Hazlett EA, Rich EL, et al: Striatal activity in borderline personality disorder with comorbid intermittent explosive disorder: sex differences. J Psychiatr Res 46:797–804, 2012

Perez-Rodriguez MM, New AS, Goldstein KE, et al: Brain-derived neurotrophic factor Val66Met genotype modulates amygdala habituation. Psychiatry Res Neuroimaging 263:85–92, 2017

Perez-Rodriguez MM, Bulbena-Cabré A, Bassir Nia A, et al: The neurobiology of borderline personality disorder. Psychiatr Clin North Am 41:633–650, 2018

Perroud N, Paoloni-Giacobino A, Prada P, et al: Increased methylation of glucocorticoid receptor gene (NR3C1) in adults with a history of childhood maltreatment: a link with the severity and type of trauma. Transl Psychiatry 1(12):e59, 2011

Perroud N, Salzmann A, Prada P, et al: Response to psychotherapy in borderline personality disorder and methylation status of the BDNF gene. Transl Psychiatry 3(1):e207, 2013

Perroud N, Zewdie S, Stenz L, et al: Methylation of serotonin receptor 3A in ADHD, borderline personality, and bipolar disorders: link with severity of the disorders and childhood maltreatment. Depress Anxiety 33:45–55, 2016

Pham TH, Philippot P: Decoding of facial expression of emotion in criminal psychopaths. J Pers Disord 24:445–459, 2010

Pietrini P, Guazzelli M, Basso G, et al: Neural correlates of imaginal aggressive behavior assessed by positron emission tomography in healthy subjects. Am J Psychiatry 157:1772–1781, 2000

Poitou P, Assicot M, Bohuon C: Soluble and membrane catechol-o-methyl transferases in red blood cells of schizophrenic patients. Biomedicine 21:91–93, 1974

Popova NK: From genes to aggressive behavior: the role of serotonergic system. Bioessays 28:495–503, 2006

Prados J, Stenz L, Courtet P, et al: Borderline personality disorder and childhood maltreatment: a genome-wide methylation analysis. Genes Brain Behav 14:177–188, 2015

Prossin AR, Love TM, Koeppe RA, et al: Dysregulation of regional endogenous opioid function in borderline personality disorder. Am J Psychiatry 167:925–933, 2010

Raine A, Lencz T, Bihrle S, et al: Reduced prefrontal gray matter volume and reduced autonomic activity in antisocial personality disorder. Arch Gen Psychiatry 57:119–127; discussion 128–129, 2000

Raine A, Lencz T, Taylor K, et al: Corpus callosum abnormalities in psychopathic antisocial individuals. Arch Gen Psychiatry 60:1134–1142, 2003

Raine A, Lee L, Yang Y, et al: Neurodevelopmental marker for limbic maldevelopment in antisocial personality disorder and psychopathy. Br J Psychiatry 197:186–192, 2010

Rautiainen M-R, Paunio T, Repo-Tiihonen E, et al: Genome-wide association study of antisocial personality disorder. Transl Psychiatry 6(9):e883, 2016

Reich J: The relationship of social phobia to avoidant personality disorder: a proposal to reclassify avoidant personality disorder based on clinical empirical findings. Eur Psychiatry 15:151–159, 2000

Reitz S, Kluetsch R, Niedtfeld I, et al: Incision and stress regulation in borderline personality disorder: neurobiological mechanisms of self-injurious behaviour. Br J Psychiatry 207:165–172, 2015

Renneberg B, Herm K, Hahn A, et al: Perception of social participation in borderline personality disorder. Clin Psychol Psychother 19:473–480, 2012

Rinne T, de Kloet ER, Wouters L, et al: Hyperresponsiveness of hypothalamic-pituitary-adrenal axis to combined dexamethasone/corticotropin-releasing hormone challenge in female borderline personality disorder subjects with a history of sustained childhood abuse. Biol Psychiatry 52:1102–1112, 2002

Ripoll LH, Triebwasser J, Siever LJ: Evidence-based pharmacotherapy for personality disorders. Int J Neuropsychopharmacol 14:1257–1288, 2011

Ripoll LH, Snyder R, Steele H, et al: The neurobiology of empathy in borderline personality disorder. Curr Psychiatry Rep 15(3):344, 2013

Rosell DR, Futterman SE, McMaster A, et al: Schizotypal personality disorder: a current review. Curr Psychiatry Rep 16(7):452, 2014

Rosell DR, Zaluda LC, McClure MM, et al: Effects of the D1 dopamine receptor agonist dihydrexidine (DAR-0100A) on working memory in schizotypal personality disorder. Neuropsychopharmacology 40:446–453, 2015

Rosenthal MZ, Kim K, Herr NR, et al: Speed and accuracy of facial expression classification in avoidant personality disorder: a preliminary study. Personal Disord 2:327–334, 2011

Roussos P, Siever LJ: Neurobiological contributions, in The Oxford Handbook of Personality Disorders. Edited by Widiger TA. Oxford, UK, Oxford University Press, 2012, pp 299–324

Roussos P, Bitsios P, Giakoumaki SG, et al: CACNA1C as a risk factor for schizotypal personality disorder and schizotypy in healthy individuals. Psychiatry Res 206:122–123, 2013

Roxo MR, Franceschini PR, Zubaran C, et al: The limbic system conception and its historical evolution. ScientificWorldJournal 11:2428–2441, 2011

Ruocco AC, Carcone D: A neurobiological model of borderline personality disorder: systematic and integrative review. Harv Rev Psychiatry 24:311–329, 2016

Ruocco AC, Amirthavasagam S, Zakzanis KK: Amygdala and hippocampal volume reductions as candidate endophenotypes for borderline personality disorder: a meta-analysis of magnetic resonance imaging studies. Psychiatry Res 201:245–252, 2012

Rüsch N, Weber M, Il'yasov KA, et al: Inferior frontal white matter microstructure and patterns of psychopathology in women with borderline personality disorder and comorbid attention-deficit hyperactivity disorder. NeuroImage 35:738–747, 2007

Sala M, Caverzasi E, Lazzaretti M, et al: Dorsolateral prefrontal cortex and hippocampus sustain impulsivity and aggressiveness in borderline personality disorder. J Affect Disord 131:417–421, 2011

Savitz J, van der Merwe L, Newman TK, et al: Catechol-o-methyltransferase genotype and childhood trauma may interact to impact schizotypal personality traits. Behav Genet 40:415–423, 2010

Schmahl C, Bohus M, Esposito F, et al: Neural correlates of antinociception in borderline personality disorder. Arch Gen Psychiatry 63:659–667, 2006

Schmahl C, Meinzer M, Zeuch A, et al: Pain sensitivity is reduced in borderline personality disorder, but not in posttraumatic stress disorder and bulimia nervosa. World J Biol Psychiatry 11:364–371, 2010

Schmitt R, Winter D, Niedtfeld I, et al: Effects of psychotherapy on neuronal correlates of reappraisal in female patients with borderline personality disorder. Biol Psychiatry Cogn Neurosci Neuroimaging 1:548–557, 2016

Schulze L, Domes G, Krüger A, et al: Neuronal correlates of cognitive reappraisal in borderline patients with affective instability. Biol Psychiatry 69:564–573, 2011

Schulze L, Schmahl C, Niedtfeld I: Neural correlates of disturbed emotion processing in borderline personality disorder: a multimodal meta-analysis. Biol Psychiatry 79:97–106, 2016

Semerari A, Colle L, Pellecchia G, et al: Metacognitive dysfunctions in personality disorders: correlations with disorder severity and personality styles. J Pers Disord 28:751–766, 2014

Sharp C, Kim S: Recent advances in the developmental aspects of borderline personality disorder. Curr Psychiatry Rep 17(4):556, 2015

Shea MT, Stout R, Gunderson J, et al: Short-term diagnostic stability of schizotypal, borderline, avoidant, and obsessive-compulsive personality disorders. Am J Psychiatry 159:2036–2041, 2002

Siegel BV, Trestman RL, O'Flaithbheartaigh S, et al: D-amphetamine challenge effects on Wisconsin Card Sort Test: performance in schizotypal personality disorder. Schizophr Res 20:29–32, 1996

Siever LJ, Davis KL: The pathophysiology of schizophrenia disorders: perspectives from the spectrum. Am J Psychiatry 161:398–413, 2004

Siever LJ, Buchsbaum MS, New AS, et al: d,l-Fenfluramine response in impulsive personality disorder assessed with [18F]fluorodeoxyglucose positron emission tomography. Neuropsychopharmacology 20:413–423, 1999

Siever LJ, Koenigsberg HW, Harvey P, et al: Cognitive and brain function in schizotypal personality disorder. Schizophr Res 54:157–167, 2002

Skodol AE, Gunderson JG, McGlashan TH, et al: Functional impairment in patients with schizotypal, borderline, avoidant, or obsessive-compulsive personality disorder. Am J Psychiatry 159:276–283, 2002a

Skodol AE, Gunderson JG, Pfohl B, et al: The borderline diagnosis I: psychopathology, comorbidity, and personality structure. Biol Psychiatry 51:936–950, 2002b

Skodol AE, Gunderson JG, Shea MT, et al: The Collaborative Longitudinal Personality Disorders Study (CLPS): overview and implications. J Pers Disord 19:487–504, 2005

Skoglund C, Tiger A, Rück C, et al: Familial risk and heritability of diagnosed borderline personality disorder: a register study of the Swedish population. Mol Psychiatry Jun 3, 2019 (Epub ahead of print)

Slavich GM, Tartter MA, Brennan PA, et al: Endogenous opioid system influences depressive reactions to socially painful targeted rejection life events. Psychoneuroendocrinology 49:141–149, 2014

Smaragdi A, Chavez S, Lobaugh NJ, et al: Differential levels of prefrontal cortex glutamate + glutamine in adults with antisocial personality disorder and bipolar disorder: a proton magnetic resonance spectroscopy study. Prog Neuropsychopharmacol Biol Psychiatry 93:250–255, 2019

Soeiro-de-Souza MG, Bio DS, David DP, et al: COMT Met (158) modulates facial emotion recognition in bipolar I disorder mood episodes. J Affect Disord 136:370–376, 2012

Soloff PH, Meltzer CC, Greer PJ, et al: A fenfluramine-activated FDG-PET study of borderline personality disorder. Biol Psychiatry 47:540–547, 2000

Soloff P, Nutche J, Goradia D, et al: Structural brain abnormalities in borderline personality disorder: a voxel-based morphometry study. Psychiatry Res 164:223–236, 2008

Soloff PH, Pruitt P, Sharma M, et al: Structural brain abnormalities and suicidal behavior in borderline personality disorder. J Psychiatr Res 46:516–525, 2012

Sonne S, Rubey R, Brady K, et al: Naltrexone treatment of self-injurious thoughts and behaviors. J Nerv Ment Dis 184:192–195, 1996

Southwick SM, Axelrod SR, Wang S, et al: Twenty-four-hour urine cortisol in combat veterans with PTSD and comorbid borderline personality disorder. J Nerv Ment Dis 191:261–262, 2003

Staebler K, Renneberg B, Stopsack M, et al: Facial emotional expression in reaction to social exclusion in borderline personality disorder. Psychol Med 41:1929–1938, 2011

Stanley B, Siever LJ: The interpersonal dimension of borderline personality disorder: toward a neuropeptide model. Am J Psychiatry 167:24–39, 2010

Stanley B, Sher L, Wilson S, et al: Non-suicidal self-injurious behavior, endogenous opioids and monoamine neurotransmitters. J Affect Disord 124:134–140, 2010

Stefanis NC, Hatzimanolis A, Avramopoulos D, et al: Variation in psychosis gene ZNF804A is associated with a refined schizotypy phenotype but not neurocognitive performance in a large young male population. Schizophr Bull 39:1252–1260, 2013

Sun Y, Zhang L, Ancharaz SS, et al: Decreased fractional anisotropy values in two clusters of white matter in patients with schizotypal personality disorder: a DTI study. Behav Brain Res 310:68–75, 2016

Suzuki M, Zhou S-Y, Takahashi T, et al: Differential contributions of prefrontal and temporo-limbic pathology to mechanisms of psychosis. Brain 128:2109–2122, 2005

Takahashi T, Suzuki M: Brain morphologic changes in early stages of psychosis: implications for clinical application and early intervention. Psychiatry Clin Neurosci 72:556–571, 2018

Takahashi T, Suzuki M, Kawasaki Y, et al: Volumetric magnetic resonance imaging study of the anterior cingulate gyrus in schizotypal disorder. Eur Arch Psychiatry Clin Neurosci 252:268–277, 2002

Takahashi T, Suzuki M, Zhou S-Y, et al: Morphologic alterations of the parcellated superior temporal gyrus in schizophrenia spectrum. Schizophr Res 83:131–143, 2006a

Takahashi T, Suzuki M, Zhou S-Y, et al: Temporal lobe gray matter in schizophrenia spectrum: a volumetric MRI study of the fusiform gyrus, parahippocampal gyrus, and middle and inferior temporal gyri. Schizophr Res 87:116–126, 2006b

Takahashi T, Wood SJ, Yung AR, et al: Progressive gray matter reduction of the superior temporal gyrus during transition to psychosis. Arch Gen Psychiatry 66:366–376, 2009

Takahashi T, Suzuki M, Zhou S-Y, et al: A follow-up MRI study of the superior temporal subregions in schizotypal disorder and first-episode schizophrenia. Schizophr Res 119:65–74, 2010

Takayanagi Y, Sasabayashi D, Takahashi T, et al: Reduced cortical thickness in schizophrenia and schizotypal disorder. Schizophr Bull 46:387–394, 2020

Tamnes CK, Agartz I: White matter microstructure in early-onset schizophrenia: a systematic review of diffusion tensor imaging studies. J Am Acad Child Adolesc Psychiatry 55:269–279, 2016

Taylor CT, Laposa JM, Alden LE: Is avoidant personality disorder more than just social avoidance? J Pers Disord 18:571–594, 2004

Tebartz van Elst L, Hesslinger B, Thiel T, et al: Frontolimbic brain abnormalities in patients with borderline personality disorder: a volumetric magnetic resonance imaging study. Biol Psychiatry 54:163–171, 2003

Teschler S, Bartkuhn M, Künzel N, et al: Aberrant methylation of gene associated CpG sites occurs in borderline personality disorder. PLoS ONE 8:e84180, 2013

Teschler S, Gotthardt J, Dammann G, et al: Aberrant DNA methylation of rDNA and PRIMA1 in borderline personality disorder. Int J Mol Sci 17(1):67, 2016

Thaler L, Gauvin L, Joober R, et al: Methylation of BDNF in women with bulimic eating syndromes: associations with childhood abuse and borderline personality disorder. Prog Neuropsychopharmacol Biol Psychiatry 54:43–49, 2014

Tielbeek JJ, Medland SE, Benyamin B, et al: Unraveling the genetic etiology of adult antisocial behavior: a genome-wide association study. PLoS ONE 7:e45086, 2012

Tiihonen J, Rossi R, Laakso MP, et al: Brain anatomy of persistent violent offenders: more rather than less. Psychiatry Res 163:201–212, 2008

Tillem S, Harenski K, Harenski C, et al: Psychopathy is associated with shifts in the organization of neural networks in a large incarcerated male sample. Neuroimage Clin 24:102083, 2019

Tomppo L, Hennah W, Miettunen J, et al: Association of variants in DISC1 with psychosis-related traits in a large population cohort. Arch Gen Psychiatry 66:134–141, 2009

Torgersen S: Genetic and nosological aspects of schizotypal and borderline personality disorders: a twin study. Arch Gen Psychiatry 41:546–554, 1984

Torgersen S: The nature (and nurture) of personality disorders. Scand J Psychol 50:624–632, 2009

Torgersen S, Lygren S, Øien PA, et al: A twin study of personality disorders. Compr Psychiatry 41:416–425, 2000

Torgersen S, Myers J, Reichborn-Kjennerud T, et al: The heritability of Cluster B personality disorders assessed both by personal interview and questionnaire. J Pers Disord 26:848–866, 2012

Trull TJ, Solhan MB, Tragesser SL, et al: Affective instability: measuring a core feature of borderline personality disorder with ecological momentary assessment. J Abnorm Psychol 117:647–661, 2008

Vandekerckhove M, Vogels C, Berens A, et al: Alterations in the fronto-limbic network and corpus callosum in borderline-personality disorder. Brain Cogn 138:103596, 2020

Velikonja T, Velthorst E, McClure MM, et al: Severe childhood trauma and clinical and neurocognitive features in schizotypal personality disorder. Acta Psychiatr Scand 140:50–64, 2019

Verona E, Sprague J, Sadeh N: Inhibitory control and negative emotional processing in psychopathy and antisocial personality disorder. J Abnorm Psychol 121:498–510, 2012

Völlm B, Richardson P, Stirling J, et al: Neurobiological substrates of antisocial and borderline personality disorder: preliminary results of a functional fMRI study. Crim Behav Ment Health 14:39–54, 2004

Vora AK, Fisher AM, New AS, et al: Dimensional traits of schizotypy associated with glycine receptor GLRA1 polymorphism: an exploratory candidate-gene association study. J Pers Disord 32:421–432, 2018

Wagner AW, Linehan MM: Facial expression recognition ability among women with borderline personality disorder: implications for emotion regulation? J Pers Disord 13:329–344, 1999

Waller R, Gard AM, Shaw DS, et al: Weakened functional connectivity between the amygdala and the ventromedial prefrontal cortex is longitudinally related to psychopathic traits in low-income males during early adulthood. Clin Psychol Sci 7:628–635, 2019

Ward J, Strawbridge RJ, Bailey MES, et al: Genome-wide analysis in UK Biobank identifies four loci associated with mood instability and genetic correlation with major depressive disorder, anxiety disorder and schizophrenia. Transl Psychiatry 7(11):1264, 2017

Weinbrecht A, Schulze L, Boettcher J, et al: Avoidant personality disorder: a current review. Curr Psychiatry Rep 18(3):29, 2016

Whalley HC, Nickson T, Pope M, et al: White matter integrity and its association with affective and interpersonal symptoms in borderline personality disorder. Neuroimage Clin 7:476–481, 2015

Williams GV, Castner SA: Under the curve: critical issues for elucidating D1 receptor function in working memory. Neuroscience 139:263–276, 2006

Williams KD, Jarvis B: Cyberball: a program for use in research on interpersonal ostracism and acceptance. Behav Res Methods 38:174–180, 2006

Wilson ST, Stanley B, Brent DA, et al: Interaction between tryptophan hydroxylase I polymorphisms and childhood abuse is associated with increased risk for borderline personality disorder in adulthood. Psychiatr Genet 22:15–24, 2012

Wingenfeld K, Driessen M, Adam B, et al: Overnight urinary cortisol release in women with borderline personality disorder depends on comorbid PTSD and depressive psychopathology. Eur Psychiatry 22:309–312, 2007

Witt SH, Streit F, Jungkunz M, et al: Genome-wide association study of borderline personality disorder reveals genetic overlap with bipolar disorder, major depression and schizophrenia. Transl Psychiatry 7(6):e1155, 2017

Wrege JS, Ruocco AC, Euler S, et al: Negative affect moderates the effect of social rejection on frontal and anterior cingulate cortex activation in borderline personality disorder. Cogn Affect Behav Neurosci 19:1273–1285, 2019

Yan Z, Schmidt SNL, Frank J, et al: Hyperfunctioning of the right posterior superior temporal sulcus in response to neutral facial expressions presents an endophenotype of schizophrenia. Neuropsychopharmacology 45:1346–1352, 2020

Yang X, Hu L, Zeng J, et al: Default mode network and frontolimbic gray matter abnormalities in patients with borderline personality disorder: a voxel-based meta-analysis. Sci Rep 6:34247, 2016

Yang Y, Raine A, Narr KL, et al: Localization of deformations within the amygdala in individuals with psychopathy. Arch Gen Psychiatry 66:986–994, 2009

Zaehringer J, Ende G, Santangelo P, et al: Improved emotion regulation after neurofeedback: a single-arm trial in patients with borderline personality disorder. Neuroimage Clin 24:102032, 2019

Zanarini MC, Frankenburg FR, Reich DB, et al: The 10-year course of physically self-destructive acts reported by borderline patients and Axis II comparison subjects. Acta Psychiatr Scand 117:177–184, 2008

Zetzsche T, Preuss UW, Frodl T, et al: Hippocampal volume reduction and history of aggressive behaviour in patients with borderline personality disorder. Psychiatry Res 154:157–170, 2007

Zimmerman M, Rothschild L, Chelminski I: The prevalence of DSM-IV personality disorders in psychiatric outpatients. Am J Psychiatry 162:1911–1918, 2005

CHAPTER 9

Longitudinal Course and Outcomes

Carlos M. Grilo, Ph.D.

Andrew E. Skodol, M.D.

In DSM-5 Section II, "Diagnostic Criteria and Codes," a personality disorder (PD) is defined as "an enduring pattern of inner experience and behavior that deviates markedly from the expectations of the individual's culture, is pervasive and inflexible, has an onset in adolescence or early adulthood, is stable over time, and leads to distress or impairment" (American Psychiatric Association 2013, p. 645). DSM-5 Section II specifies that the "enduring pattern" is manifested by problems in at least two of the following areas: cognition, affectivity, interpersonal functioning, and impulse control. The diagnostic construct of PD has evolved considerably over the past few decades, and substantial changes have occurred over time in the number and types of specific PD diagnoses and their criteria (see Skodol 1997, 2012; see also Chapter 1, "Personality Disorders: Recent History and New Directions," in this volume for a detailed ontogeny of the DSM system). Until the introduction of the Alternative DSM-5 Model for Personality Disorders in DSM-5 Section III, "Emerging Measures and Models," one central tenet—that a PD reflects a persistent, pervasive, enduring, and stable pattern—had not changed. Although the concept of stability is salient in the two major classification systems, DSM-5 and ICD-10 (World Health Organization 1992), the two systems differ somewhat in their classifications and definitions of PDs and thus demonstrate only moderate convergence for some diagnoses (Ottosson et al. 2002). Empirical evidence regarding the extent of stability of PDs, however, has historically been mixed, and thus stability over time has been the subject of debate (Grilo and McGlashan 1999; Grilo et al. 1998; Shea and Yen 2003).

The concept of stability has remained a central tenet of PDs through the various editions of DSM dating back to the first edition, published in 1952 (American Psychiatric Association 1952). In DSM-III (American Psychiatric Association 1980), PDs were placed on a separate axis (Axis II) of the multiaxial system. DSM-III indicated that the assignment to Axis II was intended, in part, to encourage clinicians to assess for additional disorders that might be overlooked when focusing on Axis I psychiatric disorders. Conceptually, this reflected, in part, the putative stability of PDs relative to the episodically unstable course of so-called Axis I psychiatric disorders (Grilo et al. 1998; Shea and Yen 2003; Skodol 1997; Skodol et al. 2002). The multiaxial system of recording diagnoses has been discontinued in DSM-5, and all mental disorders are now categorized in the same section (Section II). Although the concept of diagnostic stability of PDs persists unmodified in DSM-5 Section II, the relative stability of trait pathology and impairment in functioning is emphasized in the Section III alternative model (see also Chapter 4, "The Alternative DSM-5 Model for Personality Disorders," and Chapter 5, "Manifestations, Assessment, Diagnosis, and Differential Diagnosis," in this volume).

In this chapter, we first provide a brief review of the twentieth-century empirical literature on the stability of PDs. This period can be thought of as including the first generation (mostly clinical descriptive accounts) and the second generation (emerging findings based on attempts at greater standardization of diagnoses and assessment methods) of empirical research efforts on PDs. After reviewing the literature, we provide a brief overview of methodological problems and conceptual gaps that characterize this literature and that must be considered when interpreting ongoing research and designing future studies. We then summarize new findings from several major long-term longitudinal studies that have contributed much-needed information regarding the longitudinal course of PDs and that call into question their inherent stability.

Overview of Early Literature

Previous reviews addressing aspects of the course and outcome of PDs (e.g., Grilo and McGlashan 1999; Grilo et al. 1998; McDavid and Pilkonis 1996; Perry 1993; Ruegg and Frances 1995; Stone 1993; Zimmerman 1994), although varied, have agreed on the pervasiveness of methodological problems characterizing much of the early literature, which precluded any firm conclusions about the nature of the stability of PDs. The reviews, however, have also generally agreed that the emerging research was raising questions regarding many aspects of the construct validity of PDs (Zimmerman 1994), including their hypothesized high degree of stability (Grilo and McGlashan 1999).

The few early (pre-DSM-III-era) studies of the course of PDs reported findings that borderline PD (BPD) (e.g., Carpenter and Gunderson 1977; Grinker et al. 1968) and antisocial PD (ASPD) (Maddocks 1970; Robbins et al. 1977) were highly stable. Carpenter and Gunderson (1977), for example, reported that the impairment in functioning observed for patients with BPD was comparable to that observed for patients with schizophrenia over a 5-year period. Grilo et al. (1998) noted that the dominant clinical approach to assessing PD diagnoses based partly on treatment refractoriness naturally raises the question of whether these findings simply reflect a tautology.

The separation of PDs to Axis II in DSM-III (American Psychiatric Association 1980) contributed to increased research attention to these clinical problems (Blashfield and McElroy 1987). The development and utilization of a number of structured and standardized approaches to clinical interviewing and diagnosis during the 1980s represented notable advances (Zimmerman 1994). The greater attention paid to defining the criteria required for diagnosis in the classification systems and to developing standardized interviews greatly facilitated research efforts in this field.

In our previous reviews of DSM-III and DSM-III-R (American Psychiatric Association 1987) studies, we concluded that the available research suggested that "personality disorders demonstrate only moderate stability and that, although personality disorders are generally associated with negative outcomes, they can improve over time and can benefit from specific treatments" (Grilo and McGlashan 1999, p. 157). In our 1998 review (Grilo et al. 1998), we noted that the 20 selected studies of DSM-III-R criteria generally found low to moderate stability of any PD over relatively short follow-up periods (6–24 months). For example, studies that employed diagnostic interviews reported kappa coefficients between assessments for the presence of any PD of 0.32 (Johnson et al. 1997), 0.40 (Ferro et al. 1998), 0.50 (Loranger et al. 1994), and 0.55 (Loranger et al. 1991). Especially noteworthy is the fact that the stability coefficients for specific PD diagnoses (in the few cases they could be calculated given the sample sizes) were generally lower. Follow-up studies of adolescents diagnosed with PDs also reported modest stability; for example, Mattanah et al. (1995) reported a 50% rate of stability for any PD at 2-year follow-up, and Grilo et al. (2001) reported modest stability for dimensional PD scores in a follow-up study of psychiatrically hospitalized adolescents. Squires-Wheeler et al. (1992), as part of the New York High-Risk Project, reported low stability for schizotypal PD (STPD) and features, although the stability was higher for the offspring of patients with schizophrenia than for those of patients with mood disorders or control subjects. Subsequently, Grilo and McGlashan (1999) reviewed nine reports of longitudinal findings for PD diagnoses published from 1997 to 1998. In terms of specific diagnoses, the studies generally reported moderate stability (kappa coefficients of approximately 0.50) for BPD and ASPD. The studies in these reports, like those in most of the previous literature, had small sample sizes and infrequently followed more than one PD.

Two longitudinal studies assessed PD features using standardized interview and self-report methods to obtain complementary information on personality changes over time in nonclinical samples. In the first study, Trull et al. (1997, 1998) reported modest stability coefficients, ranging from 0.28 to 0.62, for both self-report and interview measures of BPD features using two different assessment instruments administered to a college student sample assessed twice over a 2-year period. Two-year stability coefficients for the self-report measures tended to be higher than those for interview-based measures of features. There was some heterogeneity in the borderline feature changes and reductions over time; negative affectivity, but not personal distress levels, moderated the stability of scores (Trull et al. 1998). BPD features were associated with greater academic and interpersonal difficulties at 2-year follow-up. The Longitudinal Study of Personality Disorders (LSPD; Lenzenweger 1999) assessed 250 participants drawn from Cornell University at three points over a 4-year period. Of the 250 participants, 129 had presentations that met the criteria for at least one PD, and 121 had presentations that did not meet the full criteria for any PD. Lenzenweger (1999) found that dimensional scores for the PDs were characterized by significant levels of stability both on the interview and on self-report measures of PD. Stability coefficients for total number of PD features ranged from 0.61 to 0.70, and PD dimensions showed significant declines over time, with the PD group showing more rapid declines than the group without PDs. Cluster B had the highest stability coefficients, and Cluster A had the lowest. Subsequent reanalyses of the LSPD data using individual growth curve methods revealed considerable variability in PD features across individuals over the 4-year period (Lenzenweger et al. 2004). The reanalyses also indicated that the course of PD features is heterogeneous, with different trajectories characterizing individuals considered symptomatic or with presentations meeting criteria for a diagnosis versus those with presentations not meeting criteria (Hallquist and Lenzenweger 2013).

The two nonclinical longitudinal studies (Lenzenweger 1999; Trull et al. 1997, 1998) demonstrated the value of using multiple assessment methods in repeated-measures longitudinal designs and highlighted that borderline features may be associated with poorer outcomes, even in nonclinical populations (Trull et al. 1997). These studies, however, were limited by their relatively homogeneous study groups of college students, narrow development time frames, and insufficient frequency of any specific PD diagnosis (i.e., at diagnostic caseness level), so meaningful analyses of clinical entities were not possible.

Conceptual and Methodological Issues

Previous reviews of PDs have raised various methodological concerns. Common limitations highlighted include small sample sizes; concerns about unstandardized assessments, interrater reliability, blindness to baseline characteristics, and narrow assessments; failure to consider alternative (e.g., dimensional) models of PDs; reliance on only two assessments typically over short follow-up periods; insufficient attention to the nature and effects of other co-occurring disorders; and inattention to treatment effects. Particularly striking is the absence of "relevant" comparison or control groups in the longitudinal literature. A recent review (Hopwood and Bleidorn 2018) identified six factors that affect estimates of personality and personality disorder stability and change: 1) types of stability (i.e., differential stability vs. absolute change); 2) constructs studied (i.e., personality disorders vs. personality traits); 3) sampling (i.e., at hospital admission vs. in a community); 4) assessment (i.e., self-report questionnaire vs. diagnostic interview); 5) development (i.e., adolescence or early adulthood vs. mid- or late life); and 6) other influences (i.e., genetic vs. environmental factors). We comment briefly on a few of these issues.

Reliability

Reliability of assessments represents a central issue for any study of course and outcome. The emergence of standardized instruments for collecting diagnostic data on PDs was a major development of the 1980s (Zimmerman 1994). Such instruments, however, were less-than-perfect assessment methods and have been criticized for a variety of reasons (e.g., Westen 1997; Westen and Shedler 1999). It is critical, however, to recognize that interrater reliability and test-retest reliability represent the upper limits (or ceiling) for estimating the stability of a construct.

Previous reviews of diagnostic interviews for PDs (Grilo and McGlashan 1999; Zanarini et al. 2000; Zimmerman 1994) have generally reported median interrater reliability coefficients of roughly 0.70 and short-interval test-retest reliability coefficients of 0.50 for diagnoses. These reliability coefficients compare favorably with those generally reported for diagnostic instruments for other psychiatric disorders. Similar interrater and short-term test-retest findings continued to characterize the reliability literature through DSM-IV (American Psychiatric Association 1994) and initially for DSM-5 for mental disorder diagnoses determined using various assessment methods (Regier et al. 2013). Both interrater and test-retest reliability coefficients tend to be higher for dimensional scores than for categorical diagnoses of PDs. Although technically not a "reliability issue," a related point is that even when experts administer diagnostic interviews, the degree of convergence or agreement produced by two different interviews administered only a week apart is limited (Oldham et al. 1992). Also, the degree of concordance between different diagnostic interviews, clinical interviews, and self-report methods is limited (Samuel et al. 2013). These results call into question the construct validity of PD diagnostic categories themselves.

Reliability and "Change"

Test-retest reliability is also relevant for addressing, in part, the well-known problem of "regression to the mean" in repeated-measures studies (Nesselroade et al. 1980). It has been argued that the multiwave or repeated-measures approach lessens the effects of regression to the mean (Lenzenweger 1999). This might be the case in terms of the obvious decreases in severity with time (i.e., very symptomatic participants meeting eligibility at study entry are likely to show some improvement, since by definition they are already reporting high levels of symptoms). However, other effects need to be considered whenever assessments are repeated within a study. For example, Shea and Yen (2003) noted that repeated-measures studies of both PD (Loranger et al. 1991) and other mental disorder (Robins 1985) diagnoses have found hints that participants systematically report or endorse fewer problems during repeated interviews to reduce interview time. Loranger et al. (1991), in their test-retest study of the Personality Diagnostic Examination (PDE) interview conducted between 1 and 26 weeks after baseline, observed significant decreases in PD criteria for all but two of the DSM-III-R diagnoses. The PDE, which requires skilled and trained research clinicians, has a required minimum duration stipulation of 5 years for determining persistence and pervasiveness of the criteria being assessed. Thus, the magnitude of changes observed during such a short period of time, which was shown to be unrelated to "state-trait effects," reflects some combination of the following: regression to the mean, error in either or both the baseline and repeated assessments, overreporting by patients at intake assessment, and underreporting during retest at follow-up (Gunderson et al. 2004; Loranger et al. 1991; Shea and Yen 2003). Therefore, in assessing patients for personality psychopathology, clinicians should be wary of incentives for overreporting (e.g., admission to a desirable treatment facility) and underreporting (e.g., discharge from a hospital).

Categorical Versus Dimensional Approaches

Long-standing debate regarding the conceptual and empirical advantages of dimensional models of PDs (Frances 1982; Livesley et al. 1992; Loranger et al. 1994; Skodol 2012; Widiger 1992) has accompanied the DSM categorical classification system. Overall, longitudinal studies of PDs have reported moderate levels of stability for dimensional scores for most disorders, and stability coefficients tend to be higher than for categorical or diagnostic stability (Ferro et al. 1998; Hopwood et al. 2013; Johnson et al. 1997; Klein and Shih 1998; Loranger et al. 1991, 1994; Morey et al. 2007, 2012).

Dimensional assessments of personality psychopathology (functioning and traits) are highlighted in the hybrid dimensional-categorical model of PDs in DSM-5 Section III. Recognizing that diagnostic thresholds for almost all PDs in Section II of DSM-5 are set without empirical bases, clinicians should regard "subthreshold" cases as possibly milder versions of full-blown disorders and treat the patients in these cases accordingly.

Comorbidity

Most studies have had some participants whose presentations met the criteria for multiple mental disorder diagnoses. This problem of diagnostic overlap or comorbidity represents a well-known, long-standing major challenge in working with clinical samples (Berkson 1946). One expert and critic of DSM (Tyrer 2001), in speaking of the "spectre of comorbidity," noted that "the main reason for abandoning the present classification is summed up in one word, comorbidity. Comorbidity is the nosologist's nightmare; it shouts, 'You have failed'" (p. 82). We suggest, however, that such clinical realities (multiple presenting problems that are especially characteristic of treatment-seeking patients) represent both potential confounds and potential opportunities to understand personality and dysfunctions of personality better. Comorbidity begs the question: What are the fundamental personality dimensions and disorders of personality, and how do their courses influence (and conversely, how are their courses affected by) the presence and course of other psychiatric disorders?

Continuity

A related issue pertaining to course concerns longitudinal comorbidities (Kendell and Clarkin 1992) or continuities. An obvious example is that conduct disorder during adolescence is required for the diagnosis of ASPD to be given to adults. This definitional isomorphism is one likely reason for the consistently strong associations between conduct disorder and later ASPD in the literature. This is, however, more than an artifactual relationship, because longitudinal research has documented that children and adolescents with early-onset behavior disorders have substantially elevated risk for antisocial behavior during adulthood (Moffitt 1993; Robins 1966). More generally, studies with diverse recruitment and ascertainment methods found that disruptive behavior disorders during the adolescent years prospectively predicted PDs of various types during young adulthood (Bernstein et al. 1996; Lewinsohn et al. 1997; Myers et al. 1998; Rey et al. 1995). In addition, children with conduct disorder are at risk for other externalizing and internalizing mental disorders, not only for ASPD (e.g., Kim-Cohen et al. 2003). Moreover, other childhood disorders, in addition to conduct disorder, increase the risk of ASPD (e.g., Kasen et al. 2001). Thus, the relationship between conduct disorder and ASPD is not specific. The Yale Psychiatric Institute follow-up study found that PD diagnoses in adolescent inpatients prospectively predicted greater drug use problems but not global functioning (Levy et al. 1999).

The importance of considering comorbidity is underscored in the findings of the longitudinal study by Lewinsohn et al. (1997). These authors found that the apparent longitudinal continuity for disruptive behavioral disorders during adolescence and subsequent ASPD in adulthood was predicted, in part, by the presence of other mental disorder comorbidity. More recently, analyses from the National Epidemiologic Survey on Alcohol and Related Conditions comparing adults with ASPD with adults whose presentation met all the criteria for ASPD except the requirement that conduct disorder be present before age 15 differed little in 3-year course of antisocial behaviors after adjusting for differences in psychiatric comorbidity (Goldstein and Grant 2009). A longitudinal study of young adult men found that PDs predicted the subsequent onset of psychiatric disorders during a 2-year follow-up, even after the researchers controlled for previous psychiatric history (Johnson et al. 1997).

Comorbidity and Continuity Models

Certain disorders may be associated with one another in a number of possible ways over time. A variety of models have been proposed for the possible relationships between personality and other mental disorders (e.g., Dolan-Sewell et al. 2001; Lyons et al. 1997; Shea et al. 2004; Tyrer et al. 1997). These include, for example, the predisposition, or vulnerability, model; the complication, or scar, model; the pathoplasty, or exacerbation, model; and various spectrum models. We emphasize that these models do not necessarily assume categorical entities. Indeed, an especially influential spectrum model proposed by Siever and Davis (1991) posits four psychobiological dimensions to account for all types of psychopathology. The Cloninger et al. (1993) psychobiological model of temperament and character represents another valuable approach that considers dimensions across personality and other psychopathology. More broadly, Krueger (1999; Krueger and Tackett 2003) noted that although most research has focused on pairs of constructs (i.e., personality and other disorder associations), it seems important to examine the "multivariate structure of the personality-psychopathology domain" (p. 109).

Age (Early Onset)

As stressed by Widiger (2003), PDs need to be more clearly conceptualized and carefully characterized as having an early onset. However, the validity of PDs in adolescents remains controversial (Krueger and Carlson 2001). It can be argued, for example, that determining early onset of PDs is impossible because adolescence is a period of profound changes and flux in personality and identity. A critical review of the longitudinal literature on personality traits throughout the life span revealed that personality traits are less stable during childhood and adolescence than they are later in life (Roberts and DelVecchio 2000). Roberts and DelVecchio's (2000) meta-analysis of data from 152 longitudinal studies of personality traits revealed that rank-order consistency for personality traits increased steadily throughout the life span; test-retest correlations (over 6.7-year time intervals) increased from 0.31 during childhood to 0.54 during college, to 0.64 at age 30, to a high of 0.74 at ages 50–70.

Nonetheless, if childhood precursors of PDs could be identified (as in the case of early-onset conduct disorder for ASPD), they could become part of the diagnostic criteria, creating some degree of longitudinal continuity in the diagnostic system. More generally, temperamental vulnerabilities or precursors to PDs have been posited as central in a variety of models (e.g., Cloninger et al. 1993; Siever and Davis 1991). Specific temperamental features evident in childhood have been noted to be precursors for diverse PDs (Paris 2003; Rettew et al. 2003; Wolff et al. 1991), as well as for differences in interpersonal functioning (Newman et al. 1997) in adulthood. For example, studies have noted early odd and withdrawn patterns preceding STPD in adults (Wolff et al.

1991) and shyness preceding avoidant PD (AVPD) (Rettew et al. 2003). Speaking more generally, although the degree of stability for personality traits is higher throughout adulthood than throughout childhood and adolescence (Roberts and DelVecchio 2000), longitudinal analyses of personality data have revealed that the transition from adolescence to adulthood is characterized by greater personality continuity than change (Roberts et al. 2001). (See also Chapter 10, "Early Identification and Prevention of Personality Pathology: An AMPD-Informed Model of Clinical Staging," in this volume for a detailed consideration of age-at-onset issues and their potential clinical utility.)

Age and the Aging Process

Another age issue concerns the aging process. Considerable research suggests that personality remains relatively stable through adulthood (Heatherton and Weinberger 1994; Roberts and DelVecchio 2000) and is highly stable after age 50 (Roberts and DelVecchio 2000). Little is known, however, about PDs in older persons (Abrams et al. 1998), although this topic has recently become the focus of increasing research attention (Oldham and Skodol 2013).

A 12-year follow-up of PDs as part of the Nottingham Study of Neurotic Disorder (Seivewright et al. 2002) documented substantial changes in trait scores based on blind administration of a semistructured interview. Seivewright et al. (2002) reported that two Cluster B PD diagnoses (antisocial, histrionic) showed significant improvements, whereas diagnoses in Cluster A (schizoid, schizotypal, paranoid) and Cluster C (obsessional, avoidant) appeared to worsen with age. The Seivewright et al. (2002) findings, however, are limited by the two-point cross-sectional assessment, which could not address the nature of changes during the intervening period. These findings echo somewhat the results of the seminal Chestnut Lodge follow-up studies (McGlashan 1986a, 1986b), which found that decreases in impulsivity and interpersonal instability but increases in avoidance occur with age. There exist other reports of diminished impulsivity with increasing age in patients with BPD (Paris and Zweig-Frank 2001; Stevenson et al. 2003), although this was not observed in a prospective analysis of individual borderline criteria (McGlashan et al. 2005). Galione and Oltmanns (2013), using data from a large-scale epidemiological study, reported significant associations between BPD and major depression in older adults and found that a history of major depression is particularly associated with stable BPD features related to distress, which are more common than acute behavioral features among older adults. Schuster et al. (2013), in another large epidemiological study, found that PDs are both common and strongly associated with various forms of disability and medical/psychiatric comorbidities among older adults. A recent study of 998 individuals ages 55–64 in the St. Louis Personality and Aging Network (SPAN) study showed that personality traits of neuroticism, impulsivity, and agreeableness predicted physical health problems following stressful life events that were dependent, at least in part, on the person's behavior (i.e., personality-generated stressful life events), but not following independent life events (Iacovino et al. 2016). Cruitt and Oltmanns (2018), in their recent review, concluded that personality disorder features are linked to suicidal ideation, poorer physical health, and cognitive decline in later life and recommended use of the Alternative DSM-5 Model for Personality Disorders (AMPD) with older adults.

Clinicians may have to adjust their thresholds for diagnosis of PDs in elders, because some of the standard criteria may not be applicable because of life events (e.g., death of a spouse) or changing life circumstances (e.g., retirement). The DSM-5 Section III personality functioning and trait-based criteria may be easier to use in assessing the elderly, because these criteria do not depend as heavily on specific exemplars, which are often age dependent, as do the Section II criteria.

Summary and Implications

To resolve the various complex issues discussed in this section, complementary research efforts are required with large samples of both clinical and community samples. Prospective longitudinal studies with repeated assessments over time are needed to understand the course of PDs. Such studies must consider (and cut across) different developmental eras, broad domains of functioning, and multimodal approaches to personality and PDs. These approaches have, in fact, been performed with personality traits (Roberts et al. 2001) and with other forms of psychiatric problems, such as in the National Institute of Mental Health (NIMH)–funded multisite longitudinal study of depression, the Collaborative Depression Study (NIMH-CDS; Katz et al. 1979), and have yielded invaluable insights. Over the past two decades, such advances have come to characterize the PD longitudinal literature, to which we turn next.

Review of Major Empirical Advances and Understanding of Stability

Of particular relevance for our literature review are three large-scale long-term prospective studies on the longitudinal course of PDs funded by the National Institutes of Health throughout the 1990s and continuing into the twenty-first century. The three studies are the multisite Collaborative Longitudinal Personality Disorders Study (CLPS; Gunderson et al. 2000); the McLean Study of Adult Development (MSAD; Zanarini et al. 2003); and the Children in the Community Study (CICS; Brook et al. 2002; Cohen et al. 2005b), a community-based prospective longitudinal study of personality, psychopathology, and functioning of children/adolescents and their mothers that began in 1983. These long-term studies, which corrected for many of the limitations that characterized the previous literature, have provided invaluable data for understanding the natural life course of persons with PDs. They have utilized standardized assessment methods, carefully considered training and reliability, and— perhaps most notably—employed multiwave repeated assessments that are essential for determining longitudinal change. They have employed, to varying degrees, multiple assessment methods and have considered both "personality" and PDs, as well as other mental disorders and psychosocial functioning. Collectively, these studies have provided crucial insights into the complexities of personality (features, traits, and disorders) and its vicissitudes over time.

Collaborative Longitudinal Personality Disorders Study

The CLPS (Gunderson et al. 2000; McGlashan et al. 2000; Skodol et al. 2005b) is a prospective longitudinal repeated-measures study designed to examine the natural course and outcome of PDs, with a primary focus on patients whose presentation met DSM-IV criteria for one of four specific PDs: STPD, BPD, AVPD, or obsessive-compulsive

PD (OCPD). The CLPS also includes a comparison group of patients with major depressive disorder (MDD) without any PD. This comparison group was selected because of the purported episodic and fluctuating course of MDD (thought to distinguish what were called Axis I from Axis II disorders in DSM-III through DSM-IV) and because MDD has been carefully studied in similar longitudinal designs (e.g., the NIMH-CDS; Katz et al. 1979; Solomon et al. 1997). The CLPS employed multimodal assessments (Gunderson et al. 2000; Zanarini et al. 2000) to prospectively follow and capture various aspects of the fluctuating nature of PDs and dimensions (both interviewer based and self-report, representing different conceptual models) (Morey et al. 2007, 2012; Samuel et al. 2011), other psychiatric disorders and symptoms (Cain et al. 2012; Grilo et al. 2005, 2007), psychosocial functioning (Markowitz et al. 2007; Skodol et al. 2005a, 2005c), and treatment utilization (Bender et al. 2006, 2007).

Studies of the longitudinal course and outcome of many disorders have generally employed concepts of *remission* or *recovery* (Frank et al. 1991), although these concepts have not, until recently, been applied much in PD research, likely because of the "presumption of stability" (Skodol 2012). Frank et al. (1991) defined *remission* as a brief period of improvement with no more than minimal symptoms and *recovery* as improvement lasting for an indefinite amount of time, implying recovery from the disorder. The CLPS (e.g., Grilo et al. 2004) employed the concept of *remission* using two definitions in order to allow direct comparison of the PD groups to the group of patients with MDD without PD, given the established methodology in the depression literature used by the NIMH-CDS (Solomon et al. 1997). To parallel the NIMH-CDS conventions, one definition of *remission* required at least 8 consecutive weeks (2 months) with two or fewer criteria of the diagnosis being present, and one definition required a substantially longer time requirement of 12 consecutive months with no more than two criteria of the diagnosis being present. The latter 12-month definition was adopted to provide a much more stringent definition of *remission* to reflect a more clinically significant change in PD psychopathology. The CLPS adopted a parallel definition of *relapse*, defined as the return to diagnostic threshold for at least 2 consecutive months for PDs and all other disorders, again to parallel the NIMH-CDS conventions. The CLPS prospectively evaluated time to remission and relapse using a PD interview assessment modeled after the Longitudinal Interval Follow-up Evaluation (LIFE; Keller et al. 1987) methodology used in the NIMH-CDS (Solomon et al. 1997), which was also used by the CLPS to prospectively evaluate MDD and other mental disorders.

The CLPS has reported on different concepts of categorical and dimensional stability of the four PDs over 12 months (Shea and Yen 2003), 24 months (Grilo et al. 2004), and 10 years (Gunderson et al. 2011), using prospective data obtained for 668 patients recruited from diverse settings at four universities. Shea et al. (2002) reported that a significantly greater proportion of patients in each of the four PD groups (BPD, STPD, AVPD, and OCPD) remained at diagnostic threshold throughout the first 12 months of follow-up than did those in the MDD group; the majority of patients with PDs, however, did not consistently remain above diagnostic threshold. Grilo et al. (2004) reported that on the basis of the traditional test-retest approach, blinded repeated administration of a semistructured interview conducted 24 months after baseline revealed remission rates (based solely on falling below DSM-IV diagnostic thresholds) ranging from 50% (AVPD) to 61% (STPD). Grilo et al. (2004), using life table survival analyses of prospective data regarding time to remission for the PD and MDD groups (based on parallel definitions of 2 consecutive months with minimal symptoms), found that compared with the four PD groups, the MDD group had significantly shorter time to—and higher rates of—remission. These findings represent the first definitive empirical demonstration of the central tenet that PDs are characterized by a greater degree of stability than the hypothesized episodic course of other mental disorders (see Shea and Yen 2003). Surprisingly, however, although PDs were more "stable" than MDD, a substantial number of remissions occurred during the 24 months of follow-up. When the 2-month definition of remission was used, rates ranged from 33% (STPD) to 55% (OCPD). Importantly, even when the stringent definition of 12 consecutive months with two or fewer criteria was used, remission rates ranged from 23% (STPD) to 38% (OCPD). These early CLPS findings highlighted that substantial improvements in PD psychopathology are not uncommon, even when stringent criteria for improvement are applied.

Gunderson et al. (2011) reported the primary CLPS 10-year outcome findings regarding both diagnostic stability and psychosocial functioning. In this report, two definitions of remission were considered: 1) a 12-month duration at two or fewer criteria for comparing BPD with other PDs (OPDs, comprising AVPD and OCPD) and 2) a 2-month duration for comparing BPD with MDD. By 10 years, 85% of patients with BPD had attained remission using the 12-month duration definition and 91% had attained a remission using the 2-month definition; most changes occurred during the first 2 years (Grilo et al. 2004). Remission of BPD was significantly slower than remission of MDD and significantly, albeit less markedly, slower than remission of OPDs. Only 12% of patients with BPD had experienced a relapse, and this rate was lower, and the time to relapse slower, than that observed for MDD and for OPD. Gunderson et al. (2011) also reported that all BPD criteria declined at similar rates over time. Importantly, and in sharp contrast to the substantial and durable reductions in BPD-specific psychopathology over time, social functioning measures continued to evidence severe impairment, with only modest clinical, albeit statistically significant, improvements over time. Social functioning in patients with BPD remained persistently more impaired than that observed in both the MDD and OPD groups. Collectively, these findings—based on 10 years of prospective yearly multimethod follow-up—indicate that the course of BPD is characterized by high rates of diagnostic (i.e., symptomatic) remission and low rates of relapse (return to diagnostic threshold), but severe and enduring social functioning impairment (Gunderson et al. 2011).

The CLPS also provided complementary analyses using various dimensional approaches and alternative models for PD psychopathology for 12-month (Shea and Yen 2003), 24-month (Grilo et al. 2004; Samuel et al. 2011), 5-year (Morey et al. 2007), and 10-year (Hopwood et al. 2013; Morey et al. 2012) follow-ups. Grilo et al. (2004) documented a significant decrease in the mean proportion of criteria met in each of the PD groups over 2 years, later confirmed and extended through 10 years (Gunderson et al. 2011), which is suggestive of sustained decreased severity. However, when the relative stability of individual differences was examined across the multiwave assessments (at baseline and at 6-, 12-, and 24-month time points), a high level of consistency was observed, as evidenced by correlation coefficients ranging from 0.53 to 0.67 for proportion of criteria met between baseline and 24 months. Grilo et al. (2004) concluded that patients with PDs are consistent in terms of their rank order of PD criteria (i.e., that individual differences in PD features are stable), although there may be fluctuations in the severity or number of features over time. McGlashan et al. (2005) found that individual criteria across the four PDs studied in the CLPS had varied patterns of stability and change over time. Overall, within PDs, the relatively fixed (least changeable) criteria were generally more trait-like (and attitudinal), whereas the more fluctuating criteria were generally behavioral (or reactive). McGlashan et al. (2005) posited that perhaps PDs are hybrids of traits and symptomatic behaviors, and that it is the interaction of these over time that helps to define the observable diagnostic stability versus instability.

Hopwood et al. (2013) extended these findings in several notable ways through 10 years of follow-up by testing the rank-order stability of normal traits, pathological traits, and PD dimensions, while correcting for both test-retest dependability and internal consistency. Dependability-corrected stability estimates ranged from 0.60 to 0.90 for normal/abnormal traits but only 0.25 to 0.65 for PDs. Hopwood and colleagues suggested that the relatively lower stability observed for PD symptoms could reflect differences between unstable/episodic PD pathology and more stable normal traits. Such findings highlight the need to consider both personality traits and symptoms for a fuller understanding of the longitudinal course of personality and personality disturbances (Hopwood et al. 2013). Warner et al. (2004) used a series of latent longitudinal models to test whether changes in specific traits prospectively predicted changes in relevant PDs and reported significant cross-lagged relationships between changes in specific traits and subsequent (later) changes for STPD, BPD, and AVPD, but not for OCPD. Morey et al. (2007, 2012) compared alternative models for PDs (Five-Factor Model, Schedule for Nonadaptive and Adaptive Personality, and DSM-IV PDs) for predicting important clinical outcomes (e.g., functioning, Axis I psychopathology, medication use) over time. Morey et al. (2007, 2012) reported that approaches that integrate both normative traits and PD pathology show the greatest predictive utility. Sanislow et al. (2009) examined the latent structure and stability of the four CLPS PDs and reported that they became less differentiated over time as their mean levels decreased and stability increased. Sanislow and colleagues suggested that the higher correlations among the constructs over time might reflect a greater shared base of pathology common to all PDs.

Pursuing the common characteristics of PDs in the CLPS, Hopwood et al. (2011) found that generalized severity, represented by a count of the total number of PD criteria met (regardless of the diagnosis), was the most important single predictor of concurrent and prospective (three-year) impairment in psychosocial functioning, compared with stylistic PD elements unrelated to severity and to normative personality traits. Stylistic elements did, however, increment severity in predicting functional impairment, suggesting validity for both components of PD pathology. Furthermore, using bi-factor analyses of CLPS 10-year follow-up data, Wright et al. (2016) estimated structural models that separated general (i.e., shared among PDs) variance in PD features from specific (i.e., not shared) variance, examined patterns of change in general and specific features over time, and established concurrent and dynamic longitudinal associations of PD features and external validators such as psychosocial functioning. General PD features had much lower absolute stability but were more strongly related to broad markers of psychosocial functioning, both concurrently and longitudinally, than specific features. Specific features, on the other hand, had much higher mean stability and more circumscribed associations with functioning. These results tend to support the hybrid model of personality functioning and personality traits that forms the basis of the AMPD (see Chapter 4, "The Alternative DSM-5 Model for Personality Disorders," in this volume). In another study of the 10-year CLPS follow-along data, Conway et al. (2018) dissected borderline psychopathology into time-invariant (i.e., trait) and time-varying (i.e., state) components. Less than half of the components (approximately 45%) were time-invariant or stable over the course of the study. This component, called "borderline proneness," was very closely related ($r = .81$) to a five-factor model (FFM) depiction of borderline traits. The trait components were also more strongly related to reported childhood maltreatment—putative etiological factors for BPD—suggesting discriminant validity for the different features of a hybrid model of personality pathology.

In contrast to their symptomatic improvement, however, patients with PDs showed less significant and more gradual improvement in their functioning (Gunderson et al. 2011), and this seemed particularly so for social relationships (Markowitz et al. 2007; Skodol et al. 2005d). Because personality psychopathology usually begins in adolescence or early adulthood, the potential for delays in occupational and interpersonal development is great, and even after symptomatic improvement, it might take time to overcome deficits and make up the necessary ground to achieve "normal" functioning. However, Shea et al. (2009) found that although age was not associated with differential improvement in BPD criteria over 6 years of prospective follow-up, age was significantly associated with differential course in functioning, with older patients with BPD showing some declines in functioning over time.

Several reports from the CLPS are also relevant here in regard to the issue of longitudinal comorbidities and continuities. Shea et al. (2004) examined the time-varying (longitudinal) associations between PDs and psychiatric disorders, in part guided by the Siever and Davis (1991) model of cross-cutting psychobiological dimensions. The course of BPD demonstrated significant associations with the course of certain other mental disorders (MDD and posttraumatic stress disorder), whereas the course of AVPD was significantly associated with the course of two anxiety disorders (social phobia and obsessive-compulsive disorder). Although these findings were consistent with predictions based on the Siever and Davis (1991) model, OPDs did not demonstrate significant longitudinal associations. Gunderson et al. (2004) followed up on the Shea et al. (2004) findings regarding changes in BPD and MDD by performing a more fine-grained analysis of specific changes in the two disorders using 3 years of longitudinal data. Changes (reductions) in BPD severity preceded improvements in MDD, but not vice versa (Gunderson et al. 2004). Studies of the predictive significance of PDs for other mental disorder psychopathology over time revealed complex and mixed findings. PDs predicted a significantly worse course for MDD (Grilo et al. 2005, 2010) and for some but not other anxiety disorders (Ansell et al. 2011), but not for eating disorders (Grilo et al. 2007). Collectively, comorbid PDs appear to be negative prognostic indicators of many important psychiatric disorders (Grilo et al. 2010). These findings have since been extended to an epidemiological sample and confirmed particularly for the negative impact of BPD on MDD persistence (Skodol et al. 2011) and of a variety of PDs, in addition to indicators of PD severity (i.e., multiple PDs, mean number of PD criteria met, mean number of PDs diagnosed, presence of BPD, STPD), on the persistence of generalized anxiety disorder, social and specific phobias, and panic disorder (Skodol et al. 2014).

In studies of the dynamic relationships of CLPS patients with BPD, MDD, and bipolar I and bipolar II disorders over 10 years, Gunderson et al. (2014) found that BPD and MDD had strong reciprocal effects on each other's course, delaying time to remission and accelerating time to relapse, suggesting overlap in their psychopathologies. BPD and bipolar disorders were largely independent with respect to course effects. In a similar study of BPD and the course of anxiety disorders, BPD negatively affected the course of generalized anxiety disorder, social phobia, and PTSD, but other than PTSD, anxiety disorders had little effect on BPD's course (Keuroghlian et al. 2015). The direction of effects of one disorder on another may suggest that prioritizing the disorder with the stronger effect may be a productive treatment strategy.

Case Example

Roberta is a 23-year-old single white female whose first psychiatric hospitalization occurred during her freshman year in college at a large state university. She had been an average student in a medium-sized high school, somewhat isolated from most of her peers except for a small group of friends who shared similar interests in goth clothing, music, and books. Her only ostensible problems in high school resulted from alcohol and marijuana use, which caused her to be truant frequently, leading to angry rows with her parents and to her being "grounded" for periods of time. Roberta attributed her use of substances, however, to seeking relief from unpredictable "bad moods" and her tendency to "blow up" in the face of disappointments or perceived slights from her friends. She had had a few "counseling" sessions on a number of occasions while in high school, at the instigation of her parents, but would stop therapy after a few weeks because she felt misunderstood by the therapists, who did not "get" her, and she believed that the therapy was "not helping."

Within the first months of college, Roberta became significantly depressed. She felt that she did not fit in with her average fellow student. She became increasingly isolated, attended classes only sporadically, and, after a rebuff from the only boy with whom she had become friends and to whom she had proposed "hooking up," began to abuse substances more frequently, and ended up taking an overdose of over-the-counter sleeping pills. Following a brief 3-day hospitalization, she took a leave of absence from college and returned home to live with her parents. She entered a self-help treatment program for substance abuse and outpatient treatment with a psychiatrist, who prescribed antidepressant medications. For the next 4 years, she lived at home and tried to work at various retail sales positions, which she would continue for several months at a time before quitting out of anger at an "asshole" customer or from "boredom." Initially, she had little sense of herself beyond her identification with a couple of former high school friends she clung to, who had never left town; she had no long-term plans or goals of her own, she remained very sensitive to perceived slights by her friends or at her jobs, and she became temporarily "obsessed" with a couple of men she met at bars, only to feel rejected and abandoned by them after sleeping with them when they did not call her immediately on the next day. She frequently thought about suicide but did not make another suicide attempt.

Roberta remained in therapy, however, because she believed that her psychiatrist at least "tried to understand" her. Although initially diagnosed as having BPD, she went long stretches of time not meeting full criteria, because she curtailed her substance use and did not attempt suicide. Her depression gradually improved and her moodiness stabilized over the initial years of treatment. Her tendencies to be insecurely attached to others and to fear abandonment were more persistent, however. In addition, she became more socially isolated, not wanting to risk rejection, and less inclined to try to find work. After 4 years of therapy, she was "in remission" from her personality disorder but was completely dependent financially on her parents and continued to live at home.

This case illustrates improvement in BPD psychopathology (and depression), persistence of problematic borderline "traits," and a disconnect between remission of personality psychopathology and the persistence of poor psychosocial functioning.

McLean Study of Adult Development

The MSAD (Zanarini et al. 2003, 2005a) is an ongoing prospective longitudinal study comparing the course and outcome of hospitalized patients with BPD to those with "other" PDs utilizing repeated assessments performed every 2 years (Zanarini et al. 2003) and has reported outcomes through 6 (Zanarini et al. 2003, 2005a, 2005b), 10 (Zanarini et al. 2010b), 16 (Zanarini et al. 2012, 2013, 2014, 2015, 2016), 20 (Zanarini et al. 2018), and 24 (Temes et al. 2019) years of follow-up. Zanarini et al. (2003) assessed PDs in 362 inpatients (290 with BPD and 72 with other PDs) with two complementary semistructured diagnostic interviews for personality pathology administered reliably, and administered other assessments to characterize other psychiatric disorders, psychosocial functioning domains, and treatment utilization. The authors reported remission rates for BPD of 35%, 49%, and 74% by years 2, 4, and 6, respectively. Reporting on findings consistent with those in the early CLPS reports, Zanarini et al. (2003) concluded that "symptomatic improvement is both common and stable, even among the most disturbed borderline patients, and that the symptomatic prognosis for most, but not all, severely ill borderline patients is better than previously recognized" (p. 274). Zanarini and colleagues also reported, on the basis of findings that were generally consistent with findings from the NIMH-CDS, that personality traits and BPD psychopathology both had predictive prospective utility (Hopwood and Zanarini 2010), and that BPD had negative prognostic significance for some other mental disorders, although they later reported that other mental disorders are less common over time in patients with BPD, particularly among those whose BPD remits (Zanarini et al. 2004). The MSAD also found BPD to be associated with significant psychosocial impairment (Zanarini et al. 2009); however, in contrast to findings from the CLPS, much of the impairment was associated with vocational rather than social impairment (Zanarini et al. 2009, 2010a). Consistent with findings regarding persistent vocational impairment, patients with BPD were found to be three times more likely to receive Social Security disability income over 10 years than the other PD comparisons (Zanarini et al. 2009) and less likely to occupy a higher income group (Niesten et al. 2016).

Increases in cumulative body mass index (BMI) over 10 years of follow-up were associated with numerous adverse symptomatic, functional, and medical outcomes, such as self-mutilation and dissociation; having no life partner, a poor work or school history, being on disability, having a Global Assessment of Functioning (GAF) score in the fair to poor range, and having low income; and having two or more medical conditions and using costly forms of medical care (Frankenburg and Zanarini 2011). Despite better social functioning in the patients with BPD, interpersonal problems such as intolerance of aloneness and conflicts over dependency persisted (Choi-Kain et al. 2010).

In their report of 16 years of prospective follow-up, Zanarini et al. (2012) showed that patients with BPD were significantly slower to achieve remission (defined as no longer meeting criteria for BPD according to two assessment instruments during a 2-year follow-up interval) than the comparison group with other PDs. After 16 years, however, remission rates ranged from 78% to 99% for patients with BPD and from

97% to 99% for patients with other PDs, but those with BPD had lower recovery (defined in the MSAD as good social and vocational functioning, in addition to minimal PD symptoms) rates (40%–60%) than those with other PDs (75%–85%). Relapses occurred significantly faster and at a higher rate among patients with BPD than among those with other PDs. Zanarini et al. (2012) concluded that remission is more common than recovery from BPD and that recovery is more difficult to sustain for patients with BPD than for those with other PDs. Two-year recovery at 16 years of follow-up was predicted by six variables in multivariate analyses: no prior psychiatric hospitalizations, higher IQ, good full-time vocational record for the 2 years preceding the index hospital admission, absence of a comorbid Cluster C PD, and high FFM trait agreeableness (Zanarini et al. 2014). Stable functioning as a spouse/partner and as a parent were strongly associated with recovery status for borderline patients at 16 years of follow-up (Zanarini et al. 2015). Excellent recovery (the definition of recovery above plus the addition of the absence of an impairing Axis I disorder) at 20-year follow-up was achieved by 39% of patients with BPD compared with 73% of patients with other PDs. Predictors of excellent recovery were higher IQ, good childhood school history, good adult work history, lower FFM trait neuroticism, and higher FFM trait agreeableness (Zanarini et al. 2018). Collectively, these findings suggest that personality strengths and competencies might be important for optimizing outcomes in BPD.

Not all symptoms of BPD had the same trajectory over time in the MSAD. Over 16 years, patients with BPD had more disturbed cognitions than patients with other PDs, which declined significantly over time but continued to be problematic (Zanarini et al. 2013), and had acute symptoms, such as self-mutilation and suicide attempts, that were more likely to remit than temperamental symptoms, such as chronic anger or intolerance of aloneness, and were less likely to recur (Zanarini et al. 2016). Identity disturbance was three times higher in BPD patients but declined over time, especially among those who achieved recovery over 20 years (Gad et al. 2019). Social isolation, however, remained an unfortunate outcome for a considerable minority of borderline patients (Pucker et al. 2019). It was predicted by lower childhood competence, lower trait extraversion, and lower trait agreeableness, again highlighting the importance of personality traits in longitudinal outcomes. By the 24-year follow-up, MSAD data revealed that patients with BPD are at elevated risk for premature death: 5.9% of borderline patients and 1.4% of other PD patients had died by suicide, and 14% of those with BPD, compared with 5.5% of those with other PDs, had died from other causes. Male sex and more prior psychiatric hospitalizations predicted premature death. Most patients with BPD who died by either suicide or other causes had not attained recovery before death (Temes et al. 2019).

Patients with BPD should engage with psychotherapy over the long term to pursue symptomatic remission, to guard against relapse, to develop personality strengths and coping skills, and to help improve psychosocial functioning.

Children in the Community Study

The CICS (Brook et al. 2002; Brook et al. 1995; Cohen et al. 2005a, 2005b) is an especially impressive ongoing longitudinal effort that has already provided a wealth of information about the course of personality and behavioral traits, psychiatric problems, substance abuse, and adversities. The CICS is a prospective study of nearly 1,000 families with children ages 1–10 years when originally recruited in 1975 in New York State using a random sampling procedure. The CICS researchers have performed repeated multimodal assessments and followed more than 700 participants through the developmental eras of childhood, adolescence, and early adulthood. This landmark study—which has reported 20-year outcomes (Crawford et al. 2008)—has provided data that address the critical issues of longitudinal comorbidities and continuities. In a series of papers, the collaborating researchers have documented important findings that speak to many issues raised in this review, but especially to the critical issues of continuity of risk and functioning across developmental eras. Important findings include 1) documentation of the validity of certain forms of dramatic-erratic PDs in adolescents (Crawford et al. 2001a, 2001b); 2) age-related changes in PD symptoms, including their moderate levels of stability throughout adolescence and early adulthood (Crawford et al. 2008; Johnson et al. 2000a, 2000b, 2005); 3) the association between PD psychopathology in adolescents and impairments in educational achievement (Cohen et al. 2005a; Johnson et al. 2005) and more interpersonal and partner conflicts (Chen et al. 2004); 4) indications that early forms of behavioral disturbances predict PD in adolescents and that PDs during adolescence, in addition to demonstrating significant levels of continuity into adulthood, also predict other mental disorders and suicidality (Johnson et al. 1996), as well as violent and criminal behavior (Johnson et al. 2000b) during young adulthood; and 5) adolescent PDs are associated with pain, physical illness, poorer general physical health (Chen et al. 2009), and obesity (Chen et al. 2015) in early adulthood (see Chapter 23, "Personality Disorders in the Medical Setting," in this volume for a more detailed account of the relationship of personality pathology to physical illness). The continuity of persistent forms of impairment associated with PD pathology into young and middle adulthood has also been reported by the CICS. Skodol et al. (2007) reported that young adults (mean age 33 years) with persistent forms of PD had significantly poorer functioning and greater impairment than those whose PD had gone into remission. Comorbidity between other mental disorders and PDs in early adolescence has particularly pernicious effects on both physical health (Chen et al. 2009) and psychosocial functioning (Crawford et al. 2008) 20 years later.

Collectively, these findings support the continuity and persistence of personality disturbances and their effects, although their mutual developmental pathways are not yet understood (Cohen et al. 2005b; Crawford et al. 2001a, 2001b; Johnson et al. 2000a, 2000b; Skodol et al. 2007). Although many children and adolescents with personality psychopathology may be expected to improve, the most severely affected are likely to have problems in later life and should be followed closely. They may require ongoing treatment to prevent the development of poor physical health and later impairments in functioning. All PDs in DSM-5 Section II and Section III can be diagnosed in children or adolescents except ASPD, which requires a minimum age of 18.

Conclusion

We have reviewed the literature regarding the stability, course, and outcome of PDs, focusing particular attention on recent findings from three methodologically rigorous prospective longitudinal studies with periods of follow-up ranging from 10 to 24 years. We conclude that PDs as defined in Section II of DSM-5 demonstrate only moderate stability and that they can improve over time, with the reductions in pathology persisting in many cases. We also conclude that PDs represent negative prognostic factors for many types of other psychiatric disorders and are associated with persistent impairments in psychosocial functioning. These conclusions are offered with more confidence than in our previous reviews, given the notable methodological advances in the empirical literature on the clinical course and outcome of PDs.

The results of the studies reviewed here have had implications for the AMPD presented in Section III of DSM-5. First, the longitudinal course of PDs is described as "relatively" stable in the revised general criteria for personality disorder in the alternative model, to allow for the likelihood of a more fluctuating course in patients diagnosed with PDs. Second, individual PDs are redefined in Section III by typical impairments in core elements of personality functioning shared by all PDs, and by sets of pathological personality traits derived from the Five Factor Model of personality and the Personality Psychopathology Five. Both personality functioning and personality traits are dimensional in nature, and traits especially are expected from the longitudinal research reviewed here to be more stable than traditional diagnostic categories of PDs, whose criteria are amalgams of symptoms, traits, and consequences. Third, elements of personality functioning and personality traits are expected to increment each other in predicting important clinical outcomes over time. Fourth, by representing PDs in terms of a broad hierarchical trait structure known to underlie most of psychopathology (i.e., internalizing, externalizing, and their lower-order factors), the ubiquitous comorbidity and homotypic continuity between PDs and other psychiatric disorders become understandable on the basis of shared liabilities (for more details of the AMPD and its derivation, see Chapter 4 in this volume). Future longitudinal studies should compare the stability of Section III PD conceptualizations both with traditional categorical definitions and with other types of dimensional or hybrid representations of personality psychopathology.

References

Abrams RC, Spielman LA, Alexopoulos GS, et al: Personality disorder symptoms and functioning in elderly depressed patients. Am J Geriatr Psychiatry 6:24–30, 1998

American Psychiatric Association: Diagnostic and Statistical Manual: Mental Disorders. Washington, DC, American Psychiatric Association, 1952

American Psychiatric Association: Diagnostic and Statistical Manual of Mental Disorders, 3rd Edition. Washington, DC, American Psychiatric Association, 1980

American Psychiatric Association: Diagnostic and Statistical Manual of Mental Disorders, 3rd Edition, Revised. Washington, DC, American Psychiatric Association, 1987

American Psychiatric Association: Diagnostic and Statistical Manual of Mental Disorders, 4th Edition. Washington, DC, American Psychiatric Association, 1994

American Psychiatric Association: Diagnostic and Statistical Manual of Mental Disorders, 5th Edition. Arlington, VA, American Psychiatric Association, 2013

Ansell EB, Pinto A, Edelen MO, et al: The association of personality disorders with the prospective 7-year course of anxiety disorders. Psychol Med 41:1019–1028, 2011

Bender DS, Skodol AE, Pagano ME, et al: Prospective assessment of treatment use by patients with personality disorders. Psychiatr Serv 57:254–257, 2006

Bender DS, Skodol AE, Dyck IR, et al: Ethnicity and mental health treatment utilization by patients with personality disorders. J Consult Clin Psychol 75:992–999, 2007

Berkson J: Limitations of the application of fourfold table analysis to hospital data. Biometrics Bulletin 2:47–53, 1946

Bernstein DP, Cohen P, Skodol AE, et al: Childhood antecedents of adolescent personality disorders. Am J Psychiatry 153:907–913, 1996

Blashfield RK, McElroy RA: The 1985 journal literature on the personality disorders. Compr Psychiatry 28:536–546, 1987

Brook DW, Brook JS, Zhang C, et al: Drug use and the risk of major depressive disorder, alcohol dependence, and substance use disorders. Arch Gen Psychiatry 59:1039–1044, 2002

Brook JS, Whiteman M, Cohen P, et al: Longitudinally predicting late adolescent and young adult drug use: childhood and adolescent precursors. J Am Acad Child Adolesc Psychiatry 34:1230–1238, 1995

Cain NM, Ansell EB, Wright AG, et al: Interpersonal pathoplasticity in the course of major depression. J Consult Clin Psychol 80:78–86, 2012

Carpenter WT, Gunderson JG: Five-year follow-up comparison of borderline and schizophrenic patients. Compr Psychiatry 18:567–571, 1977

Chen H, Cohen P, Johnson JG, et al: Adolescent personality disorder and conflict with romantic partners during the transition to adulthood. J Pers Disord 18:507–525, 2004

Chen H, Cohen P, Crawford TN, et al: Impact of early adolescent psychiatric and personality disorder on long-term physical health: a 20-year longitudinal follow-up study. Psychol Med 39:865-874, 2009

Chen H, Huang Y, Kasen S, et al: Impact of adolescent personality disorders on obesity 17 years later. Psychosom Med 77:921–926, 2015

Choi-Kain LW, Zanarini MC, Frankenburg FR, et al: A longitudinal study of the 10-year course of interpersonal features in borderline personality disorder. J Pers Disord 24:365–376, 2010

Cloninger CR, Svrakic DM, Przybeck TR: A psychobiological model of temperament and character. Arch Gen Psychiatry 50:975–990, 1993

Cohen P, Chen H, Kasen S, et al: Adolescent cluster A personality disorder symptoms, role assumptions in the transition to adulthood, and resolution or persistence of symptoms. Dev Psychopathol 17:549–568, 2005a

Cohen P, Crawford TN, Johnson JG, et al: The Children in the Community Study of developmental course of personality disorder. J Pers Disord 19:466–486, 2005b

Conway CC, Hopwood CJ, Morey LC, et al: Borderline personality disorder is equally trait-like and state-like over ten years in adult psychiatric patients. J Abnorm Psychol 127:590–601, 2018

Crawford TN, Cohen P, Brook JS: Dramatic-erratic personality disorder symptoms, I: continuity from early adolescence into adulthood. J Pers Disord 15:319–335, 2001a

Crawford TN, Cohen P, Brook JS: Dramatic-erratic personality disorder symptoms, II: developmental pathways from early adolescence to adulthood. J Pers Disord 15:336–350, 2001b

Crawford TN, Cohen P, First MB, et al: Comorbid Axis I and Axis II disorders in early adolescence: outcomes 20 years later. Arch Gen Psychiatry 65:641–648, 2008

Cruitt PJ, Oltmanns TF: Age-related outcomes associated with personality pathology in later life. Curr Opin Psychol 21:89–93, 2018

Dolan-Sewell RT, Krueger RF, Shea MT: Co-occurrence with syndrome disorders, in Handbook of Personality Disorders: Theory, Research, and Treatment. Edited by Livesley WJ. New York, Guilford, 2001, pp 84–104

Ferro T, Klein DN, Schwartz JE, et al: 30-month stability of personality disorder diagnoses in depressed outpatients. Am J Psychiatry 155:653–659, 1998

Frances A: Categorical and dimensional systems of personality diagnosis: a comparison. Compr Psychiatry 23:516–527, 1982

Frank E, Prien RF, Jarrett RB, et al: Conceptualization and rationale for consensus definitions of terms in major depressive disorder. Arch Gen Psychiatry 48:851–855, 1991

Frankenburg FR, Zanarini MC: Relationship between cumulative BMI and symptomatic, psychosocial, and medical outcomes in patients with borderline personality disorder. J Pers Disord 25:421–431, 2011

Gad MA, Pucker HE, Hein KE, et al: Facets of identity disturbance reported by patients with borderline personality disorder and personality-disordered comparison subjects over 20 years of prospective follow-up. Psychiatry Res 271:76–82, 2019

Galione JN, Oltmanns TF: The relationship between borderline personality disorder and major depression in later life: acute versus temperamental symptoms. Am J Geriatr Psychiatry 21:747–756, 2013

Goldstein RB, Grant BF: Three-year follow-up of syndromal antisocial behavior in adults: results from the Wave 2 National Epidemiologic Survey on Alcohol and Related Conditions. J Clin Psychiatry 70:1237–1249, 2009

Grilo CM, McGlashan TH: Stability and course of personality disorders. Curr Opin Psychiatry 12:157–162, 1999

Grilo CM, McGlashan TH, Oldham JM: Course and stability of personality disorders. J Pract Psychiatry Behav Health 4:61–75, 1998

Grilo CM, Becker DF, Edell WS, et al: Stability and change of personality disorder dimensions in adolescents followed up two years after psychiatric hospitalization. Compr Psychiatry 42:364–368, 2001

Grilo CM, Shea MT, Sanislow CA, et al: Two-year stability and change in schizotypal, borderline, avoidant, and obsessive-compulsive personality disorders. J Consult Clin Psychol 72:767–775, 2004

Grilo CM, Sanislow CA, Shea MT, et al: Two-year prospective naturalistic study of remission from major depressive disorder as a function of personality disorder comorbidity. J Consult Clin Psychol 73:78–85, 2005

Grilo CM, Pagano ME, Skodol AE, et al: Natural course of bulimia nervosa and of eating disorder not otherwise specified: 5-year prospective study of remissions, relapses, and the effects of personality disorder psychopathology. J Clin Psychiatry 68:738–746, 2007

Grilo CM, Stout RL, Markowitz JC, et al: Personality disorders predict relapse after remission from an episode of major depressive disorder: a six-year prospective study. J Clin Psychiatry 71:1629–1635, 2010

Grinker RR, Werble B, Drye RC: The Borderline Syndrome. New York, Basic Books, 1968

Gunderson JG, Shea MT, Skodol AE, et al: The Collaborative Longitudinal Personality Disorders Study, I: development, aims, designs and sample characteristics. J Pers Disord 14:300–315, 2000

Gunderson JG, Morey LC, Stout RL, et al: Major depressive disorder and borderline personality disorder revisited: longitudinal associations. J Clin Psychiatry 65:1049–1056, 2004

Gunderson JG, Stout RL, McGlashan TH, et al: Ten-year course of borderline personality disorder: psychopathology and function from the Collaborative Longitudinal Personality Disorders Study. Arch Gen Psychiatry 68:827–837, 2011

Gunderson JG, Stout RL, Shea MT, et al: Interactions of borderline personality disorder and mood disorders over 10 years. J Clin Psychiatry 75:829–834, 2014

Hallquist MN, Lenzenweger MF: Identifying latent trajectories of personality disorder symptom change: growth mixture modeling in the longitudinal study of personality disorders. J Abnorm Psychol 122:138–155, 2013

Heatherton TF, Weinberger JL (ed): Can Personality Change? Washington, DC, American Psychological Association, 1994

Hopwood CJ, Bleidorn W: Stability and change in personality and personality disorders. Curr Opin Psychol 21:6–10, 2018

Hopwood CJ, Zanarini MC: Borderline personality traits and disorder: predicting prospective patient functioning. J Consult Clin Psychol 78:58–66, 2010

Hopwood CJ, Malone JC, Ansell EB, et al: Personality assessment in DSM-5: empirical support for rating severity, style, and traits. J Pers Disord 25:305–320, 2011

Hopwood CJ, Morey LC, Donnellan MB, et al: Ten-year rank-order stability of personality traits and disorders in a clinical sample. J Pers 81:335–344, 2013

Iacovino JM, Bogdan R, Oltmanns TF: Personality predicts health declines through stressful life events during late mid-life. J Pers 84:536–546, 2016

Johnson JG, Williams JB, Goetz RR, et al: Personality disorders predict onset of Axis I disorders and impaired functioning among homosexual men with and at risk of HIV infection. Arch Gen Psychiatry 53:350–357, 1996

Johnson JG, Williams JBW, Goetz RR, et al: Stability and change in personality disorder symptomatology: findings from a longitudinal study of HIV+ and HIV– men. J Abnorm Psychol 106:154–158, 1997

Johnson JG, Cohen P, Kasen S, et al: Age-related change in personality disorder trait levels between early adolescence and adulthood: a community-based longitudinal investigation. Acta Psychiatr Scand 102:265–275, 2000a

Johnson JG, Cohen P, Smailes E, et al: Adolescent personality disorders associated with violence and criminal behavior during adolescence and early adulthood. Am J Psychiatry 157:1406–1412, 2000b

Johnson JG, First MB, Cohen P, et al: Adverse outcomes associated with personality disorder not otherwise specified in a community sample. Am J Psychiatry 162:926–932, 2005

Kasen S, Cohen P, Skodol AE, et al: Childhood depression and adult personality disorder: alternative pathways of continuity. Arch Gen Psychiatry 58:231–236, 2001

Katz MM, Secunda SK, Hirschfeld R, et al: NIMH Clinical Research Branch Collaborative Program on Psychobiology of Depression. Arch Gen Psychiatry 36:765–771, 1979

Keller MB, Lavori PW, Friedman B, et al: The Longitudinal Interval Follow-Up Evaluation: a comprehensive method for assessing outcome in prospective longitudinal studies. Arch Gen Psychiatry 44:540–548, 1987

Kendell PC, Clarkin JF: Introduction to special section: comorbidity and treatment implications. J Consult Clin Psychol 60:833–834, 1992

Keuroghlian AS, Gunderson JG, Pagano ME, et al: Interactions of borderline personality disorder and anxiety disorders over 10 years. J Clin Psychiatry 76:1529–1534, 2015

Kim-Cohen J, Caspi A, Moffitt TE, et al: Prior juvenile diagnoses in adults with mental disorder: developmental follow-back of a prospective-longitudinal cohort. Arch Gen Psychiatry 60:709–717, 2003

Klein DN, Shih JH: Depressive personality: associations with DSM-III-R mood and personality disorders and negative and positive affectivity, 30-month stability, and prediction of course of axis I depressive disorders. J Abnorm Psychol 107:319–327, 1998

Krueger RF: The structure of common mental disorders. Arch Gen Psychiatry 56:921–926, 1999

Krueger RF, Carlson SR: Personality disorders in children and adolescents. Curr Psychiatry Rep 3:46–51, 2001

Krueger RF, Tackett JL: Personality and psychopathology: working toward the bigger picture. J Pers Disord 17:109–128, 2003

Lenzenweger MF: Stability and change in personality disorder features: the Longitudinal Study of Personality Disorders. Arch Gen Psychiatry 56:1009–1015, 1999

Lenzenweger MF, Johnson MD, Willet JB: Individual growth curve analysis illuminates stability and change in personality disorder features: the Longitudinal Study of Personality Disorders. Arch Gen Psychiatry 61:1015–1024, 2004

Levy KN, Becker DF, Grilo CM et al: Concurrent and predictive validity of the personality disorder diagnosis in adolescent inpatients. Am J Psychiatry 156:1522–1528, 1999

Lewinsohn PM, Rohde P, Seeley JR, et al: Axis II psychopathology as a function of Axis I disorder in childhood and adolescence. J Am Acad Child Adolesc Psychiatry 36:1752–1759, 1997

Livesley WJ, Jackson DN, Schroeder ML: Factorial structure of traits delineating personality disorders in clinical and general population samples. J Abnorm Psychol 101:432–440, 1992

Loranger AW, Lenzenweger MF, Gartner AF, et al: Trait-state artifacts and the diagnosis of personality disorders. Arch Gen Psychiatry 48:720–728, 1991

Loranger AW, Sartorius N, Andreoli A, et al: The International Personality Disorder Examination (IPDE). Arch Gen Psychiatry 51:215–224, 1994

Lyons MJ, Tyrer P, Gunderson J, et al: Special feature: heuristic models of comorbidity of Axis I and Axis II disorders. J Pers Disord 11:260–269, 1997

Maddocks PD: A five-year follow-up of untreated psychopaths. Br J Psychiatry 116:511–515, 1970

Markowitz JC, Skodol AE, Petkova E, et al: Longitudinal effects of personality disorders on psychosocial functioning of patients with major depressive disorder. J Clin Psychiatry 68:186–193, 2007

Mattanah JJ, Becker DF, Levy KN, et al: Diagnostic stability in adolescents followed up 2 years after hospitalization. Am J Psychiatry 152:889–894, 1995

McDavid JD, Pilkonis PA: The stability of personality disorder diagnoses. J Pers Disord 10:1–15, 1996

McGlashan TH: The Chestnut Lodge Follow-Up Study, part III: long-term outcome of borderline personalities. Arch Gen Psychiatry 42:20–30, 1986a

McGlashan TH: The Chestnut Lodge Follow-Up Study, part VI: schizotypal personality disorder. Arch Gen Psychiatry 43:329–334, 1986b

McGlashan TH, Grilo CM, Skodol AE, et al: The Collaborative Longitudinal Personality Disorders Study: baseline Axis I/II and II/II diagnostic co-occurrence. Acta Psychiatr Scand 102:256–264, 2000

McGlashan TH, Grilo CM, Sanislow CA, et al: Two-year prevalence and stability of individual DSM-IV criteria for schizotypal, borderline, avoidant and obsessive-compulsive personality disorders: toward a hybrid model of Axis II disorders. Am J Psychiatry 162:883–889, 2005

Moffitt TE: Adolescence-limited and life-course-persistent antisocial behavior: a developmental taxonomy. Psychol Rev 100:674–701, 1993

Morey LC, Hopwood CJ, Gunderson JG, et al: Comparison of alternative models for personality disorders. Psychol Med 37:983–994, 2007

Morey LC, Hopwood CJ, Markowitz JC, et al: Comparison of alternative models for personality disorders, II: 6-, 8-, and 10-year follow-up. Psychol Med 42:1705–1713, 2012

Myers MG, Stewart DG, Brown SA: Progression from conduct disorder to antisocial personality disorder following treatment for adolescent substance abuse. Am J Psychiatry 155:479–485, 1998

Nesselroade JR, Stigler SM, Baltes PB: Regression toward the mean and the study of change. Psychol Bull 88:622–637, 1980

Newman DL, Caspi A, Moffitt TE, et al: Antecedents of adult interpersonal functioning: effects of individual differences in age 3 temperament. Devel Psychol 33:206–217, 1997

Niesten IJ, Karan E, Frankenburg FR, et al: Description and prediction of the income status of borderline patients over 10 years of prospective follow-up. Personal Ment Health 10:285–292, 2016

Oldham JM, Skodol AE: Personality and personality disorders and the passage of time. Am J Geriatr Psychiatry 21:709–712, 2013

Oldham JM, Skodol AE, Kellman HD, et al: Diagnoses of DSM-III-R personality disorders by two structured interviews: patterns of comorbidity. Am J Psychiatry 149:213–230, 1992

Ottosson H, Ekselius L, Grann M, et al: Cross-system concordance of personality disorder diagnoses of DSM-IV and diagnostic criteria for research of ICD-10. J Pers Disord 16:283–292, 2002

Paris J: Personality disorders over time: precursors, course and outcome. J Pers Disord 17:479–488, 2003

Paris J, Zweig-Frank H: A 27-year follow-up of borderline patients. Compr Psychiatry 42:482–487, 2001

Perry JC: Longitudinal studies of personality disorders. J Pers Disord 7(suppl):63–85, 1993

Pucker HE, Temes CM, Zanarini MC: Description and prediction of social isolation in borderline patients over 20 years of prospective follow-up. Personal Disord 10:383–388, 2019

Regier DA, Narrow WE, Clarke DE, et al: DSM-5 field trials in the United States and Canada, part II: test-retest reliability of selected categorical diagnoses. Am J Psychiatry 170:59–70, 2013

Rettew DC, Zanarini MC, Yen S, et al: Childhood antecedents of avoidant personality disorder: a retrospective study. J Am Acad Child Adolesc Psychiatry 42:1122–1130, 2003

Rey JM, Morris-Yates A, Singh M, et al: Continuities between psychiatric disorders in adolescents and personality disorders in young adults. Am J Psychiatry 152:895–900, 1995

Robbins E, Gentry KA, Munoz RA, et al: A contrast of the three more common illnesses with the ten less common in a study and 18-month follow-up of 314 psychiatric emergency room patients, III: findings at follow-up. Arch Gen Psychiatry 34:285–291, 1977

Roberts BW, DelVecchio WF: The rank-order consistency of personality traits from childhood to old age: a quantitative review of longitudinal studies. Psychol Bull 126:3–25, 2000

Roberts BW, Caspi A, Moffitt TE: The kids are alright: growth and stability in personality development from adolescence to adulthood. J Pers Soc Psychol 81:670–683, 2001

Robins LN: Deviant Children Grown Up: A Sociological and Psychiatric Study of Sociopathic Personality. Baltimore, MD, Williams & Wilkins, 1966

Robins LN: Epidemiology: reflections on testing the validity of psychiatric interviews. Arch Gen Psychiatry 42:918–924, 1985

Ruegg R, Frances A: New research in personality disorders. J Pers Disord 9:1–48, 1995

Samuel DB, Hopwood CJ, Ansell EB, et al: Comparing the temporal stability of self-report and interview assessed personality disorder. J Abnorm Psychol 120:670–680, 2011

Samuel DB, Sanislow CA, Hopwood C, et al: Convergent and incremental predictive validity of clinician, self-report, and structured interview diagnoses for personality disorders over 5 years. J Consult Clin Psychol 81:650–659, 2013

Sanislow CA, Little TD, Ansell EB, et al: Ten-year stability and latent structure of DSM-IV schizotypal, borderline, avoidant, and obsessive-compulsive personality disorders. J Abnorm Psychol 118:507–519, 2009

Schuster JP, Hoertel N, Le Strat Y, et al: Personality disorders in older adults: findings from the national epidemiologic survey on alcohol and related conditions. Am J Geriatr Psychiatry 21:757–768, 2013

Seivewright H, Tyrer P, Johnson T: Change in personality status in neurotic disorders. Lancet 359:2253–2254, 2002

Shea MT, Yen S: Stability as a distinction between Axis I and Axis II disorders. J Pers Disord 17:373–386, 2003

Shea MT, Stout RL, Gunderson JG, et al: Short-term diagnostic stability of schizotypal, borderline, avoidant, and obsessive-compulsive personality disorders. Am J Psychiatry 159:2036–2041, 2002

Shea MT, Stout RL, Yen S, et al: Associations in the course of personality disorders and Axis I disorders over time. J Abnorm Psychol 113:499–508, 2004

Shea MT, Edelen MO, Pinto A, et al: Improvement in borderline personality disorder in relation to age. Acta Psychiatr Scand 119:143–148, 2009

Siever LJ, Davis KL: A psychobiological perspective on the personality disorders. Am J Psychiatry 148:1647–1658, 1991

Skodol AE: Classification, assessment, and differential diagnosis of personality disorders. J Pract Psychiatry Behav Health 3:261–274, 1997

Skodol AE: Personality disorders in DSM-5. Annu Rev Clin Psychol 8:317–344, 2012

Skodol AE, Siever LJ, Livesley WJ, et al: The borderline diagnosis II: biology, genetics, and clinical course. Biol Psychiatry 15:951–963, 2002

Skodol AE, Grilo CM, Pagano ME, et al: Effects of personality disorders on functioning and well-being in major depressive disorder. J Psychiatr Pract 11:363–368, 2005a

Skodol AE, Gunderson JG, Shea MT, et al: The Collaborative Longitudinal Personality Disorders Study (CLPS): overview and implications. J Pers Disord 19:487–504, 2005b

Skodol AE, Oldham JM, Bender DS, et al: Dimensional representations of DSM-IV personality disorders: relationships to functional impairment. Am J Psychiatry 162:1919–1925, 2005c

Skodol AE, Pagano ME, Bender DS, et al: Stability of functional impairment in patients with schizotypal, borderline, avoidant, or obsessive-compulsive personality disorder over two years. Psychol Med 35:443–451, 2005d

Skodol AE, Johnson JG, Cohen P, et al: Personality disorder and impaired functioning from adolescence to adulthood. Br J Psychiatry 190:415–420, 2007

Skodol AE, Grilo CM, Keyes KM, et al: Relationship of personality disorder to the course of major depressive disorder in a nationally representative sample. Am J Psychiatry 168:257–264, 2011

Skodol AE, Geier T, Grant BF, et al: Personality disorders and the persistence of anxiety disorders in a nationally representative sample. Depress Anxiety 31:721–728, 2014

Solomon DA, Keller MB, Leon AC, et al: Recovery from major depression: a 10-year prospective follow-up across multiple episodes. Arch Gen Psychiatry 54:1001–1006, 1997

Squires-Wheeler E, Skodol AE, Erlenmeyer-Kimling L: The assessment of schizotypal features over two points in time. Schizophr Res 6:75–85, 1992

Stevenson J, Meares R, Comerford A: Diminished impulsivity in older patients with borderline personality disorder. Am J Psychiatry 160:165–166, 2003

Stone MH: Long-term outcome in personality disorders. Br J Psychiatry 162:299–313, 1993

Temes CM, Frankenburg FR, Fitzmaurice GM, Zanarini MC: Deaths by suicide and other causes among patients with borderline personality disorder and personality-disordered comparison subjects over 24 years of prospective follow-up. J Clin Psychiatry 80:18m12436, 2019

Trull TJ, Useda D, Conforti K, et al: Borderline personality disorder features in nonclinical young adults, 2: two-year outcome. J Abnorm Psychol 106:307–314, 1997

Trull TJ, Useda JD, Doan B-T, et al: Two-year stability of borderline personality measures. J Pers Disord 12:187–197, 1998

Tyrer P: Personality disorder. Br J Psychiatry 179:81–84, 2001

Tyrer P, Gunderson J, Lyons M, et al: Special feature: extent of comorbidity between mental state and personality disorders. J Pers Disord 11:242–259, 1997

Warner MB, Morey LC, Finch JF, et al: The longitudinal relationship of personality traits and disorders. J Abnorm Psychol 113:217–227, 2004

Westen D: Divergences between clinical and research methods for assessing personality disorders: implications for research and the evolution of Axis II. Am J Psychiatry 154:895–903, 1997

Westen D, Shedler J: Revising and assessing Axis II, part 2: toward an empirically based and clinically useful classification of personality disorders. Am J Psychiatry 156:273–285, 1999

Widiger TA: Categorical versus dimensional classification: implications from and for research. J Pers Disord 6:287–300, 1992

Widiger TA: Personality disorder and Axis I psychopathology: the problematic boundary of Axis I and Axis II. J Pers Disord 17:90–108, 2003

Wolff S, Townshend R, McGuire RJ, et al: Schizoid personality in childhood and adult life, II: adult adjustment and the continuity with schizotypal personality disorder. Br J Psychiatry 159:620–629, 1991

World Health Organization: International Statistical Classification of Diseases and Related Health Problems, 10th Revision. Geneva, World Health Organization, 1992

Wright AG, Hopwood CJ, Skodol AE, et al: Longitudinal validation of general and specific structural features of personality pathology. J Abnorm Psychol 125:1120–1134, 2016

Zanarini MC, Skodol AE, Bender D, et al: The Collaborative Longitudinal Personality Disorders Study: reliability of Axis I and II diagnoses. J Pers Disord 14:291–299, 2000

Zanarini MC, Frankenburg FR, Hennen J, et al: The longitudinal course of borderline psychopathology: 6-year prospective follow-up of the phenomenology of borderline personality disorder. Am J Psychiatry 160:274–283, 2003

Zanarini MC, Frankenburg FR, Hennen J, et al: Axis I comorbidity in patients with borderline personality disorder: 6-year follow-up and prediction of time to remission. Am J Psychiatry 161:2108–2114, 2004

Zanarini MC, Frankenburg FR, Hennen J, et al: The McLean Study of Adult Development (MSAD): overview and implications of the first six years of prospective follow-up. J Pers Disord 19:505–523, 2005a

Zanarini MC, Frankenburg FR, Hennen J, et al: Psychosocial functioning of borderline patients and Axis II comparison subjects followed prospectively for six years. J Pers Disord 19:19–29, 2005b

Zanarini MC, Jacoby RJ, Frankenburg FR, et al: The 10-year course of social security disability income reported by patients with borderline personality disorder and Axis II comparison subjects. J Pers Disord 23:346–356, 2009

Zanarini MC, Frankenburg FR, Reich DB, et al: The 10-year course of psychosocial functioning among patients with borderline personality disorder and axis II comparison subjects. Acta Psychiatr Scand 122:103–109, 2010a

Zanarini MC, Frankenburg FR, Reich DB, et al: Time to attainment of recovery from borderline personality disorder and stability of recovery: a 10-year prospective follow-up study. Am J Psychiatry 167:663–667, 2010b

Zanarini MC, Frankenburg FR, Reich DB, et al: Attainment and stability of sustained symptomatic remission and recovery among patients with borderline personality disorder and axis II comparison subjects: a 16-year prospective follow-up study. Am J Psychiatry 169:476–483, 2012

Zanarini MC, Frankenburg FR, Wedig MM, et al: Cognitive experiences reported by patients with borderline personality disorder and axis II comparison subjects: a 16-year prospective follow-up study. Am J Psychiatry 170:671–679, 2013

Zanarini MC, Frankenburg FR, Reich DB, et al: Prediction of time-to-attainment of recovery for borderline patients followed prospectively for 16 years. Acta Psychiatr Scand 130:205–213, 2014

Zanarini MC, Frankenburg FR, Reich DB, et al: The course of marriage/sustained cohabitation and parenthood among borderline patients followed prospectively for 16 years. J Pers Disord 29:62–70, 2015

Zanarini MC, Frankenburg FR, Reich DB, et al: Fluidity of the subsyndromal phenomenology of borderline personality disorder over 16 years of prospective follow-up. Am J Psychiatry 173:688–694, 2016

Zanarini MC, Temes CM, Frankenburg FR, et al: Description and prediction of time-to-attainment of excellent recovery for borderline patients followed prospectively for 20 years. Psychiatry Res 262:40–45, 2018

Zimmerman M: Diagnosing personality disorders: a review of issues and research methods. Arch Gen Psychiatry 51:225–245, 1994

PART III

Treatment

CHAPTER 10

Early Identification and Prevention of Personality Pathology

An AMPD-Informed Model of Clinical Staging

Carla Sharp, Ph.D.

Sophie Kerr, B.A.

Andrew M. Chanen, M.B.B.S., Ph.D., FRANZCP

The publication of the Alternative DSM-5 Model for Personality Disorders (AMPD) in DSM-5 Section III (American Psychiatric Association 2013) ushered in the possibility of conceiving personality pathology in novel ways. In particular, the AMPD allows us, for the first time, to elaborate maladaptive personality in developmentally sensitive ways. The AMPD achieves this, first, by legitimizing a dimensional trait perspective of personality pathology (Criterion B), which lends itself well to developmental considerations, given that dispositional personality traits are already observable in small children. Moreover, dimensional approaches to understanding psychopathology have long been a preferred approach to conceptualizing the nature and phenomenology of child and adolescent psychiatric problems. Guided by a developmental psychopathology approach, dimensionality allows for the description of heterotypic and homotypic continuity to explain the waxing, waning, and morphing of psychopathology as children and young people pass through developmental changes relative to the impact of specific environmental contexts. The AMPD also promotes a more developmentally sensitive elaboration of personality pathology by explicitly formulating personality pathology in terms of maladaptive self and interpersonal functioning (Criterion A) for the first time. By placing (especially) self functioning front and center in personality pathology, the AMPD allows for the integration of more than 50 years of research on identity functioning into our conceptualization of maladaptive personality functioning. Importantly, Criterion A is also conceptualized dimensionally. Using the Level of Personality Functioning Scale, a clinician rates aspects of identity, self-direction, intimacy, and empathy on a severity scale from 0 to 4 (5-point scale; see DSM-5 Section III, pp. 775–778). By introducing trait dimensionality and self and interpersonal functioning, the AMPD 1) provides a framework for understanding why the transition from childhood to adulthood appears to be a sensitive period for the development of personality pathology, and 2) facilitates a developmentally sensitive clinical staging approach to prevention of and early intervention for personality pathology.

To illustrate the above points, we focus this review on borderline personality disorder (BPD) for both pragmatic and substantive reasons. Pragmatically, there now exists a large body of research on BPD in young people. Substantively, BPD, and no other traditional personality disorder (PD) type, has been suggested to represent prototypical personality pathology more generally (Clark and Ro 2014; Kernberg 1967; Sharp and Fonagy 2015; Sharp and Wall 2018). This idea has been supported by research showing substantial co-occurrence ("comorbidity") between categorically defined PDs (Clark 2007), thereby spawning interest in the existence of a common factor that might account for the covariance among different psychopathologies. Consistent with expectations, and analogizing from the construct of intelligence, which has long understood the structure of mental ability to comprise general (i.e., "g") and specific (i.e., "s") skills, BPD has been shown to load onto the general ("g") factor of personality pathology (Clark and Ro 2014; Sharp et al. 2015; Williams et al. 2018; Wright et al. 2016). In other words, of all the PDs, BPD appears to capture the core of personality pathology or might be most representative. Therefore, in reviewing literature on BPD (thus conceptualized), one can tentatively and carefully consider generalization of this literature to what is common to personality pathology (Criterion A), beyond the diagnostic category of BPD itself. Moreover, while maladaptive traits (Criterion B) have been studied extensively in children and adolescents (for reviews, see De Clercq 2018; De Clercq et al. 2014a; Sharp and De Clercq 2020; Shiner and Tackett 2014), traits alone do not optimize novel approaches to assessment and intervention, as exemplified in a clinical staging approach. For that, Criterion A functioning must be considered in addition to traits, because it is Criterion A functioning that captures the process by which prepubertal maladaptive traits morph into adolescent PD (Sharp 2020; Sharp and Wall 2018; Sharp et al. 2018).

Furthermore, the developmental model presented in this chapter draws on research that has identified a distinct developmental period, extending from puberty (operationally defined as ages 10–12 years) beyond the traditional age of adolescence (12–18 years) to around 25 years of age ("young people") in economically developed societies, that is believed to support the acquisition of the culturally embodied knowledge, skills, and self-regulatory capacities that are needed to achieve independent adult role functioning and integration into society (Dahl et al. 2018; Sawyer et al. 2018). This developmental period also represents a period of vulnerability and coincides with the peak period of clinical onset for the major mental disorders, including PD (Chanen and Thompson 2019). Recognition of this distinct developmental period, its associated vulnerabilities, and blends of emerging psychopathology has led to the emergence of youth mental health as an overarching construct to guide prevention and early intervention (Malla et al. 2016; McGorry and Mei 2018). This focus on young people is conceptually coherent, with a focus on assisting young people to better navigate the transition to adulthood. However, the PD field has been slow to embrace this concept (Chanen 2015). Psychopathology during this developmental period has the potential to disrupt the transition to adulthood, derailing the acquisition of essential skills, and this is manifestly the case for young people with PD (Chanen and Thompson 2018; Cohen et al. 2005; Sharp and Wall 2018; Winograd et al. 2008). Importantly, personality pathology does not occur in isolation from other forms of psychopathology (Krueger et al. 2018). The concept of clinical staging and the "at-risk mental state," first applied to the identification of youth at ultra-high risk of developing psychosis (McGorry 2010; McGorry et al. 2018), has been expanded. One example is the meta-diagnostic Clinical High at Risk Mental State (CHARMS), which includes borderline (severe) personality pathology. CHARMS aims to identify help-seeking young people experiencing clinical distress due to subthreshold symptoms (McGorry et al. 2018). This approach acknowledges that although symptoms might follow a heterotypic course, they have independent, proximal effects on current functioning and development, often well before reaching the threshold for the "adult" mental disorder syndromes.

To provide background and context for the arguments we wish to elaborate in the current chapter, we begin with a historical overview of the establishment of the borderline diagnosis in youth.

Breaking Down the Myths

Case Example

Sarah is a 15-year-old who was admitted to an inpatient unit after she made a serious threat to kill herself. Sarah's parents got divorced when she was 4 years old, and she has been spending alternate weekends with her father. On the day she was admitted to the hospital, Sarah's father brought her to the meeting point (a park) where he was going to drop off Sarah to be picked up by her mother. When he began to leave, Sarah clung to him and started to cry. Sarah has had a tendency in the past to engage in dramatic displays to stop her parents or good friends from leaving her. This time, Sarah told her father that living with her mother had become unbearable and that if he did not stay with her, she would kill herself. During the past 2 years, Sarah had often threatened to kill herself. Her father tried to calm her down, but she shouted that he was not hearing her, and she pulled up her skirt to reveal significant cuts and burns on her thighs. Her father was shocked. Since childhood, Sarah had always been highly emotional and reactive. Recently, her father had become concerned about Sarah's alcohol intake and the fact that she was caught shoplifting a few times, but he had not been aware of any self-harm. Sarah disclosed that she has been cutting and burning herself for at least 2 years. By this time Sarah was sobbing angrily and accusing her father of never being there for her and choosing a life with his new family instead of her. When her father tried to hold her to comfort her, she punched him in the face and started running away. When a car nearly ran her over, she collapsed and her father was able to catch up with her to take her to the hospital. On admission, Sarah appeared completely calm and said that she felt separated from her body—a feeling that she said she often has when she becomes stressed. She kept scratching herself. She did not want her mother to come to the hospital. (Sharp and Fonagy 2015, p. 1258)

Although a diagnosis cannot be made on the basis of a single paragraph, for the sake of illustration, it is clear that the symptoms represented in the vignette broadly mirror at least seven of the nine BPD criteria, as outlined in Section II of DSM-5. These include abandonment fears, self-harm and suicidality, affective instability and reactivity, impulsivity, aggressive behavior, dissociation, and relationship problems (emptiness and identity disturbance are not well represented in the vignette). Given that DSM-5 Section II requires only five out of nine criteria to be present in order to reach the threshold for diagnosis, it is reasonable to argue that Sarah might be suffering from BPD. However, in routine clinical care, studies have shown that despite a fivefold increase in the studies of BPD in youth over the last decade (Sharp and Tackett 2014), clinicians still hesitate to assign the diagnosis to young people, especially those younger than 18 years. For example, in a survey of 52 British child and adolescent psychiatrists, about 80% supported the validity of the BPD diagnosis in adults, while less than 40% found the diagnosis valid in adolescents and less than 25% reported using the diagnosis for that age group in practice (Griffiths 2011). Similarly, despite nearly 60% of a sample of 556 Dutch psychologists reporting that PDs exist in adolescence, less than 10% reported diagnosing PDs in adolescents (Laurenssen et al. 2013). Thus, the accumulating evidence from the last 10–15 years does not yet appear to have gained wide acceptance in routine clinical care. Many practitioners continue to approach the diagnosis of PD in young people, especially in those younger than 18 years, with hesitation. This reluctance stems from several beliefs and/or myths about adolescent personality pathology, including the beliefs that 1) psychiatric nomenclature does not allow for adolescent PD diagnosis and BPD cannot be reliably assessed or diagnosed in young people, 2) certain features reflect normative development and the syndrome of BPD may not be present in adolescence, 3) adolescent personalities are too unstable and therefore cannot warrant diagnosis if maladaptive, 4) adult and adolescent BPD have different associated clinical features, and causal models for adult BPD might not extend to adolescent BPD, 5) symptoms are better explained by internalizing or externalizing disorders, and 6) the label is stigmatizing (Chanen and McCutcheon 2013; Sharp 2017; Shiner and Tackett 2014).

Below, we review the evidence that challenges these beliefs, with the ultimate goal of providing support for the assessment, diagnosis, and treatment of BPD in young people. This conclusion is in accordance with a recent position paper published by the Global Alliance for Prevention and Early Intervention for Borderline Personality Disorder (Chanen et al. 2017), in which we reviewed the evidence for BPD in young people as an important new public health priority.

Myth 1: BPD Cannot Be Reliably Assessed or Diagnosed in Young People

One reason that practitioners do not routinely diagnose personality pathology in adolescents is because of the misconception that diagnostic criteria require individuals to be at least 18 years of age. Laurenssen et al. (2013) found that 26% of 556 surveyed psychologists believed that DSM-IV (American Psychiatric Association 1994) did not allow for adolescent (<18 years old) PD diagnosis. In fact, PD diagnosis has never been disallowed in young people since the introduction of the modern concept of PD in DSM-III (American Psychiatric Association 1987). In DSM-5 Section II, the criteria are the same across adolescents and adults, although the necessary duration is only 1 year in adolescents, compared with 2 years in adults (American Psychiatric Association 2013), which is likely to be too short to reliably distinguish "state" from "trait" phenomena. The categorical diagnostic system does, however, urge caution, explaining that the diagnosis should only be given in adolescents in "relatively unusual instances" in which the "maladaptive personality traits appear to be pervasive, persistent, and unlikely to be limited to a particular developmental stage or another mental disorder" (American Psychiatric Association 2013, p. 647). Section III of DSM-5 does not include any cautionary notes and does not require symptoms to be present for 1 year; rather, it requires them to be "relatively stable across time" (American Psychiatric Association 2013, p. 761). There are no age-related caveats for PD diagnosis in the ICD-11 nomenclature or in national clinical guidelines for the treatment of BPD in the United Kingdom or Australia.

Clearly, the belief that diagnostic manuals do not allow for diagnosis of BPD in adolescents is unfounded. Additionally, a variety of measures have been validated over the past two decades to assess for BPD, as defined by DSM-5 Section II. These include tools originally developed for use in adults, which have been adapted for young people (see Sharp and Fonagy 2015 for a review), as well as measures designed to be developmentally appropriate. For instance, the Childhood Interview for DSM-IV Borderline Personality Disorder (CI-BPD; Zanarini 2003) was specifically developed to assess young people. It has been evaluated in clinical and community samples and demonstrates adequate internal consistency, high interrater agreement between self- and parent reports, and convergent validity with clinician diagnosis and questionnaire measures of BPD (Sharp et al. 2012; Zanarini et al. 2011). Self-report measures have also been validated. One example is the Borderline Personality Features Scale for Children (BPFS-C; Crick et al. 2005), which was adapted from the Personality Assessment Inventory—Borderline Subscale (PAI-BOR; Morey 1991) and has shown excellent criterion and concurrent validity (Chang et al. 2011; Crick et al. 2005; Sharp et al. 2011). The scale has also been adapted for parent report (BPFS-P) and demonstrated good psychometric properties (Sharp et al. 2011). Through the use of item response theory, the BPFS-C was shortened from 24 to 11 items to create the BPFS-C-11, which has shown excellent criterion validity in terms of sensitivity and specificity (Sharp et al. 2014). The PAI-BOR adolescent version (Morey 2007), also derived from the adult version of the PAI-BOR (Morey 1991), from which the BPPFC, BPFS-C-P, and BPFS-C-11 were developed, has also shown good psychometric properties in independent validation studies (Venta et al. 2018). Table 10–1 provides greater detail on the psychometric properties of available interview and self-report tools for DSM Section II and Section III assessment of BPD. Further research is needed to define the optimal setting and sequence for these assessments and to validate their use in the older age range of young people (18–25 years). However, given the existence of these validated tools, practitioners should take advantage of self-report measures to identify and screen for PD, as well as in-depth structured and unstructured clinical interviews to guide and assist clinical evaluation.

Using the measures described in Table 10–1, researchers have examined the factor structure of BPD in adolescence. To be considered a valid diagnostic entity, a coherent combination of symptoms should "hang together," evidenced by a single latent trait accounting for covariation among criteria (Robins and Guze 1970). Studies have gen-

TABLE 10–1. Assessment tools with psychometric properties for DSM 5 Section II and III borderline personality disorder (BPD) in adolescents

Measure	Internal consistency	Inter-rater reliability	Factor structure	External validity
DSM-5 Section II BPD measures				
Childhood Interview for DSM-IV Borderline Personality Disorder (CI-BPD)				
Sharp et al. 2012	0.80	0.89	Unidimensional	Associations with PAI-BOR, clinician diagnosis, BPFS-C, BPFS-P, internalizing and externalizing problems; κ=0.34 with clinician diagnosis
Michonski et al. 2013	0.78	Not reported	Unidimensional	N/A
Borderline Personality Severity Index–IV—Adolescent Version (BPDSI-IV-Adolescent)				
Marieke Schuppert et al. 2012	Adolescent: 0.94 Parent: 0.90	Not reported	Not reported	*Adolescent:* Associations with parent report and other related instruments Sensitivity: 0.92 Specificity: 0.82 *Parent:* Associations with youth report and other related instruments Sensitivity: 0.89 Specificity: 0.92
Borderline Personality Features Scale for Children (BPFS-C)				
Crick et al. 2005	0.76	N/A	Not reported	Associations with relational aggression, cognitive sensitivity, emotional sensitivity, friend exclusivity
Chang et al. 2011	0.88	N/A	Not reported	Sensitivity: 0.85 Specificity: 0.84
Haltigan and Vaillancourt 2016	Intra- and interpersonal preoccupation (α=0.82) and impulsivity/reactivity (α=0.76) scales	N/A	Two-factor latent structure: intra- and interpersonal preoccupation factor and impulsivity/reactivity factor	Associations with child-reported self-esteem and parent-reported child impulsivity

TABLE 10–1. Assessment tools with psychometric properties for DSM 5 Section II and III borderline personality disorder (BPD) in adolescents *(continued)*

Measure	Internal consistency	Inter-rater reliability	Factor structure	External validity
Borderline Personality Features Scale for Children, 11-Item Version (BPFS-C-11)				
Sharp et al. 2011	0.90	N/A	Not reported	Correlation with BPFS-C, internalizing and externalizing problems
Fossati et al. 2019	0.78	N/A	Confirmatory factor analysis did not support a one-factor model of the BPFS-C-11 items, but a bi-factor model showed that all BPFS-C-11 items loaded significantly onto a general common factor, with two specific factors largely capturing residual variance.	Confirmation and extension of findings by Sharp et al. (2014) Association with PDQ-4-BPD scale
Vanwoerden et al. 2019	0.86, 0.85, 0.86, and 0.90 (years 1–4)	N/A	Unidimensional	N/A
Borderline Personality Features Scale for Children—Parent Report (BPFS-P)				
Sharp et al. 2011	0.90	N/A	Not reported	Correlation with BPFS-C, internalizing and externalizing problems
Borderline Personality Questionnaire (BPQ)				
Chanen et al. 2008b	0.92	ICC=0.92	Not reported	Identification of SCID-II BPD: Sensitivity: 0.68 Specificity: 0.90 NPV=0.91; PPV=0.65 κ=0.57

TABLE 10–1. Assessment tools with psychometric properties for DSM 5 Section II and III borderline personality disorder (BPD) in adolescents (*continued*)

Measure	Internal consistency	Inter-rater reliability	Factor structure	External validity
DSM-5 Section II BPD measures (*continued*)				
McLean Screening Instrument for Borderline Personality Disorder (MSI-BPD)				
Chanen et al. 2008b	0.78	N/A	Not reported	Identification of SCID-II BPD: Sensitivity: 0.68 Specificity: 0.75 NPV=0.89 κ=0.35
Noblin et al. 2014	0.73	N/A	Not reported	Sensitivity: 0.71 Specificity: 0.66
Van Alebeek et al. 2017	0.79	N/A	N/A	Convergent validity with PDQ-4-BPD, SCID-II-PQ, and SCID-II BPD Using cutoff score of 5: Sensitivity: 0.94 Specificity: 0.73
Personality Assessment Inventory for Adolescents—Borderline Features Scale (PAI-A-BOR)				
Morey 2007	0.85–0.87	N/A	Four-factor	Association with range of other BPD-relevant pathology
Venta et al. 2018	Clinical sample: BOR, 0.88 BOR-A, 0.74 BOR-I, 0.65 BOR-N, 0.69 BOR-S, 0.73 Forensic sample: BOR, 0.82 BOR-A, 0.67 BOR-I, 0.56 BOR-N, 0.62 BOR-S, 0.67	N/A	Confirmatory factor analysis indicated poor fit of the four-factor structure proposed by the measure's authors.	Association with presence of symptoms on the CI-BPD Sensitivity: 0.77 Specificity: 0.79

TABLE 10–1. Assessment tools with psychometric properties for DSM 5 Section II and III borderline personality disorder (BPD) in adolescents (continued)

Measure	Internal consistency	Inter-rater reliability	Factor structure	External validity
Shedler-Westen Assessment Procedure for Adolescents, Version II, BPD scale (SWAP-II-A-BPD)				
DeFife et al. 2013	0.70–0.90	ICC=0.60	Not reported	Association with DSM-5 symptom count AUC for ROC identifying DSM-5 diagnosis: 0.84
DSM-5 Section III BPD measures				
Criterion A				
Assessment of Identity Development in Adolescence (AIDA)				
Goth et al. 2012	Scales: 0.86–0.94 Subscales: 0.73–0.86	Not reported	Unidimensional	Significant mean difference between school sample and PD subsample (determined by the SCID-II) on all scales and subscales (d=1.04–2.56)
Kassin et al. 2013	Scales: 0.85–0.94 Subscales: 0.70–0.83	Not reported	Unidimensional	Significant mean difference between school samples combined and delinquent subsample on all scales except consistency and autonomy subscales (d=0.22–1.29)
Lind et al. 2019	0.95	Not reported	Not reported	Identity diffusion and narrative coherence associated with BPFS-C
Inventory of Personality Organization for Adolescents (IPO-A), initial version				
Biberdzic et al. 2018b	0.90	Not reported	Five-factor structure	Associations with psychodynamically oriented measures of function
Biberdzic et al. 2018a	Not reported	Not reported	Cluster analysis identified three levels of personality organization	Sensitivity: 0.81–0.94 Specificity: 0.81–0.95

TABLE 10–1. Assessment tools with psychometric properties for DSM 5 Section II and III borderline personality disorder (BPD) in adolescents (*continued*)

Measure	Internal consistency	Inter-rater reliability	Factor structure	External validity
DSM-5 Section III BPD measures (*continued*)				
Criterion A (*continued*)				
Levels of Personality Functioning Questionnaire for Adolescents From 12 to 18 (LOPF-Q 12–18)				
Goth et al. 2018	Total Scale: 0.97 Scales: 0.88–0.95 Subscales: 0.76–0.91	Not reported	Four-factor structure	Association with BPFS-C ROC identifying SCID-II BPD: Sensitivity 0.81 Specificity 0.84 ROC identifying BPFS-C BPD: Sensitivity 0.81 Specificity 0.83 ROC identifying PD patients: Sensitivity: 0.75 Specificity: 0.59
Criterion B				
Personality Inventory for DSM-5 (PID-5)				
De Clercq et al. 2014b	Good ($\alpha > 0.8$) for 16 of 25 facets Poor (0.58) for Suspiciousness Moderate for 8 facets (0.68–0.79)	N/A	Suggests that the structural nature of personality pathology across adolescence and adulthood can be conceptualized within a single hierarchical framework of five basic dimensions. However, notable facet-level differences between the adolescent and adult PID-5 structures were found (may be developmental issue).	Convergent validity with age-specific facets of personality pathology was generally supported, but discriminant validity appeared low.

TABLE 10–1. **Assessment tools with psychometric properties for DSM 5 Section II and III borderline personality disorder (BPD) in adolescents** *(continued)*

Measure	Internal consistency	Inter-rater reliability	Factor structure	External validity
Personality Inventory for DSM-5 (PID-5) *(continued)*				
Somma et al. 2016	With exception of Suspiciousness, all other scales adequate (all α≥0.70; most ≥0.80)	N/A	Not reported	Associations with dimensionally assessed DSM-5 Section II PDs support construct validity.
Personality Inventory for DSM-5—Brief Form (PID-5-BF)				
Fossati et al. 2017	Domains: 0.59–0.77 Total score: 0.83	Average domain scores and total scores did not differ between baseline and retest	Five-factor structure	Association with scales of the MDPF

Note. AUC=area under the curve; MDPF=Measure of Disordered Personality Functioning; NPV=Negative Predictive Value; PAI-BOR=Personality Assessment Inventory—Borderline Features Scale; PD=personality disorder; PDQ-4-BPD=Personality Diagnostic Questionnaire–4 BPD Scale; PPV=Positive Predictive Value; ROC=receiver operating characteristic; SCID-II=Structured Clinical Interview for DSM-IV Axis II Disorders; SCID-IIBPD=Structured Clinical Interview for DSM-IV Axis II Disorders—Borderline Personality Disorder Scale; SCID-II-PQ=Structured Clinical Interview for DSM-IV Axis II Disorders—Personality Questionnaire.

erally supported a unidimensional factor structure for the CI-BPD in both clinical and population-based community samples (Michonski et al. 2013; Sharp et al. 2012). Studies of self-report measures have found similar results. For instance, despite the purported four-factor structure suggested for the PAI-BOR-A, results from a recent investigation in an inpatient adolescent sample and justice system–involved adolescent sample demonstrated poor fit of the four factors and superiority for a unidimensional factor structure (Venta et al. 2018). Similarly, the BPFFC-11 demonstrated a unidimensional factor structure in a large community sample. In another study, although confirmatory factor analysis did not support a simple unidimensional factor model in an Italian adolescent community sample, all items loaded significantly onto a general common factor, and the two specific factors largely captured residual variance (Fossati et al. 2019; Sharp et al. 2014; Vanwoerden et al. 2019). Additionally, Leung and Leung (2009) found an acceptably fitting unidimensional solution using the McLean Screening Instrument for Borderline Personality Disorder, a brief self-report measure used for screening assessment, in a large sample of Chinese high school students. Other factor structures have been demonstrated, such as the two-factor (intra- and interpersonal preoccupation and impulsivity/reactivity) model of the BPFS-C shown by Haltigan and Vaillancourt (2016); however, taken together, the evidence is most consistent with a unidimensional conceptualization (Michonski 2014). Unidimensionality of BPD should not be implied as support for the taxonicity of BPD. Haslam et al. (2012) clearly showed no evidence for taxonicity of BPD. Moreover, when BPD criteria or symptoms are modeled alongside symptoms of other PDs, no evidence for a BPD dimension emerges (see, e.g., Sharp et al. 2015).

Myth 2: BPD Cannot Be Reliably Distinguished From Typical Adolescent Development Before Age 18

Few would believe that individuals suddenly develop five or more criteria of BPD when they turn 18 years old. However, some argue that BPD features observed during adolescence reflect normative developmental features of this period rather than personality disturbance. Indeed, Laurenssen et al. (2013) found that about 40% of their sample of psychologists would not diagnose BPD in adolescence because they believed that personality problems during that developmental stage reflect the "storm and stress" of adolescence.

A key assumption underlying the idea that BPD cannot be reliably distinguished from typical adolescent development is the erroneous belief that relevant developmental processes, including personality development, identity formation, and executive functioning, are confined to the period before age 18 years. There is now extensive research, mentioned above, indicating that these processes extend well into the third decade of life and some extend even beyond this time period (Newton-Howes et al. 2015). Hence, the argument regarding distinguishing normal from abnormal development is not confined to the traditional notion of adolescence (12–18 years) but also applies to other developmental epochs across the lifespan (Newton-Howes et al. 2015).

It is true that some behaviors that are relatively common in adolescence resemble BPD features (e.g., affective instability, impulsivity, identity disturbance), and this makes it important to disentangle pathology from typical adolescent emotional experiences (Fossati et al. 2014). However, such behaviors exist on a dimension, and cross-sectional studies consistently demonstrate that the extent and severity of BPD features in young people, such as impulsivity (Lawrence et al. 2010), substance use (Scalzo et al. 2018), sexual behavior (Penner et al. 2019; Thompson et al. 2019a), and psychosocial functioning (Kramer et al. 2017), make them non-normative (Chanen 2017). Research also supports that identity disturbance in adolescence resembles identity disturbance in adults and is a clinically meaningful construct related to personality pathology across age (Westen et al. 2011). Evidence also suggests that a small proportion of adolescents portray a level of severity (deviation from normality) that would necessitate a categorical PD diagnosis (Venta et al. 2014).

Longitudinal studies suggest that BPD emerges in early adolescence, peaks in midadolescence, and declines into early adulthood (Arens et al. 2013; Cohen et al. 2005; Stepp et al. 2010). However, a subgroup of young people had a developmental trajectory that deviated from the normative decline. The Children in the Community Study (CICS) first established this trajectory (Cohen et al. 2005). The researchers found that despite the overall decline in PD symptoms across an epidemiological sample of 800 youths, about 20% demonstrated increased symptoms throughout adulthood (Cohen et al. 2005). Similarly, De Clercq et al. (2009) found that although maladaptive traits (disagreeableness, impulsivity, and compulsivity) declined over a 2-year follow-up of 477 young adolescents, the decline was less substantial in children with high scores.

The next question to address is whether this subgroup with persistently elevated symptoms prior to age 18 might meet the diagnostic threshold for BPD. Indeed, studies using the measures described in Table 10-1 have found that adolescent prevalence rates generally mirror those in adult samples (Ha et al. 2014; Leung and Leung 2009; Zanarini et al. 2011). This suggests that these young people had symptoms that would meet the threshold for categorical diagnosis. In a cross-sectional study with adolescent inpatients with BPD, psychiatrically healthy adolescents, and adult inpatients with BPD, the adolescent patients showed similar rates and severity of BPD symptoms to the adults, suggesting that they were experiencing BPD above diagnostic thresholds rather than emerging symptoms of the disorder (Zanarini et al. 2017). BPD features were not uncommon among the psychiatrically healthy adolescents, with about one-quarter of the group reporting 9 or more of the 24 measured BPD symptoms. The symptoms that they reported showed continuity with normal development (e.g., anger, anxiety and emptiness, and general impulsivity). However, the DSM threshold for a categorical diagnosis is arbitrary. There is evidence that the presence of subthreshold features of BPD is clinically significant among young people and adults (Thompson et al. 2019b). It seems likely that symptoms with greater discriminatory value, such as "quasi-psychotic thought," self-mutilation, and help-seeking suicide threats, which were reported by 3% or less of the psychiatrically healthy adolescents in Zanarini et al.'s (2017) study, are markers of more severe disorder. This is consistent with clinical studies showing that psychotic symptoms are a marker of more severe BPD in young people (Cavelti et al. 2019). Therefore, it is true that some features of BPD are common in adolescence, but severe symptoms that meet diagnostic thresholds are distinguishable from adolescent "storm and stress" and mirror those that occur in adults with PD in both form and severity, but with higher prevalence.

In summary, clinicians should consider the developmental context of the individual patient when assessing whether personality features represent an acute and transient behavior pattern or pervasive personality impairment. This context should take account of contemporary evidence regarding an expanded and more inclusive definition of adolescence, extending to the mid-20s. When there is evidence of pervasive personality impairment, clinicians should not refrain from making a PD diagnosis. Moreover, it should also be recognized that pathological personality features not reaching the threshold for a categorical diagnosis might also be clinically important. Finally, it has been suggested that given the natural course of the disorder, described above, BPD might be better conceived of as a disorder of young people (Chanen et al. 2008b).

Myth 3: Adolescent Personality Is Too Unstable to Warrant a Diagnosis of BPD

Similar to the belief that features of personality pathology in adolescence reflect normative development is the belief that PD cannot be diagnosed in adolescents because their personalities are transient and still developing. In this sense, adolescents who display BPD features might "grow out" of them as they age and therefore should not be diagnosed with BPD during this period. This belief stems from ideas that adolescent personalities are *uniquely unstable* and that PD is *very stable* in adults, leading to the conclusion that adultlike stability of PD would need to be demonstrated to validate diagnosis in adolescents (Chanen et al. 2008b; Miller et al. 2008).

In fact, research suggests that children (<10 years old) manifest remarkably stable differences in negative and positive emotion and in self and behavior regulation (Shiner 2009) and that there is substantial overlap in the psychological content covered across the domains of temperament, normal-range child personality, and child personality pathology. For instance, there is good evidence that the same five-factor conceptual framework explains variation in temperament, normal-range child personality, and child personality pathology (De Clercq et al. 2006; Shiner 2009; Tackett et al. 2013). These traits associate with later personality traits, suggesting continuity in the traits that underlie PD. For example, in a large longitudinal study that assessed girls at ages 5–8 and later at ages 14–22, temperament and symptoms reported by teachers and parents in childhood predicted BPD onset in adolescence and early adulthood, with emotionality representing the strongest predictor (Stepp and Lazarus 2017). Similarly, Cramer (2016) found that childhood traits assessed at age 11 characterized by two underlying personality dimensions (impulsivity and nonconformity, aggression) predicted adult BPD features. Another study found that over 30% of self-mutilating adult inpatients with BPD reported that they had begun engaging in self-harm prior to age 12, and these individuals reported more severe and persistent self-harm than those with a later onset (Zanarini et al. 2006). In addition to demonstrating the stability of personality, these studies hold great implications for early detection of children at risk for eventually developing PD and, again, suggest that BPD is a disorder of young people (Chanen and Thompson 2018; Chanen et al. 2008b; Kaess et al. 2014).

The CICS, which demonstrated the general pattern of onset in early adolescence, peak in mid-adolescence, and decline into early adulthood, was also the first to provide evidence that BPD demonstrates moderate to strong rank-order stability in adolescents, with coefficients in the 0.4 to 0.7 range (Cohen et al. 2005). This stability is similar to that seen with normal personality traits in adults and children and to that seen in PD in adults. The findings are mirrored in a large longitudinal twin study in which mean-level BPD traits declined from adolescence to adulthood but rank-order stability remained high, with coefficients ranging from 0.53 to 0.73 (Bornovalova et al. 2009). Additionally, an outpatient adolescent sample demonstrated a rank-order stability index of 0.54 over 2 years for BPD (Chanen et al. 2004). These studies collectively suggest that maladaptive personality traits among young people are moderately stable over time, showing similar stability to that among adults.

Despite moderate dimensional stability in both adolescents and adults, categorical diagnosis is less stable. High rates of change and "remission" have been reported in adult samples, refuting traditional beliefs that BPD is a persistent and unremitting disorder (Zanarini 2006; Zanarini et al. 2012). However, regardless of categorical and symptom instability, functional impairment persists. For example, in the CIC cohort, adolescent BPD predicted lower academic and occupational attainment, less partner involvement, fewer attained adult developmental milestones, and general impairment in adulthood despite symptom decline with age and independent of other disorders (Winograd et al. 2008). In an adult sample of hospital patients and outpatients, the 10-year course of BPD was characterized by high rates of remission (defined as having manifestations of no more than two BPD criteria present for either 2 or 12 consecutive months) and low rates of relapse (meeting at least five BPD criteria again), but also severe and persistent impairment in psychosocial functioning (Gunderson et al. 2011). In a sample of 64 outpatients with BPD in Spain, social and occupational functioning remained largely unchanged at 10-year follow-up despite significant improvements on BPD domains (Alvarez-Tomás et al. 2017). Adolescent borderline features at age 11–12 years have also been shown to predict psychotic, hypomanic, and depressive symptoms at age 22–23 years (Winsper et al. 2019), and elevated levels of borderline features at a mean age of 14 years predict poorer functioning over the subsequent two decades of follow-up (Winograd et al. 2008). Outcomes included poor role and social functioning, life satisfaction, and academic and occupational attainment, and fewer attained adult developmental milestones.

In summary, adolescent personality pathology is more stable and adult personality pathology is less stable than was once thought, such that adolescent and adult PDs show similar levels of stability over similar time intervals. Additionally, functional impairment persists long after individuals no longer have symptoms that meet the diagnostic threshold for categorically defined disorder.

Myth 4: Adult BPD and Adolescent BPD Have Different Associated Clinical Features, and Causal Models for Adult BPD Might Not Extend to Adolescent BPD

It has long been established that BPD is associated with immense suffering, impairment, and burden placed on self, others, and society (Gunderson et al. 2011; Oldham 2006; Soeteman et al. 2008a, 2008b). Comparable to adults, adolescents with BPD present with high rates of comorbidity and severe psychosocial problems. Studies report that adolescents with BPD report symptoms as severe as those reported by adults, as well as higher rates of Axis I and II comorbidity and significantly greater psychosocial impairment compared with adolescents with other psychiatric disorders (Chanen et al. 2007; Ha et al. 2014; Kaess et al. 2014). Similar to adults, adolescent inpatients with BPD also demonstrate significantly higher rates of complex comorbidity, defined as having any mood or anxiety disorder plus a disorder of impulsivity, compared with adolescent inpatients with other psychiatric disorders (Ha et al. 2014). Adolescent BPD is also associated with high rates of treatment utilization and hospitalization, higher medical expenses, and greater number of medication trials (Cailhol et al. 2013; Feenstra et al. 2012). Some evidence suggests that the costs and burden associated with adolescent BPD are even higher than those associated with BPD in adults (Hutsebaut et al. 2013; Soeteman et al. 2008a). Furthermore, quality of life is very low in adolescents with BPD and is comparable to that in their adult counterparts (Soeteman et al. 2008b). This striking degree of suffering and burden, as well as evidence that earlier onset of BPD denotes even poorer outcomes, has led to advocacy for the recognition of adolescent BPD as a public health priority (Chanen et al. 2007, 2017).

Though further research is required, evidence suggests that risk factors and etiological models of BPD from adult studies extend to adolescents. For example, in two independent community samples of youth, carriers of the short allele of the serotonin transporter promoter gene (5-HTTLPR) exhibited the highest levels of BPD traits, mirroring previous genetic associations in adults (Hankin et al. 2011). Chanen and colleagues (2008c) presented the first evidence that orbitofrontal (but not medial temporal lobe) alterations found in adult samples are already present early in the course of BPD; this finding was later replicated by two other groups (Brunner et al. 2010; Goodman et al. 2011). Though we will not discuss etiology in depth in this chapter, evidence has been most consistent with both Linehan's biosocial or stress-diathesis model (Crowell et al. 2009, 2014) and Fonagy and colleagues' mentalization-based developmental model (Fonagy and Bateman 2008; Sharp and Fonagy 2008). Extensions of adult etiological models include a longitudinal twin study that found independent and interactive inherited and environmental contributions to BPD pathology in youth (Belsky et al. 2012). Additionally, a recent study in adolescents diagnosed with BPD and psychiatrically healthy controls found that high levels of childhood neglect, low levels of childhood competence, and high levels of trait neuroticism were each associated with BPD in adolescents (Zanarini et al. 2020).

While keeping these similarities in mind, studies have found differences in symptomatology and presentation of BPD across age groups. Within a developmental psychopathology model, these differences might be attributable to heterotypic continuity, meaning the continuity of a coherent underlying organization or meaning of behaviors rather than continuity at the level of observable behaviors (Sharp et al. 2018). In other words, underlying traits can differ in how they are behaviorally manifested across developmental contexts (Courtney-Seidler et al. 2013). Studies suggest that underlying BPD symptomatology might be expressed as externalizing behavior in younger age groups, and that adolescents explicitly display more acute symptoms, including self-harm and excessive risk taking (Stepp et al. 2012). As individuals age, internalizing symptoms become more prominent, while externalizing features decrease into early adulthood and then are retained. Such age-related differences might be due to the developmental trajectory of impulsivity, which decreases from adolescence to young adulthood and then remains relatively stable (Arens et al. 2013). A cross-sectional study in which patients with BPD rated their affective state using e-diaries suggests that affective instability declines with age, irrespective of comorbidity and BPD severity (Santangelo et al. 2017). Taken together, these differences suggest not that adolescents are suffering from a different underlying pathology than adults but rather that psychopathology presents differently across developmental contexts. In a recent study, Sharp and colleagues (2018) investigated whether Section II DSM criteria operate similarly across adolescents and adults to determine if developmental adjustment for DSM criteria was needed. Three age cohorts were recruited: adolescents (ages 12–17 years; $n=484$), young adults (ages 18–25 years; $n=442$), and adults (age≥26 years; $n=953$). Item response theory methods were used to evaluate differential item (or criterion) functioning (DIF) of BPD criteria across adolescents and adults. Qualitative analyses were then used to evaluate the potential sources of DIF. Item response theory results demonstrated DIF across adolescents and adults for all DSM BPD criteria. Qualitative analyses suggested that the source of DIF was most likely rater/interviewer bias. Results also suggested that behavioral criteria might represent the heterotypic features of BPD, while intra- and interpersonal criteria represent the homotypic features of the disorder. Therefore, while the BPD construct can be readily extended downward to younger age groups, it is still crucial to consider developmental aspects when approaching personality pathology assessment and treatment when considering individual criteria.

Myth 5: Adolescent BPD Cannot Be Distinguished From Internalizing and Externalizing Disorders

Clinicians might also choose to exclude adolescents from PD diagnosis because of a belief that the symptoms are better explained by internalizing or externalizing disorders. This might become even more pronounced as hierarchical taxonomy of psychopathology (HiTOP) formulations of psychopathology (Kotov et al. 2017) begin to permeate the literature. According to the developmental personality-psychopathology spectrum approach, personality begins with temperamental traits already observable during infancy and toddlerhood, which make up the entirety of personality during the early years (Shiner 2003; Tackett 2006). As children mature, early temperamental traits develop into broader, more inclusive higher-order personality traits that map onto the Big Five (Shiner 2003). Consistent with the HiTOP model, these trait domains help to explain comorbidity among childhood disorders (Tackett 2006). The implication of this developmental model of personality-psychopathology spectrum is that personality pathology represents extreme manifestations of internalizing-externalizing spectra (Tackett et al. 2016). It is well established that adolescent and adult BPD commonly co-occur (are "comorbid") with anxiety, depression, and externalizing disorders (Chanen et al. 2007; Ha et al. 2014; Kaess et al. 2013). However, factor analytic studies suggest that internalizing and externalizing disorders do not fully account for the variability in BPD features (Eaton et al. 2011).

Adolescent PD diagnosis also provides important clinical information beyond comorbid disorders. For example, BPD provided incremental predictive value for suicidal outcomes over and above internalizing pathology in a sample of adolescent inpatients (Sharp et al. 2012). Because BPD is a highly interpersonal disorder, unique associations with BPD are particularly strong in interpersonal domains. In a sample of adolescent outpatients, BPD was a significant predictor over and above Axis I disorders and PDs for psychopathology, general functioning, peer relationships, self-care, and family and relationship functioning (Chanen et al. 2007). BPD symptoms also demonstrated moderate to strong associations with every domain of psychosocial functioning and unique associations with self-perception, social skills, and sexual behavior in a large longitudinal study (Wright et al. 2016). Furthermore, personality pathology appears to be more stable than internalizing and externalizing pathology in adolescence (Cohen et al. 2005). In a community sample of Flemish children, externalizing problems demonstrated a steeper decline over time than did indices of personality pathology, suggesting a developmental trajectory in which children "grow out" of externalizing behavior but personality pathology persists (De Clercq et al. 2009). These findings might still support a model in which personality pathology merely represents extreme variants of the internalizing-externalizing spectra. However, because these traits are already observable during infancy and early childhood, and found to be moderately stable, these results cannot explain why PD has an onset in adolescence or why certain adolescents do or do not diverge from the normative decline in maladaptive traits (C. Sharp, S. Vanwoerden, K. Schmeck, et al., "An Evaluation of Age-Group Latent Mean Differences in Maladaptive Identity in Adolescence," unpublished manuscript). Thus, attributing the symptoms of personality pathology to other comorbidities does not provide a comprehensive framework for understanding the individual. Additionally, an internalizing or externalizing conceptualization ignores the problems in self and interpersonal functioning that are key to personality pathology and provide immediate and important treatment targets (Livesley 2011; Luyten and Blatt 2013).

Rather than fully accounting for personality pathology, it appears that internalizing and externalizing disorders are a stepping-stone on the path to BPD. Results from a longitudinal twin study suggest that BPD traits in adulthood might be best understood as being preceded by inherited vulnerability for internalizing and externalizing disorders (Bornovalova et al. 2013). In another large twin study, BPD characteristics at age 12 were associated with internalizing and externalizing disorders earlier in childhood (Belsky et al. 2012). The converse is unsupported: there is no evidence that BPD precedes internalizing and externalizing disorders (Bornovalova et al. 2013; Lazarus et al. 2017). As individuals age, externalizing and internalizing problems become subsumed within personality pathology, as evidenced by shared risk factors and high rates of comorbidity throughout the lifespan. This is supported by a recent review describing nearly identical risk profiles for borderline pathology and a broad range of internalizing and externalizing disorders (Stepp et al. 2016).

We have established that adolescent BPD is not better explained by comorbid disorders. However, it might be difficult to disentangle symptoms that present similarly. When differentiating between BPD and internalizing or externalizing disorders, practitioners should carefully consider self-other (Criterion A) functioning, because it is central to personality pathology and will be more discriminating (Sharp et al. 2018). We also reiterate here that BPD is a legitimate differential diagnosis of common mental disorders in young people (Chanen 2015).

Myth 6: To Avoid Stigma, It Is Better to Not Diagnose Personality Pathology in Young People

The final argument used against the assessment, diagnosis, and treatment of BPD in adolescents is that it might be stigmatizing to label a young person with the disorder. In part, this argument rests on mistaken assumptions that PD is both chronic and untreatable. Clinical experience also suggests that some clinicians avoid the diagnosis in order to "protect" their patients from discrimination and mistreatment by other clinicians.

We have reviewed evidence above that the BPD diagnosis is not as stable as once believed, and one of the longest follow-along studies to date (Zanarini 2006) demonstrated that BPD features "remit" in almost all patients. Evidence from systematic reviews and meta-analyses supports the effectiveness of a range of specialized treatments for reducing borderline features and related problems in adults (Cristea et al. 2017). Given mounting evidence that BPD has its onset and represents a valid diagnosis in adolescence, attention has turned to tailoring treatment for younger populations (Temes and Zanarini 2019). Tables 10–2 and 10–3 summarize studies evaluating treatment of BPD in adolescent samples. Table 10–2 provides specifics about the study groups, study design, study inclusion criteria, and sample characteristics, including participants ages and diagnoses. Table 10–3 presents details on the study intervention; comparison condition(s); outcome variables; duration, measurement points, and statistical model; findings; and, if applicable, follow-up time and findings.

Treatments initially developed for adult BPD have been adapted for adolescents, including dialectical behavior therapy (DBT-A), mentalization-based therapy (MBT-A), cognitive analytic therapy (CAT), and emotion regulation training (ERT). DBT-A follows a framework similar to dialectical behavior therapy for adults but includes family members in skills groups as well as a separate family therapy component. A trial with adolescents who reported recent self-harm and at least two BPD criteria found that DBT-A was superior to enhanced usual care in reducing borderline and depressive symptoms and that DBT-A remained superior in reducing self-harm, but not other measures, at 3-year follow-up (Mehlum et al. 2014, 2019). A recent study found that DBT-A was more effective than individual and group supportive therapy in reducing self-harm, suicide attempts, and nonsuicidal self-injury in adolescents with elevated suicide risk and three or more BPD criteria (McCauley et al. 2018). MBT-A is also similar to its adult counterpart but adds a family therapy component and explicitly focuses on impulsivity and affect regulation given the developmental demands of adolescents. In adolescents with recent self-harm (73% having symptoms that met BPD criteria), the MBT-A treatment group demonstrated a greater reduction in self-harm and depressive symptoms, and fewer in the treatment group met criteria for BPD at 12 months compared with the control group (Rossouw and Fonagy 2012). In addition, group-based MBT-A in adolescents who had symptoms meeting four BPD criteria led to clinically significant change in BPD pathology, mentalizing, and trust (Bo et al. 2017). A pilot randomized controlled trial (RCT) of MBT-A group therapy furthermore demonstrated positive results relative to treatment as usual (Griffiths et al. 2019), although no treatment effects were detected in a recently conducted Danish RCT (Beck et al. 2020). Transference-focused psychotherapy, a manualized psychodynamic treatment, has also been adapted for use in adolescents, but this adaptation has yet to be evaluated in a randomized clinical trial (Normandin et al. 2014). When interpreting these results, readers should keep in mind that the inclusion criteria targeted elevated BPD symptoms, rather than requiring BPD diagnosis, and that most trials have used inadequately characterised comparison treatments that are variations on treatment as usual and/or have not reported treatment fidelity. (See also Chapters 12 through 15 in Part III, "Treatment," of this volume for expanded discussions of psychotherapies effective in the treatment of BPD.)

TABLE 10–2. Interventions for adolescent borderline personality disorder (BPD): study design, inclusion criteria, and sample characteristics

Study	Groups	Study design	Inclusion criteria	Sample characteristics (age, diagnosis)
Cognitive analytic therapy				
Chanen et al. 2008a, 2009	CAT=41 Control=37 Historical control=32	RCT, based in Helping Young People Early clinic (for 15- to 18-year-olds) specialized for BPD	Ages 15–18; at least three DSM-IV criteria for BPD; at least one childhood risk factor; referred from the community; no psychotic illness	Mean age 17 years, 81% female, mean number of DSM criteria met: 4.5
Dialectical behavior therapy				
Cooney et al. 2010, 2012	DBT=14 Control=15	RCT, 6 months of DBT vs. uncontrolled TAU in a naturalistic setting	Ages 13–19; history of suicide attempt or self-injury in previous 3 months; one responsible caregiver	Mean age 16 years, 76% female, mean number of self-harm acts: 6
McCauley et al. 2018	DBT=72 IGST=65	RCT, comparing DBT with IGST for reducing suicide attempts, NSSI, and self-harm in high-risk youth recruited through ED, inpatient, outpatient, and community programs	Ages 12–18; at least one lifetime suicide attempt, elevated past-month suicidal ideation (≥24 on the SIQ-JR), self-injury repetition (≥three lifetime self-harm episodes, including one in the prior 12 weeks), three or more BPD criteria; IQ≥70; no primary psychosis, mania, anorexia, or life-threatening condition	Mean age 14.9 years, 94.8% female
Mehlum et al. 2014, 2019	DBT=39 EUC=38	RCT, comparing DBT with EUC, based in a metropolitan community psychiatric clinic, referred for current self-harm	Ages 12–18; history of at least two episodes of self-harm (at least one within the past 16 weeks); at least two DSM-IV BPD criteria (plus the self-destructive criterion) or at least one DSM-IV BPD criterion plus at least two subthreshold-level criteria; no diagnosis of bipolar I, psychotic disorder, intellectual disability, or Asperger's syndrome	Mean age 16 years, 88% female

TABLE 10–2. Interventions for adolescent borderline personality disorder (BPD): study design, inclusion criteria, and sample characteristics *(continued)*

Study	Groups	Study design	Inclusion criteria	Sample characteristics (age, diagnosis)
Rathus and Miller 2002	DBT=29 Control=82	Quasi-experimental study of consecutive admissions; patients selected for DBT if they had a recent suicide attempt and three or more BPD criteria compared with other admissions	Suicide attempt in the past 16 weeks; diagnosis of BPD by SCID-II	Mean age 16.1 years (DBT) vs. 15 years (control), 93% (DBT) vs. 73% (control) female, BPD: 88% of the DBT group vs. 6% of the comparison group
Mentalization-based treatment				
Beck et al. 2020	MBT-G=56 TAU=56	RCT, comparing MBT-G vs. TAU in outpatient setting	Age ≤14–17; at least four DSM-5 BPD criteria, above clinical cut-off on BPFS-C; no pervasive developmental disorder, learning disability, anorexia, psychosis, antisocial PD, or primary diagnosis other than BPD	Mean age 15.8 years, 99% female, 95% met BPD criteria
Bo et al. 2017	N=34 in group-based MBT	Group-based MBT in three outpatient clinics	Ages 15–18; at least four DSM-5 BPD criteria; parents' or parent substitutes' commitment to participate in MBT-Parents program	Mean age 16.4 years, 100% female
Rossouw and Fonagy 2012	MBT-A=40 Control=40	RCT of MBT-A or TAU, based in three community clinics, consecutive referrals of young people who self-harm	Ages 12–17; at least one episode of self-harm within the past month; referred from the community because of history of intentional self-harm; no psychotic disorder	Mean age 15 years, 85% female, 97% depressed, 73% with symptoms meeting criteria for BPD

TABLE 10–2. Interventions for adolescent borderline personality disorder (BPD): study design, inclusion criteria, and sample characteristics (*continued*)

Study	Groups	Study design	Inclusion criteria	Sample characteristics (age, diagnosis)
Mentalization-based treatment (*continued*)				
Laurenssen et al. 2014	MBT-A=11 No control group	Pilot study of MBT-A, independent of the treatment developers, based in one mental health center offering specialized inpatient treatment for adolescent personality disorders; referrals to the center	Ages 14–18; at least two DSM-IV BPD criteria; no psychotic or organic brain disorder	Mean age 16.5 years, 100% female
Emotion regulation training				
Schuppert et al. 2009	ERT=23 Control=20	RCT based in five mental health centers; feasibility study testing randomization of young people with BPD symptoms to ERT+TAU or TAU alone	Ages 14–19; at least two DSM-IV BPD criteria (mood instability plus at least one of the following: impulsivity, recurrent suicidality/ self-harm, or anger)	Mean age 16 years, 88% female
Marieke Schuppert et al. 2012	ERT=54 Control=55	RCT testing addition of ERT to TAU, based in five mental health centers, consecutive referrals for self-harm and other BPD symptoms	Ages 14–19; at least two DSM-IV BPD criteria; score of ≥15 on total scale BPDSI	Mean age 16 years, 96% female, 73% with symptoms meeting BPD criteria, 63% depressed

Note. BPDSI=Borderline Personality Disorder Severity Index; BPFS-C=Borderline Personality Features Scale for Children; CAT=cognitive analytic therapy; DBT=dialectical behavior therapy; ED=emergency department; ERT=emotion regulation training; EUC=enhanced usual care; IGST=individual and group supportive therapy; MBT=mentalization-based treatment; MBT-A=mentalization-based treatment for adolescents; MBT-G=mentalization-based group treatment; NSSI=nonsuicidal self-injury; RCT=randomized controlled trial; SCID-II=Structured Clinical Interview for DSM-IV Axis II Disorders; SIQ-JR=Suicidal Ideation Questionnaire—Junior; TAU=treatment as usual.

TABLE 10–3. Interventions for adolescent borderline personality disorder (BPD): intervention decription, findings, and follow-up

Study	Intervention	Comparison condition(s)	Outcome variables	Duration, measurement points, and statistical model	Findings	Follow-up time and findings
Cognitive analytic therapy						
Chanen et al. 2008a, 2009	CAT: median of 13 CAT sessions; also available to both CAT and control groups: pharmacotherapy, activity groups, crisis teams	(a) Standardized GCC: modular package controlling for availability, accessibility, and duration of care using a problem-solving model with modules for co-occurring problems; median of 11 sessions (b) Historical TAU	SCID-II, YSR, semi-structured para-suicidal behavior interview, SOFAS	43-week treatment, assessed at 6, 12, and 24 months; mixed-effects regression models	Both groups showed significant positive effects. CAT was faster on externalizing. Both CAT and GCC were superior to historical TAU.	Up to 24 months from baseline: CAT had greatest median improvement, but effect sizes were small; biggest effect was on externalizing. CAT was superior to historical TAU on internalizing and externalizing at 24 months. GCC was superior to TAU on internalizing and parasuicidal behaviors.
Dialectical behavior therapy						
Cooney et al. 2010, 2012	DBT; individual therapy (weekly) and multifamily group skills training (110 min)	TAU (including CBT, MI focused on substance abuse, narrative-oriented family therapy)	SASII, RFL-A, BSSI	6-month treatment, baseline and posttreatment assessment; nonparametric models	Fewer people in TAU attempted suicide, but there was no difference in self-harm ED visits or substance use between groups.	N/A

TABLE 10–3. Interventions for adolescent borderline personality disorder (BPD): intervention description, findings, and follow-up *(continued)*

Study	Intervention	Comparison condition(s)	Outcome variables	Duration, measurement points, and statistical model	Findings	Follow-up time and findings
Dialectical behavior therapy *(continued)*						
McCauley et al. 2018	DBT: 6 months, weekly individual therapy, multifamily group skills training, youth and parent telephone coaching, and weekly therapist team consultation. Parents seen individually in session 1 and offered 7 or more family sessions.	IGST: 6 months, individual sessions, adolescent supportive group therapy, as-needed parent sessions (≤7 sessions), and weekly therapist team consultation	Suicide attempts, NSSI, and self-harm (SASII); suicidal ideation (SIQ-JR)	6-month treatment, assessments at baseline and 3, 6, 9, and 12 months; mixed-model analysis of variance; nonlinear and hierarchical linear models	Significant advantages were found for DBT on all primary outcomes after treatment (suicide attempts, NSSI, self-harm). Treatment completion rates were higher for DBT than for IGST, but pattern-mixture models indicated that this difference did not informatively affect outcomes.	Rates of self-harm decreased through 1-year follow-up. The advantage of DBT decreased, with no statistically significant between-group differences from 6 to 12 months.

TABLE 10–3. **Interventions for adolescent borderline personality disorder (BPD): intervention decription, findings, and follow-up** *(continued)*

Study	Intervention	Comparison condition(s)	Outcome variables	Duration, measurement points, and statistical model	Findings	Follow-up time and findings
Mehlum et al. 2014, 2019	Treatment: 19 weeks, DBT, 14 individual therapy sessions, 11 skills training group sessions, 3 family sessions	11 individual sessions, 6 family sessions, 1 group session	LPC, Short MFQ, BHS, MADRS, SIQ	19-week treatment, assessments at 8, 15, and 19 weeks; mixed-effect multiple regression	Significant drop in self-harm was found in DBT but not in EUC; differences emerged in the last third of the trial period. DBT had greater benefits on borderline symptoms and depression.	Three-year follow-up: DBT remained superior in reducing self-harm. A substantial proportion (70.8%) of the effect of DBT on self-harm frequency over the long-term was mediated through a reduction in hopelessness during the trial phase. More than 3 months follow-up treatment after the trial was associated with further enhanced outcomes in DBT.

TABLE 10–3. Interventions for adolescent borderline personality disorder (BPD): intervention decription, findings, and follow-up *(continued)*

Study	Intervention	Comparison condition(s)	Outcome variables	Duration, measurement points, and statistical model	Findings	Follow-up time and findings
Dialectical behavior therapy *(continued)*						
Rathus and Miller 2002	DBT: 12 weeks, twice weekly, including parents in the skills training group and also in some individual therapy sessions	TAU: 12 weeks, twice weekly individual and family sessions, supportive psychodynamic therapy	HASS, BDI, LPI, BSSI	12-week intervention, assessed at baseline and posttreatment; chi-square and other univariate statistics	Fewer hospital admissions occurred in the DBT condition, but there was no difference in suicide attempts. More participants in the DBT group completed treatment compared with the TAU group (62% vs. 40%).	N/A
Mentalization-based treatment						
Beck et al. 2020	MBT in groups (MBT-G) including 3 introductory, psychoeducation sessions, 37 weekly group sessions, 5 individual case formulation sessions, and 6 group sessions for caregivers	TAU with at least 12 monthly individual supportive sessions	Primary: BPFS-C Secondary: BPFS-P, BDI-Y, RTSHI-A, YSR, CGAS, ZAN-BPD, CBCL	1-year duration, outcome assessments at baseline, after 10, 20, and 30 weeks, and at end of treatment.	No significant group differences on primary or secondary outcome measures; BPFS-C mean at end of treatment was 71.3 (SD= 15.0) in MBT-G group and 71.3 (SD=15.2) in TAU group (adjusted mean difference 0.4 units in favor of MBT-G, P=0.91).	N/A

TABLE 10–3. Interventions for adolescent borderline personality disorder (BPD): intervention decription, findings, and follow-up *(continued)*

Study	Intervention	Comparison condition(s)	Outcome variables	Duration, measurement points, and statistical model	Findings	Follow-up time and findings
Bo et al. 2017	1-year program including 2 individual case formulation sessions (1 hour), 6 group-based MBT-I sessions (1.5 hours), then 34 MBT group therapy sessions (1.5 hours)	None	BPFS-C, YSR, BDI-Y, RTSHI, IPPA-R, RFQ-Y	12-month intervention, assessed at baseline and 12 months; paired sample t-tests to evaluate within-person change from baseline to end of treatment; assessment of clinically meaningful change	Significant reduction in BPFS-C score, from 84.5 to 64.6, was noted. Significant improvements were found for general psychopathology, mentalizing, peer and parent attachment, self-harm, and depressive features. No significant improvements were noted for externalizing psychopathology and risk-taking behavior. Clinically significant change occurred for borderline pathology, mentalizing, peer trust, and parent trust.	N/A

TABLE 10–3. Interventions for adolescent borderline personality disorder (BPD): intervention description, findings, and follow-up (*continued*)

Study	Intervention	Comparison condition(s)	Outcome variables	Duration, measurement points, and statistical model	Findings	Follow-up time and findings
Mentalization-based treatment (*continued*)						
Rossouw and Fonagy 2012	MBT-A: individual session once per week, plus family session once a month	TAU: NICE-recommended evidence-based interventions	RTSHI, CI-BPD, MFQ, BPFS-C	12-month intervention, assessed at 3, 6, 9, and 12 months; mixed-effects regression and logistic regression models	Significant decrease in mean number of self-harm attempts ($d = 0.3$) and number of individuals self-harming (56% vs. 82%) at 9–12 months; significant improvement in depression. At 12 months, 58% of the TAU group and only 33% of the MBT-A group had symptoms that met criteria for BPD.	N/A

TABLE 10–3. **Interventions for adolescent borderline personality disorder (BPD): intervention description, findings, and follow-up (*continued*)**

Study	Intervention	Comparison condition(s)	Outcome variables	Duration, measurement points, and statistical model	Findings	Follow-up time and findings
Laurenssen et al. 2014	MBT-A: Four group sessions plus one individual session per week, plus one weekly session each of art therapy, writing therapy, and mentalizing cognitive therapy; psychiatric consultation, social work, and psychosocial coaching also available	None	BSL, SIPP-118, EuroQol EQ-5D	12-month intervention, assessed at baseline and 12 months; paired-samples t-tests	Significant decrease in symptomatic distress ($P < .001$, $d = 1.46$) reported; there was marked improvement in personality functioning; significant improvement in quality of life ($P < .05$, $d = 1.11$); 91% of the adolescents showed reliable change, and 18% moved to normal functioning.	N/A
Emotion regulation training						
Schuppert et al. 2009	17 weekly sessions (each 105 min) of ERT, group-based self-control CBT psychoeducation, plus TAU	TAU: medication, individual psychotherapy, systemic therapy, psychiatric care tailored to individual needs	MERLC, YSR	17 weeks, assessed at baseline and posttreatment; repeated measures ANOVA	No additional benefit was seen from ERT; internal locus of control increases with ERT; more subjects in ERT were lost to follow-up than in TAU.	N/A

TABLE 10–3. Interventions for adolescent borderline personality disorder (BPD): intervention decription, findings, and follow-up *(continued)*

Study	Intervention	Comparison condition(s)	Outcome variables	Duration, measurement points, and statistical model	Findings	Follow-up time and findings
Emotion regulation training *(continued)*						
Marieke Schuppert et al. 2012	17 weekly sessions (each 105 min) of ERT, group-based self-control CBT psychoeducation	TAU: medication, individual CBT	SCID-II, K-SADS, BPDSI, SCL-90-R, YQL-R; LPI; MERLC	6-month treatment, assessment at baseline, posttreatment, and 12-month follow-up; mixed-effects models	Symptoms decreased regardless of treatment condition; there were no subgroup benefits specifically; attrition rate was low.	6 months: improvements maintained

Note.   ANOVA=analysis of variance; BDI=Beck Depression Inventory; BDI-Y=Beck Depression Inventory—Youth; BHS=Beck Hopelessness Scale; BPDSI=Borderline Personality Disorder Severity Index; BPFS-C=Borderline Personality Features Scale for Children; BPFS-P=Borderline Personality Features Scale for Parents; BSI=Brief Symptom Inventory; BSSI=Beck Scale for Suicidal Ideation; CAT=cognitive analytic therapy; CBCL=Child Behavior Checklist; CBT=cognitive-behavioral therapy; CGAS=Children's Global Assessment Scale; CI-BPD=Childhood Interview for DSM-IV Borderline Personality Disorder; DBT=dialectical behavior therapy; DBT-A=dialectical behavior therapy for adolescents; ED=emergency department; ERT=emotion regulation training; EUC=enhanced usual care; GCC=good clinical care; HASS=Harkavy–Asnis Suicide Survey; IGST=individual and group supportive therapy; IPPA-R=Inventory of Parent and Peer Attachment—Revised; K-SADS=Schedule for Affective Disorders and Schizophrenia for School-Age Children; LPC=Lifetime Parasuicide Count; LPI=Life Problems Inventory; MADRS=Montgomery–Åsberg Depression Rating Scale; MBT=mentalization-based treatment; MBT-A=mentalization-based treatment for adolescents; MBT-G=mentalization-based group treatment; MBT-I=mentalization-based introductory-group treatment; MERLC=multidimensional emotion regulation locus of control; MFQ=Mood and Feelings Questionnaire; MI=motivational interviewing; N/A=not applicable; NICE=National Institute for Health and Clinical Excellence; NSSI=nonsuicidal self-injury; RFL-A=Reasons for Living Inventory for Adolescents; RFQ-Y=Reflective Functioning Questionnaire for Youth; RTSHI=Risk-Taking and Self-Harm Inventory; RTSHI-A=Risk-Taking and Self-Harm Inventory for Adolescents; SASII=Suicide Attempt—Self-Injury Interview; SCID-II=Structured Clinical Interview for DSM-IV Axis II Disorders; SCL-90-R=Symptom Checklist-90—Revised; SIPP-118=Severity Indices of Personality Problems; SIQ=Suicidal Ideation Questionnaire; SIQ-JR=Suicidal Ideation Questionnaire—Junior; SOFAS=Social and Occupational Functioning Assessment Scale; TAU=treatment as usual; YQL-R=Youth Quality of Life—Research Version; YSR=Youth Self-Report; ZAN-BPD= Zanarini Rating Scale for Borderline Personality Disorder.

Other early interventions have been specifically created for adolescent personality pathology and aim for indicated prevention by targeting adolescents with early BPD features rather than those whose symptoms meet diagnostic thresholds. The Helping Young People Early (HYPE) program is a comprehensive prevention and early intervention program that involves use of CAT, a time-limited psychotherapy that integrates elements of psychoanalytic object relations theory and cognitive psychology (Chanen et al. 2009, 2014). In adolescents ages 15–18 with at least one childhood risk factor and at least three BPD criteria, CAT demonstrated effectiveness and more rapid recovery compared with treatment as usual, though differences were less marked at 2-year follow-up (Chanen et al. 2008a, 2009). Inclusion criteria for HYPE have changed to allow for adolescents without childhood risk factors, and ongoing research continues to evaluate its efficacy (Chanen et al. 2015).

Finally, the Dutch ERT treatment program was developed as a relatively brief group training for adolescents with two or more BPD criteria. ERT was adapted from Systems Training for Emotional Predictability and Problem Solving (STEPPS) and combines systems components with cognitive-behavioral elements and dialectical behavior therapy skills training. A randomized clinical trial found that symptoms decreased and remained so at 6-month follow-up, but that ERT did not demonstrate additional benefits compared with treatment as usual, consisting of individual pharmacotherapy and psychotherapy with a cognitive-behavioral orientation (Marieke Schuppert et al. 2012; Schuppert et al. 2009).

Though replications and further research are needed, particularly for understanding long-term outcomes, existing evidence supports the effectiveness of treatments specifically tailored for adolescent BPD. These treatments demonstrate reductions not only in BPD symptoms, including self-harm and suicidality, but also in important clinical features including risky behaviors and need for hospitalization. Though they stem from different theoretical orientations and include a variety of techniques, these treatments have 10 factors in common (Sharp and Fonagy 2015):

1. Effort to maintain engagement in treatment through validation and an emphasis on the need to address treatment-interfering behavior
2. Explanation of a valid and evidence-based model of pathology in a way that is experienced as relevant to the patient
3. Maintenance of an active therapist stance
4. Facilitation and reinforcement of epistemic trust
5. Focus on emotion processing and connecting action and feeling
6. Inquiry about mental states using behavioral analysis, clarification, and challenge
7. Structure that provides increased activity, proactivity, and self-agency
8. Monitored adherence to a manualized structure
9. Commitment of the therapist and client to the approach
10. Supervision to identify deviation from the manualized structure and provide support for adherence

Perhaps the most important feature to emphasize is that through intervening early, there is potential to reduce or even prevent a lifetime of suffering.

It is not surprising that practitioners are concerned with the stigma accompanying a BPD diagnosis, as it is arguably the most stigmatized psychiatric disorder. Indeed, one study found that adolescents with PDs experienced greater stigma than adolescents with other severe psychiatric disorders and that BPD was the strongest predictor of experiences of stigma (Catthoor et al. 2015). The impact of this stigma, particularly in such a vulnerable population, should not be underestimated. However, avoiding diagnosis can perpetuate negative stereotypes by further implying that the diagnosis would be devastating and unchanging. In view of the evidence for validity of the diagnosis and effectiveness of treatment, nondiagnosis can be described as discriminatory, because it denies the opportunity to make informed treatment decisions and excludes BPD from health care policy and implementation (Chanen et al. 2017). Practitioners often refrain from sharing a BPD diagnosis with patients and their families as they would for other psychiatric problems. However, in the common case that patients receive numerous diagnoses and treatments before learning that their symptoms reflect personality pathology, diagnosis might validate the patient's experience and instill hope for change. In fact, preliminary evidence supports the idea that receiving a diagnosis of BPD is helpful to adolescents (Courtney and Makinen 2016). Therefore, we argue that refraining from diagnosis further perpetuates stigma and, instead, BPD should be approached in the same way as other psychiatric disorders in this age group, opening the door to relevant treatment.

The research reviewed here establishes that BPD has an onset in adolescence and represents a valid diagnostic entity prior to adulthood. As in adults, adolescent personality pathology is associated with immense suffering, impairment, and cost. While further research is needed to inform and improve treatments, it is time for practitioners to reevaluate their reluctance toward acknowledging adolescent BPD and to integrate assessment, diagnosis, and treatment into routine clinical care.

AMPD Sets the Stage for a Clinical Staging

The research reviewed in the previous section was critical in challenging the myths that have perpetuated the underdiagnosis of personality pathology in youth. We have contributed to this literature, and we fully acknowledge that the BPD diagnosis in youth has been central to promoting awareness of the existence and magnitude of this important, but neglected, public health problem (Chanen et al. 2017). However, the BPD diagnosis struggles to fulfill its key purpose of guiding treatment selection and predicting outcomes, especially in youth mental health. This difficulty is due partly to the limitations of the traditional DSM-IV or DSM-5 Section II nosological classification systems, which are characterized by high comorbidity in symptoms of disorders and artificial divisions based on cross-sectional symptom sets, which are infused and confused with course-of-illness variables—especially in the developmental context (Chanen et al. 2016; McGorry and van Os 2013). It is well known that clinical features are not differentiated from those that become apparent as a disorder persists. Adding to the problem is the fact that diagnostic concepts are typically derived from samples of patients with chronic illness in tertiary care settings, where the impression of stability and validity is enhanced (Chanen et al. 2016; McGorry 2013). Consistent with a developmental psychopathology approach (Cicchetti 2006), in youth, mental disorders often do not come to clinical attention fully formed (Chanen et al. 2016). Rather, young people frequently present with nonspecific and evolving mixtures of symptoms that may or may not consolidate neatly into a categorically defined mental disorder. Diagnostic precision is frequently possible only in retrospect (Chanen et al. 2016). Nevertheless, even without a categorically defined diagnosis, youth and families experience significant distress that disrupts developmental milestones with far-reaching consequences for education, family and peer relationships (Chanen et al. 2007). In this section of the chapter, we explain how and why the AMPD facilitates a more developmentally sensitive approach to understanding, preventing, and intervening early with personality pathology through a Clinical Staging approach. (See Chapter 4, "The Alternative DSM-5 Model for Personality Disorders," in this volume for a detailed discussion of the AMPD and its development.)

To do this, we begin by offering an integrated model, based on the literature reviewed earlier, for how personality pathology evolves—a model for the developmental course of personality pathology in the context of other pathology. To recap, our literature review of BPD research in youth revealed that PD has its onset in adolescence, but not before—a sentiment expressed in all versions of DSM since PD was included in the DSM-III (C. Sharp, S. Vanwoerden, K. Schmeck, et al., "An Evaluation of Age-Group Latent Mean Differences in Maladaptive Identity in Adolescence," unpublished manuscript). However, maladaptive traits are readily observable in pre-adolescents and appear to be moderately stable throughout childhood, adolescence, and adulthood. Internalizing pathology and externalizing pathology appear to precede BPD symptoms, but not the other way around. Although clearly being antecedents of adolescent personality pathology and remaining present throughout development, internalizing psychopathology and externalizing psychopathology are neither necessary nor sufficient for BPD. Together, this research suggests that adolescence is a sensitive period for the onset of BPD. To the extent that BPD represents the general or common features of personality pathology (Criterion A), it follows that adolescence is a sensitive period for the onset of problems in the domain of Criterion A functioning (self, identity, intimacy, and empathy). In this model, which we present in Figure 10–1, Criterion B is really nothing other than internalizing-externalizing spectra symptoms, an idea suggested and empirically validated through the personality-psychopathology spectrum model (Shiner 2003; Tackett 2006). Developmentally, maladaptive trait function (Criterion B) lays the foundation in pre-adolescence upon which maladaptive self and interpersonal functioning (Criterion A) is built.

But maladaptive Criterion A function cannot come online until adolescence because adolescence affords the individual, for the first time, the metacognitive capacity to build a narrative identity (McAdams 1995; McAdams et al. 2004). McAdams highlighted a structural difference in personality function between "traits and stories." Dispositional traits (e.g., the Big Five) represent the broad, decontextualized, nonconditional aspects of individual variation, while narrative identity represents the stories people tell about themselves in the context of their significant life experiences (Adler et al. 2016; McAdams 1995). These stories do not simply chronicle events, but also reflect meaning-making of those events in the context of an individual's traits. By placing traits within a narrative, individuals create "an internalized, evolving, integrative story of the self" (McAdams 2008, pp. 242–243). Past, present and future are meaningfully connected, and individuals create a sense of unity over time. Narratives therefore provide coherence to identity by organizing it for the individual (Adler et al. 2016; Habermas and Bluck 2000). Erikson (1950) was the first to suggest the develop-

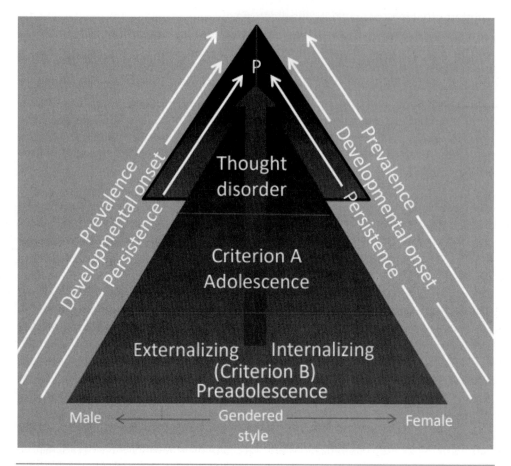

FIGURE 10–1. A developmental psychopathology model for personality pathology.

Criterion A refers to the DSM-5 Section III AMPD criterion shared by all personality disorders and defined as maladaptive self and interpersonal functioning. *P* refers to the psychopathology (or severity) factor as suggested by Caspi et al. (2014).

Source.   Adapted from Sharp and Wall 2018.

mental task of adolescence to be identity consolidation. McAdams agreed that it is during adolescence that the "binding" of the personality begins, because, for the first time, metacognitive capacities are mature enough to handle the work of holding in balance different views of the self-in-relation-to-others (C. Sharp, S. Vanwoerden, K. Schmeck, et al., "An Evaluation of Age-Group Latent Mean Differences in Maladaptive Identity in Adolescence," unpublished manuscript)—in AMPD terms, Criterion A function. In support of these ideas, we have shown that borderline features correlated with both identity diffusion and lower levels of narrative coherence, even when the identity components of the relevant borderline measure were removed from the analyses (Lind et al. 2020). Moreover, we have shown that narrative coherence was negatively related to age such that coherence increased with age (Lind et al. 2020).

This model fits well with other developmental research reviewed by Hutsebaut, Debbané, and Sharp (2020). Research suggests that hormonally and neurobiologically driven symptoms of affect and impulse dysregulation will emerge early in the course of personality pathology, with typical first clinical expressions of mood instability, anger problems, or risky behavior (Videler et al. 2019). These symptoms map well onto internalizing and externalizing types of symptoms. In contrast, symptoms related to interpersonal and social functioning often emerge only after puberty develops (Debast et al. 2017), possibly because of the increasing demand on autonomy and the associated need to relate to and learn from peers, coinciding with a renegotiation of attachment relationships with parents.

With this developmental model of the course of personality pathology in mind, we can now introduce the clinical staging approach to prevention and early intervention of personality pathology.

An AMPD-Informed Model of Clinical Staging

Clinical staging is a heuristic strategy to describe the stage of progression of a disease according to its duration and extent, and to select treatments proportionate to that stage (McGorry and van Os 2013). Consistent with a dimensional view of psychopathology, as reflected in the AMPD, clinical staging allows a refinement of diagnosis and presents a more dimensional and dynamic approach to the assessment and treatment of diseases (Scott et al. 2013; Hutsebaut et al. 2020). Originating from oncology and originally adapted for treatment of psychosis (McGorry et al. 2008), clinical staging describes the progression of disorder through five stages, ranging from the "at risk," asymptomatic Stage 0 to the late, or end, stage of disorder (Stage 4). Stages might, but do not necessarily, map onto age. Although it is unlikely that an 8-year-old will reach Stage 4 of schizophrenia or BPD, it is possible for a 13-year-old to move from Stage 0 to Stage 4 in one year, while another might take several years, and yet another might never progress beyond early-stage disorder. The important points to grasp here are 1) that interventions should be differentiated according to the stage of progression of disorder—in this case, personality impairment—and 2) that progression to later stages of disorder is not inevitable and regressions to earlier-stage disorder are common.

Three staging models have been presented related to personality pathology. The first of these (Chanen et al. 2016) was based on the well-established finding of "comorbidity" between BPD and mood disorders, including both bipolar and unipolar depression. Chanen and colleagues (2016) pointed out that the reification of these categorical DSM-based syndromes leads clinicians to miss obvious cases, mistakenly apply the wrong treatment, or withhold needed treatment. Reification and withholding of treatment occur when clinicians view these disorders as separate domains of risk, especially when symptoms are subthreshold, while in actual fact, much research has shown that subthreshold symptoms are as predictive of negative outcomes as symptoms above clinical threshold. To address this issue, Chanen et al. (2016) suggested a cross-diagnostic clinical staging approach for BPD and mood disorders in which diagnostic categories and arbitrary age restrictions are eschewed in favor of a focus on the severity and persistence of symptoms, the need for care, and the proportionality of any intervention.

In the second adaptation of a clinical staging model for personality pathology, Hutsebaut et al. (2019) argued, similarly to Sharp and colleagues (Sharp and Wall 2018; Sharp et al. 2018), that BPD features represent the generic markers of (severely) impaired personality development. These features are seen as the outcome of partly innate, partly developmentally determined dysregulations in self and interpersonal functioning, which might develop early in life and be expressed in poor attention and affect regulation, impaired impulse control, insecure attachment style, or poor regulation of frustrations. These preadolescent manifestations of personality pathology are said to lay the foundations for the more specific PD-like symptoms emerging in adolescence. In their model, Stage 0 is associated with problems in self-regulation (irritability, hypersensitivity, and excessive need for self-soothing) and interpersonal functioning (relational aggression). Stage I manifests as subthreshold BPD, including affective and impulsive symptoms (self-injurious behavior, mood swings, and temper outbursts), but symptoms are limited in extent, duration, and severity. Stage II represents the first episode of full BPD, with significant problems in four core areas, including affect regulation, impulsivity, identity, and interpersonal functioning. Stage III reflects enduring (>2 years) BPD above clinical threshold or recurring episodes of partial remission and relapse, interpersonal dysfunction, loneliness, and emptiness. Finally, Stage IV is enduring BPD, with severe problems in all areas.

Hutsebaut et al.'s (2019) model also includes descriptions of co-occurring psychopathology and areas of disability for each stage. Stage I is associated with nonspecific problems and no clinical diagnosis and might affect school and social functioning (e.g., concentration, peer contact, and social anxiety). Stage II is associated with depressive, anxiety, and conduct symptoms and imminent developmental arrest (absence from school and destructive peer group). Stage III is associated with co-occurring mental disorders, but the symptoms are limited in severity, and there is moderate to severe impact on social and school functioning. Stage IV is associated with enduring and severe co-occurring disorders and medical problems and severe and enduring impairment in social and occupational functioning, with no or limited recovery. Stage V is associated with multiple co-occurring mental state disorders, possibly including psychotic disorders, and virtually no participation in social and professional life. Hutsebaut et al.'s model extends the scope of BPD stage beyond mere symptoms of BPD, to include associated psychopathology and areas of disability to determine the stage of BPD progression. In a third, more recent extension of this model (Hutsebaut et al. 2020), the authors add specific mentalizing interventions that can be applied at each level of disease progression.

The model that we present here builds on both the Chanen et al. (2016) and Hutsebaut et al. (2019, 2020) models by more fully acknowledging the extent of co-occurring psychopathology and overlap between psychiatric problems and by supporting a clinical staging approach more broadly. However, our model is informed more directly by the empirically based developmental model presented in Figure 10–1, which also uses AMPD language to describe the development of personality pathology. The AMPD-informed clinical staging model is summarized in Table 10–4.

Stage 0 is defined as increased risk for disorder but no current symptoms. However, young people might display high levels of Criterion B maladaptive traits. These children, who are temperamentally more reactive and sensitive, are the children who have been shown in longitudinal studies to be at increased risk for the development of later personality pathology (De Clercq 2018; De Clercq et al. 2014a, 2017). They are likely to have inherited dispositional traits, or they might experience early adversity that negatively affects the development of typical stress responses to the environment, or an interaction of these. Preventative interventions available in the community that

TABLE 10–4. An AMPD-informed clinical staging model for lifespan personality pathology

Stage	Stage definition	Target population	Clinical presentation	Potential intervention and unit of care
0	Increased risk of disorder No current symptoms	For example: first-degree relatives Youth in adverse contexts Infancy, preschool age, elementary school age, adolescence	Above average scores on Criterion B maladaptive traits (or Big Five variants): negative affectivity (neuroticism), detachment (introversion), antagonism (low agreeableness), disinhibition (low conscientiousness), and psychoticism (openness) No functional impairment	Mental health literacy Self-help Community-based intervention
1a	Mild or nonspecific symptoms Mild functional change or decline	Community screening Preschool age, elementary school age, adolescence	Symptoms of both internalizing and externalizing disorder/high scores on Criterion B traits Mild issues in social and school functioning that can be handled by parents or teachers	Mental health literacy Family psychoeducation, parenting skills, supportive counseling/problem solving Community-based intervention
1b	Ultra-high risk: moderate but subthreshold symptoms	Referrals from primary care Elementary school age, adolescence, early adulthood	Confluence of internalizing and/or externalizing disorder/high scores on Criterion B traits Escalation in social and educational challenges; may struggle in peer group	Stage 1a interventions PLUS time-limited evidence-based intervention (e.g., CBT) Outpatient services
2	First episode of threshold disorder with moderate to severe symptoms and functional decline	Referrals from primary and specialist care Early, middle, late adolescence; early adulthood; adulthood	High levels of Criterion A dysfunction: maladaptive self and interpersonal functioning Internalizing and externalizing disorder/high levels of Criterion B traits maintained Moderate to severe problems in social, educational, and/or work functioning; problems in maintaining mutually rewarding relationships	Stage 1b interventions PLUS case management, educational/vocational intervention/rehabilitations, family psychoeducation and support, time-limited psychotherapy, targeted psychopharmacotherapy Outpatient services

TABLE 10–4. An AMPD-informed clinical staging model for lifespan personality pathology (*continued*)

Stage	Stage definition	Target population	Clinical presentation	Potential intervention and unit of care
3a	Recurrence of subthreshold symptoms	Referrals from primary and specialist care Early, middle, late adolescence; early adulthood; adulthood	Recurrence of internalizing and/or externalizing disorder/high levels of Criterion B traits Challenges in social and educational settings return	Stage 2 interventions PLUS emphasis on maintenance medication and psychosocial strategies for full remission Outpatient services
3b	First threshold relapse of disorder	Referrals from primary and specialist care Early, middle, late adolescence; early adulthood; adulthood	First threshold relapse of Criterion A dysfunction Internalizing and externalizing disorder/high levels of Criterion B traits Moderate to severe problems in social, educational, and/or work functioning; problems in maintaining mutually rewarding relationships	Stage 3a interventions PLUS relapse prevention strategies Outpatient services; intensive outpatient services
3c	Multiple relapses of disorder	Referrals from specialist care Early, middle, late adolescence; early adulthood; adulthood	Multiple relapses of Criterion A function, as well as internalizing and externalizing disorder/high levels of Criterion B traits Near chronic levels of social, relationship, educational, and/or work impairment	Stage 3b intervention PLUS intensive stabilization Intensive outpatient services; inpatient treatment
4	Persistent, unremitting disorder	Referrals from specialist care Early, middle, late adolescence; early adulthood; adulthood	Persistent, unremitting Criterion A dysfunction and comorbid internalizing and externalizing disorder/high levels of Criterion B traits No participation in social and professional life	Stage 3c interventions PLUS intensive psychosocial intervention (e.g., DBT/MBT) and psychopharmacological intervention Intensive outpatient services

Note. CBT = cognitive-behavioral therapy; DBT = dialectical behavior therapy; MBT = mentalization-based therapy.

strengthen resilience and quality of relationships might be important for Stage 0 populations in order to prevent progression to Stage 1 through development of overt symptoms. While the typical trajectory for the development of BPD in particular has been described as one in which BPD is preceded by a reactive and sensitive temperament during infancy and the preschool and elementary school years, it is also possible that high levels of maladaptive trait function (Criterion B) might manifest for the first time at puberty or thereafter. It is unusual, though, for elevated maladaptive traits to manifest for the first time in young adulthood.

Risk for disorder progresses to Stage 1a if the necessary "scaffolding" was not provided for a sensitive and reactive temperament. Symptoms of anxiety, oppositionality, and irritability might emerge. Children or young people might be thought of as having pleomorphic problems, presenting with attenuated (or subthreshold) features of attention-deficit/hyperactivity disorder, mood disorder, or anxiety disorder. Parents and teachers begin to struggle to manage the young person but can do so without referral to specialist services. At this stage of disorder progression, indicated prevention using supportive counseling and/or parenting skill interventions in the context of community-based settings should provide the right dosage of intervention. During Stage 1b, traits and symptoms have consolidated into disorder and a marked escalation in social and educational/vocational challenges is observed, often warranting a referral to more specialized services. From what we know of the development of BPD, Stage 1 might commonly map onto the prepubertal years, but it is also possible that the confluence of internalizing and externalizing problems might occur for the first time in the peripubertal or postpubertal period. However, as in Stage 0, it is very unlikely that the confluence of internalizing and externalizing disorder on the pathway to personality pathology would first emerge in young adulthood.

Stage 2 is where we typically see the onset of traditionally defined PD. In our model, this is when Criterion A (maladaptive self and interpersonal functioning) first comes online, usually in the pubertal or postpubertal period through to young adulthood. "Complex comorbidity" (Ha et al. 2014; Zanarini et al. 1998) (i.e., a high burden of internalizing and externalizing psychopathology) is the norm (Chanen et al. 2007) and is associated with significant impairment in relationships and vocational functioning. It is not unusual that young people in this stage drop out of school, college, or work. Relationships are nonsatisfactory, and young people begin to fall behind on developmental milestones. Outpatient, time-limited psychosocial intervention and possible pharmacotherapy for co-occurring psychopathology are indicated at this stage of the disorder.

During Stage 3a, there is a relief or partial remission from the first episode of the disorder. Stage 3b is reached if subthreshold symptoms are maintained, with further relapse into full-blown disorder. Stage 3c is characterized by multiple relapses of Criterion A function. This is usually the phase of the disorder that clinicians will recognize as prototypical, characterized by multiple admissions and readmissions to the hospital, suicide attempts, and enduring levels of social, relationship, educational, and employment breakdown. If untreated, this pattern might develop into a persistent, unremitting presentation of the disorder. As shown in Table 10–4, with the move to Stage 3, the intensity of treatment increases, in terms of both dosage and types, with intensive outpatient services becoming relevant. At Stage 4, the disorder has become chronic and persistent. While highly specialized interventions like dialectical behavior therapy or mentalization-based therapy might be indicated in addition to all other forms of intervention that preceded this stage, many individuals at this stage seek help but do not seek or engage with individual psychotherapy. Therefore, clinical case management, risk management, and the prevention of iatrogenic and other harms might become the mainstay of treatment.

Conclusion

Over the last 15 years, there has been a proliferation of research on the developmental aspects of personality pathology. Here, we reviewed this literature with several goals in mind. First, we wanted to put to rest any remaining myths regarding PD in young people. To this end, we reviewed evidence demonstrating that 1) BPD can be reliably assessed and diagnosed in young people, 2) BPD can be reliably distinguished from typical adolescent development before the age of 18, 3) personality pathology in young people is stable enough to warrant a diagnosis of BPD, 4) BPD in young people has similar associated clinical features and fits causal models documented for adult BPD, 5) BPD in young people can be reliably distinguished from internalizing and externalizing disorders, and, finally, 6) it would be stigmatizing to avoid diagnosing PD in young people, because doing so perpetuates erroneous claims that the disorder is long-lasting and treatment resistant.

Second, on the basis of a literature review, we presented a model for the course of personality pathology that takes into account AMPD formulations of Criterion A and Criterion B. This model suggests that dispositional traits (Criterion B) can be readily identified and recognized already in prepubertal children. Although children as young as infancy may evidence extreme scores on temperamental measures indicative of maladaptive trait function, they are not diagnosed with PD before adolescence, because until adolescence, there is a limited meta-cognitive capacity to allow for the "binding" of personality that occurs through the establishment of a coherent and integrated sense of self. In addition, until adolescence, there is limited requirement placed on children to acquire the new level of knowledge, skills, and cultural competence needed to successfully transition to an independent adult role. Taken together, our developmental model suggests that maladaptive trait function (Criterion B) lays the foundation in preadolescence on which maladaptive self and interpersonal functioning (Criterion A) is built.

Third, we presented a clinical staging model that maps onto the model of developmental course, thus providing an AMPD-informed model of clinical staging. This heuristic model is useful not only to stimulate further research but also to guide clinicians in stage-appropriate clinical decision making. As such, the model offers a potentially cost-effective and empirically informed framework for the prevention, early identification, and treatment of personality pathology in young people.

References

Adler JM, Lodi-Smith J, Philippe FL, Houle I: The incremental validity of narrative identity in predicting well-being: a review of the field and recommendations for the future. Pers Soc Psychol Rev 20:142–175, 2016

Alvarez-Tomás I, Soler J, Bados A, et al: Long-term course of borderline personality disorder: a prospective 10-year follow-up study. J Pers Disord 31:590–605, 2017

American Psychiatric Association: Diagnostic and Statistical Manual of Mental Disorders, 3rd Edition, Revised. Washington, DC, American Psychiatric Association, 1987

American Psychiatric Association: Diagnostic and Statistical Manual of Mental Disorders, 4th Edition. Washington, DC, American Psychiatric Association, 1994

American Psychiatric Association: Diagnostic and Statistical Manual of Mental Disorders, 5th Edition. Arlington, VA, American Psychiatric Association, 2013

Arens EA, Stopsack M, Spitzer C, et al: Borderline personality disorder in four different age groups: a cross-sectional study of community residents in Germany. J Pers Disord 27:196–207, 2013

Beck E, Bo S, Jørgensen MS, et al: Mentalization-based treatment in groups for adolescents with borderline personality disorder: a randomized controlled trial. J Child Psychol Psychiatry 61:594–604, 2020

Belsky DW, Caspi A, Arseneault L, et al: Etiological features of borderline personality related characteristics in a birth cohort of 12-year-old children. Dev Psychopathol 24:251–265, 2012

Biberdzic M, Ensink K, Normandin L, Clarkin JF: Empirical typology of adolescent personality organization. J Adolesc 66:31–48, 2018a

Biberdzic M, Ensink K, Normandin L, Clarkin JF: Psychometric properties of the Inventory of Personality Organization for Adolescents. Adolesc Psychiatry 7:127–151, 2018b

Bo S, Sharp C, Beck E, et al: First empirical evaluation of outcomes for mentalization-based group therapy for adolescents with BPD. Personal Disord 8:396–401, 2017

Bornovalova MA, Hicks BM, Iacono WG, McGue M: Stability, change, and heritability of borderline personality disorder traits from adolescence to adulthood: a longitudinal twin study. Dev Psychopathol 21:1335–1353, 2009

Bornovalova MA, Hicks BM, Iacono WG, McGue M: Longitudinal twin study of borderline personality disorder traits and substance use in adolescence: developmental change, reciprocal effects, and genetic and environmental influences. Personal Disord 4:23–32, 2013

Brunner R, Henze R, Parzer P, et al: Reduced prefrontal and orbitofrontal gray matter in female adolescents with borderline personality disorder: is it disorder specific? NeuroImage 49:114–120, 2010

Cailhol L, Jeannot M, Rodgers R, et al: Borderline personality disorder and mental healthcare service use among adolescents. J Pers Disord 27:252–259, 2013

Caspi A, Houts RM, Belsky DW, et al: The p factor: one general psychopathology factor in the structure of psychiatric disorders? Clin Psychol Sci 2:119–137, 2014

Catthoor K, Hutsebaut J, Schrijvers D, et al: Adolescents with personality disorders suffer from severe psychiatric stigma: evidence from a sample of 131 patients. Adolesc Health Med Ther 6:81–89, 2015

Cavelti M, Thompson KN, Hulbert C, et al: Exploratory comparison of auditory verbal hallucinations and other psychotic symptoms among youth with borderline personality disorder or schizophrenia spectrum disorder. Early Interv Psychiatry 13:1252–1262, 2019

Chanen AM: Borderline personality disorder in young people: are we there yet? J Clin Psychol 71:778–791, 2015

Chanen A: Borderline personality disorder is not a variant of normal adolescent development. Personal Ment Health 11:147–149, 2017

Chanen AM, McCutcheon L: Prevention and early intervention for borderline personality disorder: current status and recent evidence. Br J Psychiatry Suppl 54:s24–s29, 2013

Chanen AM, Thompson KN: Early intervention in personality disorder. Curr Opin Psychol 21:132–135, 2018

Chanen AM, Thompson KN: The age of onset of personality disorders, in Age of Onset of Mental Disorders: Etiopathogenetic and Treatment Implications. Edited by de Girolamo G, McGorry PD, Sartorius N. Cham, Switzerland, Springer International Publishing, 2019, pp 183–201

Chanen AM, Jackson HJ, McGorry PD, et al: Two-year stability of personality disorder in older adolescent outpatients. J Pers Disord 18:526–541, 2004

Chanen AM, Jovev M, Jackson HJ: Adaptive functioning and psychiatric symptoms in adolescents with borderline personality disorder. J Clin Psychiatry 68:297–306, 2007

Chanen AM, Jackson HJ, McCutcheon LK, et al: Early intervention for adolescents with borderline personality disorder using cognitive analytic therapy: randomised controlled trial. Br J Psychiatry 193:477–484, 2008a

Chanen AM, Jovev M, McCutcheon LK, et al: Borderline personality disorder in young people and the prospects for prevention and early intervention. Curr Psychiatry Rev 4:48–57, 2008b

Chanen AM, Velakoulis D, Carison K, et al: Orbitofrontal, amygdala and hippocampal volumes in teenagers with first-presentation borderline personality disorder. Psychiatry Res 163:116–125, 2008c

Chanen AM, McCutcheon LK, Germano D, et al: The HYPE clinic: an early intervention service for borderline personality disorder: J Psychiatr Pract 15:163–172, 2009

Chanen AM, McCutcheon L, Kerr IB: HYPE: a cognitive analytic therapy based prevention and early intervention programme for borderline personality disorder, in Handbook of Borderline Personality Disorder in Children and Adolescents. Edited by Sharp C, Tackett JL. New York, Springer, 2014, pp 361–383

Chanen AM, Jackson H, Cotton SM, et al: Comparing three forms of early intervention for youth with borderline personality disorder (the MOBY study): study protocol for a randomised controlled trial. Trials 16:476, 2015

Chanen AM, Berk M, Thompson K: Integrating early intervention for borderline personality disorder and mood disorders. Harv Rev Psychiatry 24:330–341, 2016

Chanen AM, Sharp C, Hoffman P; Global Alliance for Prevention and Early Intervention for Borderline Personality Disorder: Prevention and early intervention for borderline personality disorder: a novel public health priority. World Psychiatry 16:215–216, 2017

Chang B, Sharp C, Ha C: The criterion validity of the borderline personality features scale for children in an adolescent inpatient setting. J Pers Disord 25:492–503, 2011

Cicchetti D: Development and psychopathology, in Development and Psychopathology. Edited by Cicchetti D, Cohen JD. New York, Wiley, 2006, pp 1–23

Clark LA: Assessment and diagnosis of personality disorder: perennial issues and an emerging reconceptualization. Annu Rev Psychol 58:227–57, 2007

Clark LA, Ro E: Three-pronged assessment and diagnosis of personality disorder and its consequences: personality functioning, pathological traits, and psychosocial disability. Personal Disord 5:55–69, 2014

Cohen P, Crawford TN, Johnson JG, Kasen S: The Children in the Community Study of developmental course of personality disorder. J Pers Disord 19:466–486, 2005

Cooney E, Davis K, Thompson K, et al: Feasibility of evaluating DBT for self-harming adolescents: a small randomised controlled trial. Auckland, New Zealand, Te Pou o Te Whakaaro Nui, 2010

Cooney E, Davis K, Thompson P, Wharewera-Mika J, et al: Feasibility of comparing dialectical behavior therapy with treatment as usual for suicidal and self-injuring adolescents: follow-up data from a small randomized controlled trial. Paper presented at the Association of Behavioral and Cognitive Therapies 46th Annual Convention, 2012

Courtney DB, Makinen J: Impact of diagnosis disclosure on adolescents with borderline personality disorder. J Can Acad Child Adolesc Psychiatry 25:177–184, 2016

Courtney-Seidler EA, Klein D, Miller AL: Borderline personality disorder in adolescents. Clin Psychol Sci Pract 20:425–444, 2013

Cramer P: Childhood precursors of adult borderline personality disorder features: a longitudinal study. J Nerv Ment Dis 204:494–499, 2016

Crick NR, Murray-Close D, Woods K: Borderline personality features in childhood: a short-term longitudinal study. Dev Psychopathol 17:1051–1070, 2005

Cristea IA, Gentili C, Cotet CD, et al: Efficacy of psychotherapies for borderline personality disorder: a systematic review and meta-analysis. JAMA Psychiatry 74:319–328, 2017

Crowell SE, Beauchaine TP, Linehan MM: A biosocial developmental model of borderline personality: elaborating and extending Linehan's theory. Psychol Bull 135:495–510, 2009

Crowell SE, Kaufman EA, Beauchaine TP: A biosocial model of BPD: theory and empirical evidence, in Handbook of Borderline Personality Disorder in Children and Adolescents. Edited by Sharp C, Tackett JL. New York, Springer, 2014, pp 143–157

Dahl RE, Allen NB, Wilbrecht L, Suleiman AB: Importance of investing in adolescence from a developmental science perspective. Nature 554:441–450, 2018

Debast I, Rossi G, Feenstra D, Hutsebaut J: Developmentally sensitive markers of personality functioning in adolescents: age-specific and age-neutral expressions. Personal Disord 8:162–171, 2017

De Clercq B: Integrating developmental aspects in current thinking about personality pathology. Curr Opin Psychol 21:69–73, 2018

De Clercq B, De Fruyt F, Van Leeuwen K, Mervielde I: The structure of maladaptive personality traits in childhood: a step toward an integrative developmental perspective for DSM-V. J Abnorm Psychol 115:639–657, 2006

De Clercq B, Van Leeuwen K, Van den Noortgate W, et al: Childhood personality pathology: dimensional stability and change. Dev Psychopathol 21:853–869, 2009

De Clercq B, Decuyper M, De Caluwé E: Developmental manifestations of borderline personality pathology from an age-specific dimensional personality disorder trait framework, in Handbook of Borderline Personality Disorder in Children and Adolescents. Edited by Sharp C, Tackett JL. New York, Springer, 2014a, pp 81–94

De Clercq B, De Fruyt F, De Bolle M, et al: The hierarchical structure and construct validity of the PID-5 trait measure in adolescence. J Pers 82:158–169, 2014b

De Clercq B, Hofmans J, Vergauwe J, et al: Developmental pathways of childhood dark traits. J Abnorm Psychol 126:843–858, 2017

DeFife JA, Malone JC, DiLallo J, Westen D: Assessing adolescent personality disorders with the Shedler-Westen Assessment Procedure for Adolescents. Clin Psychol Sci Pract 20:393–407, 2013

Eaton NR, Krueger RF, Keyes KM, et al: Borderline personality disorder co-morbidity: relationship to the internalizing–externalizing structure of common mental disorders. Psychol Med 41:1041–1050, 2011

Erikson E: Childhood in Society. New York, WW Norton, 1950

Feenstra DJ, Hutsebaut J, Laurenssen EMP, et al: The burden of disease among adolescents with personality pathology: quality of life and costs. J Pers Disord 26:593–604, 2012

Fonagy P, Bateman A: The development of borderline personality disorder—a mentalizing model. J Pers Disord 22:4–21, 2008

Fossati A, Gratz KL, Maffei C, Borroni S: Impulsivity dimensions, emotion dysregulation, and borderline personality disorder features among Italian nonclinical adolescents. Borderline Personal Disord Emot Dysregul 1:5, 2014

Fossati A, Somma A, Borroni S, et al: The Personality Inventory for DSM-5 Brief Form: evidence for reliability and construct validity in a sample of community-dwelling Italian adolescents. Assessment 24:615–631, 2017

Fossati A, Sharp C, Borroni S, Somma A: Psychometric properties of the Borderline Personality Features Scale for Children–11 (BPFSC-11) in a sample of community dwelling Italian adolescents. Eur J Psychol Assess 35:70–77, 2019

Goodman M, Hazlett EA, Avedon JB, et al: Anterior cingulate volume reduction in adolescents with borderline personality disorder and co-morbid major depression. J Psychiatr Res 45:803–807, 2011

Goth K, Foelsch P, Schlüter-Müller S, et al: Assessment of identity development and identity diffusion in adolescence—theoretical basis and psychometric properties of the self-report questionnaire AIDA. Child Adolesc Psychiatry Ment Health 6(1):27, 2012

Goth K, Birkhölzer M, Schmeck K: Assessment of personality functioning in adolescents with the LoPF–Q 12–18 self-report questionnaire. J Pers Assess 100:680–690, 2018

Griffiths M: Validity, utility and acceptability of borderline personality disorder diagnosis in childhood and adolescence: survey of psychiatrists. The Psychiatrist 35:19–22, 2011

Griffiths H, Duffy F, Duffy L, et al: Efficacy of mentalization-based group therapy for adolescents: the results of a pilot randomised controlled trial. BMC Psychiatry 19(1):167, 2019

Gunderson JG, Stout RL, McGlashan TH, et al: Ten-year course of borderline personality disorder: psychopathology and function from the Collaborative Longitudinal Personality Disorders Study. Arch Gen Psychiatry 68:827–837, 2011

Ha C, Balderas JC, Zanarini MC, et al: Psychiatric comorbidity in hospitalized adolescents with borderline personality disorder. J Clin Psychiatry 75:e457–e464, 2014

Habermas T, Bluck S: Getting a life: the emergence of the life story in adolescence. Psychol Bull 126:748–769, 2000

Haltigan JD, Vaillancourt T: The Borderline Personality Features Scale for Children (BPFS-C): factor structure and measurement invariance across time and sex in a community-based sample. J Psychopathol Behav Assess 38:600–614, 2016

Hankin BL, Barrocas AL, Jenness J, et al: Association between 5-HTTLPR and borderline personality disorder traits among youth. Front Psychiatry 2:6, 2011

Haslam N, Holland E, Kuppens P: Categories versus dimensions in personality and psychopathology: a quantitative review of taxometric research. Psychol Med 42:903–920, 2012

Hutsebaut J, Feenstra DJ, Luyten P: Personality disorders in adolescence: label or opportunity? Clin Psychol Sci Pract 20:445–451, 2013

Hutsebaut J, Videler AC, Verheul R, Van Alphen SPJ: Managing borderline personality disorder from a life course perspective: clinical staging and health management. Personal Disord 10:309–316, 2019

Hutsebaut J, Debbané M, Sharp C: Designing a range of mentalizing interventions for young people using a clinical staging approach to borderline pathology. Borderline Personality Disorder and Emotion Dysregulation 7:1–10, 2020

Kaess M, Von Ceumern-Lindenstjerna I-A, Parzer P, et al: Axis I and II comorbidity and psychosocial functioning in female adolescents with borderline personality disorder. Psychopathology 46:55–62, 2013

Kaess M, Brunner R, Chanen A: Borderline personality disorder in adolescence. Pediatrics 134:782–93, 2014

Kassin M, De Castro F, Arango I, Goth K: Psychometric properties of a culture-adapted Spanish version of AIDA (Assessment of Identity Development in Adolescence) in Mexico. Child Adolesc Psychiatry Ment Health 7:25, 2013

Kernberg O: Borderline personality organization. J Am Psychoanal Assoc 15:641–85, 1967

Kotov R, Krueger RF, Watson D, et al: The hierarchical taxonomy of psychopathology (HiTOP): a dimensional alternative to traditional nosologies. J Abnorm Psychol 126:454–477, 2017

Kramer U, Temes CM, Magni LR, et al: Psychosocial functioning in adolescents with and without borderline personality disorder. Personal Ment Health 11:164–170, 2017

Krueger RF, Kotov R, Watson D, et al: Progress in achieving quantitative classification of psychopathology. World Psychiatry 17:282–293, 2018

Laurenssen EMP, Hutsebaut J, Feenstra DJ, et al: Diagnosis of personality disorders in adolescents: a study among psychologists. Child Adolesc Psychiatry Ment Health 7:3, 2013

Laurenssen EMP, Smits ML, Bales DL, et al: Day hospital mentalization-based treatment versus intensive outpatient mentalization-based treatment for patients with severe borderline personality disorder: protocol of a multicentre randomized clinical trial. BMC Psychiatry 14:301, 2014

Lawrence KA, Allen JS, Chanen AM: Impulsivity in borderline personality disorder: reward-based decision-making and its relationship to emotional distress. J Pers Disord 24:786–99, 2010

Lazarus SA, Beardslee J, Pedersen SL, Stepp SD: A within-person analysis of the association between borderline personality disorder and alcohol use in adolescents. J Abnorm Child Psychol 45:1157–1167, 2017

Leung S-W, Leung F: Construct validity and prevalence rate of borderline personality disorder among Chinese adolescents. J Pers Disord 23:494–513, 2009

Lind M, Vanwoerden S, Penner F, Sharp C: Inpatient adolescents with borderline personality disorder features: identity diffusion and narrative incoherence. Personal Disord 10:389–393, 2019

Lind M, Vanwoerden S, Penner F, Sharp C: Narrative coherence in adolescence: relations with attachment, mentalization, and psychopathology. J Pers Assess 102:380–389, 2020

Livesley J: Tentative steps in the right direction. Personal Ment Health 5:263–270, 2011

Luyten P, Blatt SJ: Interpersonal relatedness and self-definition in normal and disrupted personality development: retrospect and prospect. Am Psychol 68:172–183, 2013

Malla A, Iyer S, McGorry P, et al: From early intervention in psychosis to youth mental health reform: a review of the evolution and transformation of mental health services for young people. Soc Psychiatry Psychiatr Epidemiol 51:319–26, 2016

Marieke Schuppert H, Timmerman ME, Bloo J, et al: Emotion regulation training for adolescents with borderline personality disorder traits: a randomized controlled trial. J Am Acad Child Adolesc Psychiatry 51:1314–1323.e2, 2012

McAdams DP: What do we know when we know a person? J Pers 63:365–396, 1995

McAdams DP: Personal narratives and the life story, in Handbook of Personality: Theory and Research. Edited by John O, Robins RW, Pervin LA. New York, Guilford, 2008, pp 241–261

McAdams DP, Anyidoho NA, Brown C, et al: Traits and stories: links between dispositional and narrative features of personality. J Pers 72:761–784, 2004

McCauley E, Berk MS, Asarnow JR, et al: Efficacy of dialectical behavior therapy for adolescents at high risk for suicide: a randomized clinical trial. JAMA Psychiatry 75:777–785, 2018

McGorry PD: Risk syndromes, clinical staging and DSM V: new diagnostic infrastructure for early intervention in psychiatry. Schizophr Res 120:49–53, 2010

McGorry PD: Early clinical phenotypes, clinical staging, and strategic biomarker research: building blocks for personalized psychiatry. Biol Psychiatry 74:394–395, 2013

McGorry PD, Mei C: Early intervention in youth mental health: progress and future directions. Evid Based Ment Health 21:182–184, 2018

McGorry PD, van Os J: Redeeming diagnosis in psychiatry: timing versus specificity. Lancet 381:343–345, 2013

McGorry PD, Killackey E, Yung A: Early intervention in psychosis: concepts, evidence and future directions. World Psychiatry 7:148–156, 2008

McGorry PD, Hartmann JA, Spooner R, Nelson B: Beyond the "at risk mental state" concept: transitioning to transdiagnostic psychiatry. World Psychiatry 17:133–142, 2018

Mehlum L, Tørmoen AJ, Ramberg M, et al: Dialectical behavior therapy for adolescents with repeated suicidal and self-harming behavior: a randomized trial. J Am Acad Child Adolesc Psychiatry 53:1082–1091, 2014

Mehlum L, Ramleth R-K, Tørmoen AJ, et al: Long term effectiveness of dialectical behavior therapy versus enhanced usual care for adolescents with self-harming and suicidal behavior. J Child Psychol Psychiatry 60:1112–1122, 2019

Michonski JD: The underlying factor structure of DSM criteria in youth BPD, in Handbook of Borderline Personality Disorder in Children and Adolescents. Edited by Sharp C, Tackett JL. New York, Springer, 2014, pp 35–48

Michonski JD, Sharp C, Steinberg L, Zanarini MC: An item response theory analysis of the DSM-IV borderline personality disorder criteria in a population-based sample of 11- to 12-year-old children. Personal Disord 4:15–22, 2013

Miller AL, Muehlenkamp JJ, Jacobson CM: Fact or fiction: diagnosing borderline personality disorder in adolescents. Clin Psychol Rev 28:969–981, 2008

Morey L: Personality Assessment Inventory. Odessa, FL, Psychological Assessment Resources, 1991

Morey LC: Personality Assessment Inventory—Adolescent Professional Manual. Odessa, FL, Psychological Assessment Resources, 2007

Newton-Howes G, Clark LA, Chanen A: Personality disorder across the life course. Lancet 385:727–734, 2015

Noblin JL, Venta A, Sharp C: The validity of the MSI-BPD among inpatient adolescents. Assessment 21:210–217, 2014

Normandin L, Ensink K, Yeomans FE, Kernberg OF: Transference-focused psychotherapy for personality disorders in adolescence, in Handbook of Borderline Personality Disorder in Children and Adolescents. Edited by Sharp C, Tackett JL. New York, Springer, 2014, pp 333–359

Oldham JM: Borderline personality disorder and suicidality. Am J Psychiatry 163:20–26, 2006

Penner F, Wall K, Jardin C, et al: A study of risky sexual behavior, beliefs about sexual behavior, and sexual self-efficacy in adolescent inpatients with and without borderline personality disorder. Personal Disord 10:524–535, 2019

Rathus JH, Miller AL: Dialectical behavior therapy adapted for suicidal adolescents. Suicide Life Threat Behav 32:146–157, 2002

Robins E, Guze SB: Establishment of diagnostic validity in psychiatric illness: its application to schizophrenia. Am J Psychiatry 126:983–987, 1970

Rossouw TI, Fonagy P: Mentalization-based treatment for self-harm in adolescents: a randomized controlled trial. J Am Acad Child Adolesc Psychiatry 51:1304-1313.e3, 2012

Santangelo PS, Koenig J, Funke V, et al: Ecological momentary assessment of affective and interpersonal instability in adolescent non-suicidal self-injury. J Abnorm Child Psychol 45:1429–1438, 2017

Sawyer SM, Azzopardi PS, Wickremarathne D, Patton GC: The age of adolescence. Lancet Child Adolesc Health 2:223–228, 2018

Scalzo F, Hulbert CA, Betts JK, et al: Substance use in youth with borderline personality disorder. J Pers Disord 32:603–617, 2018

Schuppert HM, Giesen-Bloo J, van Gemert TG, et al: Effectiveness of an emotion regulation group training for adolescents: a randomized controlled pilot study: effectiveness of an emotion regulation group training for adolescents. Clin Psychol Psychother 16:467–478, 2009

Scott J, Leboyer M, Hickie I, et al: Clinical staging in psychiatry: a cross-cutting model of diagnosis with heuristic and practical value. Br J Psychiatry 202:243–245, 2013

Sharp C: Bridging the gap: the assessment and treatment of adolescent personality disorder in routine clinical care. Arch Child 102:103–108, 2017

Sharp C: Adolescent personality pathology and the Alternative Model for Personality Disorders: self development as nexus. Psychopathology 53:198–204, 2020

Sharp C, De Clercq B: Personality pathology in youth, in The Cambridge Handbook of Personality Disorders. Edited by Lejuez CW, Gratz KL. Cambridge, UK, Cambridge University Press, 2020, pp 74–90

Sharp C, Fonagy P: Social cognition and attachment-related disorders, in Social Cognition and Developmental Psychopathology. Edited by Sharp C, Fonagy P, Goodyer IM. Oxford, UK, Oxford University Press, 2008, pp 271–302

Sharp C, Fonagy P: Practitioner review: borderline personality disorder in adolescence—recent conceptualization, intervention, and implications for clinical practice. J Child Psychol Psychiatry 56:1266–1288, 2015

Sharp C, Tackett JL: An idea whose time has come, in Handbook of Borderline Personality Disorder in Children and Adolescents. Edited by Sharp C, Tackett JL. New York, Springer, 2014, pp 3–8

Sharp C, Wall K: Personality pathology grows up: adolescence as a sensitive period. Curr Opin Psychol 21:111–116, 2018

Sharp C, Mosko O, Chang B, Ha C: The cross-informant concordance and concurrent validity of the Borderline Personality Features Scale for Children in a community sample of boys. Clin Child Psychol Psychiatry 16:335–349, 2011

Sharp C, Ha C, Michonski J, et al: Borderline personality disorder in adolescents: evidence in support of the Childhood Interview for DSM-IV Borderline Personality Disorder in a sample of adolescent inpatients. Compr Psychiatry 53:765–774, 2012

Sharp C, Steinberg L, Temple J, Newlin E: An 11-item measure to assess borderline traits in adolescents: refinement of the BPFSC using IRT. Personal Disord 5:70–78, 2014

Sharp C, Wright AGC, Fowler JC, et al: The structure of personality pathology: both general ('g') and specific ('s') factors? J Abnorm Psychol 124:387–398, 2015

Sharp C, Vanwoerden S, Wall K: Adolescence as a sensitive period for the development of personality disorder. Psychiatr Clin North Am 41:669–683, 2018

Shiner RL: Personality differences in childhood and adolescence: measurement, development, and consequences. J Child Psychol Psychiatry 44:2–32, 2003

Shiner RL: The development of personality disorders: perspectives from normal personality development in childhood and adolescence. Dev Psychopathol 21:715–734, 2009

Shiner RL, Tackett JL: Personality disorders in children and adolescents, in Child Psychopathology. Edited by Mash EJ, Barkley RA. New York, Guilford, 2014, pp 848–896

Soeteman DI, Hakkaart-van Roijen L, Verheul R, Busschbach JJV: The economic burden of personality disorders in mental health care. J Clin Psychiatry 69:259–265, 2008a

Soeteman DI, Verheul R, Busschbach JJV: The burden of disease in personality disorders: diagnosis-specific quality of life. J Pers Disord 22:259–268, 2008b

Somma A, Fossati A, Terrinoni A, et al: Reliability and clinical usefulness of the personality inventory for DSM-5 in clinically referred adolescents: a preliminary report in a sample of Italian inpatients. Compr Psychiatry 70:141–151, 2016

Stepp SD, Lazarus SA: Identifying a borderline personality disorder prodrome: implications for community screening. Personal Ment Health 11:195–205, 2017

Stepp SD, Pilkonis PA, Hipwell AE, et al: Stability of borderline personality disorder features in girls. J Pers Disord 24:460–472, 2010

Stepp SD, Burke JD, Hipwell AE, Loeber R: Trajectories of attention deficit hyperactivity disorder and oppositional defiant disorder symptoms as precursors of borderline personality disorder symptoms in adolescent girls. J Abnorm Child Psychol 40:7–20, 2012

Stepp SD, Lazarus SA, Byrd AL: A systematic review of risk factors prospectively associated with borderline personality disorder: taking stock and moving forward. Personal Disord 7:316–323, 2016

Tackett JL: Evaluating models of the personality-psychopathology relationship in children and adolescents. Clin Psychol Rev 26:584–99, 2006

Tackett JL, Kushner SC, De Fruyt F, Mervielde I: Delineating personality traits in childhood and adolescence: associations across measures, temperament, and behavioral problems. Assessment 20:738–51, 2013

Tackett JL, Hertzhoff K, Balsis S, Cooper L: Toward a unifying perspective on personality pathology across the lifespan, in Developmental Psychopathology, Vol 3: Maladaptation and Psychopathology. Edited by Cichetti DC. New York, Wiley, 2016, pp 1039–1078

Temes CM, Zanarini MC: Recent developments in psychosocial interventions for borderline personality disorder. F1000Res 8, Apr 26, 2019

Thompson KN, Betts J, Jovev M, et al: Sexuality and sexual health among female youth with borderline personality disorder pathology. Early Interv Psychiatry 13:502–508, 2019a

Thompson KN, Jackson H, Cavelti M, et al: The clinical significance of subthreshold borderline personality disorder features in outpatient youth. J Pers Disord 33:71–81, 2019b

Van Alebeek A, Van der Heijden PT, Hessels C, et al: Comparison of three questionnaires to screen for borderline personality disorder in adolescents and young adults. Eur J Psychol Assess 33:123–128, 2017

Vanwoerden S, Garey L, Ferguson T, et al: Borderline Personality Features Scale for Children–11: measurement invariance over time and across gender in a community sample of adolescents. Psychol Assess 31:114–119, 2019

Venta A, Herzoff K, Cohen P, Sharp C: The longitudinal course of borderline personality disorder in youth, in Handbook of Borderline Personality Disorder in Children and Adolescents. Edited by Sharp C, Tackett JL. New York, Springer, 2014, pp 229–246

Venta A, Magyar M, Hossein S, Sharp C: The psychometric properties of the Personality Assessment Inventory—Adolescent's Borderline Features Scale across two high-risk samples. Psychol Assess 30:827–833, 2018

Videler AC, Hutsebaut J, Schulkens JEM, et al: A life span perspective on borderline personality disorder. Curr Psychiatry Rep 21:51, 2019

Westen D, Betan E, DeFife JA: Identity disturbance in adolescence: associations with borderline personality disorder. Dev Psychopathol 23:305–313, 2011

Williams TF, Scalco MD, Simms LJ: The construct validity of general and specific dimensions of personality pathology. Psychol Med 48:834–848, 2018

Winograd G, Cohen P, Chen H: Adolescent borderline symptoms in the community: prognosis for functioning over 20 years. J Child Psychol Psychiatry 49:933–941, 2008

Winsper C, Wolke D, Scott J, et al: Psychopathological outcomes of adolescent borderline personality disorder symptoms. Aust N Z J Psychiatry 54:308–317, 2019

Wright AGC, Zalewski M, Hallquist MN, et al: Developmental trajectories of borderline personality disorder symptoms and psychosocial functioning in adolescence. J Pers Disord 30:351–372, 2016

Zanarini MC: Childhood Interview for DSM-IV Borderline Personality Disorder (CI-BPD). Belmont, MA, McLean Hospital, 2003

Zanarini MC: Prediction of the 10-year course of borderline personality disorder. Am J Psychiatry 163:827–832, 2006

Zanarini MC, Frankenburg FR, Dubo ED, et al: Axis I comorbidity of borderline personality disorder. Am J Psychiatry 155:1733–1739, 1998

Zanarini MC, Frankenburg FR, Ridolfi ME, et al: Reported childhood onset of self-mutilation among borderline patients. J Pers Disord 20:9–15, 2006

Zanarini MC, Horwood J, Wolke D, et al: Prevalence of DSM-IV borderline personality disorder in two community samples: 6,330 English 11-year-olds and 34,653 American adults. J Pers Disord 25:607–619, 2011

Zanarini MC, Frankenburg FR, Reich DB, Fitzmaurice G: Attainment and stability of sustained symptomatic remission and recovery among patients with borderline personality disorder and Axis II comparison subjects: a 16-year prospective follow-up study. Am J Psychiatry 169:476–483, 2012

Zanarini MC, Temes CM, Magni LR, et al: Prevalence rates of borderline symptoms reported by adolescent inpatients with BPD, psychiatrically healthy adolescents and adult inpatients with BPD: BPD symptoms in adolescence. Personal Ment Health 11:150–156, 2017

Zanarini MC, Temes CM, Magni LR, et al: Risk factors for borderline personality disorder in adolescents. J Pers Disord 34 (suppl B):17–24, 2020

CHAPTER 11

Therapeutic Alliance

Donna S. Bender, Ph.D., FIPA

Any patient beginning treatment enters a relationship, whether it is for a short time during a hospital stay or over many years in long-term psychotherapy. This relationship with the clinician has the potential for improving the patient's quality of life, perhaps through the alleviation of symptoms, but more profoundly through meaningful shifts in internal mental landscape and character structure. It is sometimes uncertain a priori who will benefit from what treatment with whom, but one factor—therapeutic alliance—has stood out in the research literature as a robust predictor of outcome (Flückiger et al. 2018; Horvath et al. 2011; Safran et al. 2011).

Because establishing a productive alliance occurs within the matrix of a relationship between patient and therapist, personality serves as a central mediating factor. Characteristic ways of thinking about oneself and others, including capacities such as self-reflection, empathy, and emotion regulation, will be central in shaping the course and outcome of the treatment process. Moreover, many who present for treatment have elements of personality psychopathology that are associated in some way with significant impairment in self perceptions and interpersonal relations (Bender et al. 2011; Signer et al. 2019). Several studies have shown that the preexisting quality of the patient's relationships is what most affects the quality of the therapeutic alliance (Cookson et al. 2012; Gibbons et al. 2003; Gómez Penedo et al. 2019; Hersoug et al. 2002; Piper et al. 1991). For example, it has been suggested that patients' attachment styles and internal working models of therapy expectations significantly influence the process of alliance development (Diener and Monroe 2011; Hatcher 2010). Other authors (e.g., Alberti 2018; Dimaggio and Overholser 2019) have asserted that maladaptive schemas about self and others are at the heart of personality psychopathology, necessitating the establishment of a sound alliance as a basic foundation for therapeutic work. Improvements in patient self-esteem over the course of treatment have been linked to the presence of a secure alliance (Doorn et al. 2019), and ambivalence and resistance are intertwined with the alliance and require careful attention (Urmanche et al. 2019).

Consequently, the clinician must consider an individual's patterns of relating so that appropriate interventions can be employed to effectively retain and involve the patient in the treatment, regardless of modality or whether a formal personality disorder (PD) diagnosis is made. Forming an alliance is often difficult, however, particularly in work with patients with severely narcissistic, borderline, or paranoid proclivities, because troubled interpersonal attitudes and behaviors will also infuse the patient's engagement with the therapist. For example, narcissistically impaired patients may not be able to allow the therapist to act as a separate, thinking person for quite a long time, whereas someone with borderline issues may exhibit wildly fluctuating emotions, attitudes, and behaviors, thwarting the potential helpfulness of the clinician.

Definition of Therapeutic Alliance

The concept of the therapeutic alliance is often traced back to Freud, who observed very early in his work the need to convey interest in and sympathy to the patient to foster engagement in a collaborative treatment endeavor (Meissner 1996; Safran and Muran 2000). Freud (1912/1958) also delineated an aspect of the transference—the unobjectionable positive transference, which is an attachment that should not be analyzed because it serves as the motivation for the patient to collaborate: "The conscious and unobjectionable component of [positive transference] remains, and brings about the successful result in psychoanalysis as in all other remedial methods" (p. 319). This statement is an early precursor to the modern empirical evidence showing that alliance is related to treatment outcome across modalities.

Several contemporary definitions of *alliance* might be useful to further this discussion of treating patients with personality psychopathology. One conceptualization, using psychoanalytic language, was posited by Gutheil and Havens (1979): The patient's ability to form a rational alliance arises from "the therapeutic split in the ego which allows the analyst to work with the healthier elements in the patient against resistance and pathology" (p. 479). This definition is useful vis-à-vis personality psychopathology in two regards: 1) the recognition that there will be pathological parts of the patient's personality functioning that may serve to thwart the attempted helpfulness of the clinician, and 2) the need for the clinician to be creative in enlisting whatever adaptive aspects of the patient's character may avail themselves for the work of the treatment.

Another definition that was developed in an attempt to transcend theoretical traditions is Bordin's (1979) identification of three interdependent components of the alliance: bond, tasks, and goals. The *bond* is the quality of the relationship formed in the treatment dyad that then mediates whether the patient will take up the *tasks* inherent in working toward the *goals* of a particular treatment approach. At the same time, the clinician's ability to negotiate the tasks and goals with the patient will also affect the nature of the therapeutic bond. This multifaceted view of the alliance underscores the complexity of the factors involved (Safran and Muran 2000).

Arguably, if the goal of treatment is fundamental character change, the Bordin (1979) definition specifies necessary, but not sufficient, elements of alliance. Adler (1980) observed that patients with borderline and narcissistic difficulties may not be able to establish a mature working alliance until much later in a successful treatment. Others who typically work with more disturbed patients have noted that establishing a therapeutic alliance may be one of the primary goals of the treatment and that there may be different phases in alliance development as treatment progresses. Gunderson (2000) observed the following alliance stages in the course of conducting long-term psychotherapy with patients with borderline PD:

> 1) Contractual (behavioral): initial agreement between the patient and therapist on treatment goals and their roles in achieving them (Phase I); 2) Relational (affective/empathic): emphasized by Rogerian client-centered relationships; patient experiences the therapist as caring, understanding, genuine, and likable (Phase II); 3) Working (cognitive/motivational): psychoanalytic prototype; patient joins the therapist as a reliable collaborator to help the patient understand herself or himself; its development represents a significant improvement for borderline patients (Phases III–IV). (p. 41)

Progression through these stages, if successful, typically takes a number of years. The implication is that to reach a point at which work leading to substantive and enduring personality change can occur may require a lengthy initial alliance-building period. Establishing and maintaining a basic level of trust is a central part of the process (Kamphuis and Finn 2018). As Bach (2016) noted:

> Perhaps the primary problem in engaging the difficult patient is to build and retain what Ellman (1991) has called analytic trust....These patients have lost their trust not only in people but also in the environment as a reliable place that will hold them safely. So one task we have is to restore this faith, and to rebuild it again and again as it inevitably gets lost in the vicissitudes of the transference. (p. 217)

Alliance Strains and Ruptures

Although a strong positive alliance can predict a successful treatment outcome, the converse is also true: problems in the treatment alliance may lead to premature termination if not handled in a sensitive and timely manner. Evidence has shown that strains and ruptures in the alliance are often related to unilateral termination (Safran et al. 2011); conversely, attention to these types of incidents and careful, empathic interventions can strengthen the relationship and enhance clinical progress (Eubanks et al. 2018). Thus, negotiating ruptures in the alliance is another issue that has garnered increasing attention in the psychotherapy literature. For example, Strauss et al. (2006) demonstrated that skillfully addressing ruptures strengthens the alliance, leading to better treatment outcome for a group of patients with avoidant or obsessive-compulsive PD.

Disruptions in the alliance are inevitable and occur more frequently than may be readily apparent to the clinician (Hill 2010; Safran et al. 2011). In one study (Hill et al. 1993), patients were asked to report about thoughts and feelings that they were not expressing to their therapists. Most things that were not discussed were negative, and even the most experienced therapists were aware of uncommunicated negative material only 45% of the time. It has also been suggested, however, that therapist awareness of patients' negative feelings may actually create problems; therapists, rather than being open and flexible in response, may at times become defensive and negative or may become more rigid in applying treatment techniques (Hill 2010).

Safran and Muran (2000) outlined a model specifying two subtypes of ruptures: withdrawal and confrontation. Withdrawals are sometimes fairly subtle. One example is a therapist who assumes that treatment is progressing but may be unaware that a patient is withholding important information because of lack of trust or fear of feeling humiliated. Other types of withdrawal behaviors include intellectualizing, talking excessively about other people, or changing the subject. Withdrawal behaviors may be more common in patients who are overly compliant at times, such as those with dependent or obsessive-compulsive personality tendencies or those who are uncomfortable about interpersonal relations, such as patients who are excessively avoidant.

Confrontations, on the other hand, are usually more overt, such as complaining about various aspects of therapy or criticizing the therapist. Some may be rather dramatic, as with a patient who storms out of session in a rage or leaves an angry message on the therapist's answering machine. Confrontation ruptures are likely to be more frequently experienced with more brittle patients, such as those with borderline, narcissistic, or paranoid personalities. In any event, clinicians are best served by being alert to ruptures and adopting the attitude that these are often excellent opportunities to engage the patient in a collaborative effort to observe and learn about that patient's own style (Eubanks-Carter et al. 2010).

Personality Functioning, Traits, Diagnoses, and Alliance Considerations

DSM-5 (American Psychiatric Association 2013) includes a long-needed innovation in personality psychopathology nosology: the Alternative DSM-5 Model for Personality Disorders (AMPD). The AMPD is organized around the conceptual framework that personality dysfunction emanates from disturbances in self and interpersonal capacities. This approach to assessing personality psychopathology adds a functioning/severity of impairment scale (Level of Personality Functioning Scale) and a set of 25 trait dimensions to more broadly and flexibly represent the range of psychopathology that might occur in the personality realm. Six specific PDs are also featured, comprising relevant aspects of functioning and constituent traits. Personality diagnosis can be specified by designating 1) the level of personality functioning impairment and 2) the presence of one or more pathological traits or a specific PD that best characterizes the individual's presentation. (For more detailed consideration of this model, see Chapter 3, "Articulating a Core Dimension of Personality Pathology," and Chapter 4, "The Alternative DSM-5 Model for Personality Disorders," in this volume.)

In practical terms, it must be understood that personality is a complex amalgam of characteristic ways of mentally representing self and self-in-relation-to-others, which in turn drive adaptation and influence behavior. Thus, the most important data for understanding one's patients in forging an alliance is how an individual typically thinks about self and other people. Whether using PD diagnostic categories or assessing aspects of personality functioning or dominant traits, a clinician considering salient elements of the therapeutic alliance should determine which aspects of a patient's personality pathology are dominant or in ascendance at intake and at various points over the course of treatment. It has been suggested that the nature of the alliance established early in the treatment is an especially powerful predictor of outcome (Gómez

Penedo et al. 2019; Horvath and Luborsky 1993). One example of the relationship of early alliance and outcome regarding PDs was demonstrated in a study of long-term psychotherapy with a group of patients with borderline PD: therapist ratings of the alliance at 6 weeks predicted subsequent dropouts (Gunderson et al. 1997). As Horvath and Greenberg (1994) noted, "It seems reasonable to think of alliance development in the first phase of therapy as a series of windows of opportunity, decreasing in size with each session" (p. 3).

In the AMPD, personality functioning—based on characteristic mental representations of self and others—is assessed using the Level of Personality Functioning Scale, with levels defined by aspects of identity, self-direction, empathy, and intimacy. Personality functioning can be determined independently to inform thinking about the therapeutic alliance, used in concert with the traits to establish one of the six PDs or "PD trait-specified," or prominent problematic traits can be considered in determining salient aspects of patients' personality profiles, whether a PD diagnosis is assigned or not. Table 11–1 presents the AMPD personality diagnoses with corresponding self and interpersonal functioning elements and traits from the new model. For each diagnosis, tendencies that may serve to challenge early collaboration building are presented, as well as points of possible engagement. In what follows, I discuss each PD, along with several examples of other styles that may need to be carefully navigated in alliance formation given the presence of personality psychopathology.

Alliance Considerations for AMPD Personality Disorder Types

Schizotypal

Schizotypal phenomena are thought by some to lie on the schizophrenia spectrum, given the associated disordered cognitions and bizarre beliefs. Because it is almost always the case that individuals with such cognitions have one or no significant others outside family members, it is often assumed that individuals with schizotypal PD have no desire to become involved in relationships. However, in many cases, it is more a matter of being excruciatingly uncomfortable around people than a lack of interest in connection. This discomfort may not be readily apparent, so establishing an alliance with such patients may require being attentive to clues about what is not being said. The therapist may be a player in some elaborated fantasy that is making it difficult for the patient to find some minimum level of comfort. Bender et al. (2003) assessed various attributes of how patients with PD think about their therapists. Interestingly, results showed that patients with schizotypal PD had the highest level of mental involvement with therapy outside the session, missing their therapists and wishing for friendship while also feeling aggressive or negative. One man with schizotypal PD (who had also become attached to the female research assistant) revealed the following view of his therapist:

> Very beautiful and attractive in a sense that I yearn to have a sexual relationship with her. She's very smart and educated. She knows what she wants out of life and I wish I were working for I could take her out to the movies and dinner. She turns me on and I

TABLE 11–1. Alliance-relevant aspects of Alternative DSM-5 Model for Personality Disorders (AMPD) personality disorder (PD) styles

AMPD PD style	AMPD self and interpersonal functioning	AMPD traits	Alliance challenges	Points of possible engagement in treatment
Schizotypal	*Identity:* Confused boundaries between self and others; distorted self-concept; emotional expression often not congruent with context or internal experience. *Self-direction:* Unrealistic or incoherent goals; no clear set of internal standards. *Empathy:* Pronounced difficulty understanding impact of own behaviors on others; frequent misinterpretations of others' motivations and behaviors. *Intimacy:* Marked impairments in developing close relationships, associated with mistrust and anxiety.	Cognitive and perceptual dysregulation Unusual beliefs and experiences Eccentricity Restricted affectivity Withdrawal Suspiciousness	Suspiciousness/ paranoia Profound interpersonal discomfort Bizarre thinking	Possible motivation for human connection: Therapist may become a key support for a person who lacks a social network. Helping the patient feel heard, appreciated, and understood in spite of off-putting presentation offers an experience different from daily encounters.
Antisocial	*Identity:* Egocentrism; self-esteem derived from personal gain, power, or pleasure. *Self-direction:* Goal setting based on personal gratification; absence of prosocial internal standards associated with failure to conform to lawful or culturally normative ethical behavior. *Empathy:* Lack of concern for feelings, needs, or suffering of others; lack of remorse after hurting or mistreating another. *Intimacy:* Incapacity for mutually intimate relationships, as exploitation is a primary means of relating to others, including by deceit and coercion; use of dominance or intimidation to control others.	Manipulativeness Callousness Deceitfulness Hostility Risk taking Impulsivity Irresponsibility	Controlling Tendency to lie and manipulate No empathy or regard for others Use of pseudo-alliance to gain some advantage	Possible attendance at treatment if in self-interest or if symptoms such as depression cause sufficient distress: • Points of engagement may at first be found in speaking to the patient's immediate personal benefit. It is important to communicate in a straightforward and honest manner, addressing reality, keeping a firm handle on frame issues such as session time and fee, and being consistent and nonpunitive.

TABLE 11–1. Alliance-relevant aspects of Alternative DSM-5 Model for Personality Disorders (AMPD) personality disorder (PD) styles *(continued)*

AMPD PD style	AMPD self and interpersonal functioning	AMPD traits	Alliance challenges	Points of possible engagement in treatment
Borderline	*Identity:* Markedly impoverished, poorly developed, or unstable self-image, often associated with excessive self-criticism; chronic feelings of emptiness; dissociative states under stress. *Self-direction:* Instability in goals, aspirations, values, or career plans. *Empathy:* Compromised ability to recognize the feelings and needs of others associated with interpersonal hypersensitivity (i.e., prone to feel slighted or insulted); perceptions of others selectively biased toward negative attributes or vulnerabilities. *Intimacy:* Intense, unstable, and conflicted close relationships, marked by mistrust, neediness, and anxious preoccupation with real or imagined abandonment; close relationships often viewed in extremes of idealization and devaluation and alternating between overinvolvement and withdrawal.	Emotional lability Anxiousness Separation insecurity Depressivity Impulsivity Risk taking Hostility	Unstable emotional and cognitive states Extremely demanding Proneness to acting out	Relationship seeking, responding to warmth and support: • Understanding the suffering, vulnerability, and inherent loneliness of a patient with borderline problems can help the therapist tolerate emotional storms and alliance ruptures. It is important to express ongoing appreciation of the patient's experience through communicating empathically and maintaining a supportive stance, and to assist the patient in reflecting on his or her thoughts, emotions, and needs.

TABLE 11–1. Alliance-relevant aspects of Alternative DSM-5 Model for Personality Disorders (AMPD) personality disorder (PD) styles (*continued*)

AMPD PD style	AMPD self and interpersonal functioning	AMPD traits	Alliance challenges	Points of possible engagement in treatment
Narcissistic	*Identity:* Excessive reference to others for self-definition and self-esteem regulation; exaggerated self-appraisal may be inflated or deflated, or may vacillate between extremes; emotion regulation mirrors fluctuations in self-esteem. *Self-direction:* Goal setting is based on gaining approval from others; personal standards are unreasonably high in order to see oneself as exceptional, or too low based on a sense of entitlement; often unaware of own motivations. *Empathy:* Impaired ability to recognize or identify with the feelings and needs of others; excessively attuned to reactions of others, but only if perceived as relevant to self; over- or underestimation of own effect on others. *Intimacy:* Relationships largely superficial and exist to serve self-esteem regulation; mutuality constrained by little genuine interest in others' experiences and predominance of a need for personal gain.	Grandiosity Attention seeking	Need for constant positive regard Contempt for others Grandiose sense of entitlement	Response over time to empathy and affirmation: • Narcissistic problems stem from a significant impoverishment of the self that is coped with by looking to others for approval. Patience, affirmation, and empathic mirroring of the patient's experience are important components of the treatment.

TABLE 11–1. Alliance-relevant aspects of Alternative DSM-5 Model for Personality Disorders (AMPD) personality disorder (PD) styles *(continued)*

AMPD PD style	AMPD self and interpersonal functioning	AMPD traits	Alliance challenges	Points of possible engagement in treatment
Avoidant	*Identity:* Low self-esteem associated with self-appraisal as socially inept, personally unappealing, or inferior; excessive feelings of shame. *Self-direction:* Unrealistic standards for behavior associated with reluctance to pursue goals, take personal risks, or engage in new activities involving interpersonal contact. *Empathy:* Preoccupation with, and sensitivity to, criticism or rejection, associated with distorted inference of others' perspectives as negative. *Intimacy:* Reluctance to get involved with people unless they are certain of being liked; diminished mutuality within intimate relationships because of fear of being shamed or ridiculed.	Anxiousness Withdrawal Anhedonia Intimacy avoidance	Expectations of criticism or rejection Proneness to shame and humiliation Reluctance to disclose information	Response to warmth/empathy, desiring relationships in spite of vulnerabilities: • If the therapist is very cognizant of the patient's vulnerability to shame, a sensitive approach to discussing the patient's longing for connection may be effectively pursued. Patience must be employed toward the patient's reluctance to open up. Expressed appreciation of the patient's difficulties is important, and attunement to possible perceived slights is essential.

TABLE 11–1. Alliance-relevant aspects of Alternative DSM-5 Model for Personality Disorders (AMPD) personality disorder (PD) styles *(continued)*

AMPD PD style	AMPD self and interpersonal functioning	AMPD traits	Alliance challenges	Points of possible engagement in treatment
Obsessive-compulsive	*Identity:* Sense of self derived predominantly from work or productivity; constricted experience and expression of strong emotions. *Self-direction:* Difficulty completing tasks and realizing goals, associated with rigid and unreasonably high and inflexible internal standards of behavior; overly conscientious and moralistic attitudes. *Empathy:* Difficulty understanding and appreciating the ideas, feelings, or behaviors of others. *Intimacy:* Relationships seen as secondary to work and productivity; rigidity and stubbornness negatively affect relationships with others.	Rigid perfectionism Perseveration Intimacy avoidance Restricted affectivity	Need for control Perfectionistic toward self and others Fear of criticism from therapist Restricted affect Stubbornness	Conscientious and will try to be a "good patient": • Clinicians should be tolerant of the patient's need for control and should resist becoming embroiled in power struggles or becoming a critical authority figure. A kind and playful acceptance of nonperfection may help the patient develop greater trust. • Appreciate the patient's intellectualizing stance, while eventually gently encouraging consideration of emotions.

desperately want to make love to her eternally. She's my life and knowing she doesn't feel the same, I live in dreams. (Bender et al. 2003, p. 231)

Antisocial

Antisocial personality is associated with ongoing violation of society's norms, manifested in such behaviors as theft, intimidation, violence, or making a living in an illegal fashion such as by fraud or selling drugs. Also narcissistic by definition, people with antisocial PD have little or no regard for the welfare of others. Clearly, this PD is found extensively among inmates within the prison system. Stone (1993) suggested that there are gradations of the antisocial style, with the milder forms being more amenable to treatment. However, within the broader label of antisocial is a subset of individuals who are considered to be psychopathic. Those who are psychopathic are sadistic and manipulative pathological liars; show no empathy, compassion, or remorse for hurting others; and take no responsibility for their actions. The most dramatic form is manifested by individuals who torture or murder their victims. Those who perpetrate such violence reside on the extreme end of the spectrum of antisocial behavior and would be the most difficult to treat (see Chapter 22, "Antisocial Personality Disorder and Other Antisocial Behavior," in this volume for more detail).

In keeping with the notion that there is a spectrum of antisocial psychopathology, empirical evidence shows that some patients with antisocial PD are capable of forming a treatment alliance resulting in a positive outcome (Gerstley et al. 1989). Consequently, it has been recommended by some that a trial treatment of several sessions be applied with these patients who may typically be assumed to be untreatable. However, there is always the risk that such patients, particularly within an institutional context (e.g., a hospital or prison), may exhibit a pseudo-alliance to gain certain advantages (Gabbard 2014). For example, there could be a disingenuous profession of enhanced self-understanding and movement toward reform as an attempt to manipulate the therapist into recommending inappropriate privileges.

There is some indication that depression serves as a moderator in the treatment of patients with antisocial PD. One study demonstrated that depressed patients with antisocial PD are more likely to benefit from treatment compared with nondepressed patients with antisocial PD (Shea et al. 1992). Thus, the presence of depression may serve as motivation for these patients to seek and comply with treatment.

Borderline

Kernberg (1967) described the borderline personality as being riddled with aggressive impulses that constantly threaten to destroy positive internal images of the self and others. According to this model, the person with borderline PD does not undergo the normal developmental process of psychological integration. Rather, as a defensive attempt to deal with aggression resulting from caregiver misattunements or failures, this person creates "splits" in the mind to protect the good images from the bad. This splitting leads to a fractured self-concept and the identity problems associated with this disorder. Thus, a therapist can expect the alliance-building work to be rather rocky because these patients frequently exhibit pronounced emotional upheaval, self-destructive acting out, and views of the therapist that alternate between idealization and denigration. Within relationships, such individuals are very needy and demanding, often straining the boundaries of the treatment relationship and exerting pressure on clinicians to behave in ways they normally would not. Research has demonstrated that such pressures can impair the clinician's ability to reflect on his or her mental states and those of the patient (Diamond et al. 2003). Furthermore, clinicians who work with such patients must be able to tolerate and productively discuss anger and aggression. However, because patients with borderline PD are, in most cases, relationship seeking, this is a positive indicator for engagement in treatment.

One treatment study of patients with borderline personality examined alliance development over time (Waldinger and Gunderson 1984). Psychodynamic psychotherapy was employed using largely noninterpretive interventions in the initial alliance-building period (the issue of intervention choice is discussed later in the section "Alliance Considerations Within Different Treatment Paradigms"). The authors observed that a strong alliance and good treatment outcome were linked to two factors: 1) a solid commitment by the participating therapist to remain engaged in the treatment until significant gains had been made by the patients and 2) special emphasis on facilitating the patients' expression of aggression and rage without fear of retaliation. Other studies that have undertaken detailed analysis of alliance ruptures in the treatment of patients with borderline PD have demonstrated the importance of the therapist vigilantly attending to the alliance (e.g., Bennett et al. 2006; Horwitz et al. 1996). As Horwitz et al. (1996) noted, "Clinical observation of our cases revealed that the repair of moment-to-moment disruptions in the alliance often was the key factor in maintaining the viability of the psychotherapy" (p. 173). Bateman and Fonagy (2012) have outlined specific techniques for maintaining the integrity of the alliance through tracking and responding to fluctuations in patients' mentalizing status—the ability to reflect on the mental and emotional states of self and others (see Chapter 12, "Psychodynamic Psychotherapies," in this volume for more information on this approach to treatment).

Narcissistic

Narcissistic character traits have received considerable attention in the clinical literature. Kohut (1977) described individuals in whom there is a fundamental deficit in the ability to regulate self-esteem without resorting to omnipotent strategies of overcompensation or overreliance on admiration by others. People who are narcissistically vulnerable have difficulty maintaining a cohesive sense of self because of ubiquitous shame, resulting from a sense that they fundamentally fall short of some internal ideal. They look for constant reinforcement from others to bolster their fragile self-image. This combination of traits has been referred to alternatively as *vulnerable, deflated*, or *covert narcissism*.

On the other side of the narcissistic "coin"—what the DSM-5 Section II narcissistic PD diagnosis captures—are tendencies toward intense grandiosity and attempts to maintain self-esteem through omnipotent fantasies and defeating others. Needing others is defended against by maintaining fusions of ideal self, ideal other, and actual self-images. Thus, there is an illusion maintained whereby this manifestation of narcissism is associated with a sense that because he or she is perfect, love and admiration will be received from other "ideal people," and thus there is no need to associate with inferiors. In its most extreme form, this manifestation of character pathology has been referred to as *malignant narcissism* (Kernberg 1984). The AMPD provides the ability to indicate trait specifiers to further characterize narcissism, such as manipulativeness, deceitfulness, and callousness traits for more grandiose or malignant presentations, or traits such as anxiousness and depressivity for vulnerable narcissistic styles (American Psychiatric Association 2013).

It is important to note that narcissism is not necessarily exhibited in distinctive or rigid inflated or deflated types (Bender 2012; Levy 2012). Self-esteem oscillation is associated with pathological narcissism more generally, and both grandiose and vulnerable styles can be observed within the same individual. Moreover, there is evidence that narcissistic difficulties are dimensional—that is, they vary in severity or degree—and are present across all personality psychopathology (Morey and Stagner 2012).

In any event, it is obvious that narcissistic personality traits pose significant challenges in alliance building (Ronningstam 2012). It is often the case that the patient will need to keep the therapist out of the room, so to speak, for quite a long time by not allowing the therapist to voice anything that represents an alternative view to that of the patient. For such patients, other people, including the therapist, exist not as separate individuals but merely as objects for gratifying needs. The clinician must tolerate this state of affairs, at times for a lengthy period of time. As Meissner (1996) observed, "Establishing any degree of trust with such patients may be extremely difficult, but not impossible, for a consistent respect for their vulnerability and a recognition of their need not to trust may in time undercut their defensive need" (p. 228).

Avoidant

The individual with avoidant personality is extremely interpersonally sensitive, afraid of being criticized, and constantly concerned about saying or doing something foolish or humiliating. In spite of an intense desire to connect with others, an avoidant person does not let anyone get close unless absolutely sure the person likes him or her. Because of this acute sensitivity, there is some evidence that some patients with avoidant personality are somewhat difficult to retain in treatment. One study showed that patients with avoidant PD were significantly more likely than patients with obsessive-compulsive PD to drop out of a short-term supportive-expressive treatment (Barber et al. 1997). Clinicians who work with patients with avoidant personality need to be constantly mindful of the potentially shaming effects of certain comments, but can also work with the patients' underlying hunger for attachment to enlist them in building an alliance.

Furthermore, preliminary evidence supports the notion that at least some patients diagnosed with avoidant PD are actually better characterized as demonstrating vulnerable narcissist tendencies. These patients covertly crave admiration to bolster their fragile self-esteem and secretly or unconsciously feel entitled to it, rather than simply being afraid of not being liked or accepted (Dickenson and Pincus 2003). Gabbard (2014) referred to this style as *hypervigilant narcissism*, emphasizing extreme interpersonal sensitivity, other-directedness, and shame proneness. An underlying unrecognized narcissism in avoidant PD has significant treatment implications, changing the nature of the forces affecting the alliance as well as shaping the types of treatment interventions that are indicated.

Obsessive-Compulsive

The obsessive-compulsive character is associated with more stable interpersonal relationships than some other styles, but typical defenses are centered on repression, with patterns of highly regulated gratification and ongoing denial of interpersonal and intrapsychic conflicts (Shapiro 1965). Self-willed and obstinate, with a constant eye toward rules and regulations, individuals with obsessive-compulsive attributes guard against any meaningful consideration of their impulses toward others. Maintaining control over internal experience and the external world is a top priority, so rigidity is often a hallmark of this character type. Except in its most severe manifestations, obsessive-compulsive character pathology is less impairing than some of the others and more readily ameliorated by treatment. Although stubborn and controlling and averse to considering emotional content, individuals with obsessive-compulsive PD also generally try to be "good patients" and therefore can be engaged in a constructive alliance that is less rocky than that with patients who have other types of PD.

Case Example 1

Quentin, a 25-year-old graduate student in philosophy, began twice-weekly psychotherapy. His presenting complaint was difficulty with completing work effectively, particularly writing tasks, because of excessive anxiety and obsessionality (his personality functioning met criteria for obsessive-compulsive PD and generalized anxiety disorder). When he came for treatment, he was struggling to make progress on his master's thesis. Although Quentin socialized quite a bit, he reported that intimate relationships often felt "wooden." He was usually overcommitted, with an endless list of "shoulds" that he would constantly mentally review and that triggered thoughts of how much he was failing to satisfy his obligations. A central theme throughout treatment was his tendency to be self-denigrating, loathing himself as a person deserving of punishment in some way yet being extremely provocative (sadomasochistic trends). He also held very strong political beliefs, sure that his way of viewing things was superior to that of others.

Establishing a productive alliance with Quentin was not easily accomplished at first. In the early phase of treatment, he was extremely controlling and challenging in sessions, talking constantly and tangentially, often losing the core point of his statements because of a need to present excessive details. Any statement the therapist made was experienced as an intrusion or interruption. For example, if the therapist attempted to be empathic using a word Quentin had not used, such as saying, "That sounds difficult," he would respond, "Difficult? I don't know if I'd choose the word difficult. Challenging, maybe, or daunting, but not difficult." Thus, for a number of months in the initial phase of the treatment, the therapist chose her words carefully, which eventually paved the way for increased dialogue about his problems. Quentin also began to tolerate a discussion of his emotional life, a topic that previously had been very threatening to him.

Quentin's case is also an example of the limitations of categorical diagnosis. Although Quentin's personality functioning ostensibly meets the diagnostic criteria for obsessive-compulsive PD, there are also clear indications of narcissistic disturbance. His problems tolerating his therapist's presence and interventions and his unreasonably high personal standards are consonant with a narcissistic level of personality functioning. The sadomasochistic inclination to behave in ways that invite some kind of punishing response also presents a challenge to the clinician to manage reactions to protect the alliance and effectively intervene around enactments. (Sadomasochism is discussed more at length below.)

Examples of Alliance Considerations With Prominent Traits or Styles

As mentioned above, there are many times when none of the six PD diagnoses are relevant or adequate. It may be more effective or preferable to use personality functioning and/or prominent traits to best characterize the presentation of a particular patient. In addition, over the course of treatment, aspects of personality functioning may vary and evolve, and the manifestation of certain traits may wax and wane. Consequently, it is important to meet the patient where he or she is in terms of self-concept and interpersonal relatedness. The following are examples of how to approach the alliance through conceptualizing the presence of pronounced traits or styles using the AMPD model.

Paranoia

The "paranoid" label speaks largely for itself. Individuals with prominent paranoid tendencies are incessantly loaded for bear and see bears where others do not—that is, they are vigilantly on the lookout for perceived slights, finding offense in even the most benign of circumstances. Alliance-building challenges are obvious. Identity is associated with distortions in sense of self, which is organized around defending against perceived mistreatment (e.g., attacks on his or her character or reputation that are not apparent to others). The dominant affect is reactive anger, which may be accompanied by aggression. Goal setting is reactive rather than proactive, oriented toward self-protection rather than productivity, and thus lacks coherence and/or stability. Thoughts and actions may be confused, and capacity to reflect on internal experience is compromised by a firmly held view that life is dangerous. Empathy is significantly impaired, as a self-focused perspective in the service of harm avoidance significantly compromises the ability to appreciate and understand others' motivations and perceptions (e.g., the individual frequently believes, without sufficient basis, that others are exploiting or deceiving him or her). Relationships are significantly limited by the individual's reluctance to confide in others because of unwarranted fear that the information will be used maliciously against him or her; relationships and even cooperative efforts are disrupted due to persistent, unjustified doubts about the loyalty or trustworthiness of friends or associates, including suspicions regarding the fidelity of spouse or partner. However, it has also been noted that paranoid individuals are often acting in defense of an extremely fragile self-concept and may possibly be reached over time in treatment with an approach that includes unwavering affirmation and careful handling of the many possible ruptures (Benjamin 1993).

Maladaptive Dependency

Fearing abandonment, individuals with pronounced dependent presentations tend to be very passive, submissive, and needy of constant reassurance. They go to great lengths not to offend others, even at great emotional expense, agreeing with others' opinions when they really do not or volunteering to do unsavory chores to stay in someone's good graces. Identity definition and emotion regulation are excessively predicated on the presence of reassuring others, frequently with compromised boundary delineation. There is pronounced difficulty establishing, pursuing, or achieving personal goals without significant support from others; inability to make everyday decisions or to initiate or sustain projects without an excessive amount of advice or reassurance; and a need for others to assume responsibility for most major areas of an individual's life. Hyperattunement to the experience of others may be apparent, but predominantly with excessive emphasis on fulfilling one's own needs for care, attention, or approval. Intimate relationships are largely based on unrealistic expectations of being completely cared for by others, while feelings about intimate involvement with others are centered around extreme fear of rejection and desperate desire for connection. In the context of treatment, patients with overdependency are easily engaged, at least superficially, but often withhold a great deal of material for fear of alienating the therapist in some way. The following is an example of how this might play out:

> A patient [with pronounced dependent features] was chronically depressed, and the doctor tried her on a new antidepressant. She did not improve and had a number of side effects but did not mention them to the doctor. Fortunately, the doctor remembered to ask for the specific side effects. The patient acknowledged the signs, and the doctor wrote a prescription for a different antidepressant. The patient was willing to acknowledge the signs of problems…, but she did not offer the information spontaneously. The doctor asked her why she did not say anything. She explained, "I thought that maybe they were just part of the way the drug worked.…I figured you would know what was best." (Benjamin 1993, p. 405)

Benjamin (1993) also observed that one difficulty in working in psychotherapy with such patients is the reinforcement gained by the patient's behavior. That is, because the passivity and submissiveness usually result in being taken care of, despite the associated cost, patients with dependent personality are loath to see the value in asserting some independence. Furthermore, there is a deeply ingrained assumption by these patients that they are not capable of functioning more independently and that being more assertive will be experienced by others as alienating aggressiveness. Thus, a therapist must be very alert to the withdrawal types of strains and ruptures, such as withholding information, and to the challenge to the alliance that may occur when the therapist attempts to encourage more independence.

Sadomasochistic Character

Cases in which difficult patients take a prominent role in orchestrating situations to sabotage a potentially helpful treatment are ubiquitous in the clinical literature. This type of dynamic points to an additional element commonly overlooked in treatments in general but of particular relevance when one is trying to establish and maintain an alliance with patients with character pathology: sadomasochism (Bach 2016; Drapeau et al. 2012; Rosegrant 2012). Most dramatically overt in patients with borderline, narcissistic, and/or antisocial issues, relational tendencies that range from tinged to saturated by sadomasochistic trends span the spectrum of personality pathology. The presence of sadomasochistic patterns means not that overt sexual perversions will be present, although they may be, but rather that the patient has characteristic ways of engaging others in a struggle in which one party is suffering at the hands of the other. Patients with a sadomasochistic approach to relationships make it very difficult for the clinician working in any modality to be a helpful agent of change. Furthermore, it is sometimes the case with such patients that at the foundation of the alliance is a very subtle, or not so subtle, sadomasochistic enactment.

For example, a patient may, on the surface, be agreeing with the therapist's observations but actually be experiencing them as verbal assaults while masochistically suffering in silence and showing no improvement in treatment. Another patient may be highly provocative, attempting to bait the therapist into saying and doing things that may prove to be counterattacks. There are also patients who act out in apparently punishing ways, such as by attempting suicide using a newly prescribed medication, when it seemed as though the treatment had been progressing.

Bach (2016) described a sadomasochistic way of relating as arising as "a defense against and an attempt to repair some traumatic loss that has not been adequately mourned" (p. 166). This trauma could have come in the form of an actual loss of a parent, loss of love as a result of abuse or neglect, or some experience of loss of the self, due to such things as childhood illness or circumstances leading to overwhelming anxiety. From this perspective, the cruel behavior of the sadist may, for instance, be an attempt to punish the object for threatened abandonment. The masochistic stance involves a way of loving someone who gives ill treatment—the only way of maintaining a connection is through suffering. Early in development, this way of loving is self-preservative—the sadism of the love object is turned on the self as a way of maintaining a needed relationship. However, in an adult, this masochistic solution, with its always attendant aggressive-sadistic elements, serves to cause significant interpersonal dysfunction.

Case Example 2

Elena, a single woman in her 40s, was referred for psychotherapy after she had gone to see four or five other therapists, staying with each for no more than several sessions because she found them all to be incompetent in some way. An avid reader of self-help literature, she considered herself an expert on the helping professions. Highly intelligent and extremely articulate, Elena was aspiring to be a filmmaker. She had gone through a series of "day jobs" with corporations, reporting that her women supervisors were predictively untalented, unreasonable, and critical of her. Her interpersonal relations were always tumultuous, her moods were very unstable, and it was apparent that she had been grappling with narcissistic and borderline personality issues for decades.

Sadomasochistic trends became apparent very quickly. In the first meeting, Elena launched the first of many critiques, reporting that she had found the therapist's greeting to be too upbeat but then also criticizing the therapist for not reassuring her that she would have a successful treatment. She ultimately announced that the therapist was "gifted," so she would continue with this treatment, but there were many sessions in which she would find fault or deliver lectures on technique and theory. At the same time, she was extremely brittle and incapable of reflecting on this type of behavior, feeling as a victim if there was any vague hint that she might be doing something questionable. Thus, while attacking the therapist, she was doing it in the service of collecting grievances. [As Berliner (1947) observed about such patients, she "would rather be right than happy" (p. 46).] Hence, both the sadistic and masochistic sides of the same coin were in evidence.

With patients such as Elena, it is very important to be able to tolerate the expression of aggression. Consequently, to maintain an alliance with this very difficult woman, the therapist had to constantly assess whether the attacks represented a rupture in the alliance that had to be addressed or whether Elena simply needed to give voice to some of her tremendous anger at the world. When judging that the alliance was in jeopardy, the therapist would discuss Elena's reaction to the therapist's interventions, acknowledging Elena's distress and telling Elena that further thought would be given to what had led the therapist to make the comments that had upset her. Elena usually found great relief in this approach, appreciating the therapist's willingness to reflect on the situation.

What is central is that the therapist withstood being portrayed as bad or incompetent in the patient's mind without retaliating as though it were true. If the therapist had had a different psychology, it would have been rather easy to take up the role of sadist, perhaps wrapped in the flag of "interpreting the patient's aggression"; however, Elena and this therapist were a good match, because such retributive behavior would have been a sadomasochistic enactment and would have caused Elena to make a hasty departure.

Alliance Considerations Within Different Treatment Paradigms

Clearly, no matter what treatment paradigm one adopts for working with patients who have personality pathology, attention to the alliance is of utmost importance. Thoughts and feelings on the part of the therapist must be monitored closely, because interactions with many patients may often be provocative, inducing reactions that must be carefully managed. (See Chapter 19, "Boundary Issues," in this volume for a discussion of some of the most serious consequences of treatments gone awry.) Although this topic is usually discussed as countertransference in the psychoanalytic/psychodynamic tradition, it is also quite applicable across all treatments (Gabbard 1999).

Treatment approach and technique must be flexible so that interventions can be made appropriate to each individual patient's style. Otherwise, the alliance may be jeopardized and the patient will not benefit or may leave treatment altogether. For example, Spinhoven et al. (2007) found an interaction between alliance and therapeutic techniques that influenced course and outcome in a group of patients with borderline PD. Furthermore, it is likely that noticeable improvements in symptoms and functioning in patients with personality pathology will require a significantly longer period of treatment than is required for patients with no character pathology. Although the application of specific treatment approaches is discussed at length in other chapters of this book, it is worth mentioning here a few alliance-relevant considerations pertaining to each broad treatment context.

Psychodynamic Psychotherapies and Psychoanalysis

One long-standing issue within the psychodynamic psychotherapy tradition involves the application of particular techniques. Interpretation of the transference was long considered the heart of the psychoanalytic approach. One example of a contemporary treatment where focusing on the transference is central to working with patients with personality psychopathology is *transference-focused psychotherapy* (TFP). Practitioners of TFP are trained to be very mindful of the state of the alliance and to effectively address ruptures, which can be frequent and pronounced in more significantly impaired patients (Caligor et al. 2018). This approach is discussed more extensively in Chapter 12 ("Psychodynamic Psychotherapies").

As psychoanalysis and psychodynamic treatments in general evolved and clinicians gained more experience with more disturbed patients—most notably those with borderline and narcissistic trends—it became apparent that in many cases, transference interpretations with such patients are often counterproductive. Refraining from making deep, interpretive interventions early on is consistent with notions of writers such as Winnicott (1965) and Kohut (1984), who asserted that certain patients cannot tolerate such interpretations in the initial phase of treatment.

Gabbard (2014) stressed the importance of understanding that there is usually a mixture of supportive and expressive (interpretive) elements in every analysis or psychodynamic psychotherapy. That is, the expressive, insight-oriented mode of assisting patients in uncovering unconscious conflicts, thoughts, or affects through interpretation or confrontation may be appropriate at times, whereas a more supportive approach of bolstering the patient's defenses and coping abilities is preferable in other circumstances.

For instance, it may be difficult to focus on more insight-oriented interventions with a patient with borderline impairments until that patient is assisted in achieving a safe, more stable alliance. Similarly, the patient with severe narcissistic impairment may not be able to accept the analyst's interpretations of his or her unconscious motivations for quite a long time, so that supportive, empathic communications may be more effective interventions in building an alliance by helping the patient feel heard and understood. Conversely, some obsessional patients may benefit earlier in treatment by interpretations of the repressed conflicts that may underlie the symptoms.

The results of the Psychotherapy Research Project of the Menninger Foundation, which included patients with PDs, led Wallerstein (1986) to conclude that both expressive and supportive interventions can lead to character change. At the same time, there is empirical evidence supporting the notion that a fairly solid alliance must be present to effectively utilize transference interpretations per se. Bond et al. (1998) demonstrated with a group of patients with PDs in long-term treatment that for those patients whose alliance was weak, transference interpretations caused further impairment to the alliance. Conversely, when already solidly established, the alliance was strengthened by transference interpretations. At the same time, supportive interventions and discussions of defensive operations resulted in moving the therapeutic work forward with both the weak- and strong-alliance patient groups.

These findings are consistent with a study conducted by Horwitz et al. (1996) exploring the effect of supportive and interpretive interventions on the therapeutic alliance with a group of patients with borderline PD. The authors concluded that although therapists are often eager to pursue transference interpretations, such interventions are "high-risk, high-gain" and need to be employed carefully. These interventions may damage the alliance with patients who are vulnerable and prone to feelings of shame and humiliation. Therefore, the therapist must be flexible in adjusting technique according to the dynamics of a particular patient at a particular time, taking into account the patient's capacities and vulnerabilities, and appropriately balance both supportive and expressive interventions.

Case Example 3

Rebecca sought treatment when she was in her early 30s. She was referred for psycho-therapy from her graduate school's counseling center. Rebecca presented in a major de-pressive episode, and her presentation clearly met criteria for borderline PD. The initial phase of the twice-weekly psychodynamic treatment focused on her depression and on helping her to stabilize her sometimes devastating affective instability. She also re-ported intermittent, but not life-threatening, instances of cutting herself, particularly af-ter some unsatisfactory encounter with a friend or colleague.

Rebecca's lack of object constancy, her affective instability, and a fragmented sense of self contributed to great variations in the nature of her presence in sessions. At times she would be overwhelmed by fatigue, whereas at other times she would be engaging, funny, and analytical. She would often defend against undesirable thoughts or emo-tions by spending the session recounting her day-to-day life in great detail. The disjunc-tions in self states made it difficult at times to maintain continuity in the process, because Rebecca did not remember what happened from session to session.

A Kernbergian formulation (Kernberg 1967) of this patient was theoretically infor-mative in describing some of her dynamics (defensive splitting had been one promi-nent theme in the treatment). However, the technical implications of this particular approach, with its direct confrontation of aggression in the transference early in the treatment (Kernberg 1987), would have endangered the sometimes-fragile working alliance being forged. In fact, a few times when transference interpretations were at-tempted in the first phase of treatment, Rebecca became confused and distressed, quickly changing the subject away from a discussion of her relationship with the ther-apist, talking about ending treatment, or becoming very sleepy and shut down for several sessions. On one occasion early on, when the therapist attempted to address something in their relationship, Rebecca became very angry and said, "Why is any of this about here? These are my problems and I don't see what any of this has to do with you!" (Clearly, in the beginning phase of treatment with some patients, one needs a dif-ferent way of entering the patient's psychic world [Ellman 1998].) However, Rebecca was responsive to gentle interpretations of her defenses, such as the therapist's point-ing out to her that her self-harm behaviors were a way of "being mean" to herself in-stead of channeling anger toward those who had upset her.

Thus, for most of the first 3–4 years of this treatment, the therapist's primary tasks were to develop a working alliance and establish a "holding environment" (Winnicott 1965) within which Rebecca could begin to feel safe to explore her history, her feel-ings, and her own mind. This approach paid off, because it eventually became possi-ble to uncover, in ways that were meaningful and transformative to Rebecca, some of the split-off rage and despair underlying the identity instability and distorted cogni-tive functioning. Deeper experience and exploration of these feelings paved the way for further integration and less disjunctive experiences in her life and from session to session, and working with the transference increasingly became both possible and very productive. Rebecca has not been depressed for years, and borderline criteria are no longer met.

Cognitive-Behavioral Therapies

In recent years, work has been done to apply to personality psychopathology the cog-nitive and cognitive-behavioral treatments that have typically been used to treat symptoms such as depression and anxiety. However, Tyrer and Davidson (2000) observed that the approaches generally taken in these therapies for "mental state disorders" cannot be simply transferred to treating personality psychopathology without certain adjustments. Most cognitive and cognitive-behavioral therapies are based prominently on a therapist-patient collaboration that is assumed to be present from very early in the treatment. Such a collaboration, which revolves around the patient undertaking specific activities and assignments, depends on the establishment of a solid working alliance; however, it is sometimes very difficult to engage certain patients with personality psychopathology in the therapeutic tasks. Facilitating this alliance with patients with such challenges requires work that directly addresses patient-therapist collaboration with clearly set boundaries and that focuses on the therapeutic relationship itself when appropriate, as well as lengthier periods to complete these treatments (Tyrer and Davidson 2000). Muran et al. (2018) demonstrated that specific alliance-focused training for novice therapists improved the interpersonal process with patients in cognitive-behavioral therapy for PDs.

For example, regarding the use of the initial sessions of dialectical behavior therapy to begin establishing a working relationship, Linehan (1993) observed, "These sessions offer an opportunity for both patient and therapist to explore problems that may arise in establishing and maintaining a therapeutic alliance" (p. 446). Even though dialectical behavior therapy is a manualized treatment with clearly elaborated therapeutic tasks, it is quickly evident, particularly in working with patients with borderline PD, that a great deal of flexibility must be maintained within this paradigm to achieve an alliance (see Chapter 14, "Cognitive-Behavioral Therapy," in this volume). More specifically, there may be frequent occurrences of therapy-interfering behaviors ranging from ambivalence causing missed sessions to multiple suicide attempts that prevent the treatment from progressing as the method outlines.

Case Example 4

Lourdes, a young woman with significant dependent tendencies, was referred for behavioral treatment of a phobia of all forms of transportation (her other issues were already being addressed in an ongoing psychotherapy). The behavior therapist spent several sessions with Lourdes outlining the exposure techniques recommended for treating her phobia, but the patient was resistant to beginning any of the activities described. At the same time, while trying to pursue a classically behavioral approach, the therapist realized that it was very important for Lourdes to spend some of the time talking about her life and the impact the phobia symptoms had for her. This approach helped Lourdes to feel a connection to the therapist. The therapist made this relationship-building aspect explicit with Lourdes by agreeing to take a part of each session to talk about her situation, but the therapist also made it clear that it was necessary to reserve enough time for the exposure activities. This approach fostered an alliance sufficiently to begin the behavioral tasks. By being flexible, while setting clear tasks and boundaries, the therapist was able to engage Lourdes in the treatment, and she began taking short rides with the therapist on the bus, eventually overcoming these fears completely.

Psychopharmacology Sessions

One large-scale depression study (Krupnick et al. 1996) comparing several different psychotherapies with medication and placebo showed that the quality of the alliance was significantly related to outcome for all the study groups. This finding demonstrates the importance of considering the alliance not only in psychotherapies but also in medication sessions. Gutheil (1982) suggested that there is a particular aspect of the therapeutic alliance—what he calls the *pharmacotherapeutic alliance*—that is relevant to the prescription of medications. In this formulation of the alliance, it is recommended that the physician adopt the stance of *participant prescribing*—that is, rather than adopting an authoritarian role, the clinician should make every effort to involve the patient as a collaborator who engages actively in goal setting and in observing and evaluating the experience of using specific medications. Such collaboration, like other therapeutic processes, may be affected by the patient's transference distortions of the clinician. Furthermore, a recent review of five decades of literature demonstrated the critical role that personality and styles of meaning-making have in mediating the effects of psychotropic medications (Palmieri et al. 2020).

The notion of collaborative prescribing can be more broadly applied in transtheoretical terms to personality psychopathology because it is appropriate to consider how the patient's characteristic style may influence his or her attitudes and behaviors toward taking psychiatric medications. Some patients may become upset if medication is not prescribed, feeling slighted because they think their problems are not being taken seriously. Others with paranoid tendencies may think the physician is trying to put something over on them, or worse. Some patients who are prone to somaticizing, such as those with borderline or histrionic tendencies, might be hypersensitive to any possible side effects (real or imagined) and argue with the prescriber about his or her competence. The following is another example illustrating the importance of being mindful of how patients with PD might react around issues of medication.

> A patient [diagnosed with avoidant PD] overdosed one evening on the medicine her doctor had prescribed for her persistent depression. She liked and respected him a lot. She was discovered comatose by a neighbor who wondered why her cat would not stop meowing. The neighbor was the patient's only friend. It turned out that that morning her doctor had wondered aloud whether she had a personality disorder. The patient was deeply humiliated by that idea but secretly agreed with it. She felt extremely embarrassed and was convinced that her doctor now knew she was a completely foolish person....Rather than endure the humiliation of facing him again, she decided to end it all. (Benjamin 1993, p. 411)

Psychiatric Hospital Settings

Across the spectrum of personality psychopathology, psychiatric hospitalizations—both inpatient and day treatment programs—are most common for those patients with borderline PD (Bender et al. 2001). The central consideration regarding the alliance in this treatment context is that there is always a team of individuals responsible for the patient. With patients who have borderline issues, splitting tendencies frequently are quite pronounced. That is, as a way of trying to cope with inner turmoil, the patient's mental world is often organized in black-and-white, good-and-bad polarities, and through complicated interaction patterns with various staff members, this internal world is over time replayed externally, dividing staff members against each other.

Gabbard (1989) observed that this dynamic is often set up because the patient will present one self-representation to one or several team members and a very different representation to another. One of these staff factions may be viewed as the "good" one by the patient and the other as the "bad" one—although these designations can flip precipitously in the patient's mind—and this split becomes enacted among team members as they begin to work at cross-purposes. It can be seen rather readily that trying to develop a constructive alliance with such a patient can be extremely precarious, particularly given the ever-decreasing length of hospital stays under managed care. That means that communication and close collaboration among the members of the team are vital during every phase of the hospital treatment.

Matters are complicated further at times by the need to find a productive way for hospital staff to collaborate with clinicians providing ongoing outpatient psychotherapy and/or psychopharmacology treatments. Although the hospitalization may represent a significant rupture in the outpatient treatment alliance, this rupture does not necessarily indicate that the outpatient treatment was ineffective and must be terminated, but rather demonstrates that work will be needed to reestablish the continuity of the treatment relationship. However, it is not uncommon for the hospital staff, seeing the patient's current condition, to conclude that the outpatient clinicians were somehow not doing a competent job (this conclusion may, of course, be fueled by further splitting on the part of the patient). Moreover, at times it may be obvious that the outpatient treatment was inadequate or inappropriate. In any event, it becomes rather dicey for all parties concerned to sort out the proper role of hospital staff versus outpatient staff over the course of the inpatient or day treatment program.

Case Example 5

Meghan, a young woman diagnosed with borderline PD, was admitted to a psychiatric inpatient unit after coming to the emergency department reporting acute suicidal ideation. This patient had been hospitalized several times previously, worked in the mental health field, and "knew the ropes" quite well. She had been assigned a psychiatrist who was responsible for overall case management and a psychologist who was to provide short-term psychotherapy on the unit.

The initial psychotherapy session was extremely difficult, with Meghan refusing to speak very much and regarding the therapist with rageful contempt. However, after several more encounters, there was some softening by Meghan and she began to discuss the upsetting circumstances that led to her hospitalization. It appeared there might be the beginnings of a working alliance. Indeed, as she opened up more about her life, she reported feeling slightly more hopeful and less fragmented.

However, at the same time, she had created quite a bit of trouble with the rest of the staff by being very demanding and uncooperative and attempting to initiate discharge procedures even while refusing to deny that she would kill herself. Having reached a point of needing to take some action in the courts to keep Meghan hospitalized, the psychiatrist hastily called a meeting that included himself, the psychologist, and the patient. Having had no opportunity to confer with other team members on the matter, the psychiatrist proceeded to tell Meghan that he was initiating legal proceedings to keep her in the hospital. Mindful of the splitting tendencies of such patients, the psychiatrist was careful to make it clear that he represented the viewpoint of the entire team, including the psychologist. However, he unwittingly created another split. Meghan, feeling betrayed, stared hatefully at the psychologist, the fragile working alliance was shattered, and she subsequently refused to participate in psychotherapy or any other therapeutic activities for the rest of the hospitalization. It is possible this rupture could have been ameliorated had there been adequate consultation among treatment team members so that a less alienating approach could have been formulated.

Conclusion

Establishing an alliance in any treatment paradigm requires a great deal of empathy and attunement to the core features of a patient's personality—their characteristic ways of seeing themselves and others. Individuals may present with problematic self-assessments linked with disturbed patterns of interpersonal relations, which pose treatment challenges and opportunities that must be navigated skillfully. Research has shown not only the importance of building an alliance but also the vital role this alliance plays in the earliest phase of treatment. One cannot rigidly pursue the dictates of one's treatment paradigm without being prepared to make frequent adjustments to address the various ruptures that may occur. Gleaning clues from the patient's accounts of their relationships can serve to guide the clinician's general interpersonal stance. Furthermore, monitoring the therapeutic alliance in response to clinical interventions is a useful way to assess the effectiveness of one's approach and is informative in determining appropriate modifications in the style and content of the therapist's interactions with the patient.

References

Adler G: Transference, real relationship and alliance. Int J Psychoanal 61:547–558, 1980

Alberti GG: Psychotherapy by alliance and corrective experiences: a possible general model. J Psychother Integr 28:31–45, 2018

American Psychiatric Association: Diagnostic and Statistical Manual of Mental Disorders, 5th Edition. Arlington, VA, American Psychiatric Association, 2013

Bach S: On treating the difficult patient, in Chimeras and Other Writings: Selected Papers of Sheldon Bach. Astoria, NY, International Psychoanalytic Books, 2016, pp 217–228

Barber JP, Morse JQ, Krakauer ID, et al: Change in obsessive-compulsive and avoidant personality disorders following time-limited supportive-expressive therapy. Psychotherapy 34:133–143, 1997

Bateman A, Fonagy P (eds): Handbook of Mentalizing in Mental Health Practice. Washington, DC, American Psychiatric Publishing, 2012

Bender DS: Mirror, mirror on the wall: reflecting on narcissism. J Clin Psychol 68:877–885, 2012

Bender DS, Dolan RT, Skodol AE, et al: Treatment utilization by patients with personality disorders. Am J Psychiatry 158:295–302, 2001

Bender DS, Farber BA, Sanislow CA, et al: Representations of therapists by patients with personality disorders. Am J Psychother 57:219–236, 2003

Bender DS, Morey LC, Skodol AS: Toward a model for assessing level of personality functioning in DSM-5, part I: a review of theory and methods. J Pers Assess 93:332–346, 2011

Benjamin LS: Interpersonal Diagnosis and Treatment of Personality Disorders. New York, Guilford, 1993

Bennett D, Parry G, Ryle A: Resolving threats to the therapeutic alliance in cognitive analytic therapy of borderline personality disorder: a task analysis. Psychol Psychother 79:395–418, 2006

Berliner B: The role of object relations in moral masochism. Psychoanal Q 27:38–56, 1947

Bond M, Banon E, Grenier M: Differential effects of interventions on the therapeutic alliance with patients with personality disorders. J Psychother Pract Res 7:301–318, 1998

Bordin ES: The generalizability of the psychoanalytic concept of the working alliance. Psychotherapy: Theory, Research, and Practice 16:252–260, 1979

Caligor E, Kernberg OF, Clarkin JF, Yeomans FE: Psychodynamic Therapy for Personality Pathology: Treating Self and Interpersonal Functioning. Washington, DC, American Psychiatric Association Publishing, 2018

Cookson A, Daffern M, Foley F: Relationship between aggression, interpersonal style, and therapeutic alliance during short-term psychiatric hospitalization. Int J Ment Health Nurs 21:20–29, 2012

Diamond D, Stovall-McClough C, Clarkin JF, et al: Patient–therapist attachment in the treatment of borderline personality disorder. Bull Menninger Clin 67:227–259, 2003

Dickenson KA, Pincus AL: Interpersonal analysis of grandiose and vulnerable narcissism. J Pers Disord 17:188–207, 2003

Diener MJ, Monroe JM: The relationship between adult attachment style and therapeutic alliance in individual psychotherapy: a meta-analytic review. Psychotherapy 48:237–248, 2011

Dimaggio G, Overholser JC: Treatment of clients with anxious and over-controlled personality disorders: an international accord. J Contemp Psychother 49:1–6, 2019

Doorn KA-v, Kealy D, Ehrenthal JC, et al: Improving self-esteem through integrative group therapy for personality dysfunction: investigating the role of the therapeutic alliance and quality of object relations. J Clin Psychol 75:2079–2094, 2019

Drapeau M, Perry JC, Korner A: Interpersonal patterns in borderline personality disorder. J Pers Disord 26:583–592, 2012

Ellman SJ: Freud's Technique Papers: A Contemporary Perspective. Northvale, NJ, Jason Aronson, 1991

Ellman SJ: The unique contribution of the contemporary Freudian position, in The Modern Freudians. Edited by Ellman CS, Grand S, Silvan M, et al. Northvale, NJ, Jason Aronson, 1998, pp 237–268

Eubanks CF, Burckell LA, Goldfried MR: Clinical consensus strategies to repair ruptures in the therapeutic alliance. J Psychother Integr 28:60–76, 2018

Eubanks-Carter C, Muran JC, Safran JD: Alliance ruptures and resolutions, in The Therapeutic Alliance: An Evidence-Based Guide to Practice. Edited by Muran JC, Barber JP. New York, Guilford, 2010, pp 74–96

Flückiger C, Del Re AC, Wampold BE, Horvath AO: The alliance in adult psychotherapy: a meta-analytic synthesis. Psychotherapy 55:316–340, 2018

Freud S: The dynamics of transference (1912), in The Standard Edition of the Complete Psychological Works of Sigmund Freud, Vol 12. Translated and edited by Strachey J. London, Hogarth Press, 1958, pp 99–108

Gabbard GO: Splitting in hospital treatment. Am J Psychiatry 146:444–451, 1989

Gabbard GO: An overview of countertransference: theory and technique, in Countertransference Issues in Psychiatric Treatment. Edited by Gabbard GO (Review of Psychiatry Series, Vol 18; Oldham JM and Riba MB, series eds). Washington, DC, American Psychiatric Press, 1999, pp 1–25

Gabbard GO: Psychodynamic Psychiatry in Clinical Practice, 5th Edition. Washington, DC, American Psychiatric Press, 2014

Gerstley L, McLellan AT, Alterman AI, et al: Ability to form an alliance with the therapist: a possible social marker of prognosis for patients with antisocial personality disorder. Am J Psychiatry 146:508–512, 1989

Gibbons MB, Crits-Cristoph P, de la Cruz C, et al: Pretreatment expectations, interpersonal functioning, and symptoms in the prediction of the therapeutic alliance across supportive-expressive psychotherapy and cognitive therapy. Psychother Res 13:59–76, 2003

Gómez Penedo JM, Zilcha-Mano S, Roussos A: Interpersonal profiles in emotional disorders predict the importance of alliance negotiation for early treatment outcome. J Consult Clin Psychol 87:617–628, 2019

Gunderson JG: Psychodynamic psychotherapy for borderline personality disorder, in Psychotherapy for Personality Disorders. Edited by Gunderson JG, Gabbard GO (Review of Psychiatry Series, Vol 19; Oldham JM and Riba MB, series eds). Washington, DC, American Psychiatric Press, 2000, pp 33–64

Gunderson JG, Najavits LM, Leonhard C, et al: Ontogeny of the therapeutic alliance in borderline patients. Psychother Res 7:301–309, 1997

Gutheil TG: The psychology of psychopharmacology. Bull Menninger Clin 46:321–330, 1982

Gutheil TG, Havens LL: The therapeutic alliance: contemporary meanings and confusions. Int
Rev Psychoanal 6:467–481, 1979

Hatcher RL: Alliance theory and measurement, in The Therapeutic Alliance: An Evidence-
Based Guide to Practice. Edited by Muran JC, Barber JP. New York, Guilford, 2010, pp 7–28

Hersoug AG, Monsen J, Havik OE, et al: Quality of working alliance in psychotherapy: diagnoses, relationship and intrapsychic variables as predictors. Psychother Psychosom 71:18–
27, 2002

Hill CE: Qualitative studies of negative experiences in psychotherapy, in The Therapeutic Alliance: An Evidence-Based Guide to Practice. Edited by Muran JC, Barber JP. New York,
Guilford, 2010, pp 63–73

Hill CE, Thompson BJ, Cogar MC, et al: Beneath the surface of long-term therapy: therapist and
client report of their own and each other's covert processes. Journal of Counseling Psychology 40:278–287, 1993

Horvath AO, Greenberg LS (eds): The Working Alliance: Theory, Research, and Practice. New
York, Wiley, 1994

Horvath AO, Luborsky L: The role of therapeutic alliance in psychotherapy. J Consult Clin Psychol 61:561–573, 1993

Horvath AO, Del Re AC, Flückiger C, et al: Alliance in individual psychotherapy. Psychotherapy (Chic) 48:9–16, 2011

Horwitz L, Gabbard GO, Allen JG, et al: Borderline Personality Disorder: Tailoring the Psychotherapy to the Patient. Washington, DC, American Psychiatric Press, 1996

Kamphuis JH, Finn SE: Therapeutic assessment in personality disorders: toward the restoration
of epistemic trust. J Pers Assess 101:662–674, 2018

Kernberg OF: Borderline personality organization. J Am Psychoanal Assoc 15:641–685, 1967

Kernberg OF: Severe Personality Disorders: Psychotherapeutic Strategies. New Haven, CT,
Yale University Press, 1984

Kernberg OF: An ego psychology–object relations theory approach to the transference. Psychoanal Q 56:197–221, 1987

Kohut H: The Restoration of the Self. New York, International Universities Press, 1977

Kohut H: How Does Analysis Cure? Chicago, IL, University of Chicago Press, 1984

Krupnick JL, Sotsky SM, Simmens S, et al: The role of the therapeutic alliance in psychotherapy
and pharmacotherapy outcome: findings in the National Institute of Mental Health Treatment of Depression Collaborative Research Program. J Consult Clin Psychol 65:532–539,
1996

Levy KN: Subtypes, dimensions, levels and mental states in narcissism and narcissistic personality disorder. J Clin Psychol 68:886–897, 2012

Linehan MM: Cognitive-Behavioral Treatment of Borderline Personality Disorder. New York,
Guilford, 1993

Meissner WW: The Therapeutic Alliance. New Haven, CT, Yale University Press, 1996

Morey LC, Stagner BH: Narcissistic pathology as core personality dysfunction: comparing the
DSM-IV and the DSM-5 proposal for narcissistic personality disorder. J Clin Psychol
68:908–921, 2012

Muran JC, Safran JD, Eubanks CF, Gorman BS: The effect of alliance-focused training on a cognitive-behavioral therapy for personality disorders. J Consult Clin Psychol 86:384-397,
2018

Palmieri A, Zidarich S, Kleinbub JR: Symbolic meaning of drugs in psychotherapy: a psychodynamic perspective. Psychoanal Psychol 37:294–304, 2020

Piper WE, Azim HFA, Joyce AS, et al: Quality of object relations versus interpersonal functioning as predictors of therapeutic alliance and psychotherapy outcome. J Nerv Ment Dis
179:432–438, 1991

Ronningstam E: Alliance building and narcissistic personality disorder. J Clin Psychol 68:943–
953, 2012

Rosegrant J: Narcissism and sadomasochistic relationships. J Clin Psychol 68:935–942, 2012

Safran JD, Muran JC: Negotiating the Therapeutic Alliance. New York, Guilford, 2000

Safran JD, Muran JC, Eubanks-Carter C: Repairing alliance ruptures. Psychotherapy (Chic) 48:80–87, 2011

Shapiro D: Neurotic Styles. New York, Basic Books, 1965

Shea MT, Widiger TA, Klein MH: Comorbidity of personality disorders and depression: implications for treatment. J Consult Clin Psychol 60:857–868, 1992

Signer S, Estermann Jansen R, Sachse R, et al: Social interaction patterns, therapist responsiveness, and outcome in treatments for borderline personality disorder. Psychol Psychother e12254, Oct 4, 2019 (online ahead of print)

Spinhoven P, Giesen-Bloo J, van Dyck R, et al: The therapeutic alliance in schema-focused therapy and transference-focused psychotherapy for borderline personality disorder. J Consult Clin Psychol 75:104–115, 2007

Stone MH: Abnormalities of Personality. New York, WW Norton, 1993

Strauss JL, Hayes AM, Johnson SL, et al: Early alliance, alliance ruptures, and symptom change in a nonrandomized trial of cognitive therapy for avoidant and obsessive-compulsive personality disorders. J Consult Clin Psychol 74:337–345, 2006

Tyrer P, Davidson K: Cognitive therapy for personality disorders, in Psychotherapy for Personality Disorders. Edited by Gunderson JG, Gabbard GO (Review of Psychiatry Series, Vol 19; Oldham JM and Riba MB, series eds). Washington, DC, American Psychiatric Press, 2000, pp 131–149

Urmanche AA, Oliveira JT, Gonçalves MM, et al: Ambivalence, resistance, and alliance ruptures in psychotherapy: it's complicated. Psychoanal Psychol 36:139–147, 2019

Waldinger RJ, Gunderson JG: Completed psychotherapies with borderline patients. Am J Psychother 38:190–202, 1984

Wallerstein RS: Forty-Two Lives in Treatment: A Study of Psychoanalysis and Psychotherapy. New York, Guilford, 1986

Winnicott DW: The Maturational Processes and the Facilitating Environment. London, Hogarth Press, 1965

CHAPTER 12

Psychodynamic Psychotherapies

Frank E. Yeomans, M.D.
John F. Clarkin, Ph.D.
Kenneth N. Levy, Ph.D.

Psychodynamic means "the mind in motion." *Psychodynamic psychotherapy* refers to psychotherapies that stem from the psychoanalytic tradition and focus on the role of conflicting forces within the mind—competing desires, impulses, emotions, fears, and prohibitions—and their interface with external reality as sources of suffering and symptoms. The psychoanalytic tradition centers on the understanding of the mind elaborated initially by Freud (1923/1961) that emphasizes the role of unconscious aspects of mental functioning and the interaction of constitutional biological predispositions and environmental influences in psychological development. While psychodynamic therapies are primarily psychological treatments, in the course of the therapy, the therapist must continue to assess the impact of biological factors that affect the patient's condition. As psychoanalysis evolved, its focus shifted from symptoms to character pathology (Gabbard 2005). More recently, with the emphasis on evidence-based treatments, models of psychodynamic therapy to treat specific types of personality disorder (PD) have been developed and researched (Bateman and Fonagy 2012; Clarkin et al. 2006; Yeomans et al. 2015). As the field continues to evolve, the dialogue between evidence-based models and clinical analytic practice is enriching both. As part of our discussion of the psychotherapy of personality disorders, we will also review the evolving conceptualization of those disorders.

In this chapter, we summarize psychoanalytic concepts relevant to the treatment of personality disorders and describe different models of psychodynamic psychotherapy for PDs based on those concepts. Our focus is on psychodynamic therapies rather than psychoanalysis, because the former have been developed specifically to address the challenges of working with patients with PDs, whereas the practice of more traditional psychoanalysis tends not to focus on the importance of a specific diagnosis and the advisability of adjusting the application of technique to the diagnosis or the level of the severity of the personality disorder. As the field evolves, the boundary between psychoanalysis and psychodynamic therapies is becoming less precise, especially as the reality of clinical practice is to move from psychoanalysis carried out four or five times per week to psychodynamic therapy with one or two sessions per week.

Shedler (2010) listed how psychodynamic therapy differs from other therapies. In the following description, we borrow from and add to his list. Psychoanalysis and the psychodynamic therapies are characterized by 1) an emphasis on the role of unconscious mental forces (e.g., urges, fantasies, prohibitions) and the notion that an individual's conscious mind is only a slice of his or her mental activity and that unconscious forces influence the individual's feelings, thoughts, and actions in ways beyond his or her awareness; 2) an emphasis, to varying degrees, on the past and development—as filtered through and registered in the mind—as determining the individual's experience of the present; 3) a focus on containment of intense affects and expression of emotion; 4) exploration of attempts to avoid distressing feelings and thoughts; 5) identification of recurring themes and patterns to be understood; 6) a focus on interpersonal relations; 7) a focus on the therapy relationship; 8) exploration of fantasy life; and 9) the goal of deep change in the personality to improve the overall quality of the patient's life experience beyond symptom change.

Psychodynamic therapies vary along several dimensions. First, these variations reflect the fact that the categorization of therapies into distinct models that might be found in a "pure" form, such as psychodynamic and cognitive-behavioral, is somewhat artificial because most therapists practicing dynamic therapy include some elements of cognitive-behavioral therapy (CBT), and vice versa (Ablon and Jones 2002). Second, wtihin psychodynamic therapies, there is varying emphasis on different psychoanalytic elements among the models. Running through the items reviewed above is concern with internal psychological conflict: conflicts among competing urges within the mind, between urges and internal values or prohibitions, and between urges and the social reality within which one lives. We will keep these variations in mind as we review specific models of psychodynamic psychotherapy.

The principles of technical intervention within a psychoanalytic framework are fundamentally 1) interpretation, 2) transference analysis, 3) a technically neutral stance, and 4) use of countertransference awareness. Psychoanalysis and the different forms of psychodynamic therapy can be categorized according to the degree to which they employ each of these four technical principles (Kernberg 2018). In addition, one can also consider a spectrum across psychodynamic therapies, from those that stress the importance of verbal communication and interpretation as the motor of change to those that emphasize the experience of a containing and reflective relationship as the main element in change (Gabbard and Westen 2003; Winnicott 1965).

The development of a model of therapy is closely linked to the conceptualization of the disorder to be treated. Of course, the conceptualization of the disorder has an impact on the treatment approach, such as whether one addresses symptoms more directly or focuses on underlying processes. The concept of PD is complex and controversial. Personality can be thought of in terms of a set of personality traits (McCrae and Costa 1997) or in terms of a style of processing information (Mischel and Shoda 1995). PDs can be conceptualized categorically or dimensionally. Until the introduction of the Alternative DSM-5 Model for Personality Disorders (AMPD) introduced in DSM-5, Section III (American Psychiatric Association 2013), the categorical approach to classification, which has continued from DSM-IV (American Psychiatric Association 1994) into DSM-5, Section II, "Diagnostic Criteria and Codes," was characterized by considerable overlap of diagnostic categories, comorbidity, and frequent use of the "personality disorder not otherwise specified" diagnosis. The AMPD emphasizes a dimensional rather than a categorical understanding of PDs and considers PDs in terms of Criterion A, impairments in self and interpersonal functioning, and Criterion B, which describes the presence of pathological personality traits, such as negative affectivity, detachment, antagonism, disinhibition, and psychoticism (American Psychiatric Association 2013). The model goes on to consider the level of personality functioning as essential to the understanding of an individual's PD, using the Level of Personality Functioning Scale to assess severity of impairment. This understanding of PDs can guide us in our thinking about treatment, suggesting that the role of self-concept and interpersonal functioning should be considered in the course of the treatment of all PDs. (See Chapter 4, "The Alternative DSM-5 Model for Personality Disorders," in this volume for a more detailed discussion.)

The movement toward a dimensional understanding of personality disorders has been supported by studies of personality disorders (Sharp et al. 2015; Wright et al. 2016). In this emerging model, converging data point to the core defining features of PDs as the domains of self and interpersonal functioning. The AMPD describes all PDs as organized around 1) a disturbance in the self, thought of in terms of identity and self-directedness, and 2) interpersonal functioning, in terms of the capacity for intimacy and empathy. Sharp and her colleagues (2015) found, in a study of 966 inpatients diagnosed with PDs, that a general, or "g" factor, characterized all the patients, with the exception of those with narcissistic, antisocial, and schizotypal PDs. In discussing the findings, Sharp pointed out that they are compatible with Kernberg's (1984) formulation of personality pathology along a severity continuum, with the quality of an individual's mental representation of self and others (object relations) as a central component of this continuum. This "structural model" of PDs, a model that is based on psychoanalytic concepts and guides treatment techniques according to the level of the pathology (Bender et al. 2011), may offer the treatment model that corresponds best to this emerging understanding of PDs. The model will be discussed below in the subsection "Object Relations Theory."

In the overall field of psychotherapy, since the 1990s there has been an increasing emphasis on evidence-based treatments. There is a prevalent misunderstanding that the body of evidence for CBT treatments far outweighs that for psychodynamic treatments. A series of meta-analyses (see Shedler 2010 for a review) has corrected that misunderstanding. The current emphasis on evidence-based treatments has important implications for students of therapy. This emphasis has intensified divisions in the field of psychotherapy between researchers and clinicians. Some researchers have raised questions about the neglect of science by practitioners (Baker et al. 2008). Some clinicians have experienced researchers as imposing findings from studies that do not represent real-world clinical settings and have called for more clinically relevant research. Among psychotherapy researchers, there are divisions between those who narrowly construe evidence as consisting of findings exclusive to randomized controlled trials (Chambless and Ollendick 2001) and those who seek to broaden what is considered evidence to a range of findings from diverse data (see Norcross 2011). These researchers point out that narrow conceptions of evidence usually include nongeneralizable samples in which patients lack the complexity usually experienced in psychotherapy practice (Westen and Morrison 2001). Another area of tension within psychotherapy research is the use of treatment manuals. Some researchers criticize manuals for promoting rigid therapies that do not respect either the complexity of the patient as an individual or therapy as a process unique to each patient-therapist dyad. These authors tend to espouse clinically based models of treatment that are difficult to study empirically because they are not manualized. An argument for manualizing a treatment, in addition to providing systematic guidelines for therapists, includes the fact that it makes it possible to demonstrate adherence to the model across therapists. Some applaud such efforts, saying they lead to clearer and more effective delivery of services, whereas others criticize this approach, saying that it ties the hands of the therapist. A moderate position sees evidence-based psychodynamic therapies as principle driven so that the therapist can use his or her best clinical judgment within the structure and principles of the therapy.

Psychotherapy research is a broad field. The most well-known studies to date involve randomized controlled trials designed to compare a model of treatment with a control to establish the efficacy of treatment. However, an emerging area of research investigates the impact of specific elements within a therapy. An example of this is Høglend et al.'s (2008) work that studied transference interpretations in contrast to interpretations that did not address the transference. His findings turned traditional clinical thinking, which posited that transference interpretations would work best with higher-functioning, "psychologically minded" patients, on its head: transference interpretations were found to have the greatest impact on patients who were at a lower level of self-other relatedness. This research supports the utility of thinking in terms of level of pathology and the implications for clinical practice. It also challenges the conventional wisdom that psychodynamic therapies are only helpful to those who are psychologically minded. It seems that in working with lower-level patients, basing interpretations on the experience shared by the patient and therapist can make tangible those aspects of the patient's psychological functioning that had previously been beyond his or her grasp. Further research is consistent with Høglend et al.'s findings in that transference-focused psychotherapy (TFP), a transference-based psychotherapy described below (see subsection "Object Relations Theory"), was found to be particularly good for patients with low mentalizing capacities as compared with dialectical behavior therapy (DBT) or supportive psychotherapy (Levy et al. 2012).

In this chapter, as we explore different psychodynamic models in terms of their understanding of PDs and then describe the application of these models in treatment, we emphasize those therapies that have an evidence base. The psychodynamic literature has historically focused more on describing the underlying dynamics of PDs than on describing treatment techniques in a detailed and methodical way. This tendency has begun to change with the introduction of manualized treatments. Traditionally, as in classical psychoanalysis, psychodynamic therapists tended to follow the patient's associations, keeping the treatment open-ended, with little attention to specific diagnosis, specific treatment goals, or any sense of a treatment plan. Early psychodynamic literature often assumed that the therapist could use the psychoanalytic method of free association and interpretation to achieve an understanding of the unconscious conflicts in a patient with a given PD that would bring about symptomatic change. However, psychodynamic therapists and analysts who treat patients with severe character pathology have increasingly realized that effective treatment of PDs requires specific treatment modifications of general analytic technique. The trend of a more precise focus on technique and the development of treatment manuals began with the detailed description of psychodynamic treatments for patients with interpersonal difficulties (Luborsky 1984; Strupp and Binder 1984) and recently has been expanded with descriptions of psychodynamic treatments for those with severe PDs (Bateman and Fonagy 2012; Caligor et al. 2018; Choi-Kain and Gunderson 2019; Yeomans et al. 2015).

Psychoanalytic explorations of character pathology not only predate but also attempt to go beyond the descriptive focus on signs and symptoms of DSM-III (American Psychiatric Association 1980) and its successors. The AMPD in DSM-5 connects with some of this thinking. DSM-III started the trend of taking the American Psychiatric Association's diagnostic system away from a conceptual understanding of psychiatric illnesses toward one based on signs and symptoms, with the goal of increasing the reliability of diagnosis. However, a side effect of this approach has been to increase the number of personality disorder diagnoses per patient. From the phenomenological vantage point of DSM-IV, there are 10 different and supposedly distinct PDs. We do not think it is conceptually valid, however, to describe psychodynamic treatments for each of the 10 PDs as if they are separate and distinct. Many patients with PD who appear for evaluation have multiple PD diagnoses according to DSM-IV, and their functioning might be better conceptualized by considering the overall severity of their personality dysfunction as laid out in the AMPD and the research described above. In most cases, it is not clinically relevant to think of assessment and treatment for one of the 10 PDs as separate from the others. We will therefore consider how a psychodynamic therapy addresses the underlying psychological structures that subtend many of the PDs and their specific symptoms.

Psychodynamic Perspectives on the Nature of Personality Pathology

Psychoanalysis has spawned many branches. The psychodynamic models of psychological developments most relevant to the treatment of character pathology are 1) ego psychology, 2) object relations theory, and 3) attachment theory. These psychodynamic models can be contrasted with and complemented by other models of pathology, such as the cognitive, interpersonal, evolutionary, and neurocognitive models (Lenzenweger and Clarkin 2005). Psychodynamic approaches do not espouse a purely "psychological" understanding of psychopathology and do incorporate brain findings as research advances. Psychodynamic concepts such as affects and drives have a clear grounding in biology (Valzelli 1981). What distinguishes a psychodynamic approach is the further elaboration of mental functioning that focuses on both the conscious and unconscious meanings of experience as biological forces interact with interpersonal (social, cultural, and linguistic) influences. Beyond these commonalities, the various schools of psychodynamic thinking lend different emphases to libidinal/affiliative drives or to aggressive drives, to drives as a whole or to defenses, and to the role of conflict among intrapsychic forces in contrast to deficits in the development of psychic structures and psychological capacities. Most of these differences are not either/or debates but rather "degree of emphasis" debates.

Ego Psychology

Although the ego psychology school of psychoanalysis does not offer a specific model of therapy for personality disorders, its concepts are included, to some degree, in most applications of psychoanalytic techniques. Ego psychology stems directly from the Freudian "structural model" (Freud 1923/1961). In this model the id, ego, and superego are the key psychic structures that interact in ways that lead either to successful or to unsuccessful resolution of conflicts between competing forces in the mind. Unsuccessful resolution of these internal conflicts—for example, between an aggressive impulse and an internal prohibition against acting aggressively—can result in psychopathology such as anxiety, depressive affect, obsessive symptoms, or sexual inhibition. The id is seen as the seat of pleasure seeking and aggressive drives and strives for their immediate satisfaction. The ego is the more largely conscious system that mediates contact with the constraints of reality, involving perception and the use of reason, judgment, and other "ego functions." The ego also includes defense mechanisms, which are unconscious ways of attempting to resolve or deal with the anxiety stemming from the conflicts between the competing psychic agencies. Certain defense mechanisms are more mature and successful, whereas others are more primitive and provide a suboptimal decrease in anxiety and/or a reduction in anxiety that is at the expense of successful adaptation to life. If the defense mechanism is "mature"—as with humor or sublimation—the conflict may be dealt with in a way that does not interfere with the individual's functioning or feeling state. However, less mature, or neurotic, defense mechanisms, such as repression or reaction formation, tend to result in psychological symptoms, such as anxiety or impaired functioning, and related behaviors, such as compulsive behaviors. The most primitive defenses, such as splitting or projective identification, characterize the rigid and distortion-prone psychological structures found in severe PDs. Splitting involves internal dissociation of opposing aggressive and libidinal (affiliative and sexual) aspects of the mind that prevents the individual from achieving an integrated sense of self and leads to disruptive discontinuity in the patient's life experience. The superego is the largely unconscious set of rules (a combination of prohibitions and ideals) that often oppose the strivings of the id for unbridled drive satisfaction. Broadly speaking, ego psychology addresses the question of what are the individual's psychological resources—ego functions and defenses—for adapting to internal and external demands. It views character pathology as the result of the habitual use of maladaptive defense mechanisms, with corresponding problems in functioning such as impulsive behavior, poor affect control, and an impaired capacity for accurate self-reflection.

Object Relations Theory

With object relations theory, psychoanalysis transitioned from a one-person system concerned primarily with drive forces and prohibitions against them to a more complex system considering the drives in relation to their objects—that is, the object of the positive or negative affect related to the drive (Fairbairn 1952; Jacobson 1964; Kernberg 1980, 1995; Klein 1946/1975). Within this model, internalized representations of relationships are referred to as "object relation dyads." Each dyad constitutes a particular image of the self, as it experiences an affect connected to a libidinal or aggressive drive, in relation to a particular image of the other who is the object of that affect. An example is the contented, satisfied self in relation to a nurturing other linked by an affect of warmth and love. An opposite example is the abandoned self in relation to the neglectful other linked by an affect of fear and anger. In the course of development, opposing experiences of gratification or frustration with others are internalized, and these dyads, laid down as memory traces, become the building blocks of psychic structure that then influence the individual's perceptions of the world and, in particular, of relationships.

In normal psychological development, representations of self and others become increasingly differentiated and complex to better correspond to the individuality of real external objects (others) and become integrated so that they better match the complexity of real beings. These mature, integrated representations allow for the realistic blending of good and bad, positive and negative emotions, and the tolerance of ambivalence, difference, and contradiction in oneself and others. For Kernberg (1984), the degree of differentiation and integration of these representations of self and other determines the level of personality organization. He describes a range of PDs from neurotic to high-level borderline to low-level borderline. Borderline organization—which is a broader concept than the DSM-5 borderline PD but fits with the AMPD and the levels of severity—is a psychological structure based on simplistic representations of self and other divided into purely good and purely negative segments, in contrast to more integrated and complex representations of self and other that characterize healthier personality organization and better functioning in the world.

Given the fragmented nature of this psychological makeup, all personality disorders at the borderline organization are characterized by three features: 1) the use of primitive defense mechanisms (e.g., splitting, projective identification, dissociation), 2) identity diffusion (a fragmented and inconsistent view of self and others in contrast to a coherent one), and 3) generally intact but unstable reality testing (the risk of experiencing a situation in relation to an internal representation [e.g., the abandoning other] that does not accurately correspond to the real situation). This dimensional view of a borderline level of psychological organization includes the categories of paranoid, schizoid, schizotypal, borderline, narcissistic, antisocial, histrionic, and dependent PDs of DSM-5 Section II, as well as other categories of personality disorders not included in the DSM system: sadomasochistic, hypochondriacal, cyclothymic, and hypomanic (Kernberg 1996). In this system of classification, the obsessive-compulsive, hysterical, and depressive-masochistic PDs are considered to be at the more highly organized neurotic level; they are characterized by a more integrated sense of self and others, defense mechanisms based on repression rather than splitting, and accurate reality testing. This classification system has treatment implications: those PDs organized at the neurotic level may be treated by psychoanalysis or a modified psychoanalytic psychotherapy (Caligor et al. 2007, 2018), whereas those organized at a borderline level need a more structured form of psychodynamic therapy such as TFP (Clarkin et al. 2006; Yeomans et al. 2015) or mentalization-based therapy (MBT) (Bateman and Fonagy 2012).

To understand how psychic structure leads to symptoms, one can consider the primitive defense mechanisms that devolve from the split psychic structure: splitting, idealization-devaluation, primitive denial, projective identification, and omnipotent control. These defense mechanisms are attempts to wall off intense feelings, affects, and impulses that the individual has difficulty accepting in himself or herself. This walling off does not eliminate these feelings; instead it leads to dealing with them in ways that interfere with functioning. Since these feelings are not integrated into the conscious experience of self, the person with the disorder cannot make conscious decisions about how to manage these affects, in action or in fantasy. Without conscious awareness of these affects, the individual acts them out (puts the emotion into an action without being consciously aware of it) and/or projects them and sees them in others. For instance, because the split in the psyche prevents the integration of aggressive feelings and libidinal/affectionate feelings into a more complex whole, the individual may alternate abruptly between extremely positive and extremely negative feelings toward other people in his or her life: at one moment, the other is experienced as perfectly caring, and another moment, based on a "trigger event," the experience of the other could shift to the opposite: an uncaring and cruel other. This lack of integration of these feelings underlies the instability in interpersonal relations seen in many patients with PDs. An individual may also deal with split-off feelings by subtly inducing them in another person and then experiencing an awareness of them as though they originated in the other person (projective identification). This leads to chaos and confusion in relationships as well as in the ability to deal with one's own feelings. We return to concepts of object relations in discussing the specific therapies later in this chapter.

Attachment Theory

Attachment theory, first formulated by Bowlby (1969, 1973, 1980), emerged from the object relations tradition. However, in contrast to object relations theorists who retained much of Freud's emphasis on sexual and aggressive drives and fantasies, Bowlby stressed the centrality of the affective bond developed in close interpersonal relationships. Although this perspective has led to much interesting developmental and clinical work, it has emphasized the importance of the attachment system with little attention to the other main motivational systems, such as the sexual and assertive/aggressive systems. Although Bowlby's work fell within the framework of psychoanalysis, he also turned to other scientific disciplines, including ethology, cognitive psychology, and developmental psychology, to explain affectional bonding between infants and their caregivers and the long-term effects of early attachment experiences on personality development and psychopathology.

Central to attachment theory is the concept of internal working models (IWMs) of attachment, or mental representations that are formed through repeated transactions with attachment figures (Bretherton 1987; Shaver et al. 1996). These working models subsequently act as heuristic guides in relationships, organizing personality development and the regulation of affect. They include expectations, beliefs, emotional appraisals, and rules for processing or excluding information. These IWMs are partly conscious and partly unconscious and need not be completely consistent or coherent. The reader may be reminded of the concept of the object relations dyad discussed above; indeed, the similarities speak to underlying conceptual similarities between object relations theory and attachment theory. For instance, although Bowlby (1973) stressed that IWMs "are tolerably accurate reflections of the experiences those individuals actually had" (p. 20), he also realized that these models could be distorted, as Kernberg emphasized in arguing for the centrality of transference interpretation, in which the internal relational model (whether it is considered an object relations dyad or an IWM) can be observed and reflected on as it is activated in the interaction with the therapist. Moreover, both object relations dyads and IWMs include representations of self and others that are complementary and mutually confirming and include unconscious and emotional aspects of representation. Both theories note that these representations need not be consistent or coherent and that, to the degree that multiple inconsistent representations exist, the individual will have difficulty behaving consistently. Both Kernberg and Bowlby note that these multiple and inconsistent representations could oscillate in the individual's consciousness. Finally, both authors discuss defensive processes for excluding representational information that is difficult to integrate with conscious representations of self and others; Kernberg (1984) called this *splitting*, whereas Bowlby referred to this process as *defensive exclusion*.

Bowlby (1973) postulated that insecure attachment lies at the center of disordered personality traits, and he tied the overt expression of felt insecurity to specific characterological disorders. For instance, he connected anxious ambivalent attachment to "a tendency to make excessive demands on others and to be anxious and clingy when they are not met, such as is present in dependent and hysterical personalities," and avoidant attachment to "a blockage in the capacity to make deep relationships, such as is present in affectionless and psychopathic personalities" (Bowlby 1973, p. 14). Many of the symptoms of borderline PD, such as the unstable, intense interpersonal relationships, feelings of emptiness, chronic fears of abandonment, and intolerance of aloneness, have been reinterpreted as sequelae of insecure internal working models of attachment (Blatt and Levy 2003; Diamond et al. 1999; Fonagy et al. 1995; Gunderson 1996; Levy and Blatt 1999).

The work of Fonagy and colleagues (Fonagy et al. 1995, 2003) has elaborated on attachment theory and led to the development of MBT for borderline PD. *Mentalization*, defined as the capacity to think about mental states in oneself and in others, is seen as a form of social cognition—that is, an imaginative mental activity that enables one to perceive and interpret human behavior in terms of intentional mental states, such as needs, desires, feelings, and goals (Bateman and Fonagy 2012). Fonagy and colleagues' developmental research suggests that the capacity for reflective awareness in a child's caregiver increases the likelihood of the child's secure attachment, which in turn facilitates the development of mentalization in the child. The authors proposed that a secure attachment relationship with the caregiver gives the child a chance to explore his or her own mind and the mind of the caregiver. The caregiver's reflective awareness—having the child's mind in mind—contributes to the child's understanding of himself or herself as a thinker. This model includes a fundamental hypothesis of the relationship between PDs and childhood abuse. Individuals who experience early trauma may defensively inhibit their capacity to mentalize to avoid having to think about their caregiver's harmfulness toward them. This inhibition of mentalizing is associated with an absence of adequate symbolic representations of affects and self-states and creates a subjective experience of internal chaos typical of severe PDs, with consequent difficulties in managing affects.

Failures to mentalize are seen as underlying the characteristics of borderline PD and also as central to other PDs and other types of psychopathology. In cases of maltreatment, the child internalizes the self-directed attitudes of the abusive attachment figure into the child's own self-structure. In such a case, however, the internalized other and its aggressive characteristics remain alien and unconnected to the rest of the self; the self is "colonized" by an aggressive element that is not actually a part of the self. Although lodged within the self, this "alien self" is projected outside—both because it does not match the rest of the self and because of its persecutory nature. This projection and the attempt to control the object of the projection are seen as the basis for many symptoms of borderline PD.

Fonagy and colleagues (2012) have expanded their concept of mentalization along four functional spectra that can be considered in evaluating and treating patients: 1) automatic (reflexive and implicit) to controlled (explicit, reflective) mentalizing, 2) internally focused to externally focused, 3) self oriented to other oriented, and 4) cognitive processing to affective processing.

Indications for Psychodynamic Treatment

In general, patients with the less severe PDs, such as obsessive-compulsive, hysterical, avoidant, and dependent, are suited for psychoanalytic or general psychodynamic treatment (Caligor et al. 2009, 2018; Gabbard 2005, 2014). These patients would be seen as having neurotically organized personalities, as compared with patients who have the more severe PDs with borderline organization (Kernberg 1984). Neurotic psychological organization involves a generally coherent and integrated sense of self, but with a consistently rigid repressive defensive system that does not allow for adequate integration of an element of psychological life, such as aggressive affects in the case of obsessive-compulsive PD or sexual affects in the case of hysterical PD. The decision of whether to recommend psychoanalysis or psychodynamic therapy for these disorders depends on a number of factors. One consideration is the patient's motivation for deep change influencing all areas of his or her life versus seeking more specific relief from anxiety or resolution of problems in specific areas. Other considerations include psychological mindedness,[1] propensity to regress without becoming disorganized, impulse control, frustration tolerance, and financial resources.

Patients with the more severe PDs are seen by some researchers (Bateman and Fonagy 2012; Clarkin et al. 2006; Kernberg 1984) as potentially responsive to modified, more highly structured, empirically based psychodynamic treatments (Bateman and Fonagy 1999, 2001; Clarkin et al. 2007; Levy et al. 2006). In parallel to the development of these manualized treatments, psychoanalytic practice in general is broadening to incorporate modifications in technique to work more effectively with this patient population. Kernberg (1984) cautioned, however, that borderline patients with a high level of narcissistic, paranoid, and antisocial traits, a syndrome termed *malignant narcissism*, are the most challenging to treat, and that even with a highly structured treat-

---

[1]Assessing patients for psychological mindedness may require a period of working with the patient, because apparent lack of these capacities may serve as an initial defense against insight and may change with interpretation.

ment these patients have a poorer prognosis than other patients with personality organized at the borderline level. Patients with antisocial PD (those with no capacity for remorse or for nonexploitative relationships) may be beyond the reach of psychodynamic, or any, psychotherapy.

Across the spectrum of the PDs, psychodynamic clinicians utilize nondiagnostic patient variables as indicators of psychodynamic treatment. In general, the presence and capacity for meaningful relationships and attachments to others, investment in work at the level of one's capacities and training, normal intelligence or higher, the capacity to reflect on one's experience, relatively good impulse control, absence of secondary gain of illness (i.e., lack of practical illness-related benefits such as disability payments or extra attention), and intact reality testing would be good prognostic signs for psychodynamic psychotherapy (Gabbard 2014). Lack of meaningful relations or investment in work, presence of secondary gain, and impaired impulse control or reality testing are not contraindications to psychodynamic therapy but rather require more work in establishing adequate conditions for carrying out the therapy and in monitoring the therapy's progress to avoid slipping into an endless process of supporting secondary gain of illness. Nonetheless, patients with low intelligence, those who lack psychological mindedness (in contrast to defensive nonreflectiveness), and those who will not give up secondary gain of illness may be referred to psychodynamically informed supportive treatment (Rockland 1992) in contrast to a more exploratory one.

Psychodynamic Treatments of Personality Disorders

We described the principal psychodynamic models of personality pathology earlier in this chapter in the order of their historical development. In this section, we describe both some specific treatments that have derived from these models and the more eclectic models of therapy. The most fully articulated treatments include a clinical description of the pathology, a treatment manual, and empirical research. Psychodynamic thinking about treating character pathology has historically centered on narcissistic (Kernberg 1984; Kohut 1971), borderline (Fonagy et al. 1995, 2003; Gunderson 1984; Kernberg 1980, 1984), hysterical (Kernberg 1980; Zetzel 1968), obsessive-compulsive (Reich 1972), and schizoid (Fairbairn 1952) character pathology. Others (e.g., Gabbard 2014) have more specifically addressed the individual PDs as defined by DSM-IV, sometimes gearing treatment techniques to the Cluster A, B, and C groupings of the disorders. At present, there are an increasing number of studies of psychotherapy for PDs, along with a long-standing history of case reports and a number of uncontrolled trials, all contributing to the evidence for the effectiveness of psychodynamic therapy (Abbass et al. 2014; American Psychiatric Association 2001; Leichsenring and Leibling 2003; Leichsenring and Rabung 2008; Levy et al. 2012; Shedler 2010).

It does not make sense to address treatment of all the specific DSM-5 PD diagnoses separately, because most research to date has focused on a mix of PDs, avoidant PD, or borderline BD, and because, as mentioned in the introduction to this chapter, there is extensive co-occurrence among DSM personality categories. Therefore, the therapist should have an understanding both of the basic psychological structure that underlies severe PDs as reflected in the AMPD's discussion of sense of self and quality of relations with others as core axes underlying the PDs and of the particular dynamic issues that distinguish the different disorders.

Waldinger (1987) described a set of common characteristics of dynamic therapies for patients with borderline PD, beyond the fundamental characteristics of dynamic therapies in general that were listed in the introduction to this chapter. Waldinger's list, which generalizes to those PDs with borderline organization or Cluster B disorders other than antisocial PD, includes the following characteristics: 1) emphasis on the stability of the frame of the treatment; 2) increase in the therapist's participation during sessions as compared with therapy with neurotic patients; 3) tolerance of the patient's hostility as manifested in the negative transference; 4) use of clarification and confrontation to discourage self-destructive behaviors and render them ego-dystonic and ungratifying; 5) use of interpretation to help the patient establish bridges between actions and feelings; 6) blocking of acting-out behaviors by setting limits on actions that endanger the patient, others, or the treatment; 7) focusing early therapeutic work and interpretations on the here and now rather than on material from the past; and 8) careful monitoring of countertransference feelings.

Taking into account these common modifications to general psychodynamic technique, we review below how different specific models address the treatment of PDs. While we discuss these models separately, in practice many therapists use their clinical judgment to combine elements of the different models.

Transference-Focused Psychotherapy

Among object relations models of therapy (Gabbard 2014; Strupp and Binder 1984), TFP is the most fully elaborated (Clarkin et al. 2006; Yeomans et al. 2002) and evidence based (Clarkin et al. 2007; Doering et al. 2010; Levy et al. 2006). TFP combines an emphasis on the structure of the treatment, established through the contracting process, with the exploration of the patient's internal world of representations of self and others.

The goal of TFP is to help patients with severe PDs change from a state of identity diffusion to a coherent identity, a process that involves increased reflective functioning and is accompanied by improved modulation of affects. The therapist focuses on the patient's principal contradictory representations of self and of others as they unfold in the transference and helps the patient become more consciously aware of these representations in order to then integrate them. Because patients with character pathology have chronic difficulties in tolerating their emotions in the context of relationships with others, including with the therapist, this model emphasizes the need for a clear understanding of the conditions of treatment to be established between therapist and patient before beginning the actual therapy. The verbal contract is the foundation for containing acting out, for communicating that feelings can be contained and experienced in contrast to being acted out, and for observing and interpreting the patient's interactions within a clear frame, since a patient's reaction to the treatment frame generally provides a window into his or her personality structure (characteristic way of experiencing self in relation to others).

This twice-weekly individual therapy emphasizes the therapist's empathy with the entire range of the patient's affective responses, including negative affects as they inevitably arise in the transference, with the implicit message that even the most intense and disturbing affects can be contained and reflected on. Addressing the negative transference early on is felt to create a fuller alliance with the patient by indicating that the therapist can tolerate, and help the patient tolerate, the expression of the patient's most difficult internal states in order to move on to helping integrate them with the aid of the interpretive process.

Mutative Techniques

TFP advocates early interpretation of transference as the patient stabilizes in the treatment frame. This involves elaborating the patient's experience of the therapist at different moments as it is distorted by the patient's internal representations, encouraging reflection on those experiences and the associated representations, and helping the patient develop internal representations that are richer, more nuanced, and more flexible in their ability to adapt to shifting external realities (Caligor et al. 2009). This strategy focuses on the affect experienced in the here and now with the therapist in contrast to early interpretation of the patient's past, because clinical experience has shown that interpretations have more impact when they are made in the context of the actual experience of conflict-based affects.

Transference interpretation is a process. The ground for it is set by clarification of the patient's feeling states—that is, by helping the patient symbolically and cognitively represent or describe his experience of self in relation to the therapist. The work then helps the patient observe that forms of acting out represent identifications with parts of himself—usually of an aggressive nature, but sometimes of a loving nature—that the patient sees in others but typically does not accept in himself. The therapy moves on to explore contradictions in the patient's presentation over time. These contradictions are considered reflections of the split, unintegrated internal world underlying borderline pathology that keeps positive and negative representations of self, and of others, separate. The therapist brings these contradictory dyads more fully into the patient's awareness and explores the unconscious motivations for keeping distinctly different, often opposite, dyads separated. Key moments in therapy occur when the patient becomes aware of an aspect of himself that, up to now, he had only expressed in behavior, with no awareness, and/or has projected and seen in others.

For example, when a patient was vigorously accusing and verbally attacking her therapist for being both neglectful and useless because she still experienced unfair rejection and criticism from her classmates, the therapist said, "I understand the conviction in what you're saying, but I wonder if you could take a step back and reflect on what is going on here right now." The patient paused and acknowledged that she might seem as if she were being "mean and critical" to the therapist in a way that had similarities to her experience of her classmates' behavior toward her. The therapist pointed out that the patient had every right to be critical, and even mean, if she chose to, but that she appeared to not see this aspect of herself and to see such things as coming only from others. He added that two things might happen if the patient were aware of these feelings in herself: first, she might find ways to express them in a healthier way, and second, she might be in a better position to see her contribution to difficult relations that she tended to experience as always originating in the other party. However, the therapist also expressed empathy with the fact that gaining this awareness would be a painful step. The working through of a theme such as this consists of repeatedly analyzing the dyads that appear first in the transference and then analyzing them as they appear in the patient's life outside the therapy and in the patient's past.

Mechanisms of Change

Change comes first from the therapist's capacity to contain intense affects that the patient has generally not been able to tolerate consciously. This requires awareness and containment of the therapist's countertransference. In addition, change comes both from interpretations that increase the patient's awareness of aspects of himself or herself that are split off and projected onto others and from the patient's eventual ability to experience the relationship with the therapist as different from his or her prior "repertoire" of relations and to generalize this more full-bodied experience of self and other to relationships outside the therapeutic setting.

Research has shown that, in addition to symptom change (improvement in depression, anxiety, and social functioning; decrease in suicide attempts, hospitalizations, and aggression), TFP has thus far been unique in its association with improved mentalization/reflective functioning, attachment security, and narrative coherence in patients (Clarkin et al. 2007; Doering et al. 2010; Levy et al. 2006).

Mentalization-Based Therapy

MBT, rooted in attachment theory, has been developed for Cluster B PDs; it was initially practiced as a day hospital treatment and generally combines individual sessions with group sessions. MBT was developed as a basic model of therapy to be delivered largely by nurse therapists in the U.K. National Health Service and does not aim to achieve structural personality change or to alter cognitions and schemas. Rather, its goal is to enhance mentalization so that the individual is more equipped to solve problems and manage emotional states, especially mental states stimulated in interpersonal situations (Bateman and Fonagy 2012).

The emotional instability of Cluster B disorders is seen as secondary to failures in an individual's capacity to *mentalize*—to reflect on and appreciate intentions, feelings, and motivations in self and others. It is the role of psychotherapy to challenge automatic, distorted, and simplistic assumptions about self and others and to reflect and reevaluate the assumptions in the context of the relationship between therapist and patient. In this sense, MBT shares TFP's focus on helping the patient achieve accurate, in contrast to inaccurate or distorted perceptions of self and others. However, MBT restricts its emphasis to helping the patient repair failures in mentalizing without addressing the resolution of intrapsychic conflicts, and therefore can be situated toward the cognitive end of the spectrum on psychodynamic therapies.

Failures in mentalization are believed to be related to attunement difficulties between infant and caretaker that impede the development of a secure sense of attachment. The therapist's efforts to increase the patient's capacity to mentalize help the patient move from a disorganized attachment, in which affects are volatile and unpredictable and the patient's subjectivity is vulnerable to collapse, toward a more secure attachment in which the experience of affects is less capricious and more stable. Identifying and fostering appropriate expression of affect is integral to this process. Within the range of affects, anger and aggression are seen as responses to neglect and abuse rather than primary affects that eventually need to be integrated into the self as part of treatment.

Central to the MBT process, especially with borderline patients who are seen as readily destabilized in their attachment relationships, is the ability of the therapist to titrate the shifting attachment process between therapist and patient so that the level of emotional arousal in the patient is modulated without destabilizing intensity. Contrary moves are used by the therapist so that, for example, if the patient is internally focused and self focused, the therapist inquires about how such mentation or action would affect others. A sequence of intervention is suggested, progressing from supportive and empathic clarification (i.e., clarifying the patient's perception of self in relation to others) to challenge (i.e., not to confront but to question the patient's perception) to affect focus (i.e., focus on the current affect shared by patient and therapist) to mentalizing the transference (Bateman and Fonagy 2012). *Mentalizing the transference* refers to a collaborative process of exploring alternative perspectives on the current patient-therapist relationship, seeing this as a rehearsal of mentalizing ability in other intimate relationships in the patient's life.

Mutative Techniques

The MBT technique centers on identifying moments when mentalization is lost and the patient reverts to thinking in terms of psychic equivalency, pretend mode, or teleological mode. The therapist rewinds to the moment before the break, focusing on the momentary affects between patient and therapist (e.g., love, desire, hurt, catastrophe, excitement), slowly clarifying and naming the affects, and including identification of the therapist's contribution to the break. The focus remains on the mind rather than behavior, relating affects to the current event or activity and the "mental reality," using the therapist's mind as a model, with the option of disclosure. The work may include the therapist's accepting to "hold," through projection and countertransference, aspects of the alien self (described earlier in this chapter in the attachment theory subsection of "Psychodynamic Perspectives on the Nature of Personality Pathology") so that elements of the patient's mind can be better reflected on as perceived in the therapist. Throughout the process, the therapist uses concise "sound-bite" interventions, in contrast to any lengthy interpretation, because of the patient's current absence of symbolic representation of affects (and consequent difficulty taking in interpretations) and to avoid intellectualization.

Mechanisms of Change

The mechanism of therapeutic action in MBT is based on developing the patient's ability to have an awareness of mental states and thus find meaning in his or her own and other people's behavior. Transference interpretations are avoided because of concern that 1) they excessively activate the attachment system (arouse affect to levels that interfere with cognition), and 2) direct transference interpretation, it is believed, is at too high a level of abstraction for patients with borderline PD to understand. Bateman and Fonagy (2012) therefore recommend using "transference tracers"—that is, comments that predict likely future action on the basis of the patient's previous experience in a way that heightens the patient's ability to begin to see transference patterns as they occur in the here-and-now interaction. A difference between this approach and the TFP approach described above is that the MBT therapist might complete the therapy without bringing elements of the patient's mind that are projected onto the therapist back to the patient, since the aggressive elements in the interaction are not seen as a part of the patient's mind, but rather as "alien" elements.

The core of the work in MBT is helping patients understand their emotional reactions in the context of the treatment relationship. The patient is urged to "rewind" and consider who engendered the feeling that is being experienced in the moment and how, and to ask: "What feeling may I have engendered in someone else, even if I am not conscious of it, that may have made him behave that way toward me?" An important part of this is focusing the patient's attention on the therapist's experience, with the goal of the exploration of a mind by a mind within an interpersonal context. This involves "mental closeness" in the sense of representing accurately the feeling state of the patient and its accompanying internal representations, distinguishing the state of mind of self and other, and helping the patient appreciate this distinction.

A clinical example of MBT involves a patient who came into a session looking agitated and frightened and remained silent. The therapist proposed, "You appear to see me as frightening today." The patient replied, in a challenging way, "What makes you say that?" The therapist provided the immediate evidence: "You had your head down and avoided looking at me." The patient responded, "Well, I thought that you were cross with me." The therapist then proposed to explore a bit more deeply within the patient: "I am not aware of being cross with you, so it may help if we think about why you were concerned that I was" (Bateman and Fonagy 2003, pp. 198–199). This maps to a certain degree to the work that would be done in TFP. However, the TFP model of treatment would put emphasis on the likelihood that the patient's perceiving the therapist as "cross" would not only be a misreading of the therapist but also include a projection of the patient's own unacknowledged aggressive feelings.

The strength of the MBT approach is implied by impressive outcome data, both at the end of treatment and on long-term follow-up (Bateman and Fonagy 1999, 2001). The ability of MBT to reduce symptoms, and the maintenance of that symptom reduction, would be better understood with research data showing an increase in aspects of mentalization as related to symptom change in treatment.

Supportive-Expressive and Eclectic Therapies

A number of psychodynamic-based treatments for PDs have been developed, some with an evidence base and some based on clinical experience. The most widely practiced version of psychodynamic psychotherapy of PDs is probably expressive-supportive therapy (Gabbard 2014; Gunderson and Links 2008; Luborsky 1984). Other treatment modalities that have been studied include Russell Meares' interpersonal–self-psychological approach (also known as the conversational approach) and Robert Gregory's deconstructive dynamic psychotherapy (DDP; Gregory et al. 2008). In addition, Anthony Ryle's cognitive analytic therapy (CAT; Ryle 1997) and John Gunderson's good psychiatric management (GPM; Choi-Kain and Gunderson 2019) (see also Chapter 15 in this volume) can be considered strongly influenced by psychodynamic theory.

Types of Supportive-Expressive and Eclectic Therapies

Expressive-supportive therapy. Wallerstein (1986), in analyzing the Menninger Foundation Psychotherapy Research Project, concluded that most therapy included a mix of the more formal elements of psychoanalysis, termed *expressive* (e.g., the therapist's neutrality and use of interpretation, with the goal of helping the patient become more aware of internal conflicts and resolving them to become more integrated, harmonious, and effective), and elements described as *supportive* (e.g., the therapist at times supporting rather than interpreting the patient's current defenses so that the patient makes more effective use of coping skills and relies on the healthier in contrast to the more primitive of the defenses within his or her repertoire). *Supportive-expressive therapy* refers to an eclectic therapeutic stance of selecting interventions from any of the more specific theoretical models according to what seems to be the best fit with a given patient at a given moment in the treatment. Therapeutic goals can vary from more analytic (e.g., helping the patient to gain insight and achieve resolution of internal psychological conflict, increase the cohesiveness of the self, and improve the quality of interpersonal relationships) to more supportive (e.g., helping the patient to adapt to stresses while not directly addressing the split psychological structure that underlies severe PDs). This form of therapy proposes the "expressive-supportive continuum of interventions" (Gabbard 2014). Moving from the supportive to the expressive end, this continuum includes affirmation, giving advice and praise, empathic validation, encouragement to elaborate, clarification, confrontation, and interpretation.

The expressive-supportive approach allows the therapist to modulate between more analytic exploration and more supportive involvement according to what he or she feels will be tolerated by and helpful for the patient in the moment. A risk, however, is that the therapist may unconsciously collude with the patient in avoiding certain "hot" areas by shifting from an analytic focus to a supportive one when that area comes up. Awareness of this risk, and appropriate supervision, are the best guarantees against this collusion. Supportive-expressive therapy emphasizes establishing a positive therapeutic alliance as the sine qua non of the therapeutic process, a view that is supported by research (Luborsky et al. 1980). Therefore, the central task, especially early in therapy, is primarily supportive and relationship-building, with the fostering of positive or even idealizing aspects of the transference (Buie and Adler 1982). Alliance building takes precedence over focusing on the contract and conditions of treatment out of concern that an emphasis on these latter areas might elicit negative transference or too quickly challenge the patient's defenses. Luborsky's (1984) manual for expressive-supportive therapy summarizes many aspects of the treatment. (See also Chapter 11, "Therapeutic Alliance," in this volume for a full discussion of this topic.)

Interpersonal–self-psychological approach.   Meares developed an interpersonal–self-psychological approach for the treatment of BPD guided by the Conversational Model (CM) of Hobson (1985) (also referred to as a psychodynamic interpersonal therapy [Guthrie 1999]), whose main aim is to foster the emergence of reflective consciousness that William James called *self-consciousness* (James 1890). A basic tenet of this approach is that self-consciousness is achieved through a particular form of conversation and reflects a deeper sense of relatedness. In a pre-post study that evaluated the effects of a non-manualized psychodynamic treatment for patients with BPD (Stevenson and Meares 1992), the authors found that compared to before therapy, patients at the end of treatment showed an increase in time in active employment and decreases in number of medical visits, number of self-harm episodes, and number and length of hospitalizations. In a later quasi-experimental study (Meares et al. 1999), researchers compared BPD patients treated twice weekly for 1 year with those in a treatment-as-usual wait-list control group (all waitlisted patients received their usual treatments, which consisted of supportive psychotherapy, crisis intervention only, cognitive therapy, and pharmacotherapy). Thirty percent of patients with interpersonal-psychodynamic psychotherapy no longer had symptoms that met criteria for a DSM-III (American Psychiatric Association 1980) BPD diagnosis at the end of the treatment year, whereas all of the patients receiving treatment as usual still had symptoms that met criteria for the diagnosis. These results demonstrated that psychotherapy based on psychodynamic principles is generally beneficial to patients with BPD in a naturalistic setting, having strong ecological validity in a real-world setting. A 5-year follow-up found that the improvements were maintained (Stevenson et al. 2005). A second quasi-experimental study (Korner et al. 2006) replicated these findings. A recently completed dissertation presented findings from a randomized controlled trial (RCT) comparing DBT with the CM. It found that both treatments resulted in significant improvements over a 14-month period, with no differences between treatment models (Walton 2019).

Dynamic deconstructive psychotherapy.   DDP (Gregory and Remen 2008) is a 1-year psychodynamic treatment package that addresses three neurocognitive functions distorted in individuals with BPD: *attribution* (thoughts of value or motive assigned to people and behaviors), *association* (linking symbols or language to experiences or physical characteristics), and *alterity* (the ability to realistically and objectively view the world and others accurately as separate from the self). DDP has shown efficacy for comorbid BPD and substance use disorders, which is a common but severe and refractory condition (Gregory et al. 2008). In a 12-month RCT with 30-month follow-up, DDP was compared with optimized community care—a high-intensity community treatment. DDP resulted in significant reductions in suicide attempts and self-harm, drug use, and multiple measures of psychopathology, including depression, dissociation, BPD symptoms, and perceived lack of social support (Gregory et al. 2008, 2010). In two secondary analyses, therapists' adherence to dynamic deconstructive psychotherapy techniques was highly correlated with outcome (Goldman and Gregory 2009, 2010), which suggests that the putative mechanisms of the treatment were responsible for the improvements. Findings were maintained at 18-month and 30-month follow-ups (Gregory et al. 2010). Additionally, in a naturalistic comparison with DBT and an unstructured psychotherapy control, both DBT and DDP showed significant reductions in symptoms of BPD and depression and in disability; however, DDP obtained better overall outcome than DBT.

Cognitive analytic therapy.   CAT is an integrative relational-based, time-limited psychotherapy for BPD developed by Anthony Ryle (1997) in the context of the U.K.'s National Health Service. CAT combines psychoanalytic theory with cognitive therapy–like exercises. These exercises are geared to the explication of characteristic ways of perceiving the self, other, and ways of interacting with others with a particular focus on triggers of vacillating "self-states" seen in BPD. CAT is increasingly popular in the United Kingdom and, although initially developed for BPD, has been applied to a range of disorders. CAT has been evaluated in a number of open pre-post studies (Kellett et al. 2013; Ryle and Golynkina 2000; Wildgoose et al. 2001) with adults and one RCT with adolescents (Chanen et al. 2008), in which it was shown to have comparable outcome to TAU (Chanen et al. 2008). Further research is needed to determine if CAT is a reliable, effective treatment for BPD and comparable to other BPD treatments.

Good psychiatric management (GPM). GPM for BPD (Choi-Kain and Gunderson 2019; Gunderson and Links 2014) was developed as a general basic pragmatic treatment based on established principles in the treatment of BPD patients that can be offered as a "first line" treatment to patients who do not have access to one of the more fully developed specialized treatments described above. Gunderson stated that the goals of GPM are generally less ambitious than those other treatments but that its role is to provide a basic training in good therapy for BPD patients to a broad base of practitioners (Gunderson 2016). GPM is based on a model of interpersonal hypersensitivity rooted in Bowlby's attachment theory, in which a patient is subject to an ongoing cycle that starts with a state of fragile connectedness, moving to a state of feeling threatened due to perceptions of external rejection by others, proceeding to states of aloneness and then despair if support is not forthcoming. Support only helps the patient re-achieve the state of fragile connectedness, leading to repeated cycling into feeling threatened, alone, and in despair. GPM has evolved into a more eclectic model that includes diagnostic disclosure, psychoeducation, overt support, the provision of skills, family involvement, treatment goals (prioritizing work over love), use of case management interventions, collaboration, and an expectation of progress. Although GPM includes these aspects of a variety of therapy orientations, the central focus on interpersonal hypersensitivity, based strongly on an attachment theory perspective, as well as other dynamic principles such as interpretation of anger and acting out and on mentalizing, situates it as a psychodynamic treatment. (See also Chapter 15, "Good Psychiatric Management: Generalist Treatments and Stepped Care for Borderline Personality Disorder," in this volume.)

The fact that many of the elements of GPM are present to some degree in other psychodynamic models (e.g., TFP, MBT) as well as nondynamic models (e.g., DBT) reflects a convergence of views within the community of PD specialists regarding the value of these interventions. The differences between the models consists, to some degree, in the relative emphasis given to each element. For example, GPM includes providing direct support and encouragement, while TFP involves maintaining a stance of "concerned neutrality" in which the therapist does not offer overt support because of the idea that a more neutral therapeutic setting will allow for the emergence of the negative affects (negative transference) that need to be aired, explored, and ultimately integrated into the patient's sense of self. We can consider GPM and TFP as providing a spectrum of psychodynamically informed treatment, from the more supportive end (GPM) to the more deeply exploratory end (TFP), with some overlap in interventions with patients.

GPM served as an active and credible control in an RCT examining the efficacy of DBT. In that trial, no between-group differences were found across a broad range of outcomes at end of treatment (12 months) and at 24 months postdischarge (McMain et al. 2009, 2012). The version of GPM used in that study was a once-weekly individual psychodynamic psychotherapy based on the writings of Gunderson (Gunderson and Links 2008). GPM has evolved since that original research trial to the more general frontline approach described above, with more flexibility, as, for example, in allowing the therapist to vary the frequency of sessions.

Mutative Techniques

Depending on the relative expressiveness versus supportiveness of the eclectic therapy, the therapist would either directly offer interpretations to the patient (these could address the transference, defenses, impulses, and/or the patient's past) or use the therapist's own awareness to guide an understanding of the patient while avoiding interpretation. Similarly, the therapist can choose between a more expressive approach to resistance—exploring unconscious material by interpreting and helping the patient understand the function of the resistance—and a supportive approach—bolstering resistance to disturbing material in the service of reinforcing weak defensive structures in the patient.

The supportive-expressive therapist gears interventions to the particular defensive structure of the patient. For instance, in treating a patient with paranoid PD, the therapist would be informed by an awareness of the patient's tendency to perceive attack from the therapist and thus to evoke the therapist's defensive responses (Gabbard 2014). Resisting these responses, the expressive psychodynamic therapist would leave the patient's suspicious accusations and projections "hanging," neither denying nor interpreting them. In this way, the projections of hatred and badness are contained by the therapist. The hope is that as this lack of defensiveness, combined with empathy for the patient's subjective state, creates a sense of alliance, the patient will become more open and revealing. In this process, the therapist helps the patient label feelings and distinguish better between internal emotions and reality (Meissner 1976). A more supportive intervention would involve guiding the patient's perceptions of reality by questioning his or her assumptions. ("You assumed when your friend didn't wave back from the other side of the theater that he was trying to avoid you. But are you sure that he saw you in that crowd?")

The fact that the therapist does not respond in the way anticipated, and provoked, by the patient is meant to lead the patient to a "creative doubt" (Meissner 1986) about the way the patient perceives the world. This questioning of his or her own way of thinking will help the patient develop a better capacity to accurately reflect on and perceive himself or herself in relation to others.

Mechanisms of Change

The traditional psychoanalytic principle of bringing subconscious aspects of the patient's mind into consciousness still holds. However, the expressive-supportive model emphasizes both the role of increasing the patient's understanding through interpretation and the role of the experience of a new type of relationship with the therapist as mechanisms of change. Another way to consider supportive-expressive therapy is that it promotes the therapist's independence to delve into the toolbox of the common factors of therapy elements and techniques. GPM is explicit in encouraging the therapist to be guided by what seems best in the moment rather than by an over-arching goal, such as integration of a split internal psychological structure. Judging what is the best combination for a given patient requires great skill at assessing the person's level of personality pathology in order to determine what degree of deep change and improvement versus stabilization at the current level of psychological structure can be expected.

Conclusion

Psychodynamic therapies stem from a long tradition of addressing understanding and treatment of PDs. Psychodynamic models differ in certain areas, such as the degree to which PDs are considered the result of intrapsychic conflict or of a deficit in psychic structure or self-structure. These differences reflect a number of issues, including the model's underlying conceptualization of personality and personality pathology, the modal level of pathology targeted by the particular treatment model, and the level of training that is feasible in a given health care delivery system. According to a model's position on these issues, the technical approach may put more emphasis on exploration and interpretation versus overt empathy and support. Nevertheless, it is important to keep in mind a common theme: the individual's biological temperament, in combination with aspects of development, can create a psychic structure—especially in terms of experience of and reactions to self and others—that does not adapt well to dealing with the complexities of the real world in ways that involve aspects of the person that are unconscious to him or her. Psychodynamic therapy can provide the tools to help the individual integrate or enrich that psychic structure and thereby replace failure and frustration in life with a realistic measure of satisfaction and achievement. Psychodynamic therapies will continue to evolve and enrich each other as clinical experience and research provide us with more knowledge about the brain, the creation of subjectivity in the mind, interpersonal processes, and social cognition.

References

Abbass AA, Kisely SR, Town JM, et al: Short-term psychodynamic psychotherapies for common mental disorders. Cochrane Database Syst Rev (7):CD004687, 2014

Ablon JS, Jones EE: Validity of controlled clinical trials of psychotherapy: findings from the NIMH Treatment of Depression Collaborative Research Program. Am J Psychiatry 159:775–783, 2002

American Psychiatric Association: Diagnostic and Statistical Manual of Mental Disorders, 3rd Edition. Washington, DC, American Psychiatric Association, 1980

American Psychiatric Association: Diagnostic and Statistical Manual of Mental Disorders, 4th Edition. Washington, DC, American Psychiatric Association, 1994

American Psychiatric Association: Practice guideline for the treatment of patients with borderline personality disorder. Am J Psychiatry 158 (10 suppl):1–52, 2001

American Psychiatric Association: Diagnostic and Statistical Manual of Mental Disorders, 5th Edition. Arlington, VA, American Psychiatric Association, 2013

Baker TB, McFall RM, Shoham V: Current status and future prospects of clinical psychology: toward a scientifically principled approach to mental and behavioral health care. Psychol Sci Public Interest 9:67–103, 2008

Bateman A, Fonagy P: The effectiveness of partial hospitalization in the treatment of borderline personality disorder: a randomized controlled trial. Am J Psychiatry 156:1563–1569, 1999

Bateman A, Fonagy P: Treatment of borderline personality disorder with psychoanalytically oriented partial hospitalization: an 18-month follow-up. Am J Psychiatry 158:36–42, 2001

Bateman A, Fonagy P: The development of an attachment-based treatment program for borderline personality disorder. Bull Menninger Clin 67:187–211, 2003

Bateman A, Fonagy P (eds): Handbook of Mentalizing in Mental Health Practice. Washington, DC, American Psychiatric Publishing, 2012

Bender DS, Morey LC, Skodol AE: Toward a model for assessing level of personality functioning in DSM-5, part I: a review of theory and methods. J Pers Assess 93:332–346, 2011

Blatt SJ, Levy KN: Attachment theory, psychoanalysis, personality development, and psychopathology. Psychoanal Inq 23:102–150, 2003

Bowlby J: Attachment and Loss, Vol 1: Attachment. London, Hogarth Press and Institute of Psycho-Analysis, 1969

Bowlby J: Attachment and Loss, Vol 2: Separation, Anxiety, and Anger. London, Hogarth Press and Institute of Psycho-Analysis, 1973

Bowlby J: Attachment and Loss, Vol 3: Loss: Sadness and Depression. London, Hogarth Press and Institute of Psycho-Analysis, 1980

Bretherton I: New perspectives on attachment relations: security, communication, and internal working models, in Handbook of Infant Development, 2nd Edition. Edited by Osofsky JD. Oxford, UK, Wiley, 1987, pp 1061–1100

Buie DH, Adler G: Definitive treatment of the borderline personality. Int J Psychoanal Psychother 9:51–87, 1982

Caligor E, Kernberg OF, Clarkin JF: Handbook of Dynamic Psychotherapy for Higher Level Personality Pathology. Washington, DC, American Psychiatric Publishing, 2007

Caligor E, Diamond D, Yeomans FE, et al: The interpretive process in the psychoanalytic psychotherapy of borderline personality pathology. J Am Psychoanal Assoc 57:271–301, 2009

Caligor E, Kernberg OK, Clarkin JF, Yeomans FE: Psychodynamic Therapy for Personality Pathology: Treating Self and Interpersonal Functioning. Washington, DC, American Psychiatric Press, 2018

Chambless DL, Ollendick TH: Empirically supported psychological interventions: controversies and evidence. Annu Rev Psychol 52:685–716, 2001

Chanen AM, Jackson HJ, McCutcheon LK, et al: Early intervention for adolescents with borderline personality disorder using cognitive analytic therapy: randomised controlled trial. Br J Psychiatry 193:477–484, 2008

Choi-Kain LW, Gunderson JG (eds): Applications of Good Psychiatric Management for Borderline Personality Disorder: A Practical Guide. Washington, DC, American Psychiatric Association Publishing, 2019

Clarkin JF, Yeomans FE, Kernberg OF: Psychotherapy for Borderline Personality: Focusing on Object Relations. Washington, DC, American Psychiatric Publishing, 2006

Clarkin JF, Levy KN, Lenzenweger MF, et al: Evaluating three treatments for borderline personality disorder: a multiwave study. Am J Psychiatry 164:922–928, 2007

Diamond D, Clarkin J, Levine H, et al: Borderline conditions and attachment: a preliminary report. Psychoanal Inq 19:831–884, 1999

Doering S, Hoerz S, Rentrop M, et al: Transference-focused psychotherapy v treatment by community therapists for borderline personality disorder: randomized controlled trial. Br J Psychiatry 196:389–395, 2010

Fairbairn WRD: An object-relations theory of the personality, in Psychoanalytic Studies of the Personality. London, Routledge & Kegan Paul, 1952, pp 3–179

Fonagy P, Leigh T, Kennedy R, et al: Attachment, borderline states and the representation of emotions and cognitions in self and other, in Emotion, Cognition, and Representation. Edited by Cicchetti DT, Sheree L. Rochester, NY, University of Rochester Press, 1995, pp 371–414

Fonagy P, Gergely G, Jurist E, et al: Affect Regulation, Mentalization, and the Development of the Self. New York, Other Books, 2003

Fonagy P, Bateman, AW, Luyten P: Introduction and overview, in Handbook of Mentalizing in Mental Health Practice. Edited by Bateman AW, Fonagy P. Washington, DC, American Psychiatric Publishing, 2012, pp 3–42

Freud S: The ego and the id (1923), in The Standard Edition of the Complete Psychological Works of Sigmund Freud, Vol 14. Translated and edited by Strachey J. London, Hogarth Press, 1961, pp 1–66

Gabbard GO: Psychoanalysis, in The American Psychiatric Publishing Textbook of Personality Disorders. Edited by Oldham JM, Skodol AE, Bender DS. Washington DC, American Psychiatric Publishing, 2005, pp 257–274

Gabbard GO: Psychodynamic Psychiatry in Clinical Practice, 5th Edition. Washington, DC, American Psychiatric Publishing, 2014

Gabbard GO, Westen D: Rethinking therapeutic action. Int J Psychoanal 84:823–841, 2003

Gill M: Analysis of Transference, Vol 1: Theory and Technique. New York, International Universities Press, 1982

Goldman GA, Gregory RJ: Preliminary relationships between adherence and outcome in dynamic deconstructive psychotherapy. Psychotherapy (Chic) 46:480-485, 2009

Goldman GA, Gregory RJ: Relationships between techniques and outcomes for borderline personality disorder. Am J Psychother 64:359-371, 2010

Gregory RJ, Remen AL: A manual-based psychodynamic therapy for treatment-resistant borderline personality disorder. Psychotherapy: Theory, Research, Practice, Training 45:15–27, 2008

Gregory RJ, Chlebowski S, Kang D, et al: A controlled trial of psychodynamic psychotherapy for co-occurring borderline personality disorder and alcohol use disorder. Psychotherapy (Chic) 45:28–41, 2008

Gregory RJ, Delucia-Deranja E, Mogle JA: Dynamic deconstructive psychotherapy versus optimized community care for borderline personality disorder co-occurring with alcohol use disorders: 30-month follow-up. J Nerv Ment Dis 198:292–298, 2010

Gunderson JG: Borderline Personality Disorder. Washington, DC, American Psychiatric Press, 1984

Gunderson JG: The borderline patient's intolerance of aloneness: insecure attachments and therapist availability. Am J Psychiatry 153:752–758, 1996

Gunderson JG: The emergence of a generalist model to meet public health needs for patients with borderline personality disorder. Am J Psychiatry 173:452–458, 2016

Gunderson JG, Links PS: Borderline Personality Disorder: A Clinical Guide, 2nd Edition. Arlington, VA, American Psychiatric Publishing, 2008

Gunderson JG, Links PS: Handbook of Good Psychiatric Management for Borderline Personality Disorder. Washington, DC, American Psychiatric Publishing, 2014

Guthrie E: Psychodynamic interpersonal therapy. Adv Psychiatr Treat 5(2):135–145, 1999

Hobson RF: Forms of Feeling: The Heart of Psychotherapy. London, Tavistock, 1985

Høglend P, Bogwald KP, Amlo S, et al: Transference interpretations in dynamic psychotherapy: do they really yield sustained effects? Am J Psychiatry 165:763–771, 2008

Jacobson E: The Self and the Object World. New York, International Universities Press, 1964

James W: Principles of Psychology. New York, Henry Holt, 1890

Kellett S, Bennett, D, Ryle T, Thake A: Cognitive analytic therapy for borderline personality disorder: therapist competence and therapeutic effectiveness in routine practice. Clin Psychol Psychotherapy 20:216–225, 2013

Kernberg OF: Internal World and External Reality: Object Relations Theory Applied. New York, Jason Aronson, 1980

Kernberg OF: Severe Personality Disorders: Psychotherapeutic Strategies. New Haven, CT, Yale University Press, 1984

Kernberg OF: Psychoanalytic object relations theories, in Psychoanalysis: The Major Concepts. Edited by Moore B, Fine B. New Haven, CT, Yale University Press, 1995, pp 450–462

Kernberg OF: A psychoanalytic theory of personality disorders, in Major Theories of Personality Disorder. Edited by Clarkin JF, Lenzenweger MF. New York, Guilford, 1996, pp 106–140

Kernberg OF: Treatment of Severe Personality Disorders: Resolution of Aggression and Recovery of Eroticism. Washington, DC, American Psychiatric Association Publishing, 2018

Klein M: Notes on some schizoid mechanisms (1946), in Envy and Gratitude and Other Works, 1946–1963. New York, Free Press, 1975, pp 1–24

Kohut H: The Analysis of the Self: A Systematic Approach to the Psychoanalytic Treatment of Narcissistic Personality Disorders. New York, International Universities Press, 1971

Korner A, Gerull F, Meares R, Stevenson J: Borderline personality disorder treated with the conversational model: a replication study. Compr Psychiatry 47:406– 411, 2006

Leichsenring F, Leibling E: The effectiveness of psychodynamic therapy and cognitive behavior therapy in the treatment of personality disorders: a meta-analysis. Am J Psychiatry 160:1223–1233, 2003

Leichsenring F, Rabung S: Effectiveness of long-term psychodynamic psychotherapy. JAMA 300:1551–1565, 2008

Lenzenweger MF, Clarkin JF: The personality disorders: history, classification, and research issues, in Major Theories of Personality Disorder. Edited by Clarkin JF, Lenzenweger MF. New York, Guilford, 2005, pp 1–42

Levy KN, Blatt SJ: Attachment theory and psychoanalysis: further differentiation within insecure attachment patterns. Psychoanal Inq 19:541–575, 1999

Levy KN, Meehan KB, Kelly KM, et al: Change in attachment patterns and reflective function in a randomized control trial of transference focused psychotherapy for borderline personality disorder. J Consult Clin Psychol 74:1027–1040, 2006

Levy KN, Ellison WD, Temes CM, et al: The outcome of psychotherapy for borderline personality disorder: a meta-analysis (Specific and Common Factors of Psychotherapy for Borderline Personality Disorder; Livesley J, Chair). Paper presented at the 2nd International Congress on Borderline Personality Disorder and Allied Disorders, Amsterdam, September 2012

Luborsky L: Principles of Psychoanalytic Psychotherapy: A Manual for Supportive-Expressive Treatment. New York, Basic Books, 1984

Luborsky L, Mintz J, Auerbach A, et al: Predicting the outcome of psychotherapy: findings of the Penn Psychotherapy Project. Arch Gen Psychiatry 37:471–481, 1980

McCrae RR, Costa PT Jr: Personality trait structure as a human universal. Am Psychol 52:509–516, 1997

McMain SF, Links PS, Gnam WH, et al: A randomized trial of dialectical behavior therapy versus general psychiatric management for borderline personality disorder. Am J Psychiatry 116:1365–1374, 2009

McMain SF, Guimond T, Streiner DL, et al: Dialectical behavior therapy compared with general psychiatric management for borderline personality disorder: clinical outcomes and functioning over a 2-year follow-up. Am J Psychiatry 169:650–661, 2012

Meares R, Stevenson J, Comerford A: Psychotherapy with borderline patients, I: a comparison between treated and untreated cohorts. Aust N Z J Psychiatry 33:467– 472, 1999

Meissner WW: Psychotherapeutic schema based on the paranoid process. Int J Psychoanal Psychother 5:87–114, 1976

Meissner WW: Psychotherapy and the Paranoid Process. Northvale, NJ, Jason Aronson, 1986

Mischel W, Shoda Y: A cognitive-affective system theory of personality: reconceptualizing situations, dispositions, dynamics, and invariance in personality structure. Psychol Rev 102:246–268, 1995

Norcross JC: Psychotherapy Relationships That Work, 2nd Edition. New York, Oxford University Press, 2011

Reich W: Character Analysis. New York, Farrar, Straus & Giroux, 1972

Rockland LH: Supportive Therapy for Borderline Patients: A Psychodynamic Approach. New York, Guilford, 1992

Ryle A: Cognitive Analytic Therapy and Borderline Personality Disorder: The Model and the Method. Chichester, UK, Wiley, 1997

Ryle A, Golynkina K: Effectiveness of time-limited cognitive analytic therapy of borderline personality disorder: factors associated with outcome. Br J Med Psychol 73:197–210, 2000

Sharp C, Wright AGC, Fowler JC, et al: The structure of personality pathology: both general ('g') and specific ('s') factors? J Abnorm Psychol 124:387–398, 2015

Shaver PR, Collins N, Clark CL: Attachment styles and internal working models of self and relationship partners, in Knowledge Structures in Close Relationships: A Social Psychological Approach. Edited by Fletcher J. Hillsdale, NJ, Erlbaum, 1996, pp 25–61

Shedler J: The efficacy of psychodynamic psychotherapy. Am Psychol 65:98–109, 2010

Stevenson J, Meares R: An outcome study of psychotherapy for patients with borderline personality disorder. Am J Psychiatry 149:358–362, 1992

Stevenson J, Meares, R, D'Angelo R: Five-year outcome of outpatient psychotherapy with borderline patients. Psychol Med 35:79–87, 2005

Strupp HH, Binder JL: Psychotherapy in a New Key: A Guide to Time-Limited Dynamic Psychotherapy. New York, Basic Books, 1984

Valzelli L: Psychobiology of Aggression and Violence. New York, Raven Press, 1981, pp 67–69

Waldinger RJ: Intensive psychodynamic therapy with borderline patients: an overview. Am J Psychiatry 144:267–274, 1987

Wallerstein RS: Forty-Two Lives in Treatment: A Study of Psychoanalysis and Psychotherapy. New York, Guilford, 1986

Walton CJ: A randomised clinical trial of dialectical behaviour therapy and conversational model for the treatment of borderline personality disorder: a hybrid efficacy-effectiveness study in a public sector mental health service in Australia. Doctoral dissertation, University of Newcastle, New South Wales, Australia, 2019

Westen D, Morrison K: A multidimensional meta-analysis of treatments for depression, panic, and generalized anxiety disorder: an empirical examination of the status of empirically supported therapies. J Consult Clin Psychol 69:875–899, 2001

Wildgoose A, Clarke S, Waller G: Treating personality fragmentation and dissociation in borderline personality disorder: a pilot study of the impact of cognitive analytic therapy. Br J Med Psychol 74:47–55, 2001

Winnicott DW: Maturational Processes and the Facilitating Environment: Studies in the Theory of Emotional Development. New York, International Universities Press, 1965

Wright AG, Hopwood CJ, Skodol AE, Morey LC: Longitudinal validation of general and specific structural features of personality pathology. J Abnorm Psychol 125:1120–1134, 2016

Yeomans FE, Clarkin JF, Kernberg OF: A Primer of Transference-Focused Psychotherapy for the Borderline Patient. Northvale, NJ, Jason Aronson, 2002

Yeomans FE, Clarkin JF, Kernberg OF: Transference-Focused Psychotherapy for Borderline Personality Disorder: A Clinical Guide. Washington, DC, American Psychiatric Publishing, 2015

Zetzel ER: The so-called good hysteric. Int J Psychoanal 49:256–260, 1968

CHAPTER 13

Dialectical Behavior Therapy

Barbara Stanley, Ph.D.

Beth S. Brodsky, Ph.D.

Ilana Gratch, B.A.

Dialectical behavior therapy (DBT) was developed in the late 1980s by Marsha Linehan as a treatment specifically for suicidal and self-injuring individuals with borderline personality disorder (BPD) (Linehan 1993a), a population with a broad range of serious problems in addition to suicidality (Kehrer and Linehan 1996). A form of cognitive-behavioral psychotherapy, DBT can be adapted for use in other personality disorders, particularly those in which there is significant behavioral and emotional dyscontrol (Stanley et al. 2001). Adaptations of DBT have been developed for a number of disorders, such as eating disorders (Bankoff et al. 2012) and PTSD (Harned et al. 2012), and populations, such as adolescents (Mehlum et al. 2014; Miller et al. 2006) and geriatric patients (Lynch et al. 2003).

DBT has been evaluated in several efficacy studies (Panos et al. 2014). In this chapter, we summarize DBT as described in the three published treatment manuals (Linehan 1993a, 1993b, 2014) and as implemented in efficacy studies in the literature. DBT was developed in response to the need for empirically supported psychotherapies for chronically suicidal individuals with BPD. Although originally developed for those who self-harm, it is also used in the segment of the BPD population that does not exhibit self-harm behaviors (Robins et al. 2001). Treatment retention of individuals with

This work was supported in part by National Institute of Mental Health grants R01 MH61079, MH062665, and P20AA015630 to Dr. Stanley. The authors would like to thank Alex Chapman, Ph.D., postdoctoral fellow in Behavior Research and Therapy Clinics, under the direction of Marsha Linehan, Ph.D., of the University of Washington, for his thoughtful comments on an earlier draft of this chapter.

BPD is a well-known and significant problem, as is their lack of progress and dissatisfaction with their therapies. At the time when DBT was developed, empirical support for existing therapies, including supportive and psychodynamically oriented treatment, was lacking. Cognitive-behavioral therapy (CBT) showed efficacy in patients with depression and anxiety disorders, but individuals with BPD had trouble tolerating standard CBT (Dimeff and Linehan 2001). CBT places a strong emphasis on change strategies that, by themselves, are very difficult for individuals with BPD to accept and utilize. BPD patients tend to experience an almost exclusive focus on change as criticism and invalidation of their suffering rather than its intent as helpful. This approach, in turn, exacerbates their already harsh self-criticism and contributes to their poor retention rate in therapy.

In attempting to tackle this problem, DBT explicitly emphasizes the need to balance change strategies with acceptance and validation techniques. This balance is important for two primary reasons. First, acceptance and change, in and of themselves, are important ingredients in any successful psychotherapy. Many problems and issues confronted in psychotherapy cannot be changed. An obvious example is past history and childhood experiences. Patients are sometimes entrenched in a place of nonacceptance about their past and consequently are unable to move beyond a stance that it "should not have happened." Second, acceptance and change have a dynamic interplay that creates a *dialectic*. Increased acceptance enables greater change, and more change allows for increased tolerance and acceptance of what cannot be changed.

In this chapter we describe the theoretical underpinnings of DBT, provide an overview of the components of standard DBT treatment as developed for individuals with BPD who experience self-injurious and suicidal behavior, discuss basic DBT techniques and strategies, review the empirical findings of its efficacy, and provide case material demonstrating crucial aspects of the treatment. Our intent in this chapter is to provide an overview of DBT and illustrate how it uniquely addresses the difficulties specific to the treatment and retention of individuals with BPD. For a comprehensive description of DBT, the treatment manuals (Linehan 1993a, 1993b, 2014) should be consulted.

Theoretical Perspectives

Biosocial Theory of Borderline Personality Disorder

DBT was developed from a particular theoretical perspective on the nature of BPD (Linehan 1987, 1993a). BPD is viewed as a disorder of *dysregulation*—dysregulation of behavior, affect, cognition, and interpersonal relationships. The chronic suicidal behavior characteristic of many individuals with BPD is seen as a consequence of these dysregulations. The first iteration of biosocial theory (Linehan 1993a), on which DBT rests, attributed the dysregulation to a transaction between an inborn emotional vulnerability and an emotionally invalidating childhood environment. The biologically based emotional vulnerability is characterized by an intense, quick reaction to emotionally evocative stimuli in the environment, along with a slow return to baseline after emotional arousal. The invalidating environment consists of caretakers who may punish, ignore, reject, and/or disregard the child's emotional experience and therefore do not provide conditions in which the individual can learn to regulate emotional experiences. A transaction between these two elements—in which 1) the emotional sensitivity leads to increased perception of threat in interpersonal situations and 2) the invalidating response from the environment exacerbates the emotional vulnerability—results in a propensity to dysregulation. Linehan (1993a) also applied learning theory to explain how the emotionally vulnerable individual develops self-destructive behaviors to obtain a nurturing response from the invalidating environment. As the behaviors escalate, they are intermittently reinforced, making them very difficult to unlearn.

In light of empirical discoveries in the years since the development of the biosocial theory of BPD, our understanding of BPD has since been extended to include a developmental psychopathology perspective (Crowell et al. 2009, 2014). Specifically, the extended biosocial developmental model of BPD posits that inherited, trait impulsivity emerges in the child early on, independent of emotion, and is accompanied by the development of emotional lability, formed and maintained by the familial environment. Similar to the first iteration of the biosocial theory of BPD, the reciprocal transaction between the biological vulnerabilities and environmental risk factors contributes to the propensity toward dysregulation, ultimately becoming identifiable by middle to late adolescence, exacerbating the risk for developing BPD in adulthood.

The most egregious example of an invalidating environment would be one involving sexual abuse, physical abuse, or neglect. Besides being a clear example of invalidation of the child's needs, the experience of childhood abuse and neglect is often characterized by much inconsistency and conflict as the child experiences both nurturing and abuse/neglect from the same caretaker. Given the high prevalence of reported childhood abuse among individuals with BPD (Brodsky et al. 1995; Herman et al. 1989; Ogata et al. 1990), the biosocial theory maintains that abuse cannot be ignored as contributory to the etiology of BPD. Nor is abuse thought to have been present in all individuals who develop BPD. Less explicit forms of invalidation such as repeated dismissal or denial of a child's emotional experience and reinforcement of maladaptive coping mechanisms can also lead to severe impairment in self-regulation (Stanley and Brodsky 2005). For example, if children who cry in response to disappointments are repeatedly told, "You have nothing to cry about," the result is often not what is intended—that is, to make them feel better. Instead, if it is a frequent occurrence, children begin to mistrust their inner states and become unable to read their own emotional cues. Children begin to question whether in fact there is something to cry about and become confused about their internal sense of upset and uncertain about what they are feeling. If carried forward into adulthood, their emotional experiences remain somewhat mysterious to them. Emotions are misperceived, misread, mistrusted, and experienced as an unidentifiable jumble of upset.

It is important to note that this theoretical stance does not ascribe "weights" to how much biological vulnerability and environmental invalidation is necessary to yield BPD. If an individual has a biological predisposition to emotional sensitivity, vulnerability, and reactivity, he or she is likely to be more easily hurt. Patients with preexisting vulnerability experience hurt more deeply, react more strongly, and have a greater propensity to feel invalidated. Thus, it can be challenging to provide a validating and supportive environment for the emotionally sensitive child. Finally, it is also important to underscore the fact that this theoretical perspective awaits empirical validation. Although some research has begun to examine this theory of BPD (Sharp and Kim 2015), at this point it remains largely a theoretical perspective, and it may be shown ultimately that either biological predispositions or environmental factors are the overriding determinants of BPD. Nevertheless, like other forms of psychotherapy, DBT was developed from a theoretical orientation, but its techniques and applicability are not dependent on it.

Theoretical Underpinnings of Dialectical Behavior Therapy

DBT is a theoretically and philosophically coherent treatment, with dialectical philosophy at its core, embedded within which is behavioral science (learning principles) and Zen mindfulness practice (Linehan 1993a, 2014). These perspectives have direct applicability in the treatment techniques and the understanding of patients and their problems.

Learning Principles

The predominant theoretical approach of DBT is learning principles. An exhaustive review of learning principles is beyond the scope of this review, but in brief, behaviors are understood as being maintained through either operant or classical conditioning. This distinction serves to shape the way in which behavior change should be approached. If a maladaptive behavior is understood as being maintained through operant conditioning, removal of reinforcers is called for. Alternatively, positive reinforcement of adaptive behaviors can be implemented. If a maladaptive behavior is maintained through respondent (classical) conditioning, loosening the connection between the conditioned and unconditioned stimuli is important.

Although learning principles are prominent in all forms of CBT, some forms of CBT emphasize the importance of, and therefore focus on, the role of cognitions. Other forms of CBT emphasize behavior. For example, the CBT developed by Beck emphasizes the importance of distorted cognitions (Beck et al. 2003). Exposing and examining these faulty cognitions then becomes an important focus of the treatment. Correcting them is believed to be the pathway to change. Alternatively, DBT places a greater emphasis on emotion. Given the behavioral perspective, DBT defines cognition as behavior. DBT focuses on understanding that reinforcers maintain a maladaptive behavior and attempts to loosen the links that lead to the behavior through a variety of means. This focus does not imply that DBT never examines distorted cognitions or that Beck's CBT never examines behavioral reinforcers. Instead, CBT varies in its approach to problems, as do the variety of psychodynamically oriented psychotherapies.

DBT aims to provide increased support for patients to remain safe on an outpatient basis as well as support for the therapist working with the chronically suicidal outpatient. This goal is achieved through applying learning principles to enhance capability and motivation of both patient and therapist. Patient capability is enhanced through the teaching of adaptive skillful behaviors, and motivation is enhanced through the reinforcement of progress and nonreinforcement of maladaptive behaviors. For the therapist, a DBT outpatient consultation team is a source of support and guidance as well as an aid to keep the therapist focused on the treatment goals and format.

Mindfulness Orientation

Certain aspects of Eastern philosophy are integral to DBT (Robins 2002), particularly a focus on acceptance and the importance of mindfulness practice. Linehan (1997) observed that an exclusive focus on change in behavior therapy is experienced as invalidating by traumatized or rejection-sensitive individuals and can result in early dropout or resistance to change within the treatment. Therefore, the DBT strategy involves acceptance of whatever is valid about the individual's current behaviors, viewing these behaviors as the patient's best efforts to cope with unbearable pain. However, Linehan (1997) also noted that ignoring the need for change is just as invalidating because it does not take the problems and negative consequences of the patient's behavior seriously. This can lead to hopelessness and suicidality. Thus, acceptance and validation are combined with change strategies. The balance of change with acceptance is one of the most unique aspects of the dialectical approach (described in the next subsection) and is solidly based in the Zen mindfulness perspective. Change is achieved through the tension and resolution of this essential conflict between acceptance of individuals as they are right now and the demand that they change. Thus, the dialectical strategy encourages cognitive restructuring from an "either/or" to a "yes/and" perspective—directly addressing the dichotomous thinking that is characteristic of individuals with BPD and that often leads to maladaptive behaviors (Linehan 1997).

Mindfulness practice teaches controlling the mind to stay in the present moment without judgment. This practice is extremely useful in helping patients remain in the present rather than focusing on past worries or future fears. As patients fight urges to hurt themselves, mindfulness practice is useful in helping them distract themselves from urges, and it ultimately helps them to reduce the intensity of their urges.

Dialectical Approach

DBT is based on a dialectical perspective representing a reconciliation of opposites by arriving at a synthesis of these opposites. A dialectical worldview is the overarching perspective in DBT and is manifest in the strategies and assumptions of the treatment. Therapists create a balance between accepting patients' dysfunctions and helping them modify their thinking and behavior. The dialectical philosophy leads to the following assumptions that underlie DBT. The first explicit assumption is that patients are doing the best they can. At the same time, patients want to improve, but they need to do better, try harder, and be more motivated to change. A second assumption is that patients may not have caused all of their own problems, but they have to solve them anyway. An additional assumption is that patients cannot fail in therapy; rather, if failure occurs, it is the treatment that fails (Linehan 1993a, 1997).

These philosophical assumptions serve to enhance motivation and inform the therapeutic stance at all times (Cialdini et al. 1975; Freedman and Fraser 1966). For example, the first assumption encourages a nonjudgmental approach and discourages negative thinking on the therapist's part in the face of ongoing difficult patient behavior. The second assumption validates the need for change, without blame or judgment, and promotes effective problem solving. It also underscores the belief that the therapist cannot save the patient—the patient must do most of the work with the help of the therapist. The therapist's role is to encourage self-care rather than to take care of the patient. If the patient does not make progress, gets worse, or drops out of treatment, the burden of the failure is assumed by the therapy—that is, that the therapy was not successful in enhancing motivation, and this removes blame from the patient regarding lack of motivation. This approach is particularly helpful to patients who experience tremendous, crippling self-blame that can inhibit taking chances and extending themselves in both therapy and life generally.

Treatment Components: A Two-Pronged Approach

DBT consists of two components in which patients participate: individual psychotherapy and group skills training. This approach derives from a point of view not only that individuals need to understand their maladaptive patterns of behavior as they occur in individual psychotherapy, but that they also have certain deficits that can best be overcome by developing a means of compensation and skills. These patients often report that they know *why* they "do what they do" but they "do not know what to do instead" or how to get themselves to do what they know they should do. Although the first half of this statement may be only partially correct, the second half is almost always true. A two-pronged approach to treatment acknowledges this problem by adopting a stance that patients may need to be taught coping strategies and skills in a more explicit manner than is typically done with patients who have personality disorders. Thus, this approach suggests that both an understanding of maladaptive patterns of thinking and behavior and skill development are useful in treating patients with personality disorders. Personality disorders are seen, in part, as deficits in certain skill areas that prevent the person from behaving in an effective manner. In addition to these two forms of patient contact, a consultation team for DBT therapists is considered an integral aspect of the treatment.

Individual Therapy

Patients attend at least one, sometimes two, individual therapy sessions of 50–60 minutes each week. Double sessions of 90–110 minutes can be utilized (Linehan 1993a). It is desirable, though not always possible, to have the flexibility to alter session lengths depending on the patient's needs and the task at hand. For example, patients who have difficulty opening up or who have trouble closing up at the end of sessions may benefit from longer sessions for a period of time until they develop the capacity to transition in and out of sessions. Also, there are times when the type of treatment work benefits from longer sessions. When conducting trauma exposure sessions, longer session lengths are required. Alternatively, some patients have difficulty tolerating the intense closeness that can be experienced in individual treatment for more than brief periods of time. While this capacity to tolerate closeness is being worked on with the patient, allowing briefer sessions avoids premature termination.

The individual therapy session is structured by the treatment hierarchy and a variety of behavioral techniques. Any life-threatening behaviors (target 1) are the top priority and must be addressed within an individual session if they have occurred. Therapy-interfering behaviors (target 2) are the second in priority and are the first priority in the absence of life-threatening behaviors. As long as target 1 and 2 behaviors are either absent or addressed within a session, quality-of-life issues may also be targeted within any given session. The patient is required to keep a daily record of behaviors, level of misery, and suicidal ideation on what is called a *diary card* (Linehan 1993b) (described in more detail later). Therapist and patient review the diary card together and use it to create an agenda for the session. If the patient engaged in self-injury, a behavioral analysis (described later) is required.

Skills Training

Skills training is generally based on learning theory and utilizes behavioral principles such as shaping, modeling, repeated practice, behavior rehearsal, homework, and reinforcement of socially appropriate behaviors. Behavior change is facilitated by the combination of the direct instruction of information, modeling of behaviors by role models, prompting of specific behaviors, and positive reinforcement of successive approximations toward the desired goal. The specific goal or behavior to be changed will differ depending on the patient's presenting problem. The teaching of skillful behaviors with which to replace the maladaptive ones is a major component of capacity enhancement in DBT. Attending a weekly skills training group in which skills are taught within a didactic framework, preferably by a therapist other than the individual therapist, is an essential component of the treatment. The group serves to introduce and teach the concepts of skills, and it provides an opportunity to interact with other patients who are also learning skills. A skills training manual (Linehan 1993b, 2014) describes the skills and how to teach them and contains worksheets and homework assignments to facilitate learning. In vivo skills coaching is conducted in such a way as to enhance patient capability and motivation.

The first step in the process of skills training is the assessment of the skill deficit, which in DBT takes place in the individual therapy session. Once the specific deficit has been identified, skills training may be implemented. Direct instruction on the skill to be learned begins the training. This instruction gives the patient the required knowledge to perform the skill. Next is modeling, by the therapist or skills trainer, of the skill behavior to be learned. Modeling has many functions for the patient (Spieglar and Guevremont 1998). First, the patient is taught a new behavior through observation of a model. Second, the patient is prompted to perform a behavior after observing a clinician model the behavior. Third, the patient is motivated to engage in similar behavior after observing the favorable consequences it receives, which is the concept of *vicarious reinforcement*. Lastly, after observing a person who is serving as a model safely engaging in the anxiety-provoking behavior, the patient's anxiety is decreased.

After the skill has been modeled for the patient, it is the patient's turn to perform the behavior, often referred to as *behavior rehearsal*. The first step is prompting or reminding the patient to perform a behavior. Next is the process of shaping, which is the reinforcing of components of the target behavior that are successively closer approximations of the actual target behavior. Feedback is given to the patient regarding success, and there is reinforcement of the behavior results. After the skill has been rehearsed or practiced, the patient is then asked to participate in a role-play situation that requires use of the skill. Outside of skills training sessions, patients may be asked to complete homework assignments that will require more use of the skill. Eventually, this repeated practice will lead to mastery of the targeted skill or behavior.

Linehan (1993b) outlined four specific skills training modules that target the four areas of dysregulation of BPD: mindfulness skills to address cognitive dysregulation, distress tolerance skills to address behavioral dysregulation, emotion regulation skills to address affect dysregulation, and interpersonal effectiveness skills to address dysregulation of interpersonal relationships (Table 13–1).

TABLE 13–1.	Dialectical behavior therapy skills training modules

I. Mindfulness
    A. Core mindfulness skills (the mindfulness "what" and "how" skills)
    B. Other perspectives on mindfulness
II. Distress tolerance
    A. Crisis survival skills
    B. Reality acceptance skills
    C. Skills for when the crisis is addiction
III. Emotion regulation
    A. Understanding and naming emotions
    B. Changing emotional responses
    C. Reducing vulnerability to emotions
    D. Managing extreme emotions
IV. Interpersonal effectiveness
    A. Core interpersonal effectiveness skills
    B. Building healthy relationships and ending destructive relationships (supplemental)
    C. Skills for walking the middle path

Although the modules were developed for BPD, they have broad applicability to other problems and disorders, such as avoidant, dependent, and paranoid personality disorders (Stanley et al. 2001). The individual modules have each been designed to remedy a specific dysfunction; however, they reinforce one another, thus creating a comprehensive treatment of the "whole patient."

The first module is core *mindfulness* skills training, which focuses on dysregulations of self and cognition. Mindfulness skills are based on Eastern Zen Buddhist principles. Patients are taught techniques for focusing their thoughts and attention on the present, establishing attentional control, and coupling awareness with nonjudgmental thinking. The goal is to help the patient establish a lifestyle of mental awareness and inner connectivity, along with the ability to see reality as it is. The DBT mindfulness approach encourages the synthesis of two disparate states of mind—"reasonable mind" and "emotion mind"—into a singular overarching state of "wise mind" in which emotions can be experienced in a regulated manner, in balance with and informing logical thought processes. In addition to basic DBT mindfulness skills, other spiritual and physical movement approaches to mindfulness, such as yoga, martial arts, and religious prayer, are reviewed.

The second module is *distress tolerance* skills training, which focuses on teaching skills to help the patient tolerate and deal with problems such as impulsivity and suicidal ideation. The fundamental goal of this module is learning the skills of both distracting from a distressing situation and accepting situations when they cannot be changed. Distress tolerance skills focus on how to live through a crisis situation without engaging in destructive behaviors. Crisis survival strategies include self-soothing and distracting techniques, and pros-and-cons analyses. Distress tolerance skills include the concept of "radical acceptance," providing guidance to turn the mind from fighting to accepting reality in order to accept necessary pain but reduce unnecessary suffering. The module also includes crisis survival strategies specifically targeting substance addiction, in particular, the relapse prevention concept of "dialectical abstinence," which incorporates a synthesis of absolute abstinence and harm reduction.

The third skill module is *emotion regulation*, which teaches the necessary skills to control dysregulated experiences and expressions of anger, anxiety, fear, and depression as well as dysregulated positive emotions such as love and joy. Individuals learn that each emotion has a function and is necessary for survival. Emotion regulation is about experiencing emotions in a regulated way rather than trying to "get rid" of one's emotions. Emotion regulation skills include observing and identifying emotional states, learning how to be mindful of one's current emotion, and validating and accepting one's emotional reactions. There are also techniques for decreasing vulnerability to negative emotions and increasing the experience of positive emotions. Emotion regulation skills are paired with distress tolerance skills in order to manage extreme emotions that lead someone to experience the "skills breakdown point."

Finally, the fourth module is *interpersonal effectiveness* training, which exposes borderline patients to effective strategies for mending interpersonal conflict. Interpersonal effectiveness skills include the core skills of asking for what one needs, saying no, and managing interpersonal conflicts skillfully. Additionally, interpersonal effectiveness training involves teaching how to build healthy relationships and end destructive ones through teaching skills aimed at finding potential friends, being mindful of others' needs, ending relationships, and walking the middle path. Three skill sets are part of walking the middle path: dialectics (i.e., every relationship continuously changes), validation (i.e., both providing others with validation and recovering from invalidation), and strategies for changing behaviors in others (i.e., positive and negative reinforcement, shaping, extinction, satiation, and punishment).

Case Example 1

Ms. K is a highly intelligent 28-year-old woman working as a secretary and studying for her bachelor's degree. She lives with her boyfriend of 6 years; the two were in couples therapy seeking help in deciding whether to get married. Ms. K was referred by the couples therapist to individual therapy for the treatment of binge-eating disorder; the patient's obesity and out-of-control binge eating were interfering with the couple's sex life. During the course of individual psychotherapy, it became apparent that the patient was exhibiting symptoms of BPD that were contributing to the primary difficulties in her relationship with her boyfriend. Her binge eating was an impulsive behavior that was often triggered by fears of abandonment, feelings of emptiness, and identity diffusion, and the binge eating was a self-soothing mechanism for feelings of uncontrollable rage. The patient was also having difficulties in her relationships with supervisors at work due to a tendency to idealize, and then devalue, those in authority and to feel used and victimized and view the supervisors with suspicion when under stress. The individual therapist identified the need for the patient to develop more skillful coping mechanisms to replace the binge eating and impaired interpersonal functioning and referred her for adjunct DBT skills training. Although Ms. K was not initially interested in changing her interpersonal behaviors, because she viewed her difficulties with her supervisors as external to herself, she was highly motivated to gain control over her eating and agreed to undergo skills training.

Ms. K immediately took to the skills training. She found the mindfulness skills extremely helpful in allowing her to observe and describe urges to binge, which gave her increasing control over her eating behaviors. She learned distress tolerance skills that helped her distract from and also tolerate the feelings of anger and emptiness without resorting to binge eating. She was able to use the support of the other group members to observe her interpersonal patterns, and she became more willing to try new ways of interpreting the behaviors of others. She described it thus: "Mindfulness skills helped me more clearly distinguish between my thoughts and behaviors in an interpersonal interaction and what the contribution of the other person was."

Stages of Treatment

DBT has four stages of treatment. Stage 1 specifically targets the reduction of life-threatening behavior and is therefore the most researched and of particular interest to clinicians who treat the chronic suicidality of BPD patients on an outpatient basis. Within the context of treating self-injury, other behavioral, interpersonal, cognitive, and emotional difficulties are also addressed. These include behaviors that interfere with the therapy and interpersonal difficulties. Once a patient has control over self-injurious behaviors, the patient enters into stage 2. Stage 2 in DBT helps patients increase emotional experiencing. Because many individuals with BPD have a history of childhood abuse (Brodsky et al. 1995; Herman et al. 1989), exposure-based procedures are used to treat the residue of childhood trauma (Foa 1997). Other quality-of-life issues, such as self-actualization in social and vocational arenas, become the target of treatment during stage 3. Finally, stage 4 treatment focuses on increasing joy and a sense of completeness and connectedness.

Hierarchy of Treatment Goals

A standard hierarchy of goals is built into stage 1 DBT (Table 13–2). The primary goal is the reduction of life-threatening behaviors. The first task of the clinician is to establish a commitment from the patient to accept this hierarchy of goals, particularly the primary one of reducing self-injury. The sessions in which this commitment is negotiated are considered the pretreatment phase.

A second goal in stage 1 is the reduction of therapy-interfering behaviors. Such behaviors include lateness, missed sessions (of individual and/or skills groups), failure to keep a diary card (described later), and any other behavior on the part of the patient or therapist that interferes with the therapy. The third goal is the reduction of behaviors that interfere with quality of life, such as interpersonal difficulties and problems in personal and vocational functioning.

Case Example 2

Ms. L is a 28-year-old single woman living with two roommates in a major metropolitan area. She was referred to DBT from a day program she had been attending for 3 months following hospitalization for a suicide attempt. The suicide attempt consisted of a serious overdose of her roommate's benzodiazepines, which Ms. L took impulsively after an argument with her boyfriend. She had lost consciousness, was found by her roommate, and was taken to the emergency department, where she received gastric lavage. She regained consciousness after a few hours.

At the time of the attempt, Ms. L was taking art courses and looking for a position as an office worker. In the past, after graduating from college, she had worked as an administrative assistant at a bank for about 2 years until she became depressed, somewhat paranoid, and angry. She would miss work frequently and get into altercations with co-

TABLE 13–2.	Hierarchy of dialectical behavior therapy goals in stage 1

1. Reduction of life-threatening behaviors
2. Reduction of therapy-interfering behaviors
3. Reduction of quality-of-life-interfering behaviors

workers when she was there. As she described it, "I stopped coming to work because I felt as if my boss was deliberately trying to give me a hard time." She was referred to DBT because she had been diagnosed with BPD and was intermittently suicidal. She experienced suicidal ideation, she occasionally engaged in self-injury consisting of cutting her inner arm without intent to die, her mood fluctuated from depression to anger to feelings of emptiness, and she had interpersonal difficulties due to increased guardedness and suspiciousness when she was under stress. She reported a severe history of repeated sexual abuse at the hands of her stepfather between the ages of 8 and 12. When drunk he would enter her room at night and would frighten her into having intercourse and remaining quiet about it. This abuse ended when her mother and stepfather divorced. Ms. L suspected that her mother knew about the abuse but was uncertain that this was the case. She developed an inability to trust her own perceptions and had a very conflicted relationship with her mother, whom she perceived as weak and in need of protection. Ms. L had a treatment history of not regularly attending therapy and not remaining with one particular therapy treatment for more than a few months. She reported on intake that she had never found therapy very helpful and never felt that she could allow herself to trust a therapist to understand or help her.

Following the DBT hierarchy, the therapist identified treatment goals with Ms. L. Target 1 was the reduction of life-threatening behaviors. For Ms. L, these were suicide attempts in the form of overdoses, nonsuicidal self-cutting behaviors, and suicidal ideation. Target 2 was the correction of treatment-interfering behavior; Ms. L needed to attend therapy and skills training group sessions consistently and on time and with diary card and skills homework prepared. Target 3 would attend to quality-of-life issues—in this case, finding and maintaining employment.

The main challenge was to obtain Ms. L's commitment to the goal of reducing self-injury. From the patient's perspective, the self-injury was not problematic. She would vacillate between feeling that "having to live with the horrible feelings and memories is just too much to bear and suicide feels like the only way out" and feeling that "I don't think I will do something stupid like that [overdosing on pills] again; I'm not suicidal anymore." Her stated goal for treatment was to work through her childhood trauma, which was the main cause of her unhappiness and hopelessness.

Every time the therapist asked Ms. L to commit to the goal of reducing her self-injury, she would respond, "You just don't get it," start crying, and withdraw from interaction. Ms. L was experiencing the focus on changing her behavior as invalidation of her trauma history. Thus, the therapist implemented a "foot in the door" rather than "door in the face" technique. This intervention required a major focus on validation—of the pain, the hopelessness, and the horror of her childhood abuse.

The use of validation strategies over a number of sessions allowed Ms. L to feel that the therapist understood the disruption that her trauma history caused her in all areas of her life, despite the insistence on reducing her self-injury. The therapist explained that she was very interested in working with Ms. L on healing from the trauma. However, Ms. L needed first to be able to control the life-threatening behaviors and increase her adaptive coping strategies for dealing with the painful feelings surrounding the trauma. Ms. L and the therapist eventually made a commitment to work together to reduce her self-injury.

Consistent attendance to therapy was identified as a second goal of treatment. Finding employment would be a third, a quality-of-life goal that they would work toward in the absence of self-injury or therapy-interfering behavior. Although Ms. L agreed to focus on reduction of self-injury as the primary goal, the therapist agreed to balance this focus with understanding that the suicidal feelings and self-injury were validations of Ms. L's pain. Several times during Ms. L's treatment she would miss a session only to return and insist that she needed to focus on the trauma and not on the reduction of her self-injury. Later analysis revealed that she had felt invalidated by too strong an emphasis on change in the previous session. At these times, the commitment needed to be revisited on both sides: Ms. L's commitment to reducing her behaviors, and the therapist's commitment to balancing change with validation.

This case demonstrates the DBT treatment hierarchy and how it is implemented when working with patients. In Ms. L's case, the patient was experiencing an overwhelming number of problems simultaneously. Having a treatment hierarchy provided both the patient and the therapist with a "road map" for the treatment and helped to prevent the continual sense of "putting out fires" that can characterize many treatments with BPD individuals. This latter approach often comes at the expense of working on longer-term goals and issues that will equip the individual for leading a more functional and independent life.

Major Treatment Techniques and Strategies

A broad range of techniques are employed in DBT. An exhaustive review is beyond the scope of this chapter. Instead, in this section we give some examples of the major tools and techniques to give the reader a sense of how the treatment is conducted.

Chain Analysis

A central change intervention used either in the individual session or in the group setting is the step-by-step analysis of problem behaviors (chain analysis). The dialectical approach to chain analysis is unique to DBT. The chain analysis approach rests on the notion that any behavior is the result of a series of linked components "chained" together. This approach involves identifying the vulnerability the patient brings to the situation, the precipitating event, and the reinforcing consequences of the problem behaviors. The positive consequences for the patient, such as immediate relief from unbearable emotional pain, are highlighted and validated. The patient and therapist then collaborate in reconstructing the series of events (thoughts, feelings, actions, and environmental events) that led to the behavior. The therapist asks for as much detail as possible and weaves solutions or alternative skillful behaviors the patient might have used into the thread of the analysis. Chain analysis is a useful tool for gaining an understanding of the emotional and behavioral events that lead to an unwanted behavior and for generating specific solutions. It is also built into DBT as an aversive consequence of the maladaptive behavior. The expectation of spending a good portion of the next therapy session involved in a painstaking analysis of a problem behavior often serves as a deterrent.

Crisis Management, Coaching, and Intersession Contact

Therapist availability between sessions is critical when treating suicidal patients. In DBT, in vivo skills coaching is conducted by the individual therapist to provide the necessary support for learning new behaviors "in the moment." Patients are encouraged to call or page individual therapists between sessions when they are fighting urges to self-injure and require help in implementing a substitute skillful behavior. During these phone contacts, the therapist and patient decide on a number of skillful ways of handling the current stressful situation. Skills coaching through phone consultation is also a strategy for encouraging the generalization of skillful behavior to other life situations.

Rather than resulting in constant calling by the patient, phone contacts are focused and limited to skills coaching and relationship repair. If the patient calls but is not really interested in problem solving, the therapist indicates availability when the patient is interested in skills coaching and quickly ends the contact. If skills coaching is agreed on, therapist and patient quickly review which skills the patient has already tried, and the therapist "cheerleads" and helps the patient generate a plan to try new skills. The therapist praises the patient for calling and validates the difficulty of tolerating the pain and trying a new behavior. These contacts are generally brief and goal directed, often resulting in the prevention of self-injury, and therefore are positively reinforcing for the therapist (if not the patient).

The 24-hour rule of DBT states that patients cannot call the therapist for 24 hours after they have engaged in self-injury. This rule does not apply to scheduled appointments. If a patient calls the therapist after the fact, the therapist, once ascertaining that the patient is safe from further self-harm, expresses regret that they cannot speak for the next 24 hours. The therapist wishes out loud that the patient had called sooner so he or she could have received skills coaching and support. The therapist then expresses the desire to hear from the patient as soon as the 24-hour period is past. Thus, patients are encouraged to call before they engage in self-injurious behavior, giving the therapist a chance to intervene. The rationale for this rule is to avoid reinforcement of life-threatening behavior and to provide the opportunity for reinforcement of appropriate help-seeking behavior.

If a patient uses between-session contact inappropriately and the therapist begins to feel burned-out, it is addressed as a therapy-interfering behavior—by conducting behavioral analyses, generating solutions, and applying skills to the reduction of the behavior.

Case Example 3

Ms. M is a 24-year-old woman with a history of more than 20 brief psychiatric hospitalizations for suicidality. In response to her distress, Ms. M often takes overdoses of available medications and then goes or is taken to the emergency department. These visits usually result in hospitalization, which Ms. M finds both helpful (because it gives her a rest from the troubles of her life) and disruptive (because of the negative reactions of family and friends and because she misses work and other responsibilities). Ms. M expressed a desire not to be hospitalized anymore. The therapist suggested that developing a safety plan would help in the short term while skills and strategies were being developed to handle distress.

About 6 months into Ms. M's treatment, she paged her therapist on a Sunday morning because she had taken a "handful" (10–12) of pills to help her calm down after being very upset by an interaction with her boyfriend. The patient said she could not remember exactly which pills she took. It is important to note that although the "24-hour rule" emphasizes the importance of asking for help prior to engaging in a self-injurious behavior, the safety of the patient is evaluated and a safety plan is developed at any point that the patient contacts the therapist. Ms. M's boyfriend had called her at the last minute the previous evening to cancel their plans because he wanted to see a friend first and then meet later. She became very angry with him and told him not to bother coming at all. She then felt very lonely and guilty that she had yelled at him. She became agitated, lying awake all night thinking that he would leave her. She then took the pills to help her get to sleep.

The therapist reminded the patient that it might have been helpful to have paged the therapist before taking the pills so that the therapist could have evaluated the patient's safety and could have determined, with the patient, whether or not she should have gone to the emergency department to get a medical evaluation. Ms. M expressed a desire to be admitted to the hospital because she was tired, she needed a rest and needed to "get away from things." She stated that she did not really want to kill herself but was not sure she could prevent herself from taking pills again. The therapist validated her feelings of wanting a rest but also reminded her of all that they had been working on and expressed the wish that Ms. M would stay out of the hospital so that they could have their outpatient appointment the next day. The therapist offered to do whatever she could to help the patient tolerate staying out of the hospital and not resort to taking another overdose. The therapist reminded Ms. M that it was her choice whether to present herself to the emergency department as in need of hospitalization. The therapist encouraged Ms. M to call from the emergency department so that the therapist could either coach her to stay out of the hospital or engage the hospital staff to make them aware of the treatment goals.

Ms. M called as requested—she had been medically cleared but still wanted to be hospitalized for a rest. The therapist spoke with emergency staff and asked them to evaluate her suicidality. The therapist also encouraged them to make their decision to hospitalize based on the current level of suicidality rather than the patient's desire to be hospitalized. The therapist indicated that she would be willing to see Ms. M the next day as an outpatient and work with her to keep her safe outside the hospital. Ms. M called later that day, complaining that the emergency staff had made her wait 10 hours and she just wanted to go home. The therapist let Ms. M know that she was looking forward to seeing her the next day for their appointment.

This case illustrates how a DBT approach works both to ensure the safety of a potentially suicidal patient in crisis and to encourage the patient to stay out of the hospital and continue building a life worth living. This vignette also describes the way in which DBT encourages managing the contingencies in the environment (working with the emergency department staff) in order to avoid reinforcing less skillful behavior and to promote more skillful behavior (i.e., encouraging Ms. M to figure out a way to control her suicidal urges and to stay out of the hospital and resume outpatient therapy).

Diary Cards

Diary cards are used to track behaviors to decrease and skills to increase, with the top half of the hard copy card used for the former and the bottom half used for the latter. Patients keep track of all target 1 problems (life-threatening and self-injurious behaviors as well as behaviors that have an impact on target 1 problems) on a daily basis. Some examples of these problems might be overall mood, use of nonprescribed substances, urges to self-injure, and adherence to medication regimens. The therapist and patient decide together about any other important behaviors, urges, and feelings to track. These may include eating disorders, urges to physically hurt other people, and impulsive behaviors such as shoplifting. Additionally, diary cards list skills patients are trying to increase, so that the patient can circle the skills they used each day. In recent years, diary cards have been made available via mobile web apps that support DBT, such as Pocket Skills, where patients can access past cards and more readily track their progress (Schroeder et al. 2018).

The diary card serves as the means for setting the session agenda and is reviewed with the patient at the outset of each session. These cards are particularly useful for patients who experience frequent episodes of dissociation or who tend to remember only what happened in their current mood state. The cards are also helpful for patients who feel a great deal of shame about their behaviors. If the shameful behaviors are not recorded on the card, patients often feel too embarrassed to bring them up. Surprisingly, although some patients do not record all relevant behaviors and urges on the cards, it seems easier for patients to be truthful and record these items on the cards than to take the initiative of bringing up these behaviors and urges in a session. Diary cards jog the memory of patients and often result in having available information that would never have been brought up or recollected.

Validation

Validation is a strategy that is used in many forms of psychotherapy including supportive, psychodynamic, and client-centered therapies. Linehan (1993a) presented the essence of validation in the context of DBT psychotherapy: "The therapist communicates to the client that her responses make sense and are understandable within her current life context or situation. Validation strategies require the therapist to search for, recognize, and reflect to the client the validity inherent in her response to events" (p. 223). Validation is at the core of the acceptance/change dialectic and is a crucial aspect of the therapeutic approach in DBT. Linehan therefore delineated five levels of validation: 1) listening and observing; 2) using accurate reflection; 3) articulating the unverbalized; 4) validating in terms of sufficient, but not necessarily valid, causes; and 5) validating as reasonable "in the moment."

Validation is much less frequently utilized in CBT. In DBT, discussions of the patient's emotional experiences, suffering, and difficulty with change are some of the occasions for using validation. The basic function of validation is to communicate to patients that their responses are understandable and make sense within their current life situation or context (Linehan 1993a). Validation should never be patronizing, and it should never validate that which is invalid. Validation is composed of three steps: 1) active observing of what the patient is reporting; 2) reflection of the patient's feelings, thoughts, and behaviors in a nonjudgmental and nonauthoritarian manner, whereby the therapist phrases the reflection not as a pronouncement but more as a question; and 3) direct validation of the validity and "understandability" of the patient's response.

Balancing Change and Acceptance

There is an ongoing focus on maintaining a balance between change and acceptance strategies within each intervention and over the course of the treatment. Validation and acceptance without a change focus can lead to demoralization and a sense that things will never be any different. An approach that focuses too intensely on change can make a patient feel poorly understood and criticized. This effect, in turn, can increase a patient's self-blame and lead to early treatment dropouts.

Consultation Team

An assumption of DBT is that therapists treating suicidal individuals with BPD also need support. An integral aspect of DBT is the role of the consultation team, to which therapists can bring any problems they are experiencing with their patients. The consultation team assumes a dialectic stance and provides both suggestions and support. In addition, the team provides the valuable function of helping therapists stay on track and follow the treatment hierarchy as prescribed. It is important to note that this consultation team is more like a supervision team than a patient's "treatment team." In the DBT model, team members in a day hospital or an inpatient setting tend not to have meetings jointly with the patient, in order to avoid "splitting" or to avoid presenting a unified front to patients—which can be experienced as overwhelming and intimidating to patients. Instead, each staff member's experience with the patient is treated as valid and a synthesis of their experiences is sought. Furthermore, staff members are treated in the therapy as any other person in the patient's life. Therefore, instead of intervening and talking to the other staff member about a patient's complaint or upsetting concern, the therapist coaches a patient on how to handle the complaint directly with the staff member. For example, if a patient in DBT complains bitterly to the therapist that the psychiatrist is often late to appointments and the patient finds it enraging, the therapist's first approach is to help the patient express the feelings about the lateness directly to the psychiatrist rather than the therapist discussing it with the psychiatrist.

Efficacy Data

DBT was originally tested in a randomized controlled clinical trial (Linehan et al. 1991, 1993, 1994; Shearin and Linehan 1992). The 1-year DBT treatment, compared with treatment as usual, showed significant effects in three areas: 1) suicidal behavior and self-mutilation, 2) maintenance in treatment, and 3) amount of inpatient treatment. DBT subjects engaged in significantly fewer self-injurious acts than treatment-as-usual subjects. This effect was most marked in the first 4 months of treatment. DBT patients also had significantly fewer severe self-injurious acts, in terms of medical consequences, than treatment-as-usual patients. Also, DBT patients had greater retention in individual therapy compared with treatment-as-usual patients (with 84% remaining in DBT treatment) and significantly fewer days of hospitalization per person. In addition, DBT showed a greater reduction in anger, as well as comparatively more improved functioning (Linehan et al. 1994). There were no group differences on measures of depression, hopelessness, suicidal ideation, or reasons for living. On 1-year follow-up, Linehan et al. (1993) found that DBT subjects had significantly fewer suicidal and self-mutilating behaviors, less anger, fewer psychiatric inpatient days, and better social adjustment than treatment-as-usual subjects.

Several efficacy trials have since been conducted evaluating the use of DBT in the treatment of BPD. Verheul et al. (2003) conducted a 12-month trial comparing DBT with treatment as usual in 58 women with BPD in the Netherlands. DBT was found to have a better retention rate and greater reductions in self-injury and other forms of self-damaging impulsive behavior. Suicide attempt rates were low in both groups and approached but did not reach significance, with 7% of the DBT group making suicide attempts compared with 26% of the treatment-as-usual group. In a randomized clinical trial of DBT applied to college students, Pistorello et al. (2012) found that DBT was more successful than an optimized treatment-as-usual approach in decreasing suicidality, depression, amount of nonsuicidal self-injury, and BPD symptoms, and it resulted in greater improvements in social adjustment. Koons et al. (2001), in an outpatient study of female veterans with BPD, found that those in DBT had lower rates of self-injury, suicidal ideation, hopelessness, anger, and depression when compared with a treatment-as-usual group. Carter et al. (2010) conducted a randomized controlled trial in Australia comparing DBT with treatment as usual plus waiting list in a sample of women with BPD and found that while both groups showed improvements in direct self-harm and hospitalizations, those who received DBT also showed superior improvements in measures of disability and quality of life. Similarly, McMain et al. (2009), in another randomized trial of DBT for treatment of BPD, found DBT to be equal to general psychiatric management in reducing frequency and severity of suicidal and nonsuicidal self-injurious behaviors. In a follow-up study, McMain et al. (2012) found that most treatment effects had not diminished 2 years later in either group, including the reduction of suicidal and nonsuicidal self-injurious behaviors.

In addition to standard DBT, several variations of the treatment have been tested for treatment of BPD, including DBT as a 6-month treatment (Stanley et al. 2007). Stanley et al. (2007), in a pilot study, found that individuals in DBT demonstrated decreased rates of self-injurious behavior and urges to self-injure and decreased hopelessness and subjective depression over the course of a 6-month treatment. Treatment retention was very high, with a 95% completion rate. McMain et al. (2017) conducted a randomized trial of 20 weeks of DBT skills training in suicidal patients with BPD. Compared with those in the wait-list condition, those receiving DBT skills training showed greater improvements on suicidal behaviors and nonsuicidal self-injurious behaviors between baseline and posttreatment follow-up. Those who received DBT also demonstrated superior improvement with regard to anger, distress tolerance, and emotion regulation compared with those in the control condition. Additionally, Linehan et al. (2015) conducted a randomized clinical trial comparing standard DBT (including skills training and individual therapy) to skills training/case management and individual therapy/activities groups. All treatments yielded similar decreases in frequency and severity of suicide attempts and suicidal ideation, while the skills training conditions were more successful in reducing frequency of nonsuicidal self-injurious acts.

DBT has also been adapted for inpatient settings (Bohus et al. 2004; Kröger et al. 2006; Simpson et al. 1998; Swenson et al. 2001; Turner 2000). Barley et al. (1993) conducted a partial replication of DBT's efficacy in a pre-post design by showing a reduction in rates of suicidal behavior and self-mutilation incidents with DBT. Monthly rates of self-destructive behavior on an inpatient unit were compared before and after the introduction of DBT with rates on a similar general adult inpatient unit using a non-DBT treatment. Mean monthly rates of self-injurious behavior on the DBT unit were significantly lower after the introduction of DBT, whereas rates on the non-DBT unit were not significantly altered during the same time period. Therefore, DBT appears to be effective in treating the more serious behavioral aspects of BPD, namely suicidal behavior and self-mutilation. In addition, Bohus et al. (2004), in a controlled inpatient trial of DBT, found that compared with those in treatment as usual plus waiting list, those receiving three months of DBT had made superior gains in depression, anxiety, interpersonal functioning, social adjustment, global psychopathology, and self-mutilation 4 weeks postdischarge. Kleindienst et al. (2008) followed up on those who received DBT for 21 months postdischarge and found that the improvements persisted over the course of the follow-up period.

In recent years, DBT has been adapted to treat those with posttraumatic stress disorder (PTSD) who have comorbid BPD and suicidal or nonsuicidal self-injurious behavior (Harned et al. 2012). This approach incorporates prolonged exposure (PE), including in vivo and imagined exposures, into standard outpatient DBT, and is referred to as DBT PE. In a pilot randomized controlled trial comparing DBT with DBT PE in women with BPD, PTSD, and intentional self-injury, DBT PE facilitated greater and more persistent improvements in PTSD. Those who received DBT PE were 2 times more likely to be in remission, 2.4 times less likely to attempt suicide, and 1.5 times less likely to engage in self-injurious behavior (Harned et al. 2014).

Although there are no trials of patients with other personality disorders, efficacy data have been shown for DBT with domestic violence partners (Fruzzetti and Levensky 2000) and in patients with bulimia (Safer et al. 2001), binge eating (Telch et al. 2001), hyperactivity (Hesslinger et al. 2002), and substance use disorders (Linehan et al. 1999, 2002; van den Bosch et al. 2002). Also, adaptations and efficacy in special populations have been explored, including forensic patients (McCann et al. 2000; Trupin et al. 2002), the elderly depressed (Lynch et al. 2003), and adolescents (Mehlum et al. 2014; Miller et al. 2006; Rathus and Miller 2002). A new evidence-based treatment incorporating DBT approaches, Radically Open DBT (RO-DBT), offers treatment of disorders involving excessive self-control, such as anorexia nervosa (Hempel et al. 2018). See Scheel 2000 and Robins and Chapman 2004 for a comprehensive critical review of empirical findings regarding DBT for all disorders.

Conclusion

DBT is a cognitive-behavioral treatment that has demonstrated efficacy in BPD. It has also been adapted to other disorders and specialized populations. Although it has not yet been adapted to other personality disorders, it is likely to be useful in those disorders in which impulsivity and behavioral dyscontrol are prominent. While DBT trials have promising findings, there are significant challenges associated with its dissemination and implementation. A UK-based study found that only 57% of active DBT programs provided full DBT; reasons reported for inactive programs included lack of buy-in from management, insufficient funding, and staff turnover (Swales et al. 2012). In qualitative interviews with clinicians (Carmel et al. 2014) and administrators (Herschell et al. 2009), a number of barriers to implementation were identified, including problems with staff turnover, challenges with referring appropriate clients, and lack of necessary resources. Moreover, the training required—the DBT Intensive Training Model developed by Linehan—is extensive, including two 5-day trainings with 6 months of self-guided study in between (Landes and Linehan 2012). However, the extent of training does not differ substantially from other evidence-based psychotherapies, particularly for the type of complex problems DBT addresses.

References

Bankoff SM, Karpel MG, Forbes HE, et al: A systematic review of dialectical behavior therapy for the treatment of eating disorders. Eat Disord 20:196–215, 2012

Barley WD, Buie SE, Peterson EW, et al: Development of an inpatient cognitive-behavioral treatment program for borderline personality disorder. J Pers Disord 7:232–240, 1993

Beck AT, Freeman A, Davis DD: Cognitive Therapy of Personality Disorders, 2nd Edition. New York, Guilford, 2003

Bohus M, Haaf B, Simms T, et al: Effectiveness of inpatient dialectical behavioral therapy for borderline personality disorder: a controlled trial. Behav Res Ther 42:487–499, 2004

Brodsky BS, Cloitre M, Dulit RA: Relationship of dissociation to self-mutilation and childhood abuse in borderline personality disorder. Am J Psychiatry 152:1788–1792, 1995

Carmel A, Rose ML, Fruzzetti AE: Barriers and solutions to implementing dialectical behavior therapy in a public behavioral health system. Adm Policy Ment Health 41:608–614, 2014

Carter GL, Willcox CH, Lewin TJ, et al: Hunter DBT Project: randomized controlled trial of dialectical behaviour therapy in women with borderline personality disorder. Aust N Z J Psychiatry 44:162–173, 2010

Cialdini RB, Vincent JE, Lewis SK, et al: Reciprocal concessions procedure for inducing compliance: the door-in-the-face technique. J Pers Soc Psychol 31:206–215, 1975

Crowell SE, Beauchaine TP, Linehan MM: A biosocial developmental model of borderline personality: elaborating and extending Linehan's theory. Psychol Bull 135:495–510, 2009

Crowell SE, Kaufman EA, Beauchaine TP: A biosocial model of BPD: theory and empirical evidence in Handbook of Borderline Personality Disorder in Children and Adolescents. Edited by Sharp C, Tackett JL. New York, Springer, 2014, pp 143–157

Dimeff L, Linehan M: Dialectical behavior therapy in a nutshell. The California Psychologist 34:10–13, 2001

Foa EB: Psychological processes related to recovery from a trauma and an effective treatment for PTSD. Ann NY Acad Sci 821:410–424, 1997

Freedman JL, Fraser SC: Compliance without pressure: the foot-in-the-door technique. J Pers Soc Psychol 4:195–202, 1966

Fruzzetti AE, Levensky ER: Dialectical behavior therapy for domestic violence: rationale and procedures. Cogn Behav Pract 7:435–447, 2000

Harned MS, Korslund KE, Foa EB, et al: Treating PTSD in suicidal and self-injuring women with borderline personality disorder: development and preliminary evaluation of a dialectical behavior therapy prolonged exposure protocol. Behav Res Ther 50:381–386, 2012

Harned MS, Korslund KE, Linehan MM: A pilot randomized controlled trial of dialectical behavior therapy with and without the dialectical behavior therapy prolonged exposure protocol for suicidal and self-injuring women with borderline personality disorder and PTSD. Behav Res Ther 55:7–17, 2014

Hempel R, Vanderbleek E, Lynch TR: Radically open DBT: targeting emotional loneliness in anorexia nervosa. Eat Disord 26:92–104, 2018

Herman JL, Perry JC, van der Kolk BA: Childhood trauma in borderline personality disorder. Am J Psychiatry 146:490–495, 1989

Herschell AD, Kogan JN, Celedonia KL, et al: Understanding community mental health administrators' perspectives on dialectical behavior therapy implementation. Psychiatr Serv 60(7):989–992, 2009

Herschell AD, Lindhiem OJ, Kogan JN, et al: Evaluation of an implementation initiative for embedding dialectical behavior therapy in community settings. Eval Program Plann 43:55–63, 2013

Hesslinger B, Tebartz van Elst L, Nyberg E, et al: Psychotherapy of attention deficit hyperactivity disorder in adults: a pilot study using a structured skills training program. Eur Arch Psychiatry Clin Neurosci 252:117–184, 2002

Kehrer CA, Linehan MM: Interpersonal and emotional problem-solving skills and parasuicide among women with borderline personality disorder. J Pers Disord 10:153–163, 1996

Kleindienst N, Limberger MF, Schmahl C, et al: Do improvements after inpatient dialectical behavioral therapy persist in the long term? A naturalistic follow-up in patients with borderline personality disorder. J Nerv Ment Dis 196:847–851, 2008

Koons C, Robins CJ, Tweed JL, et al: Efficacy of dialectical behavior therapy in women veterans with borderline personality disorder. Behav Ther 32:371–390, 2001

Kröger C, Schweiger U, Sipos V, et al: Effectiveness of dialectical behaviour therapy for borderline personality disorder in an inpatient setting. Behav Res Ther 44:1211–1217, 2006

Kröger C, Harbeck S, Armbrust M, et al: Effectiveness, response, and dropout of dialectical behavior therapy for borderline personality disorder in an inpatient setting. Behav Res Ther 51:411–416, 2013

Landes SJ, Linehan MM: Dissemination and implementation of dialectical behavior therapy: an intensive training model, in Dissemination and Implementation of Evidence-Based Psychological Interventions. Edited by McHugh RK, Barlow DH. Oxford, UK, Oxford University Press, 2012, pp 187–208

Linehan MM: Dialectical behavior therapy: a cognitive-behavioral approach to parasuicide. J Pers Disord 1:328–333, 1987

Linehan MM: Cognitive-Behavioral Treatment of Borderline Personality Disorder. New York, Guilford, 1993a

Linehan MM: Skills Training Manual for Treating Borderline Personality Disorder. New York, Guilford, 1993b

Linehan MM: Dialectical behavior therapy for borderline personality disorder. J Calif Alliance Ment Ill 8:44–46, 1997

Linehan MM: DBT Skills Training Manual, 2nd Edition. New York, Guilford, 2014

Linehan MM, Armstrong HE, Suarez A, et al: Cognitive-behavioral treatment of chronically parasuicidal borderline patients. Arch Gen Psychiatry 48:1060–1064, 1991

Linehan MM, Heard HL, Armstrong HE: Naturalistic follow-up of a behavioral treatment for chronically parasuicidal borderline patients. Arch Gen Psychiatry 50:971–975, 1993

Linehan MM, Tutek D, Heard HL, et al: Interpersonal outcome of cognitive-behavioral treatment for chronically suicidal borderline patients. Am J Psychiatry 5:1771–1776, 1994

Linehan MM, Schmidt H, Dimeff LA, et al: Dialectical behavior therapy for patients with borderline personality disorder and drug-dependence. Am J Addict 8:279–292, 1999

Linehan MM, Dimeff LA, Reynolds SK, et al: Dialectical behavior therapy versus comprehensive validation therapy plus 12-step for the treatment of opioid dependent women meeting criteria for borderline personality disorder. Drug Alcohol Depend 67:13–26, 2002

Linehan MM, Comtois KA, Murray AM, et al: Two-year randomized controlled trial and follow-up of dialectical behavior therapy vs. therapy by experts for suicidal behaviors and borderline personality disorder. Arch Gen Psychiatry 63:757–766, 2006

Linehan MM, Korslund KE, Harned MS, et al: Dialectical behavior therapy for high suicide risk in individuals with borderline personality disorder: a randomized clinical trial and component analysis. JAMA Psychiatry 72:478–452, 2015

Lynch TR, Morse JQ, Mendelson T, et al: Dialectical behavior therapy for depressed older adults: a randomized pilot study. Am J Geriatr Psychiatry 11:33–45, 2003

McCann RA, Ball EM, Ivanoff A: DBT with an inpatient forensic population: the CMHIP forensic model. Cogn Behav Pract 7:447–456, 2000

McMain SF, Links PS, Gnam WH, et al: A randomized trial of dialectical behavior therapy versus general psychiatric management for borderline personality disorder. Am J Psychiatry 166:1365–1374, 2009

McMain SF, Guimond T, Streiner DL et al: Dialectical behavior therapy compared with general psychiatric management for borderline personality disorder: clinical outcomes and functioning over a 2-year follow-up. Am J Psychiatry 169:650–661, 2012

McMain SF, Guimond T, Barnhart R, et al: A randomized trial of brief dialectical behaviour therapy skills training in suicidal patients suffering from borderline disorder. Acta Psychiatr Scand 135:138–148, 2017

Mehlum L, Tørmoen AJ, Ramberg M, et al: Dialectical behavior therapy for adolescents with repeated suicidal and self-harming behavior: a randomized trial. J Am Acad Child Adolesc Psychiatry 53:1082–1091, 2014

Miller AL, Rathus JH, Linehan MM: Dialectical Behavior Therapy With Suicidal Adolescents. New York, Guilford, 2006

Ogata SN, Silk KR, Goodrich S, et al: Childhood sexual and physical abuse in adult patients with borderline personality disorder. Am J Psychiatry 147:1008–1013, 1990

Panos PT, Jackson JW, Hasan O, et al: Meta-analysis and systematic review assessing the efficacy of dialectical behavior therapy (DBT). Res Soc Work Pract 24:213–223, 2014

Pistorello J, Fruzzetti AE, MacLane C, et al: Dialectical behavior therapy (DBT) applied to college students: a randomized clinical trial. J Consult Clin Psychol 80:982–994, 2012

Rathus JH, Miller AL: Dialectical behavior therapy adapted for suicidal adolescents. Suicide Life Threat Behav 32:146–157, 2002

Robins CJ: Zen principles and mindfulness practice in dialectical behavior therapy. Cogn Behav Pract 9:50–57, 2002

Robins CJ, Chapman AL: Dialectical behavior therapy: current status, recent developments, and future directions. J Pers Disord 18:73–89, 2004

Robins CJ, Ivanoff AM, Linehan MM: Dialectical behavior therapy, in Handbook of Personality Disorders: Theory, Research, and Treatment. Edited by Livesley WJ. New York, Guilford, 2001, pp 117–139

Safer DL, Telch CF, Agras WS: Dialectical behavior therapy for bulimia nervosa. Am J Psychiatry 158:632–634, 2001

Scheel KR: The empirical basis of dialectical behavior therapy: summary, critique, and implications. Clin Psychol Sci Pract 7:68–86, 2000

Schroeder J, Wilkes C, Rowan K, et al: Pocket skills: a conversational mobile web app to support dialectical behavior therapy (Paper No 398), in CHI 2018: Proceedings of the 2018 CHI Conference on Human Factors in Computing Systems. New York, ACM, 2018

Sharp C, Kim S: Recent advances in the developmental aspects of borderline personality disorder. Curr Psychiatry Rep 17:1–9, 2015

Shearin EN, Linehan MM: Patient-therapist ratings and relationship to progress in dialectical behavior therapy for borderline personality disorder. Behav Ther 23:730–741, 1992

Simpson EB, Pistorello J, Begin A, et al: Use of dialectical behavior therapy in a partial hospital program for women with borderline personality disorder. Psychiatr Serv 49:669–673, 1998

Spieglar MD, Guevremont DC: Contemporary Behavior Therapy, 3rd Edition. Pacific Grove, CA, Brooks/Cole Publishing, 1998

Stanley B, Brodsky B: Suicidal and self-injurious behavior in borderline personality disorder: the self-regulation action model, in Understanding and Treating Borderline Personality Disorder: A Guide for Professionals and Families. Edited by Gunderson JG, Hoffman PD. Washington, DC, American Psychiatric Publishing, 2005, pp 43–63

Stanley B, Bundy E, Beberman R: Skills training as an adjunctive treatment for personality disorders. J Psychiatr Pract 7:324–335, 2001

Stanley B, Brodsky B, Nelson JD, et al: Brief dialectical behavior therapy (DBT-B) for suicidal behavior and non-suicidal self-injury. Arch Suicide Res 11:337–341, 2007

Swales MA, Taylor B, Hibbs RA: Implementing dialectical behaviour therapy: programme survival in routine healthcare settings. J Ment Health 21:548–555, 2012

Swenson CR, Sanderson C, Dulit RA, et al: The application of dialectical behavior therapy for patients with borderline personality disorder on inpatient units. Psychiatr Q 72:307–324, 2001

Telch CF, Agras WS, Linehan MM: Dialectical behavior therapy for binge eating disorder. J Consult Clin Psychol 69:1061–1065, 2001

Trupin EW, Stewart DG, Beach B, et al: Effectiveness of dialectical behaviour therapy program for incarcerated female juvenile offenders. Child and Adolescent Mental Health 7:121–127, 2002

Turner RM: Naturalistic evaluation of dialectical behavior therapy-oriented treatment for borderline personality disorder. Cogn Behav Pract 7:413–419, 2000

van den Bosch LMC, Verheul R, Schippers GM, et al: Dialectical behavior therapy of borderline patients with and without substance abuse problems: implementation and long-term effects. Addict Behav 27:911–923, 2002

Verheul R, van den Bosch LMC, Koeter MWJ, et al: Dialectical behavior therapy for women with borderline personality disorder. Br J Psychiatry 182:135–140, 2003

CHAPTER 14

Cognitive-Behavioral Therapy

J. Christopher Fowler, Ph.D.

William H. Orme, Ph.D.

John M. Hart, Ph.D.

Theory, Definition, and Interventions

Cognitive-behavioral therapy (CBT) has a rich history dating back to the 1960s that emerged from the pioneering works of cognitive theorists like Aaron T. Beck and Albert Ellis; behavior theorists B.F. Skinner, Arnold Lazarus, and Joseph Wolpe; and the social learning theory of Albert Bandura. Despite inevitable ideological differences, CBT has emerged as an integrative approach to understanding human problems and advancing psychotherapy. At the heart of CBT interventions is the focus on alleviating suffering by modifying dysfunctional beliefs and helping clients acquire new coping skills. CBT, like most approaches to psychotherapy, is generally aimed at helping people function better, reduce distress, solve problems, and ultimately seek an increased sense of well-being.

The impact of Beck on CBT cannot be overstated. He began with a premise based on the stoic philosophy of Epictetus that it is not internal or external experiences that directly impact individuals' emotional, behavioral, and physiological reactions, but rather the meaning that is made from their experiences. Likewise, Ellis held that it is troublesome that people find themselves in distress, but the real issue is that people distress themselves. Ellis's cognitive model (commonly referred to as the ABC model), which includes an activating event (A), a person's beliefs (B), and resulting emotional, behavioral, and psychophysiological consequences (C), has served as the organizing basis of CBT. However, the ABC model is not linear and is conceptualized as multidimensional and interrelated (David and Freeman 2014).

Borrowing from traditional behavioral therapy, CBT practitioners emphasize identifying problems, setting goals, measuring and monitoring progress, assessing the environmental contingencies maintaining dysfunction, eliciting feedback, and developing specific effective interventions. As CBT continued to develop, it incorporated skill acquisition and building behavioral repertoires with interventions such as assertiveness training, progressive muscle relaxation, role-playing, positive reinforcement, and exposure therapy. As proponents of behavioral theories continued to build their approaches based on empirical work, it became apparent that internal events such as perceptions, expectations, values, attitudes, and evaluations needed to be accounted for within a learning framework. In reference to personality disorders (PDs), behavioral therapies treated PD symptoms not as an expression of an underlying condition but rather as learned human responses to specific or general stimuli (Goldfried and Davison 1990).

During the formative years of CBT development, the greatest emphasis was on treating depression and anxiety with relatively low dose and duration. As specific treatments for PDs began to accelerate in the early 1990s, Beck and Freeman (1990) held that a PD is identified by the dysfunctional beliefs that characterize and perpetuate it. Dysfunctional beliefs form the core component of a CBT case conceptualization and serve as a main target for intervention (Beck 1998). For example, a core dysfunctional belief for narcissistic PD would be "I'm inferior, and to compensate I have to be special." Concurrently, Young (1999) developed an attachment-based schema approach to PDs in which schemas are patterns of internal experience consisting of memories, beliefs, emotions, and thoughts that can become maladaptive when core needs are not met in childhood development. PDs are formed and maintained by a process of dysfunctional coping styles that surrender to the maladaptive schema, avoid it, or overcompensate for it.

Cognitive-behavioral therapy for individuals with PDs is an evolving process in which collaboratively planned interventions are intended to become part of the patient's way of experiencing the external world and inner experiences. Challenging maladaptive negative thoughts extends beyond examining the *content* of a belief or the truth and falsity of any particular thought to considering how the *process* of thinking functions within a person's life and the world in which he or she lives (Björgvinsson and Hart 2006). Cognitive therapy theorists generally agree that it is necessary to identify and modify core problems in interpersonal, emotional, and cognitive domains when treating individuals with PDs (Beck et al. 2004) and to view the products of these core problems as available for conscious-level psychological work (Ingram and Hollon 1986). A tripartite intervention strategy targeting schemas about the self and others, self-destructive and defeating behaviors, and affect dysregulation is assumed to be necessary to working effectively with patients with PDs. CBT is an evolving theoretical and treatment structure with the capacity to integrate interventions and concepts from a broad base of scientific disciplines.

Modern CBT incorporates a wide range of techniques (Table 14–1), including cognitive restructuring, behavior modification, exposure, psychoeducation, and skills training (Matusiewicz et al. 2010). Effective CBT for the PDs includes a careful negotiation of a therapeutic alliance with specific attention to developing an agreement on the goals of the treatment. The collaborative nature of goal setting is one of the most important features of cognitive therapy in general, although achieving an effective collaboration can be particularly challenging in this situation because patients struggling with PDs are being asked to modify their primary modes of operating and to alter their sche-

TABLE 14–1. **Components of cognitive-behavioral therapy (CBT)–based interventions for personality disorders (PDs)**

Intervention	Definition
Goal setting	An intervention that actively involves the patient in establishing clear and attainable goals for treatment. The emphasis in PD treatment is on fostering an atmosphere of collaboration in support of patient autonomy and agency.
Psychoeducation	Explicit instruction regarding case conceptualization, diagnoses, and treatment approach, including discussion of core schemas and likely etiologies. Also refers to the teaching component of skills training.
Cognitive reframing	A technique for identifying the rules, assumptions, and core beliefs that contribute to symptoms and systematically modifying distortions through collaborative evaluation and reattribution. In PD treatment, the emphasis is on shifting core beliefs about the self.
Schema modification	A key ingredient of schema therapy that consists of understanding and altering the internal template that organizes self-other perceptions (i.e., core schemas). This includes targeting the cognitive, affective, and behavioral correlates of foundational schemas through various exercises.
Behavior modification	A dedicated focus on decreasing self-defeating behaviors and increasing adaptive action. This includes monitoring daily living activities, identifying self-destructive patterns, increasing pleasurable experiences, and fostering self-care. Often includes homework involving tasks that are graded in difficulty.
Exposure	A particular behavioral intervention aimed at facilitating contact with situations that are avoided or feared while reinforcing experiential learning. Exposure happens in a graded fashion and may include both imaginal and in vivo exercises.
Behavioral experiments	Experiential activities, collaboratively developed, that are tailored to test and challenge cognitive distortions, improve flexibility, and increase awareness.
Skills training	Identification of skill deficits and a focus on building mastery in these areas. This may include the capacity for emotion regulation, mindful observation, relaxation training, assertiveness, intimacy skills, and so forth.

mas about the self and others (Beck et al. 2004). Not surprisingly, CBT for PDs requires modification of brief treatment models to bring about lasting improvement in underlying schemas, affect regulation, and behavioral patterns that frequently produce negative reinforcement such as nonsuicidal self-injury (NSSI) in order to decrease emotional distress and produce analgesic effects (Nock and Prinstein 2005).

Broadly speaking, problematic personality traits and disturbance in schemas about self and other are maintained by a combination of maladaptive beliefs about self and others and contextual factors that reinforce problematic behavior and undermine effective behavior (Beck et al. 2004; Linehan 1993). Sperry (2006) construed PDs as a disharmony in the interaction of character and temperament. Character refers to developmentally learned beliefs and values based on psychosocial influences on the individual and is commonly associated with the term *schema*. Schemas are cognitive structures consisting of basic beliefs that individuals use to organize their views of the world, the self, and the future; these implicit and explicit schemas interact with genetic factors that influence expression of personality.

Cognitive-behavioral treatments that emphasize the role of distorted schemas about self and other, along with disturbance in affect regulation and behavior, are readily integrated into the conceptualization of the alternative model for PDs appearing in DSM-5 Section III, "Emerging Measures and Models" (American Psychiatric Association 2013). According to this alternative model, the central, defining features of PDs are 1) an overarching pattern of distorted and maladaptive thinking about oneself and 2) impaired interpersonal relationships (Bender et al. 2011; Morey et al. 2011). Numerous studies indicate that maladaptive patterns of mental representations form a common substrate of core impairments across PDs (Bender and Skodol 2007). Thus, internal working models or schemas constitute an overarching domain of personality function that impacts the quality of relationships. The focus on a dimensional conceptualization of personality traits as an organizing approach to the identification of problematic areas of functioning also fits well with the philosophy of cognitive-behavioral therapies that attend to dysfunction in behavioral and interpersonal domains but do not necessarily subscribe to a view of categorical PDs.

Meta-analyses and Reviews

Randomized controlled trials (RCTs) and high-quality effectiveness studies of CBT for PDs reveal generally positive outcomes (for a review of the CBT outcome literature for PDs, see Matusiewicz et al. 2010). A series of meta-analyses on the effectiveness of psychotherapy for treatment of PDs demonstrated that cognitive-behavioral and psychodynamic psychotherapies of middle to long duration are effective in reducing depression and the burden of global psychiatric symptoms, even when co-occurring disorders are present (Leichsenring and Leibing 2003; Leichsenring and Rabung 2008). Far less evidence exists on the effectiveness of psychotherapies in the treatment of specific PDs other than borderline PD (BPD); nonetheless, evidence has emerged during the past three decades to suggest that CBT is effective in treating other PDs (Matusiewicz et al. 2010; McMain and Pos 2007).

Because the vast majority of effectiveness and efficacy studies have targeted BPD symptomatology, more is known about effective treatment for this particular disorder. The American Psychiatric Association's (2001) guideline for the treatment of patients with BPD and the subsequent guideline watch (Oldham 2005) confirm that psychotherapy represents the primary treatment for BPD, with adjunctive, symptom-targeted pharmacotherapy used to mitigate severity of core symptoms. A persuasive review of data from approximately 24 RCTs of BPD (Leichsenring et al. 2011) demonstrated clear and compelling evidence that several forms of psychotherapy, including CBT and dialectical behavior therapy (DBT), help patients with BPD decrease the frequency of self-destructive behaviors such as NSSI, as well as common secondary symptoms of depression, anxiety, and substance abuse. Recent meta-analyses continue to support the use of CBT treatments for PDs (Cristea et al. 2017; Stoffers et al. 2012), although the distinction between these treatments and treatment as usual (TAU) has become less clear in recent years, likely of because control treatments incorporating more known factors related to PD treatment effectiveness (Bateman et al. 2015). Refer to the section "New Directions" below for further discussion.

Traditional Cognitive-Behavioral Therapy

Efficacy trials of traditional CBT demonstrate generally positive results for the treatment of PDs. In the Borderline Personality Disorder Study of Cognitive Therapy (BOSCOT), individuals were randomly assigned to a TAU arm consisting of community-based medication management and emergency services ($n=52$) or to TAU+CBT ($n=54$) (Davidson et al. 2006). Treatment duration was 1 year (maximum of 30 sessions), with an average of 16 sessions attended. The active ingredients of the CBT arm included cognitive restructuring, modifying dysfunctional schemas and core beliefs, implementing behavioral change (decreasing self-defeating and self-destructive behaviors), and increasing adaptive responses to problems. Although patients in both treatment groups demonstrated improvement, those in the TAU+CBT group reported fewer suicide attempts. At treatment termination TAU+CBT subjects reported lower symptom distress, reduced anxiety, and fewer dysfunctional cognitions; however, the active treatment arm did not demonstrate superiority over TAU in number of hospitalizations, number of emergency department admissions, frequency of NSSI or psychiatric symptoms, level of interpersonal functioning, and level of global functioning at follow-up. A 6-year follow-up demonstrated durable gains for the TAU+CBT subjects (Davidson et al. 2010). A reexamination of therapist effects in the BOSCOT trial indicated that patients receiving a higher quantity and more competent delivery of CBT had two to three times greater improvement in suicide-related outcomes (Norrie et al. 2013).

An RCT of treatment of patients with BPD demonstrated equivalent outcomes between CBT and Rogerian supportive counseling on measures of anxiety, depression, dysfunctional cognitions, and suicide-related behaviors; however, patients in the CBT condition demonstrated superior outcomes at 24-month follow-up of patient- and clinician-rated global symptom severity (Cottraux et al. 2009). The latter finding must be interpreted with caution, however, because intent-to-treat analyses were not performed and dropout/loss-to-follow-up rates were high.

Another CBT designed to augment individual psychotherapy is manual assisted cognitive treatment (MACT). This six-session treatment combines components of CBT with elements of DBT, including distress tolerance and functional analysis of NSSI. In the most recent RCT for MACT (Weinberg et al. 2006), MACT+TAU demonstrated superiority to TAU in decreasing frequency and severity of NSSI but did not differ from TAU in time to the first instance of suicidal ideation or repeat suicide attempt.

Group-based cognitive-behavioral interventions specifically developed for reducing the self-defeating and self-destructive behaviors associated with BPD have demonstrated considerable promise. Systems Training for Emotional Predictability and Problem Solving (STEPPS; Blum et al. 2002) is based on the premise that individuals with BPD have limited access to specific emotion regulation and behavior management strategies. Such deficits negatively impact the emotional and interpersonal stability of relationships, thereby impairing an individual's capacity to utilize support systems (Blum et al. 2002, 2008). The active treatment consists of 20 weekly group sessions divided into four modules: 1) assembling of a support system, 2) psychoeducation about BPD for the members of the support system, 3) psychoeducation for patients to help them identify thoughts and emotions that contribute to problematic behavior, and 4) emotion management skills training for patients. STEPPS has been evaluated in three RCTs involving outpatients diagnosed with BPD who were randomly assigned to receive either TAU or TAU+STEPPS (Blum et al. 2008; Freije et al. 2002; Van Wel et al. 2006). Results from all three trials indicate the superiority of STEPPS to TAU in decreasing BPD symptom severity, negative affectivity, impulsivity, and global impairment in functioning, with gains generally maintained over 1-year follow-up. A fourth RCT comparing STEPPS plus focused individual therapy with TAU yielded similar results, showing improvements posttreatment and at 6-month follow-up in BPD symptomology and quality of life (Bos et al. 2010). Most recently, the effectiveness of STEPPS was evaluated in an uncontrolled study involving a U.K. community-based sample (Hill et al. 2016). The results indicated that even when STEPPS was implemented by novice facilitators, participants showed significant improvement in BPD symptomology and overall quality of life. Results from all studies indicate, however, that STEPPS does not appear to reduce the targeted suicide-related behaviors, NSSI, or corresponding rates of inpatient hospitalizations or emergency department visits.

A second group treatment, emotion regulation group therapy (ERGT; Gratz and Gunderson 2006), is an acceptance-based model that aims to increase the capacity of patients to control behavior while in states of distress, rather than attempting to control the experiences of emotions. The model and treatment highlight the functional aspects of emotion problem solving and the difficulties associated with attempts to control and suppress emotional experiences. A preliminary RCT involving women diagnosed with BPD who were randomly assigned to TAU ($n=10$) or weekly group sessions of ERGT+TAU ($n=14$) demonstrated a significant reduction in frequency of NSSI as well as clinically significant reductions in symptoms of depression, anxiety, stress, emotional dysregulation, experiential avoidance, and BPD criteria. The TAU group failed to demonstrate improvements in any outcomes of interest. This small RCT was followed by an open trial of ERGT treating a wider array of individuals with NSSI (Gratz and Tull 2011). Results indicated significant changes from pretreatment to posttreatment, with large effect sizes on all measures except quality of life and blatantly self-destructive behaviors (the latter demonstrated a medium-large effect size). Importantly, 55% of the ERGT group reported abstinence from NSSI during the last 2 months of the group treatment. Gratz and colleagues (2014) found continued support for the efficacy of ERGT in an RCT of outpatient women with BPD and NSSI who were randomly assigned to ERGT+TAU ($n=31$) or TAU wait-list ($n=30$). The findings showed significant effects of ERGT on NSSI, BPD symptoms, quality of life, depression, and stress levels. Treatment gains were either sustained or improved at an uncontrolled 9-month follow-up, with an impressive 47% of participants reporting continued abstinence from NSSI. ERGT has been evaluated beyond research settings to show the feasibility of implementation and effectiveness of treatment within community clinics for women with BPD and NSSI (Sahlin et al. 2017).

Effectiveness of cognitive psychotherapy for avoidant PD has been demonstrated in an RCT in which CBT proved superior to brief dynamic therapy in improving social phobia, avoidance, and obsessive symptoms (Emmelkamp et al. 2006). A 52-week open trial of CBT showed reductions in depression and personality symptoms at the end of treatment of patients with avoidant PD and patients with obsessive-compulsive PD (Strauss et al. 2006). Evidence from single case experimental designs also suggests that brief cognitive therapy consisting of 12 sessions may be potentially beneficial for individuals with avoidant PD, although additional research with larger sample sizes is needed to further clarify (Rees and Pritchard 2015).

Group CBT for patients with avoidant PD utilizes cognitive restructuring, exposure, skills training, and intimacy skills training to decrease social avoidance and anxiety. A well-designed multi-arm RCT (Alden 1989) compared three active group CBT treatments with a wait-list control group. The standard group CBT arm included exposure with limited cognitive components, the second arm consisted of standard group CBT plus general skills training, and the third consisted of the group CBT plus intimacy-focused skills training. All active treatment conditions produced reductions in depression, anxiety, and avoidant behavior, as well as improvements in social functioning, with gains maintained at 3 months posttreatment. Renneberg et al. (1990) found modest recovery rates following brief, intensive group CBT, which consisted of exposure and skills training across four full-day group sessions. At treatment completion, 40% of patients receiving group CBT were considered recovered on the basis of their fear of negative evaluation; however, much lower rates of recovery were demonstrated for depression, anxiety, social avoidance, distress, and overall social functioning. A series of studies demonstrated that exposure and skills training were sufficient to bring about significant improvement and target symptoms, whereas cognitive restructuring had minimal effect (Stravynski et al. 1982, 1994).

Thus far, CBT has demonstrated modest efficacy in the treatment of antisocial PD but has not demonstrated superiority over TAU. Davidson et al. (2009) randomly assigned men with antisocial PD to receive either CBT or TAU. In both treatment conditions, patients demonstrated a lower frequency of verbal and physical aggression at follow-up; however, there were no improvements observed in secondary symptoms such as anger, negative beliefs about others, depression, or anxiety. Black et al. (2016) found promising results in a series of two RCTs that evaluated individuals with antisocial PD and comorbid BPD versus those with BPD alone in response to the CBT-based STEPPS program. Results from both RCTs suggested that individuals with comorbid antisocial PD and BPD benefited from STEPPS as much or more than those with BPD alone in regard to impulsivity, BPD-related symptoms, and negative affectivity. The findings represent positive indicators of the potential for individuals with antisocial PD to benefit from CBT treatment. At the present time, there are no known open trials or RCTs assessing CBT for schizoid, schizotypal, paranoid, dependent, narcissistic, or histrionic PD.

Schema-Focused Therapy

Schema-focused therapy (SFT) integrates techniques from behavioral, psychodynamic, experiential, interpersonal, and cognitive-behavioral techniques (Young 1999; Young and Lindemann 2002). Its primary cognitive theoretical framework incorporates the construct of psychological schemas about the self and others and assumes that rigid patterns of avoidant and compensatory behaviors develop to avoid the triggering of underlying painful schemas. Modifying early maladaptive schemas is a primary focus of the treatment and requires individual psychotherapy treatment durations ranging from 1 to 4 years.

In a large-scale RCT, patients with BPD were randomly assigned to receive either SFT or transference-focused psychotherapy (TFP) (Giesen-Bloo et al. 2006). Patients in the SFT arm demonstrated greater improvement across BPD dimensions, including relationship impairment, identity disturbance, abandonment fears, dissociation, impulsivity, and NSSI. SFT also proved efficacious in decreasing symptomatic behaviors consisting of general symptoms, defense mechanisms, and paranoia. Improvement in these latter symptoms imply change in underlying schemas. Although both treatment arms demonstrated significant improvement in targeted symptoms and behaviors, SFT demonstrated a 66% overall gain in clinically significant change compared with 43% for TFP.

Research on SFT was extended to other PDs in a multicenter RCT conducted by Bamelis and colleagues (2014). Individuals with avoidant, dependent, obsessive-compulsive, histrionic, narcissistic, or paranoid PD were randomly assigned to receive either SFT (n=147), TAU (n=135), or clarification-oriented therapy (n=41), a specialized form of client-centered therapy for individuals with PDs. Results indicated that SFT significantly outperformed TAU and clarification-oriented therapy on the primary outcome of remission of PD symptoms. No differences were found between clarification-oriented therapy and TAU. Individuals receiving SFT also had improved global, social, and occupational functioning in comparison with TAU.

SFT has been adapted for a 30-session group format as an augmentation to individual psychotherapy. Farrell et al. (2009) randomly assigned patients with BPD to receive TAU+SFT or TAU (TAU consisted of high-quality psychodynamic psychotherapy delivered by well-trained and experienced clinicians). Compared with patients receiving TAU alone, patients receiving TAU+SFT evidenced a significantly greater decrease in BPD symptoms and in general level of psychiatric impairment and showed greater improvement in overall functioning. In another study evaluating group-based SFT, Dickhaut and Arntz (2014) performed an open trial with two small cohorts of patients with a primary diagnosis of BPD. Both cohorts received group-based SFT in conjunction with individual therapy. Results were very positive, with a large effect size (Cohen's d=2.34) for remission of BPD symptoms at a 2.5 year follow-up. Several other studies have emerged that provide additional support for group-based SFT in varying populations, including a community mental health sample (Leppänen et al. 2016), psychiatric inpatients (Reiss et al. 2014), individuals with mixed PDs (Skewes et al. 2015), and a group of outpatients with heterogeneous conditions (van Vreeswijk et al. 2012). Strong results from group-based SFT studies have spurred additional feasibility research (Fassbinder et al. 2016) and forthcoming international RCTs (Baljé et al. 2016; Van Dijk et al. 2019).

Dialectical Behavior Therapy

DBT was developed to treat patients with BPD, with a specific focus on suicide-related behaviors and NSSI (Linehan 1993) (for an extant review of DBT, see Chapter 13, "Dialectical Behavior Therapy," in this volume). DBT is the most investigated treatment for

BPD (Kliem et al. 2010) and is currently used in the treatment of multiple psychiatric conditions. Drawing from behavioral science, dialectic philosophy, and Zen practice, DBT balances acceptance and change in the pursuit of not only surviving but constructing a life worth living (Lynch et al. 2007).

Linehan (1993), in her biosocial theory of BPD, contended that the patient's emotional and behavioral dysregulation are elicited and then reinforced by the interplay between an invalidating developmental environment and a biological tendency toward emotional vulnerability and reactivity. Moreover, DBT characterizes maladaptive behaviors as natural and understandable reactions to environmental reinforcements (Linehan 1993; Lynch et al. 2007). DBT differs from traditional CBT in that it focuses on acceptance and validation of behavior as it is in the present moment, on reducing therapy-interfering behaviors, on the therapeutic alliance, and on dialectical processes (Linehan 1993). The overarching emphasis on dialectics helps patients' reconciliation of opposites in an ongoing process of synthesis. Linehan delineated three basic dialectics: 1) competence versus active passivity, 2) unrelenting crisis versus inhibiting experience, and 3) emotional vulnerability versus self-invalidation. A major treatment dialectic concerns problem solving versus acceptance.

Technical interventions focus on developing skills in core mindfulness, emotion regulation, interpersonal effectiveness, and self-management. Linehan's full-package DBT includes individual sessions with support from weekly skill-building groups, ideally led by someone other than the individual therapist. Therapy occurs in four stages: 1) focusing on reducing suicidal behaviors, therapy-interfering behaviors, and behaviors that negatively impact patients' quality of life; 2) aiding patients in moving from desperation to emotional experiencing through supportively reducing the patient's learned avoidance of aversive emotions; 3) targeting problems of living, including trauma-related issues, family, academic, and career problems, and other disorders; and 4) increasing the capacity for freedom and joy (Lynch et al. 2007).

The full package generally requires a 1-year treatment duration and has demonstrated significant improvement in BPD symptoms and self-destructive behaviors. Early RCTs varied in the quality of the TAU condition (Linehan et al. 1991; Verheul et al. 2003). Nonetheless, outcomes were quite favorable, with the DBT arm demonstrating substantial reduction in and frequency of NSSI and anger, as well as high rates of treatment retention, with durable gains maintained at 6- and 12-month follow-up (Linehan et al. 1993). In a later RCT (Linehan et al. 2006), outpatients with BPD were randomly assigned to receive either 1 year of community treatment by BPD experts (n=51) or the full-package DBT (n=52). Groups were matched for clinician characteristics, including gender, level of training, supervision, and treatment allegiance. For the 1-year outcome, the patients in the DBT condition evidenced fewer suicide attempts, emergency department contacts, and inpatient psychiatric days, and they had superior retention rates compared to those receiving treatment from community BPD experts.

Two RCTs that included a DBT arm demonstrated equivalence in outcomes between DBT and the comparator treatment. McMain et al. (2009) compared a large sample of patients randomly assigned to receive DBT (n=90) or general psychiatric management (n=90); the latter consisted of psychodynamic treatment and targeted medication management. Both treatment arms demonstrated a significant decrease in frequency of suicide attempts and NSSI, medical severity of suicide-related behaviors, number and frequency of emergency department visits, and inpatient psychiatric days; however, DBT did not prove superior—a finding counter to the study hypothesis. Clarkin et al. (2007) randomly assigned outpatients with BPD to receive 1 year of twice-weekly TFP ($n=23$), full-package DBT ($n=17$), or weekly psychodynamic supportive therapy ($n=21$). All three treatment arms demonstrated significant improvement in symptoms of depression and anxiety, social adjustment, and global functioning; however, psychodynamic supportive therapy did not impact rates of suicide-related behavior. Consistent with previous findings, DBT produced a decrease in suicide-related behaviors; however, patients in the TFP arm had fewer suicide attempts than did those in DBT. Reductions in physical assault, verbal aggression, and irritability were also demonstrated in the TFP condition.

DBT has been adapted to inpatient treatments with significant success. Barley et al. (1993) found that patients in a long-term inpatient ward who were transitioned to a DBT treatment model evidenced a decrease in NSSI and overdose attempts after the ward transitioned to DBT. The authors compared the DBT phase of treatment with TAU on another long-term general psychotherapy ward, demonstrating that NSSI decreased significantly on the DBT unit, whereas no decrease was observed on the TAU unit. An open pilot trial of inpatient DBT (Bohus et al. 2000) found similar outcomes for a 3-month inpatient DBT-based treatment, with a significant decrease in the frequency of NSSI, depression, stress, anxiety, and overall psychiatric symptoms. A subsequent trial (Bohus et al. 2004) randomly assigned women with BPD to a wait-list TAU condition ($n=31$) or inpatient DBT ($n=19$). The inpatient DBT group demonstrated decreases in NSSI, depression, anxiety, and social and global function, with gains at outcomes maintained at 1-month postdischarge. The TAU condition demonstrated no discernible improvement in any outcomes. Inpatient DBT was evaluated again (Kröger et al. 2013) in a large open trial. Significant reductions in BPD symptomology were observed over a three-month hospitalization, with small to moderate effect sizes. Approximately 45% of participants evidenced reliable improvement.

In clinical practice, subcomponents of DBT, such as skills groups or DBT individual therapy, are often implemented rather than the full treatment. Linehan et al. (2015) performed a dismantling study that tested the various subcomponents versus the full treatment. Over the course of several years, 99 women with BPD and recent suicide attempts or NSSI were randomly assigned to the full DBT treatment, DBT skills groups plus case management (DBT-S), or DBT individual therapy without skills training (DBT-I). Results indicated that all conditions showed equivalent improvements in suicidal ideation, suicide attempts, and crisis service utilization. However, interventions that included skills training (i.e., full DBT and DBT-S) appeared to be superior on outcomes of NSSI, depression, and anxiety than DBT-I alone, suggesting that the skills training component of DBT may be critical to effectiveness in clinical settings.

More recent reviews and meta-analyses (Panos et al. 2014; Stoffers et al. 2012) continue to support the efficacy of DBT in treating PDs and self-destructive behaviors. In particular, a comprehensive Cochrane review concluded that DBT had the most compelling evidence across the broadest range of outcomes relative to other treatments (Stoffers et al. 2012). In comparison with TAU, DBT was found to have moderate to very large effects for suicidal behavior, NSSI, anger, anxiety, depression, and overall mental health status. (See Chapter 13, "Dialectical Behavior Therapy," in this volume for more discussion of this psychotherapy.)

New Directions

A number of developments in the treatment of PDs have emerged in recent years. Cognitive analytic therapy is an integrative combination of cognitive therapy and psychodynamic object relations (Ryle and Kerr 2002) and as such cannot be viewed as a pure brand of CBT. Rather, the treatment model and evidence base supporting its efficacy in decreasing the symptom burden for individuals with BPD (Chanen et al. 2008; Clarke et al. 2013) point to a shift to integrated treatments with structured, well-defined interventions targeting specific personality trait pathology. Recent reviews have echoed this sentiment by noting increased interest in common factors and mechanisms of change among the specialized treatments for PDs (e.g., DBT, SFT, transference-focused psychotherapy, and mentalization-based therapy), given overall similar treatment effects (Bateman et al. 2015; Links et al. 2017). Reviewers have noted that in more recent clinical trials, well-designed control interventions that address common factors have performed as well as specialized treatments (Bateman et al. 2015; Cristea et al. 2017), highlighting the potential benefit of well-informed generalist care for individuals with PDs. This is an encouraging development given that the current need for specialized treatment of PDs far exceeds the availability of well-trained providers (Bateman et al. 2015; Linehan et al. 2015). New studies are investigating various generalist treatments, such as general psychiatric management or structured clinical management, with early positive results (Choi-Kain et al. 2017). The future of PD treatment may involve a first line of generalist treatment, offered by capable clinicians with relatively less training, followed by referral to specialists for treatment-resistant conditions or PDs complicated by complex, co-occurring disorders (Bateman et al. 2015; Temes and Zanarini 2019). (See Chapter 15, "Good Psychiatric Management: Generalist Treatments and Stepped Care for Borderline Personality Disorder," in this volume.)

Emerging CBT-informed treatments, particularly acceptance and commitment therapy (Hayes et al. 2013) and mindfulness-based treatments (Kabat-Zinn 2003), integrate interventions from a broader philosophical and treatment tradition that includes but is not exclusively focused on modifying distorted cognitions. These treatments are being modified and applied with early positive results for individuals with personality disorders (Chakhssi et al. 2015; Clarke et al. 2014; Morton et al. 2012; Sachse et al. 2011). The case example that follows highlights this integrative approach in the treatment of a young woman with avoidant PD.

Empirical Case Study

Ana is a young woman of Hispanic heritage who was admitted to the Menninger Clinic because of severe depression, anxiety, and the inability to benefit from outpatient therapy. She received twice-weekly CBT (as part of an integrated multimodal treatment package) at the clinic to address severe social anxiety and fear of being imperfect. In the years prior to this admission, Ana was a competitive athlete and excelled in academics through high school. She placed unrelenting pressure on herself to excel and constantly felt that she failed to live up to her internal standards. Ana developed a highly perfectionistic style of organizing her interests, daily tasks, and relationships to the point of being unable to complete basic tasks. Falling short of these unrelenting standards generated so much anxiety and shame that she failed to maintain any adaptive life path.

Ana developed an eating disorder and polysubstance abuse, both of which functioned to reduce stress and anxiety. Ana also experienced frequent panic attacks that were associated with feeling rejected by peers. Her rejection sensitivity led to frequent ruptures in relationships and abrupt endings. Eventually, Ana's unrelenting standards and her excessive need for autonomy and approval seeking failed, and Ana began to avoid things that mattered to her. She gave up on athletics, had many failed attempts at college, and increased her drug use. She avoided social and public events because of her self-consciousness and excessive fears of negative evaluation. Attempts at work and college were met with a similar inability to sustain functioning due to unremitting anxiety. As she became more dysfunctional, Ana was admitted to a residential treatment center for her eating disorder and substance use. This early treatment proved moderately beneficial; however, Ana's pattern of interpersonal avoidance and social anxiety interfered with outpatient treatment. After nearly 2 years of failed school attempts, short-term jobs, and intermittent drug use, she sought voluntary admission at the Menninger Clinic.

An integral part of the Menninger Clinic treatment program includes standardized research-based diagnostic assessment and routine assessment of symptomatic functioning at 2-week intervals throughout the course of treatment, with feedback provided to the patient and treatment team to aid treatment planning and monitoring of progress (Allen et al. 2009). Ana's research diagnoses at admission included dysthymic disorder, major depressive disorder (recurrent and severe), substance use disorder, eating disorder not otherwise specified, and avoidant PD with significant borderline and obsessive-compulsive traits. Her responses to the battery of psychological measures conducted at admission indicated that Ana had a broad array of severe psychiatric symptoms and significant impairments in daily functioning and emotion regulation. Ana's responses to the Patient Health Questionnaire (PHQ; Spitzer et al. 1999) indicated that she experienced severe anxiety and depressive symptoms (Figure 14–1). Results from the World Health Organization Disability Assessment Schedule 2.0 (WHODAS 2.0; World Health Organization 2013) and the five-item World Health Organization Well-Being Index (WHO-5; Bech 1997) showed that Ana had severe disability and a poor sense of well-being, respectively (Figure 14–2). According to her scores on the Difficulties in Emotion Regulation Scale (DERS; Gratz and Roemer 2004), Ana had trouble accepting her emotional responses, experienced deficits in strategies for regulating her emotions, and had problems sustaining goal-directed activity because of emotional interference (Figure 14–3). Her performance on the Acceptance and Action Questionnaire–II (AAQ-II; Bond et al. 2011) indicated that Ana struggled with experiential avoidance and lack of psychological flexibility (Figure 14–4).

During the first session of individual CBT, Ana described intense distaste for the interpersonal intensity of the social milieu on the hospital unit. She was defensive, emotionally guarded, and isolated from peers and staff. Education on the cognitive-behavioral model was introduced, with special emphasis on developing a collaborative treatment frame. Liberal use of explanations and illustrations of the principles of CBT helped to reduce her fears of failure and rejection and to begin to foster a therapeutic alliance. Ana self-rated her therapeutic alliance with the treatment team (on the Work-

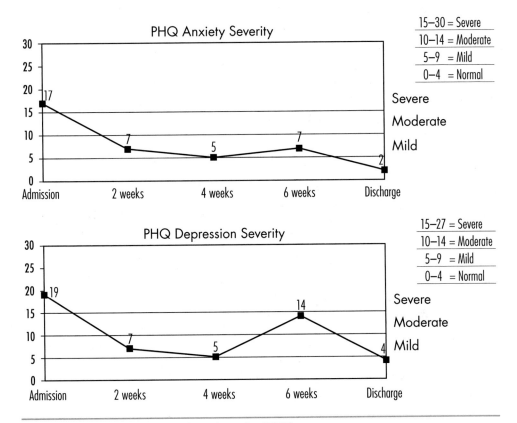

FIGURE 14–1. Patient Health Questionnaire (PHQ).

ing Alliance Inventory; Horvath and Greenberg 1989) as average to high from the outset of treatment (Figure 14–5), which was a good predictor of a positive outcome.

Upon further assessment, Ana's psychiatric disturbance was confirmed to be much broader than her presenting complaint and was more consistent with avoidant PD. There was some debate among her treating clinicians about whether social anxiety disorder (SAD) was more applicable than avoidant PD. There is a significant overlap between SAD and avoidant PD, and some researchers have concluded that avoidant PD is a more severe variant of SAD (Chambless et al. 2008; Cox et al. 2009). Others, however, have argued for a distinction between the two disorders, characterizing avoidant PD as encompassing more severe depression, introversion, and social and occupational impairment (Sanislow et al. 2012). Individuals with SAD alone tend to avoid anxiety-provoking situations for fear of doing something embarrassing or of being negatively evaluated in the moment. In contrast, individuals such as Ana have a broader pattern of avoidance that is driven by pervasive emotional avoidance, fears of rejection, and severe feelings of inadequacy. Patients with avoidant PD—whether it is a discrete entity or a severe variant of SAD—have more interpersonal fears (Perugi et al. 2001) and are more emotionally guarded than those with SAD (Marques et al. 2012). Clinically, patients with avoidant PD are less likely to accept exposure-based interventions than are those with SAD alone (Taylor et al. 2004); patients with avoidant PD tend to be less willing to tolerate the anxiety of repeated exposure because it triggers a more pervasive emotional response (Huppert et al. 2008).

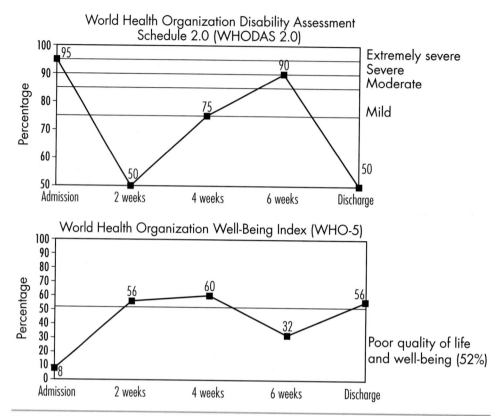

FIGURE 14–2. World Health Organization Disability Assessment Schedule 2.0 and five-item World Health Organization Well-Being Index.

A change of 10% indicates a significant alteration in sense of well-being.

In early individual therapy sessions Ana described her childhood as difficult but not overtly abusive. She felt she could never live up to her parents' expectations and felt constant disapproval from her family. The fear of disapproval was internalized and became a salient schema in her processing of information and emotional responding. To fend off self-criticism, she frequently became argumentative and would often "melt down" when corrected or challenged. She described herself as a hard worker and viewed success in sports and school as buffers against disapproval, rejection, and shame. Ana's stated goals for treatment were to "be able to go to school, be more independent, and not be so afraid of people." Several patterns were identified that needed to be addressed in order to help her reach her treatment goals: 1) effortful suppression and hiding of her anxiety, 2) self-criticism and ruminations, 3) intense rejection sensitivity, and 4) limited strategies for contending with strong emotions.

During the first 2 weeks of treatment, Ana hid her anxiety from peers and staff, believing that being anxious was a sign of weakness that would evoke disapproval from others. Like other patients with vulnerability to shame (Hejdenberg and Andrews 2011), she showed flashes of anger whenever she felt criticized. She ruminated over past events and used these to anticipate future criticism. Rumination as an emotion regulation strategy has been shown to have a strong link across several forms of psychopathology (Aldao et al. 2010), as well as a strong association with shame proneness and

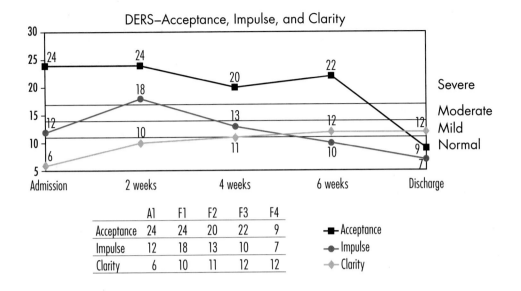

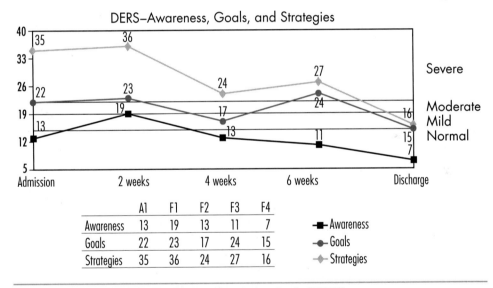

FIGURE 14–3. Difficulties in Emotion Regulation Scale (DERS).

self-criticism (Gilbert and Proctor 2006; Rector et al. 2008). Additionally, Ana frequently engaged in post-event processing. Repetitive thinking about perceived inadequacy in social interactions is related to depression and anxiety (McEvoy et al. 2010). At times Ana would externalize these feelings, but typically she would internalize anger and retreat into ruminative self-criticism and harsh self-judgment. Ana's self-criticism was intense and a potential treatment barrier. Self-criticism has been identified, for example, as an impediment to treatment with CBT for depression (Rector et al. 2000).

Ana worried excessively about a variety of themes, but primarily about becoming overwhelmed by her emotions. In individual therapy sessions she learned that worry was an insulator against overwhelming emotions—worrying about negative outcomes

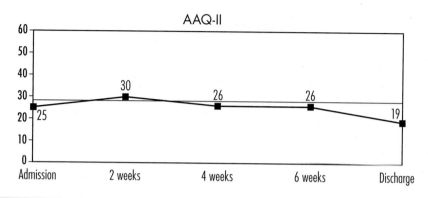

FIGURE 14–4. Acceptance and Action Questionnaire–II (AAQ-II).
Scores below 28 indicate increased psychological flexibility.

at every turn protected her from being hopeful and then disappointed. Because of the rigid and overgeneralized nature of Ana's worry, she missed opportunities for self-soothing and for developing capacities for processing underlying sadness, shame, and guilt (Newman and Llera 2011).

During early sessions the therapist shared these observations and formulations as an integral part of CBT. After feedback and education about the conceptualization of her condition, Ana reformulated her treatment goals to include work on rumination/worry, shame, anxiety in social situations, and anger. She recognized that she was plagued with rumination and saw this as a major impediment to progress in life. A functional assessment was initiated that emphasized the consequences of rumination, while analysis at the content level was necessary to help Ana modify distorted beliefs, challenge maladaptive thoughts, and correct faulty assumptions. These goals were worked on using a variety of traditional cognitive therapy interventions, such as dysfunctional thought records, pro-and-con analysis, and downward arrow exercises (Beck 2011). Many patients like Ana, however, have ongoing internal dialogues about the accuracy of their thoughts, which can be aimed at avoiding a painful emotional experience. Although useful, analysis at the content level can run the risk of providing fodder for the ruminative process. Ana said that throughout her life, family and others close to her had always tried to offer solutions and to talk her out of her negative feelings. Breaking this cycle of seeing herself as being broken and needing repair required empathic understanding by the therapist of her underlying emotions. In direct response to Ana's ruminations, the therapist asked her to reflect on how her current rumination helped her improve her life or sense of longer-term well-being. Another part of the functional analysis was to help Ana identify her underlying emotional states.

Identifying emotions was difficult for Ana. A good deal of time was spent helping her identify and define her emotions, including her response tendencies for them. Being able to identify emotions when she had them gave her greater access to a range of emotions and helped her process them more fully. Another part of the functional analysis looked at how these patterns of avoidance developed throughout her life. Ana maintained that emotions such as sadness, fear, and shame were met by her parents with attempts to solve her problems and quickly alleviate her emotions. These attempts by others to alleviate her distress led Ana to conclude that emotions were "wrong."

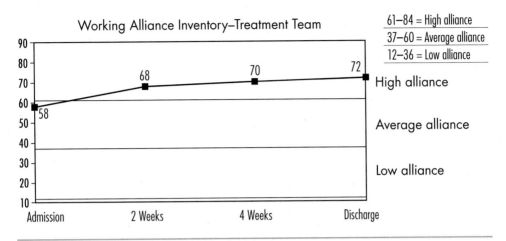

FIGURE 14–5. Working Alliance Inventory—Treatment Team.

Interventions aimed at increasing self-compassion were engaged to address her self-critical rumination and shame proneness. Increasing self-compassion has been shown to effectively address self-criticism and maladaptive levels of shame, as well as to increase a sense of well-being (Germer and Neff 2013). Particularly helpful for Ana was writing a letter of self-compassion from an "imaginary compassionate friend" in which the friend expressed compassion that was balanced and realistic but not indulgent or placating (Neff and Lamb 2009). Many self-critical patients believe that without their own criticism, they will lapse into a complete state of inadequacy. Although initially resistant to self-compassion, Ana eventually caught on to the balanced and realistic self-compassionate approach that helped her think about her deficits and flaws in a more open and accepting way so that she could change what was possible to change.

One technique that helped Ana learn to identify and process unwanted emotions was to determine the nature of a threat in situations in which she felt overwhelmed with anger and/or anxiety. Mindfulness exercises helped her develop an observer mode that mitigated against over-identification with her thoughts and feelings. Ana often found herself responding to troubling situations with emotion-driven behaviors that were characterized by avoidance and withdrawal or externalizing defensive aggression. Threats typically involved making mistakes, feeling embarrassed or exposed to perceived weaknesses, and being evaluated or judged negatively. Because of her history of emotion regulation problems, Ana had strong emotional responses to even neutral social events. In other situations, her automatic emotional response was frequently out of proportion to the event. Cognitive reappraisal helped her identify and modify maladaptive thinking patterns with the aim of increasing her flexibility in appraising various situations.

Ana's anticipatory anxiety prior to attending a group on the unit was so intense that she often decided not to go. This emotionally driven avoidance was negatively reinforced by a reduction in her anxiety; however, this short-lived reduction would be followed by guilt and shame from which a chain reaction of avoidances occurred, such as avoiding staff, missing subsequent groups and activities, and so on. Cognitive reappraisal helped Ana gain a more realistic assessment of the actual threat. Cognitive reappraisal also included skill-building interventions to help her cope with the "worst that could happen" scenario. Ana developed the capacity to reappraise and rehearse coping strategies to use in the event that her fears came to fruition. Other chances for skill building occurred in vivo, such as when she found herself in conflict with her roommate and was able to use a "Dear Man" skill from DBT (Linehan 1993)—an interpersonal approach to conflict resolution that involves 1) describing the situation of concern for the speaker, 2) expressing the emotion(s) related to the situation, 3) asserting needs or setting a boundary, 4) reinforcing the rationale behind the assertion, 5) mindfully focusing on the exchange, 6) appearing confident, and 7) negotiating the outcome. To prepare for implementing such an interpersonally challenging technique, Ana realistically appraised the potential problems and was able to realize that she could not be effective unless she was willing to feel anxious.

It was also emphasized with Ana that behavioral avoidance was a type of emotional suppression that was ineffective for adaptively regulating emotional responses and that interrupted effective emotion processing. Breaking the pattern of behavioral avoidance was essential for Ana's recovery. For most patients with avoidant PD, exposures typically need to be carried out with a clear rationale as to how these experiences fit with the rest of their treatment. Skill building and cognitive reappraisal are important, but an experiential component is also needed. In-session experiential components involved directly addressing past hurts and traumas, with allowance for Ana to experience her emotions fully. Ana responded to a mindfulness exercise that consisted of just listening to her critical voice, and she eventually constructed realistic responses to this inner voice. This exercise was in the service of helping Ana experience her distressing emotions in a safe and empathic environment.

These strategies provided a stage for increasing Ana's willingness to experience aversive emotions in more public settings. She reframed her participation in groups from a performance to an experience. This was an important factor for Ana—as she viewed it, her entire life had been a performance that she could never get right. The concept of willingness to experience was vital to her recovery as she began to realize that pursuing valued life experiences could not be done if she insisted on controlling unwanted emotions. Ana was able to set valued life experiences as goals rather than "emotional goals," which were typically managed with avoidance, rumination/worry, and suppression of thoughts and feelings. To increase her willingness to experience unwanted thoughts and feelings, Ana constructed a "what for" list, consisting of values and experiences she wanted to pursue. Constructing a list of experiences to increase motivation for change was essential for breaking maladaptive patterns, because valued patterns are individualized and are intrinsically self-reinforcing (Wilson and Dufrene 2008). Once Ana's values were established through a structured exercise, she became more cognizant of the costs of controlling and avoiding painful thoughts and feelings in contrast to the rewards of pursuing more effective and satisfying experiences.

Ana listed the following among her most important values: having relationships with family and friends, learning, helping and caring for others, and being healthy. Similarly, she became more in touch with "lost" values, such as feelings of gratitude and forgiveness. She began to make a shift from fixed, specific superlative goals to more flexible, reasonable goals guided by her identified values. In a more self-compassionate way, Ana developed a more balanced and realistic view of her strengths and flaws. Interpersonally, she began taking more risks by interacting with others without heavy reliance on externalizing or internalizing defenses.

Ana made clinically significant improvement through her treatment. At admission she had a broad range of psychiatric disturbances that required a variety of interventions, but with a focused set of therapeutic targets. CBT for her social anxiety alone was unlikely to succeed, but it was an essential component of therapy throughout the treatment. Targets for treatment were her basic core belief in her basic inadequacy, her expectation that others would ultimately reject and hurt her, and her pervasive fear of her own emotions.

As can be seen from Ana's outcome measures, her anxiety and depression levels decreased significantly (see Figure 14–1). Her overall sense of well-being increased, and her perceived severity of disability dramatically decreased (see Figure 14–2). Her ability to accept aversive internal experiences and gain psychological flexibility increased moderately (see Figure 14–4). Lastly, as shown in Figure 14–3, her ability to accept her emotional experiences (Acceptance), take a more workable look at her feeling about herself and her relationships (Awareness), set goals and commit to effective behaviors without emotionally driven interference (Goals), and construct strategies to help her effectively regulate her emotions (Strategies) improved in meaningful ways.

In examining Ana's outcome measures, it is noteworthy that during week 6 she had a spike in her self-reported depression severity (see Figure 14–1) and functional disability (see Figure 14–2), as well as a decrease in her sense of well-being (see Figure 14–2). At this juncture she admitted to secretly engaging in her eating disorder symptoms after many months of control. She felt ashamed, embarrassed, and humiliated and believed that she would be asked to leave treatment. The serious nature of this behavior was explained to her; however, she was also praised for coming forth with this information. Despite reassurance, Ana continued to believe that she had lost the confidence of those trying to help her and that she would be rejected. This "therapeutic rupture" was an important focus during the final 2 weeks of her treatment as she worked through the experience with staff and her peers (as can be seen in the precipitous decline in depression severity and the functional improvement as discharge approached).

Conclusion

Manualized cognitive-behavioral therapies, including at least one acceptance-based treatment (Gratz and Gunderson 2006), are effective in reducing symptoms associated with PDs, and particularly BPD. What is abundantly clear, however, is that more systematic efficacy and effectiveness studies must be conducted involving patients with other PDs, especially those PDs with relatively high prevalence rates, such as avoidant PD (Fowler and Oldham 2013).

References

Aldao A, Nolen-Hoeksema S, Schweizer S: Emotion-regulation strategies across psychopathology: a meta-analytic review. Clin Psychol Rev 30:217–237, 2010

Alden L: Short-term structured treatment for avoidant personality disorder. J Consult Clin Psychol 57:756–764, 1989

Allen JG, Frueh BC, Ellis TE, et al: Integrating outcomes assessment and research into clinical care in inpatient adult psychiatric treatment. Bull Menninger Clin 73:259–295, 2009

American Psychiatric Association: Practice guideline for the treatment of patients with borderline personality disorder. Am J Psychiatry 158 (10 suppl):1–52, 2001

American Psychiatric Association: Diagnostic and Statistical Manual of Mental Disorders, 5th Edition. Arlington, VA, American Psychiatric Association, 2013

Baljé A, Greeven A, van Giezen A, et al: Group schema therapy versus group cognitive behavioral therapy for social anxiety disorder with comorbid avoidant personality disorder: study protocol for a randomized controlled trial. Trials 17(1):487, 2016

Bamelis LL, Evers SM, Spinhoven P, et al: Results of a multicenter randomized controlled trial of the clinical effectiveness of schema therapy for personality disorders. Am J Psychiatry 171:305–322, 2014

Barley WD, Buie SE, Peterson EW, et al: Development of an inpatient cognitive-behavioral treatment program for borderline personality disorder. J Pers Disord 7:232–240, 1993

Bateman AW, Gunderson J, Mulder R: Treatment of personality disorder. Lancet 385:735–743, 2015

Bech P: Quality of life instruments in depression. Eur Psychiatry 12:194–198, 1997

Beck AT, Freeman A: Cognitive Therapy of Personality Disorders. New York, Guilford, 1990

Beck A, Freeman A, Davis D: Cognitive Therapy of Personality Disorders, 2nd Edition. New York, Guilford, 2004

Beck JS: Complex cognitive therapy treatment for personality disorder patients. Bull Menninger Clin 62:170–194, 1998

Beck JS: Cognitive Behavior Therapy: Basics and Beyond, 2nd Edition. New York, Guilford, 2011

Bender DS, Skodol AE: Borderline personality as a self-other representational disturbance. J Pers Disord 21:500–517, 2007

Bender DS, Morey LC, Skodol AE: Toward a model for assessing level of personality functioning in DSM-5, part I: a review of theory and methods. J Pers Assess 93:332–346, 2011

Björgvinsson T, Hart J: Cognitive behavior therapy and mentalizing, in Handbook of Mentalization-Based Treatment. Edited by Allen JG, Fonagy P. New York, Wiley, 2006, pp 157–170

Black DW, Simsek-Duran F, Blum N, et al: Do people with borderline personality disorder complicated by antisocial personality disorder benefit from the STEPPS treatment program? Personal Ment Health 10:205–215, 2016

Blum N, Pfohl B, St John DS, et al: STEPPS: a cognitive-behavioral systems-based group treatment for outpatients with borderline personality disorder—a preliminary report. Compr Psychiatry 43:301–310, 2002

Blum N, St John D, Pfohl B, et al: Systems Training for Emotional Predictability and Problem Solving (STEPPS) for outpatients with borderline personality disorder: a randomized controlled trial and 1-year follow-up. Am J Psychiatry 165:468–478, 2008

Bohus M, Haaf B, Stiglmayr C, et al: Evaluation of inpatient dialectical-behavioral therapy for borderline personality disorder—a prospective study. Behav Res Ther 38:875–887, 2000

Bohus M, Haaf B, Simms T, et al: Effectiveness of inpatient dialectical behavioral therapy for borderline personality disorder: a controlled trial. Behav Res Ther 42:487–499, 2004

Bond FW, Hayes SC, Baer RA, et al: Preliminary psychometric properties of the Acceptance and Action Questionnaire–II: a revised measure of psychological inflexibility and experiential avoidance. Behav Ther 42:676–688, 2011

Bos EH, Van Wel EB, Appelo MT, et al: A randomized controlled trial of a Dutch version of systems training for emotional predictability and problem solving for borderline personality disorder. J Nerv Ment Dis 198:299–304, 2010

Chakhssi F, Janssen W, Pol SM, et al: Acceptance and commitment therapy group-treatment for non-responsive patients with personality disorders: an exploratory study. Personal Ment Health 9:345–356, 2015

Chambless DL, Fydrich T, Rodebaugh TL: Generalized social phobia and avoidant personality disorder: meaningful distinction or useless duplication? Depress Anxiety 25:8–19, 2008

Chanen AM, Jackson HJ, McCutcheon LK, et al: Early intervention for adolescents with borderline personality disorder using cognitive analytic therapy: randomised controlled trial. Br J Psychiatry 193:477–484, 2008

Choi-Kain LW, Finch EF, Masland SR, et al: What works in the treatment of borderline personality disorder. Curr Behav Neurosci Reports 4:21–30, 2017

Clarke S, Thomas P, James K: Cognitive analytic therapy for personality disorder: randomised controlled trial. Br J Psychiatry 202:129–134, 2013

Clarke S, Kingston J, James K, et al: Acceptance and Commitment Therapy group for treatment-resistant participants: a randomized controlled trial. J Context Behav Sci 3:179–188, 2014

Clarkin JF, Levy KN, Lenzenweger MF, et al: Evaluating three treatments for borderline personality disorder: a multiwave study. Am J Psychiatry 164:922–928, 2007

Cottraux J, Note ID, Boutitie F, et al: Cognitive therapy versus Rogerian supportive therapy in borderline personality disorder: two-year follow-up of a controlled pilot study. Psychother Psychosom 78:307–316, 2009

Cox BJ, Pagura J, Stein MB, et al: The relationship between generalized social phobia and avoidant personality disorder in a national mental health survey. Depress Anxiety 26:354–362, 2009

Cristea IA, Gentili C, Cotet CD, et al: Efficacy of psychotherapies for borderline personality disorder: a systematic review and meta-analysis. JAMA Psychiatry 74:319–328, 2017

David DO, Freeman A: Overview of cognitive-behavioral therapy of personality disorders, in Cognitive Therapy of Personality Disorders, 3rd Edition. Edited by Beck AT, Davis DD, Freeman A. New York, Guilford, 2014, pp 3–18

Davidson KM, Norrie J, Tyrer P, et al: The effectiveness of cognitive behavior therapy for borderline personality disorder: results from the borderline personality disorder study of cognitive therapy (BOSCOT) trial. J Pers Disord 20:450–465, 2006

Davidson KM, Tyrer P, Tata P, et al: Cognitive behaviour therapy for violent men with antisocial personality disorder in the community: an exploratory randomized controlled trial. Psychol Med 39:569–577, 2009

Davidson KM, Tyrer P, Norrie J, et al: Cognitive therapy v. usual treatment for borderline personality disorder: prospective 6-year follow-up. Br J Psychiatry 197:456–462, 2010

Dickhaut V, Arntz A: Combined group and individual schema therapy for borderline personality disorder: a pilot study. J Behav Ther Exp Psychiatry 45:242–251, 2014

Emmelkamp PM, Benner A, Kuipers A, et al: Comparison of brief dynamic and cognitive-behavioural therapies in avoidant personality disorder. Br J Psychiatry 189:60–64, 2006

Farrell JM, Shaw IA, Webber MA: A schema-focused approach to group psychotherapy for outpatients with borderline personality disorder: a randomized controlled trial. J Behav Ther Exp Psychiatry 40:317–328, 2009

Fassbinder E, Schuetze M, Kranich A, et al: Feasibility of group schema therapy for outpatients with severe borderline personality disorder in Germany: a pilot study with three year follow-up. Front Psychol 7:1851, 2016

Fowler JC, Oldham JM: Co-occurring disorders and treatment complexity. FOCUS 11:123–128, 2013

Freije H, Dietz B, Appelo M: Borderline persoonlijkheidsstoornis met de VERS: de vaardigheidstraining emotionele regulatiestoornis. Directieve Therapie 4:367–378, 2002

Germer CK, Neff KD: Self-compassion in clinical practice. J Clin Psychol 69:856–867, 2013

Giesen-Bloo JH, van Dyck R, Spinhoven P, et al: Outpatient psychotherapy for borderline personality disorder: randomized trial of schema-focused therapy vs transference-focused psychotherapy. Arch Gen Psychiatry 63:649–658, 2006

Gilbert P, Proctor S: Compassionate mind training for people with high shame and self-criticism: overview and pilot study of a group therapy approach. Clin Psychol Psychother 13:353–379, 2006

Goldfried MR, Davison GC: Clinical Behavior Therapy. New York, Wiley, 1990

Gratz K, Gunderson J: Preliminary data on acceptance-based emotion regulation group intervention for deliberate self-harm among women with borderline personality disorder. Behav Ther 37:25–35, 2006

Gratz KL, Roemer L: Multidimensional assessment of emotion regulation and dysregulation: development, factor structure, and initial validation of the Difficulties in Emotion Regulation Scale. J Psychopathol Behavl Assess 26:41–54, 2004

Gratz KL, Tull MT: Extending research on the utility of an adjunctive emotion regulation group therapy for deliberate self-harm among women with borderline personality pathology. Personal Disord 2:316–326, 2011

Gratz KL, Tull MT, Levy R: Randomized controlled trial and uncontrolled 9-month follow-up of an adjunctive emotion regulation group therapy for deliberate self-harm among women with borderline personality disorder. Psychol Med 44:2099–2112, 2014

Hayes SC, Levin ME, Plumb-Vilardaga J, et al: Acceptance and commitment therapy and contextual behavioral science: examining the progress of a distinctive model of behavioral and cognitive therapy. Behav Ther 44:180–198, 2013

Hejdenberg J, Andrews B: The relationship between shame and different types of anger: a theory-based investigation. Pers Individ Diff 50:1278–1282, 2011

Hill N, Geoghegan M, Shawe-Taylor M. Evaluating the outcomes of the STEPPS programme in a UK community-based population; implications for the multidisciplinary treatment of borderline personality disorder. J Psychiatr Ment Health Nurs 23:347–356, 2016

Horvath AO, Greenberg LS: Development and validation of the Working Alliance Inventory. J Couns Psychol 36:223–233, 1989

Huppert JD, Strunk DR, Ledley DR, et al: Generalized social anxiety disorder and avoidant personality disorder: structural analysis and treatment outcome. Depress Anxiety 25:441–448, 2008

Ingram RE, Hollon SD: Cognitive therapy for depression from an information processing perspective, in Information Processing Approaches to Clinical Psychology. Edited by Ingram RE. San Diego, CA, Academic Press, 1986, pp 255–281

Kabat-Zinn J: Mindfulness-based interventions in context: past, present, and future. Clinical psychology: Science and Practice 10:144–156, 2003

Kliem S, Kroger C, Kosfelder J: Dialectical behavior therapy for borderline personality disorder: a meta-analysis using mixed-effects modeling. J Consult Clin Psychol 78:936–951, 2010

Kröger C, Harbeck S, Armbrust M, et al: Effectiveness, response, and dropout of dialectical behavior therapy for borderline personality disorder in an inpatient setting. Behav Res Ther 51:411–416, 2013

Leichsenring F, Leibing E: The effectiveness of psychodynamic therapy and cognitive behavior therapy in the treatment of personality disorders: a meta-analysis. Am J Psychiatry 160:1223–1232, 2003

Leichsenring F, Rabung S: Effectiveness of long-term psychodynamic psychotherapy: a meta-analysis. JAMA 300:1551–1565, 2008

Leichsenring F, Leibing E, Kruse J, et al: Borderline personality disorder. Lancet 377:74–84, 2011

Leppänen V, Hakko H, Sintonen H, et al: Comparing effectiveness of treatments for borderline personality disorder in communal mental health care: the Oulu BPD study. Community Ment Health J 52:216–227, 2016

Linehan M: Cognitive-Behavioral Treatment of Borderline Personality Disorder. New York, Guilford, 1993

Linehan MM, Armstrong HE, Suarez A, et al: Cognitive-behavioral treatment of chronically parasuicidal borderline patients. Arch Gen Psychiatry 48:1060–1064, 1991

Linehan MM, Heard HL, Armstrong HE: Naturalistic follow-up of a behavioral treatment for chronically parasuicidal borderline patients. Arch Gen Psychiatry 50:971–974, 1993

Linehan MM, Comtois KA, Murray AM, et al: Two-year randomized controlled trial and follow-up of dialectical behavior therapy versus therapy by experts for suicidal behaviors and borderline personality disorder. Arch Gen Psychiatry 63:757–766, 2006

Linehan MM, Korslund KE, Harned MS, et al: Dialectical behavior therapy for high suicide risk in individuals with borderline personality disorder: a randomized clinical trial and component analysis. JAMA Psychiatry 72:475–482, 2015

Links PS, Shah R, Eynan R: Psychotherapy for borderline personality disorder: progress and remaining challenges. Curr Psychiatry Rep 19:1–10, 2017

Lynch TR, Trost WT, Salsman N, et al: Dialectical behavior therapy for borderline personality disorder. Annu Rev Clin Psychol 3:181–205, 2007

Marques L, Porter E, Keshaviah A, et al: Avoidant personality disorder in individuals with generalized social anxiety disorder: what does it add? J Anxiety Disord 26:665–672, 2012

Matusiewicz AK, Hopwood CJ, Banducci AN, et al: The effectiveness of cognitive behavioral therapy for personality disorders. Psychiatr Clin North Am 33:657–685, 2010

McEvoy PM, Mahoney AE, Moulds ML: Are worry, rumination and post-event processing one and the same? Development of the Repetitive Thinking Questionnaire. J Anxiety Disord 24:509–519, 2010

McMain S, Pos AE: Advances in psychotherapy of personality disorders: a research update. Curr Psychiatry Rep 9:46–52, 2007

McMain SF, Links PS, Gnam WH, et al: A randomized trial of dialectical behavior therapy versus general psychiatric management for borderline personality disorder. Am J Psychiatry 166:1365–1374, 2009

Morey LC, Berghuis H, Bender DS, et al: Toward a model for assessing level of personality functioning in DSM-5, part II: empirical articulation of a core dimension of personality pathology. J Pers Assess 93:347–353, 2011

Morton J, Snowdon S, Gopold M, et al: Acceptance and commitment therapy group treatment for symptoms of borderline personality disorder: a public sector pilot study. Cogn Behav Pract 19:527–544, 2012

Neff KD, Lamb LM: Self-compassion, in Handbook of Individual Differences in Social Behavior. Edited by Leary MR, Hoyle RH. New York, Guilford, 2009, pp 561–573

Newman MG, Llera SJ: A novel theory of experiential avoidance in generalized anxiety disorder: a review and synthesis of research supporting a contrast avoidance model of worry. Clin Psychol Rev 31:371–382, 2011

Nock MK, Prinstein MJ: Contextual features and behavioral functions of self-mutilation among adolescents. J Abnorm Psychol 114:140–146, 2005

Norrie J, Davidson K, Tata P, et al: Influence of therapist competence and quantity of cognitive behavioural therapy on suicidal behaviour and inpatient hospitalisation in a randomised controlled trial in borderline personality disorder: further analyses of treatment effects in the BOSCOT study. Psychol Psychother 86:280–293, 2013

Oldham JM: Guideline watch: practice guideline for the treatment of patients with borderline personality disorder. FOCUS 3:396–400, 2005

Panos PT, Jackson JW, Hasan O, et al: Meta-analysis and systematic review assessing the efficacy of dialectical behavior therapy (DBT). Res Soc Work Pract 24:213–223, 2014

Perugi G, Nassini S, Maremmani I, et al: Putative clinical subtypes of social phobia: a factor-analytical study. Acta Psychiatr Scand 104:280–288, 2001

Rector NA, Bagby RM, Segal ZV, et al: Self-criticism and dependency in depressed patients treated with cognitive therapy or pharmacotherapy. Cognitive Therapy and Research 24:571–584, 2000

Rector NA, Antony M, Laposa J, et al: Assessing content domains of repetitive thought in the anxiety spectrum: rumination and worry in nonclinical and clinically anxious samples. Int J Cogn Ther 1:352–377, 2008

Rees CS, Pritchard R: Brief cognitive therapy for avoidant personality disorder. Psychotherapy 52:45–55, 2015

Reiss N, Lieb K, Arntz A, et al: Responding to the treatment challenge of patients with severe BPD: results of three pilot studies of inpatient schema therapy. Behav Cogn Psychother 42:355–367, 2014

Renneberg B, Goldstein A, Phillips D, et al: Intensive behavioral group treatment of avoidant personality disorder. Behav Ther 21:363–377, 1990

Ryle A, Kerr IB: Introducing Cognitive Analytic Therapy. New York, Wiley, 2002

Sachse S, Keville S, Feigenbaum J: A feasibility study of mindfulness-based cognitive therapy for individuals with borderline personality disorder. Psychol Psychother 84:184–200, 2011

Sahlin H, Bjureberg J, Gratz KL, et al: Emotion regulation group therapy for deliberate self-harm: a multi-site evaluation in routine care using an uncontrolled open trial design. BMJ Open 7(10):e016220, 2017

Sanislow CA, Bartolini EE, Zoloth EC: Avoidant personality disorder, in Encyclopedia of Human Behavior, 2nd Edition. Edited by Ramachandran VS. San Diego, CA, Academic Press, 2012, pp 257–266

Skewes SA, Samson RA, Simpson SG, et al: Short-term group schema therapy for mixed personality disorders: a pilot study. Front Psychol 5:1592, 2015

Sperry L: Cognitive Behavior Therapy of DSM-IV-TR Personality Disorders: Highly Effective Interventions for the Most Common Personality Disorders. New York, Routledge, 2006

Spitzer RL, Kroenke K, Williams JB: Validation and utility of a self-report version of PRIME-MD: the PHQ primary care study. JAMA 282:1737–1744, 1999

Stoffers JM, Völlm BA, Rücker G, et al: Psychological therapies for people with borderline personality disorder. Cochrane Database Syst Rev (8):CD005652, 2012

Strauss JL, Hayes AM, Johnson SL, et al: Early alliance, alliance ruptures, and symptom change in a nonrandomized trial of cognitive therapy for avoidant and obsessive-compulsive personality disorders. J Consult Clin Psychol 74:337–345, 2006

Stravynski A, Marks I, Yule W: Social skills problems in neurotic outpatients: social skills training with and without cognitive modification. Arch Gen Psychiatry 39:1378–1385, 1982

Stravynski A, Belise M, Marcouiller M, et al: The treatment of avoidant personality disorder by social skills training in the clinic or in real-life settings. Can J Psychiatry 39:377–383, 1994

Taylor CT, Laposa JM, Alden LE: Is avoidant personality disorder more than just social avoidance? J Pers Disord 18:571–594, 2004

Temes CM, Zanarini MC. Recent developments in psychosocial interventions for borderline personality disorder. F1000Research 8, Apr 26, 2019

Van Dijk SDM, Veenstra MS, Bouman R, et al: Group schema-focused therapy enriched with psychomotor therapy versus treatment as usual for older adults with cluster B and/or C personality disorders: a randomized trial. BMC Psychiatry 19(1):26, 2019

Van Vreeswijk MF, Spinhoven P, Eurelings-Bontekoe EHM, et al: Changes in symptom severity, schemas and modes in heterogeneous psychiatric patient groups following short-term schema cognitive-behavioural group therapy: a naturalistic pre-treatment and post-treatment design in an outpatient clinic. Clin Psychol Psychother 21:29–38, 2012

Van Wel B, Kockmann I, Blum N, et al: STEPPS group treatment for borderline personality disorder in the Netherlands. Ann Clin Psychiatry 18:63–67, 2006

Verheul R, van den Bosch LM, Koeter MW, et al: Dialectical behaviour therapy for women with borderline personality disorder: 12-month, randomised clinical trial in the Netherlands. Br J Psychiatry 182:135–140, 2003

Weinberg I, Gunderson JG, Hennen J, et al: Manual assisted cognitive treatment for deliberate self-harm in borderline personality disorder patients. J Pers Disord 20:482–492, 2006

Wilson KG, Dufrene T: Mindfulness for Two: An Acceptance and Commitment Therapy Approach to Mindfulness in Psychotherapy. Oakland, CA, New Harbinger, 2008

World Health Organization: WHO-DAS II Training Manual: A Guide to Administration. 2013. Retrieved from: www.who.int/icidh/whodas/training_man.pdf. Accessed August 29, 2013.

Young JE: Cognitive Therapy for Personality Disorders: A Schema-Focused Approach. Sarasota, FL, Professional Resource Press, 1999

Young JE, Lindemann M: An integrative schema-focused model for personality disorders, in Clinical Advances in Cognitive Psychotherapy: Theory and Application. Edited by Leahy RL, Dowd ET. New York, Springer, 2002, pp 93–109

CHAPTER 15

Good Psychiatric Management

Generalist Treatments and Stepped Care for Borderline Personality Disorder

Lois W. Choi-Kain, M.D., M.Ed.

Richard Hersh, M.D.

The development of evidence-based psychotherapies for borderline personality disorder (BPD) has powerfully paved the way for a growing sense of optimism that patients with the diagnosis can get better with appropriate clinical care (Choi-Kain et al. 2017a, 2017b). In addition, these manualized treatments, which include dialectical behavior therapy (DBT; Linehan et al. 1991), mentalization-based treatment (MBT; Bateman and Fonagy 1999), transference-focused psychotherapy (TFP; Clarkin et al. 2007), and schema-focused therapy (Giesen-Bloo et al. 2006), have revolutionized the field of psychotherapy at large by forming new brands of treatment that represent the modern era of evidence-based medicine, targeting major mental illness associated with serious morbidity (Trull et al. 2010), mortality (Paris and Zweig-Frank 2001), and costs to society (Hastrup et al. 2019; Soeteman et al. 2008). While these "brand name" evidence-based treatments for BPD yield comparable effects (Cristea et al. 2017; Stoffers et al. 2012), their differing theoretical positions on the etiology of BPD, therapeutic maneuvers, and training requirements set them apart from one another. Just like brands use "trade dress"—that is, "any material

Preparation of this manuscript was supported by the donors to the BPD Challenge Fund for expanding care to underserved populations. We would like to thank Evan Iliakis and Gabrielle Ilagan for their assistance with preparing this manuscript.

quality of a product's packaging or physical appearance that serves a branding function" and establishes the product as "distinct from other, similar products"—to give themselves an edge in a market, so too do brand-name treatments use recognizable positions on theory, practice, and training to underscore their quality and reliability (Greene and Kesselheim 2011, p. 83; see also Gunderson et al. 2018). Both the tailoring of these treatments to intervene with BPD as the major problem, and the varying trade dress of each manualized psychotherapy, have helped the clinical world learn what works in the treatment of this prevalent and sometimes life-threatening psychiatric illness.

As much as the advent of these treatment approaches has innovated the BPD care landscape, the branding and exclusivity of these treatments have perpetuated an access-to-care problem characterized by a short supply of trained treaters in the face of a monopoly on the efficacy they represent. Their intensive, comprehensive, and lengthy team-based requirements challenge broad implementation to serve the public health needs of the United States and, even more dire, any country with limited health care resources (Iliakis et al. 2019). Because of their extensive training and intensity, these specialized evidence-based psychotherapies are unlikely to be implemented by the generalist mental health clinician in most settings (i.e., inpatient units, emergency departments, general outpatient psychiatric clinics) where most patients seek care. Even more unlikely is their adaptation to primary care, where significant first-line or definitive intervention occurs. Fortunately, several generalist clinical management approaches for BPD in both young people and adults have been tested and have shown enough similarity in their outcomes when compared to gold standard treatments for BPD to be considered a *generic* variant. With enough similarity to the basic essential ingredients of effective treatment for BPD, these generalist treatments, which rely less on psychotherapeutic techniques and content, can be applied as a substitute, making good care for BPD more accessible, affordable, and sustainable for health care systems both in the United States and internationally.

The evidence basis for generalist approaches to treating BPD derives from two of the largest and most methodologically rigorous studies in the BPD treatment literature comparing DBT and MBT with protocolized, less intensive generalist approaches for BPD. The reports on these two large trials were published in the same issue of the *American Journal of Psychiatry* in 2009. Manualized by Paul Links, M.D., based on John Gunderson's landmark clinical guide (Gunderson and Links 2008), general (a.k.a. good) psychiatric management (GPM; Gunderson and Links 2014) performed as well as DBT in reducing suicidality and self-harm, BPD symptoms, and depression, while also increasing social functioning and quality of life (McMain et al. 2009). Improvement in both arms of the MBT trial occurred, with steeper improvements for MBT but nonetheless favorable outcomes for the generalist structured clinical management arm (SCM; Bateman and Fonagy 2009; Bateman and Krawitz 2013). A recent meta-analysis underscores these conclusions, finding comparable efficacy of both specialized and generalist protocolized treatments for BPD (Oud et al. 2018). These generalist approaches, GPM and SCM, were developed by leading clinical experts based on both American Psychiatric Association (APA) and National Institute for Clinical Excellence guidelines for the care of patients with BPD. Pared down to basic ingredients of effective and organized clinical management, using up-to-date medical knowledge about BPD, both GPM and SCM provide a standardization of expert care that any generalist can use as a clinical case management approach. These data argue that these approaches constitute the distillation of the essential ingredients of BPD treatment.

The rise of generalist treatments for BPD has taken form in parallel ways to the rise of generic drugs, providing the core ingredients of the innovator treatments with different packaging and lower cost. While some central ingredients of the treatments remain similar enough to brand-name psychotherapies (e.g., focus on BPD as the central problem, psychoeducation, role induction), the packaging, so to speak, or the "trade dress" (Greene and Kesselheim 2011), is what differs. An important caveat, however, is that generalist treatments do not aim to completely replace more intensive or specialized psychotherapies. Rather, the generalist treatments aim to be an initial step of care that most mental health practitioners can employ and that most patients should be able to access. Within the scope of stepped care models, which allocate different intensities of treatment for different clinical stages or situations (Chanen et al. 2016; Choi-Kain et al. 2016; Paris 2013), generalist treatments can be the first step. If these generalist models of BPD care can be widely proliferated as the new "treatment as usual," many more clinicians will be equipped to treat most patients with BPD capably, and the limited number of specialists can be reserved to lead generalist teams or to treat more severe but likely treatment-responsive patients for whom generalist approaches prove inadequate.

Brand-name advocates question the credibility and definitions of generalist approaches, thus seemingly reinforcing their claims of exclusive rights to be considered a treatment that works for the disorder (Comtois and Fruhbauerova 2019). The debates and contentiousness between brand-name and generic representatives (i.e., researchers and advocates) provide an important parallel to this current situation between stakeholders in brand-name treatments and these new generalist treatments on the rise. In the mid-twentieth century, the era of brand-name prescribing, pharmaceutical companies lobbied to prevent generic substitution, or "counterfeiting," questioning the purity and safety of generic medications. However, in the face of escalating health care costs in the latter half of the twentieth century, it became apparent that a system relying exclusively on brand-name drugs was unsustainable. While pharmaceutical companies vociferously opposed bills to mandate generic drug prescription, pharmacists staged a "generic backlash," leading to the valorization of generic drugs in the 1970s in the procedure for U.S. Food and Drug Administration bioequivalence approval (Greene 2011). Generic drugs became household items, accounting for the majority of prescriptions filled in the United States alone and easing the financial burden imposed by pharmaceutical companies on patients and the health care system more broadly (Greene 2011). Similarly, generalist or clinical management approaches to BPD have their own growing evidence base and represent the genericization of effective treatment for BPD. Hopefully, these generic variants of evidence-based treatments for BPD will infiltrate the public consciousness as just appropriate care, to strip off the marketing and business dimensions of the sale of treatments and their training as a business, rather than as health care.

In this chapter we review the essential elements of generalist treatment for BPD, with a focus on GPM as a prototype of a protocolized but flexible approach, preserving key effective elements of BPD-specific treatments, that can be delivered in a pragmatic way in the usual settings where patients with BPD seek care. Although all of the major generalist approaches are briefly reviewed in this chapter, along with the research findings that show their effectiveness, GPM is the major focus. The chapter describes the basic ingredients of GPM, using clinical vignettes to illustrate the application of this approach. Lastly, we discuss the use of various stepped care models of treatment for BPD in order to map out how clinicians can organize their recommendations to patients, care systems, and clinical resources. These stepped care algorithms provide a place for both generalist first-line BPD treatments that all clinicians should learn and a more rarified brand-name approach for those who prefer it or who need more intensive specialized care. Our hope is that GPM will equip any clinician, regardless of training or background, with fundamental and pragmatic tools to serve the patients they encounter with BPD in any clinical setting where psychiatric disorders are treated.

Generalist Care Models

General (or "Good" or "Good Enough") Psychiatric Management

In the early 2000s, Shelley McMain and her collaborators compared high-quality adherent DBT with a general psychiatric management approach (GPM) led by Paul Links (McMain et al. 2009). This study design aimed to eliminate differences in structure, BPD focus, and expertise between the two treatment arms to test whether specific ingredients involved in DBT (e.g., skills training and coaching) resulted in superior outcomes. What the two treatments had in common were 1) a theoretical basis of understanding BPD; 2) a treatment structure with once-weekly individual therapy as well as weekly clinician supervision; and 3) primary treatment strategies, including diagnostic disclosure with psychoeducation, a helpful clinical relationship, here-and-now (as opposed to childhood) focus, collaborative crisis management protocols, validation, emotion focus, and patient and clinician accountability to roles. Core components of DBT (i.e., skills training group, dialectical strategies, prioritization of focus on self-harm and suicidality, and explicit behavioral strategies such as shaping, exposure, diary cards, and behavioral analysis) were formally used in the DBT condition, and psychodynamic attentiveness to anger (and aggression), as well as to countertransference reactions, was more formally utilized in the GPM condition. The aim of using skills rather than medications in DBT was adopted as the guiding principle for medication management, whereas APA guidelines were the foundation of pharmacological prescribing in the GPM arm.

There were no differences in major outcomes between these two rigorously managed treatment arms. Patients with BPD improved significantly in both treatments in terms of borderline symptoms, depression, anger, symptom distress, frequency and severity of suicidal and non-suicidal self-injurious episodes, and health service utilization (McMain et al. 2009). These gains were sustained 2 years after treatment (McMain et al. 2012). Although DBT prioritized a focus on self-harm and suicidality and GPM emphasized interpersonal problems, the outcome measures of reduction of self-destructive behavior and improvement in interpersonal functioning did not differ. Notably, dropout rates among patients with more severe Axis I comorbidity were significantly lower with GPM, with its well-delineated guidelines for managing comorbidities and prescribing medications, among participants with high DSM-IV Axis I comorbidity (Wnuk et al. 2013). The lack of differences in major outcomes at the end of 12 months of treatment and at 2 years after the end of treatment suggests that the common factors between DBT and GPM account for more of the symptomatic change generated than did the specific divergent theoretical bases and techniques. The good news is that these simple features of good psychiatric care for any diagnosis, if employed in a systematic and supervised way, can result in significant improvement for patients with BPD without use of a highly specified and intensive treatment like DBT.

Structured Clinical Management

Other generalist care models have been developed with similar ingredients (Table 15–1). Of these, SCM (Bateman and Krawitz 2013) is the most well developed and proliferated. Like GPM, SCM integrates key ideas from effective BPD treatments (i.e. MBT, DBT, psychodynamic influences) into a pragmatic package of case management and problem-solving elements summarized in a readable concise handbook (see Choi-Kain et al. 2017a for a comparison of GPM and SCM). As mentioned earlier in this chapter, Bateman and Fonagy compared SCM with MBT in a large well-conducted outpatient randomized controlled trial, finding significant improvement in both arms. Steeper declines in suicidality, self-harm, and hospitalization were present in the MBT arm, although SCM was superior in the initial months at reducing self-harm. Subsequent analyses demonstrated that MBT was superior in outcome to SCM in cases of complex personality disorder meeting criteria for a number of different personality disorder diagnoses (Bateman and Fonagy 2013), illustrating a possible consideration for how patients can be allocated to more specialized care, such as MBT, over generalist care.

Good Clinical Care

Good clinical care (GCC; Chanen et al. 2008) is a brief manualized generalist care model developed for adolescents with emerging BPD. In a trial of early intervention for BPD, GCC was compared with cognitive analytic therapy (CAT; Ryle et al. 1997) in 24 weekly sessions with 24 months of outcome assessment. GCC was designed to be a higher quality of BPD care than treatment as usual (Chanen et al. 2008). It employed a problem-solving model, with additional sessions delivered based on co-occurring symptoms such as depression, anxiety, or anger management problems. Some interventions were based on cognitive-behavioral principles, such as linking cognitions and emotions and evaluating maladaptive thoughts. GCC also employed a team-based model with case management. Patient improvement in both the CAT and GCC arms was statistically and clinically significant, with no between-group differences in outcomes. The results of this trial of generalist care for adolescents with BPD demonstrate that early intervention can be safe and effective, with sustained improvements in BPD symptoms and externalizing behaviors, with just 6 months of organized BPD-focused care (Chanen et al. 2008).

Guideline-Informed Treatment for Personality Disorders

Guideline-informed treatment for personality disorders (GIT-PD; Aalders and Hengstmengel 2019; Hutsebaut and Kaasenbrood 2015) is a broad-based, inclusive, pantheoretical framework of treatment guidelines that synthesizes the common elements of

TABLE 15–1. Summary of generalist treatments for borderline personality disorder (BPD)

Study	Study details	Specialized treatment	Generalist comparator	N	Outcomes	Dropout
Bateman and Fonagy 2009	18-month trial at St. Ann's Hospital in London, United Kingdom	MBT	SCM	134 MBT: 71 SCM: 63	Significant improvement across outcomes in both MBT and SCM. MBT—steeper improvement and better outcomes. Differences in suicidality and self-injurious behaviors only become significant at 12 months. Self-harm improves more quickly with SCM initially.	MBT: 27% (19) SCM: 25% (16)
Chanen et al. 2008	Trial of up to 24 sessions of treatment for adolescents ages 15–18 years in Melbourne, Australia Participants followed for 2 years	CAT	GCC	78 CAT: 41 GCC: 37	Significant improvement in both CAT and GCC groups, along with lower odds of frequent self-harm. CAT yields slightly faster improvement across outcomes.	CAT: 63% (26) GCC: 57% (21)
McMain et al. 2009	12-month trial through University of Toronto teaching hospitals	DBT	GPM	180 DBT: 90 GPM: 90	No significant differences across groups. GPM better regarding retention of cases with more comorbidity. Significant improvement in suicidality, NSSI, BPD symptoms, distress, depression, anger, and interpersonal functioning in both groups. Reduction in general health care utilization.	DBT: 39% (35) GPM: 38% (34)

Note. BPD=borderline personality disorder; CAT=Cognitive analytic therapy; DBT=dialectical behavior therapy; GCC=good clinical care; GPM=general (good) psychiatric management; MBT=mentalization-based treatment; NSSI=nonsuicidal self-injury; SCM=structured clinical management.

existing specialized and generalist treatments to serve the Dutch health care system. Its guidelines are structured in such a way that they can be fulfilled from a mentalization-based framework, a skills-based framework, or an eclectic framework that maintains a focus on generalist principles (Figure 15–1). The guidelines themselves have yet to be tested in a randomized controlled trial, but they rely on the common factors of evidence-based treatments. GIT-PD shares many characteristics of GPM (see Figure 15–1), including collaborative diagnostic disclosure, psychoeducation, avoidance of polypharmacy, setting of clear goals, crisis planning, service integration, case management, avoidance of hospitalization, evaluation of effectiveness, and family involvement. However, it draws from SCM in its 1) recommendation of an SCM-style problem-solving group; 2) greater specificity on the details of how to apply GIT-PD in practice, including stipulations on team structure and caseload limitations to 20 patients; and 3) theoretical conceptualization of personality disorders as consisting of disturbances across several domains, including not only interpersonal sensitivity but also impulsivity, emotion regulation, and identity disturbance (Aalders and Hengstmengel 2019; Hutsebaut and Kaasenbrood 2015).

Training for Good Psychiatric Management

What these specified theories and techniques packaged in each specialist psychotherapy for BPD share is a coherent package or brand that therapists can organize, affiliate, and identify with as a secure base of operations in the face of the expectable intensities of working with patients with BPD. Peter Fonagy and his collaborators explain that the theory, framework, and tools of brand-name psychotherapies may themselves confer the components that breed epistemic trust—that is, trust in the knowledge conveyed—for both the clinician and the patient, in the face of the expectable symptomatic challenges involved in the clinical management of BPD (Fonagy and Allison 2014). The validation of these treatments as effective provides a rationale that gives clinicians the confidence that what they are doing is indicated, informed, and tested, counteracting usual countertransference feelings of helplessness and inadequacy, as well as the experience of feeling overwhelmed and disorganized (Colli et al. 2014) that is expectable in interactions with patients with BPD. In addition, clinical supervision incorporated as an essential feature of both specialized and generalist treatments may add an important element providing support, alternative ways of thinking about clinical problems, and direction organized around major tenets of the treatment. These treatments provide an important roadmap for navigating difficult clinical terrain, and the supervision provides helpful guidance and advisement, offering containment for practitioners so that they can in turn reliably contain the intensive process involved in the care of patients with BPD.

The confidence, support, and reassurance that evidence-based treatments provide clinicians can be generated and sustained by only a single day of training in GPM. A study of almost 300 clinicians—including clinical social workers (29.5%), psychiatrists (26.1%), nurses (22.7%), psychologists (12.5%), psychiatry residents (4.5%), primary care physicians (2.3%), and physician assistants (2.3%)—before and after the one day of training that GPM requires showed that the training itself decreases avoidance, dislike, and hopelessness regarding the care of patients with BPD and increases feelings

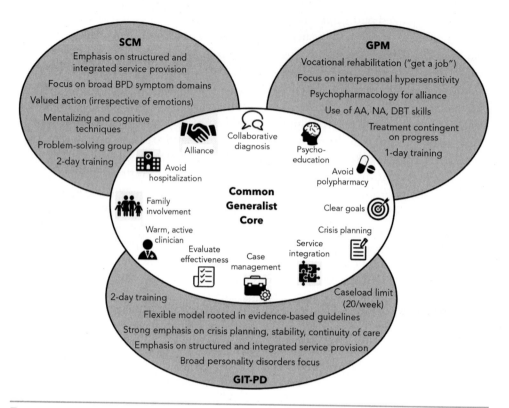

FIGURE 15–1. Common elements of generalist treatments.

AA=Alcoholics Anonymous; BPD=borderline personality disorder; GPM=good psychiatric management; DBT=dialectical behavior therapy; GIT-PD=guideline-informed treatment for personality disorders; NA=Narcotics Anonymous; SCM=structured clinical management.

of competence, belief in one's capacity to make positive differences, and belief that effective treatments exist in the care of patients with BPD (Keuroghlian et al. 2016). Importantly, younger clinicians in this sample reported greater increases in feeling competent after the training than older clinicians, who likely have learned what GPM embodies through years of clinical experience. In a separate study extending the assessment of clinician attitudes to 6 months post–GPM training, most of the changes in attitude were sustained over time, and some changes became more evident over time (Masland et al. 2018). Immediately post–GPM training, clinicians in this second study reported a decrease in preference to avoid patients with BPD as well as an increased sense of competence in treatment of patients with BPD and willingness to disclose the diagnosis to patients. These changes were sustained at 6-month follow-up. Additionally, 6 months after training, clinicians reported reductions in dislike of patients with BPD and hopelessness about its prognosis, along with increased feelings of being able to make a positive difference, capacity to feel empathy, and comfort in interactions with patients with BPD. Lastly, in the period between the training and 6-month follow-up, clinicians endorsed an increased willingness to take on new patients with BPD. Given that individuals with BPD are hypersensitive to the attitude others may have toward them, these clinician-related changes likely influence the viability of treatment and attitudes on both sides of the therapeutic alliance. Furthermore, the reduction in negative sentiments and increases in optimism, feelings of competence, and belief in their ability to make a positive difference appear to be related to an increased willingness to make BPD the central diagnosis in care, as well as to take on patients with the disorder. Therefore, GPM training appears to increase available care by encouraging generalists that they are good enough and capable of treating patients with BPD.

Generalist care models aim to encourage the practices of good care that mental health clinicians already know, reorganized around an enhanced and modernized knowledge base regarding BPD. The trainings for generalist approaches are therefore shorter and less expensive than the trainings for specialized psychotherapies for BPD (Choi-Kain et al. 2016; Iliakis et al. 2019), albeit still led by experts in the field. However, training for these generalist approaches has been less available than for the specialized psychotherapies. Since 2015, the Gunderson Personality Disorders Institute (GPDI), formerly known as the Borderline Personality Disorder Training Institute (BPDTI), at McLean Hospital has trained faculty to teach others GPM at training programs across the world. To enhance availability of training, an internet-based full-day course in GPM, filmed with faculty John Gunderson, Lois Choi-Kain, and Brian Palmer, is available through Harvard Medical School CME Online until 2022 (http://hms.harvard.edu/BPD). This course is provided for free for the first 6,000 learners (a fee of $25.00 will apply to subsequent registrants) from the Gunderson Personality Disorders Institute, McLean Hospital, thanks to a generous gift from an anonymous donor. Increasing the availability of training while decreasing costs, time, and travel requirements makes GPM accessible to all mental health clinicians who want basic tools to care for patients with BPD. Although the clinical management of BPD remains challenging, focused and structured care combines common factors of effective treatments for BPD (Gunderson and Choi-Kain 2018), facilitating the natural course of remission of symptoms and recovery observed in its longitudinal course (Zanarini et al. 2012).

Basic Components of Good Psychiatric Management

The central tenets of GPM are informed by an attitude that useful, competent treatment of patients with BPD can and should be provided by clinicians with different training backgrounds, who may not necessarily see themselves as "experts" but nevertheless can provide effective treatment. Clinicians can learn the GPM approach in one day of formal didactics, which can be replaced or enhanced by reading *Handbook of Good Psychiatric Management for Borderline Personality Disorder* (Gunderson and Links 2014), hereafter referred to as the GPM Handbook. This main text spans only 67 pages in its core instruction and is supplemented by just over 80 pages of clinical illustrations and vignettes. Here, we briefly highlight core components that all clinicians can employ immediately without elaborate psychotherapeutic techniques, extensively trained coordinated teams, or lengthy or intensive treatment. These central elements, listed in Table 15–2, are meant to orient prospective clinicians by distilling years of accumulated research and experience.

Good psychiatric management for any condition begins with a diagnosis, which is then shared objectively and unapologetically with the patient as the focus of the treat-

TABLE 15–2.	Guiding principles of good psychiatric management for borderline personality disorder

Diagnostic disclosure and psychoeducation

Goal setting (convey that change is expected)

Case management (be active, not reactive, and maintain a focus on life outside treatment)

Interpersonal hypersensitivity

Multimodality

Flexible duration and intensity

Clinician attitude (be flexible, pragmatic, and eclectic)

ment relationship. The primary function of the treatment relationship is to help the patient manage the symptoms and vulnerabilities of their illness, reducing symptoms while maximizing recovery, functionality, and quality of life. Psychoeducation provides the patient with scientific findings about and a clinical formulation of BPD as a problem of interpersonal hypersensitivity, establishing a context within which the patient, clinician, and family members can understand the patient's history and behavior patterns. By presenting the patient's challenges as reflecting a medical condition, the clinician can address others' concerns that the patient's symptoms reflect either a "manipulative" stance or the incompetence of the treater.

The medicalized model of care encourages patients and clinicians to proactively manage risk for morbidity and mortality. It also provides guidelines for managing comorbidity and medications. Importantly, it warns against iatrogenic harm related to tendencies to promote unrealistic dependency on the treatment relationship. Because of the tendency of patients with BPD to act angrily or self-destructively to get others to understand their level of need and pain, receiving more psychiatric care can often reinforce symptomatic states. Certainly, the current systems of care provide more intensive treatment for increased acuity and dangerousness, which may work against patients' motivations to improve.

To counteract these iatrogenic influences, GPM promotes the patient's responsibility for using the treatment to reach clinical and life goals. In fact, the provision of treatment is made contingent on improvement rather than acuity. GPM encourages patients to refocus their energies to build a meaningful and functional life outside of treatment, rather than remain mired in an identity as a patient. Getting a job is an important task within GPM that provides structure and interaction with others to counteract the loneliness frequently experienced by patients with BPD. It also provides a means of building self-reliance and self-esteem, which is not staked on an exclusive relationship. Although GPM therapists are encouraged to be flexible and eclectic in many ways, they should remain firm in helping the patient function in the adult world and manage usual responsibilities. While GPM integrates concepts from psychodynamic psychotherapy with more practical life management strategies and techniques, the focus on taking concrete steps to build a meaningful life should come before any exploration of the patient's developmental history. The following GPM tasks are aimed at promoting a productive treatment relationship as well as working toward the ultimate goal of building a life and identity outside of treatment.

Diagnostic Disclosure and Psychoeducation

Many clinicians fear that disclosing a diagnosis of BPD will aggravate or devastate the patient. However, secrecy around the diagnosis can increase the risk of iatrogenic harm (e.g., polypharmacy, derailing hospitalizations, aimless psychotherapies) and block the patient from receiving appropriate treatment. Zimmerman et al. (2016) recently showed that patients with BPD who are told about their diagnosis after an initial evaluation are as satisfied with the evaluation as are patients with a diagnosis other than BPD who are told their diagnosis. Zimmerman's study did not support the argument that patients cannot tolerate or react badly to the BPD diagnosis. Disclosing the BPD diagnosis informs the direction of care, allows accurate communication with colleagues, and serves as a good risk-management strategy, since it indicates a rationale for clinical decision making guided by evidence-based treatment. Diagnostic disclosure allows the clinician to speak frankly and directly with the patient and his or her family about what is driving chaotic behaviors and how to predict vulnerabilities in the future. This frank and direct approach enhances clarity in conceptualizing clinical problems and reduces indirect and vague communications that might aim to avoid undue stress or distress for the patient. By being clearer and more direct, a GPM clinician respectfully treats patients as though they can and should be responsible for themselves; this is a key message in the GPM approach.

Diagnostic disclosure can be done simply by using the DSM-5 criteria list for BPD to review ways in which the patient's history and behaviors support the diagnosis. Ideally, this process is approached collaboratively and affirmatively, encouraging patients that they are not alone, that others struggle with similar problems, and that their problems are understandable. Oftentimes, patients with BPD have been treated for comorbidities such as depression and anxiety without desired or sustainable improvement. In addition, they may have been misdiagnosed and treated with interventions that are both burdensome in their side effects and of limited utility. The BPD diagnosis can provide a reason that other treatments may have been inadequate or ineffective, and can counteract the common assumption that the patient cannot be helped or is broken beyond repair. Reframing the clinical focus of treatment on BPD can therefore have a beneficial, or even stimulating, effect, restoring morale and hope that more effective treatment may exist.

GPM is not the only intervention for BPD that prioritizes the need for proactive psychoeducation about the condition for patients and families. It does, however, stress that clinicians generally, including those without a particular expertise in treating the syndrome, should know enough about the disorder to share information about course, heritability, and response to treatments, including psychotherapies and medication. Psychoeducation about BPD is, of course, contingent on, first, the clinician's willingness to ask questions that might yield information about BPD signs and symptoms, and, then, the clinician's openness to making a BPD diagnosis. This openness to making a BPD diagnosis can occur without collateral informants if criteria are met clearly by the patient's report, even when co-occurring conditions such as mood or anxiety disorders, substance use, or eating disorders have not fully remitted. GPM advocates for starting treatment with evaluation and diagnosis to organize the therapeutic relationship and its goals. The therapist starts with asking pertinent questions about symptoms, including affective instability, unstable relationships, and suicidality, among other lines of inquiry. Then the GPM therapist should feel able to share with the patient and/or family his or her diagnostic impression.

This central tenet of GPM, first making and then disclosing a BPD diagnosis, extends to clinicians in settings other than outpatient treatment. Hong (2016) described the use of GPM principles in making and sharing a BPD diagnosis in the emergency department when appropriate; the GPM Handbook stresses the utility of using a psychiatric inpatient hospitalization to provide clarification of diagnosis for the patient and family members (Gunderson and Links 2014). These interventions can then lead to a psychoeducation process. Because BPD has significant heritability, GPM clinicians are expected to impart these facts in a medicalized, professional way to mitigate shame and stigma as part of a general approach. The clinician's professional, deliberate approach to diagnosis, along with forthright sharing of the diagnosis with patients and family, aims to underscore that BPD is a well-recognized condition and one that clinical interventions can effectively treat, as proven by a significant body of research. This communication directly addresses familiar scenarios that can include an assumption by family members or other clinicians that the patient's BPD symptoms reflect a pattern of gratuitous manipulation or a purposefully oppositional stance. Similarly, this approach can proactively counteract an assumption that the BPD patient's parents are "bad" or "abusive," thereby offering an alternative understanding than instead suggests that parents may be uninformed or lacking in skills.

The psychoeducation component can be anchored in the robust finding that there is a relatively good prognosis associated with BPD, with the caveats that 1) evidence-based treatment likely facilitates recovery; 2) the risk of suicide needs to be considered given data about significant rates of suicide completion in the BPD population; and 3) even with recovery over time, many patients with BPD will continue to have challenges engaging in meaningful work and relationships even when they technically no longer meet criteria for the disorder (Zanarini et al. 2012). Psychoeducation also includes information about evidence-based treatments available for the disorder, as well as details about the expectable morbidities associated with the condition and, as noted, the real risk of associated mortality by suicide or possibly inadvertent self-harm.

Growing evidence suggests that psychoeducation about the symptoms of BPD is a useful form of pretreatment in and of itself. An initial study of psychoeducation about BPD found a greater decline in general impulsivity and turmoil in close relationships in the intervention group than in the control group (Zanarini and Frankenburg 2008). More recently, Zanarini et al. (2018) extended the psychoeducational intervention to an online format, which includes introductory information about the history of the BPD diagnosis and the stigma associated with it, symptoms of BPD and theories of how these symptoms interact, comorbid disorders, etiology, longitudinal course, and available treatments. Female participants who completed the online psychoeducational curriculum reported a significant decline in BPD symptoms while actively participating in the intervention, with maintenance of most of this improvement during the year of follow-up. Compared with a control group who received no psychoeducational curriculum, the participants in online psychoeducation showed greater declines in symptoms of BPD in affective, interpersonal, behavioral, and cognitive sectors as well as a greater decline in symptoms overall. In a recent Italian randomized controlled trial of GPM-style psychoeducation of 96 patients in matched samples, Ridolfi and colleagues (2019) found that those who received psychoeducation on the etiology, course, and GPM treatment of BPD fared better 12 weeks after the psychoeducation intervention and at the 24-week follow-up on all sectors of BPD symptomatology (interpersonal, emotional, behavioral, cognitive) compared with those who did not receive psychoeducation.

Lastly, GPM instructs clinicians to ground their own, their patients', and their patients' family members' understanding of BPD in terms of interpersonal hypersensitivity. Interpersonal hypersensitivity is seen as a core vulnerability of BPD in which symptoms are driven by dependency, rejection sensitivity, and intolerance of aloneness (Gunderson and Lyons-Ruth 2008). The oscillation in the patient's symptoms is seen as a reaction to the responses and availability of others (as illustrated in Figure 15–2 later in this chapter) and is explained further in the interpersonal hypersensitivity section later in this chapter. Teaching this model to patients allows them the opportunity to understand their fluctuating states of emotion, behavior, and patterns of relating to others in a coherent way. As the GPM clinician and the patient with BPD together understand the intense impact that responses from others have on the patient's presentation, they come to understand interpersonal hypersensitivity as a handicap requiring special considerations.

Case Example 1

Jake is a first-year student at a large Midwestern university who started college after years of struggling with marked mood instability, periodic self-harm by cutting superficially in areas of his arms and thighs, and occasional bulimia symptoms in periods of heightened distress. Jake had sought treatment in his last year of high school and had seen a local psychologist, who told Jake she thought he might have a depressive disorder. Despite his persistent symptoms, Jake did not return for a second appointment. The stress of midterm exams during his first semester at college, and his turmoil-infused relationship with his girlfriend back home, led Jake to ask his resident advisor for help because of escalating suicidal feelings. Jake was escorted to the campus mental health center, where he was seen by Mr. Figueroa, a social worker.

The university mental health center had organized a one-day training the previous year to introduce the staff to the basic elements of GPM for BPD after the staff had asked for extra help in treating this sub-population of students. Mr. Figueroa had participated in the training and reviewed the GPM Handbook, which helped him feel he could competently and effectively treat students with BPD or BPD traits.

Mr. Figueroa saw Jake for an initial 90-minute session, during which he obtained permission and contacted the psychologist Jake had seen back at home. Mr. Figueroa then arranged a follow-up session to review his diagnostic impression with Jake. Mr. Figueroa explained to Jake the central elements of a BPD diagnosis, specifically the maladaptive coping strategies that caused Jake concern and his patterns of self-criticism and marked sensitivity to the actions of others. Mr. Figueroa reviewed with Jake the diagnostic criteria for BPD; Jake was struck by how many of the symptoms were familiar to him. He asked Mr. Figueroa whether this meant he might not have depression. Mr. Figueroa explained that BPD and depression often occur together but that their treatments were different and the likely benefit of medications was more limited without active treatment for the BPD symptoms. Mr. Figueroa also reviewed with Jake the evidence for the significant heritability of BPD and described the scientifically proven treatments available both at the campus mental health center and in the community.

Goal Setting

In GPM, setting goals is a central task that promotes agency, self-reliance, engagement in treatment, and productive collaboration rather than dependency on others. Although well-articulated long-term goals might relate to work, school, or social life, even a goal of identifying personal goals would be sufficient. In this way, the GPM clinician conveys an assumption that the patient with BPD can achieve certain improvements in behavior and functioning. Symptomatic remission is important insofar as it is the basis of having a more satisfying life outside of treatment, providing stable vocational and social/romantic functioning that more consistently fuels the development of identity, self-esteem, and trust in others. Because all personality disorders by diagnostic definition involve impairments in self-direction and functioning in relationships in general and at school, work, and leisure, any treatment for personality disorders should attend to functionality. (See Chapter 5, "Manifestations, Assessment, Diagnosis, and Differential Diagnosis," in this volume for a detailed discussion of the application of the Alternative DSM-5 Model for Personality Disorders [AMPD] to patients with personality pathology.) Specifically, vocational functioning (and more broadly, engagement in meaningful activities and relationships) has been identified by both researchers and patients as a positive prognostic factor and a key aspect of the patient's recovery journey (Ng et al. 2019), especially since long-term deficits in vocational functioning are prevalent in this population (Caruana et al. 2018; Ng et al. 2016; Zanarini et al. 2010, 2012).

However, within the treatment relationship, improvement in BPD symptoms, through improved behavioral control and capacity for reflective thinking, is emphasized as an expectation if the treatment is working. Case management strategies can help guide the patient toward necessary life skills that can be achieved in the short term, such as making a budget, going to the gym, or maintaining hygiene. These shorter-term goals allow patients to witness their own growing ability to diminish the self-esteem problems that promote dependency and withdrawal from life. Patients with BPD may not intentionally seek attention through their symptoms, but symptomatic states may be reinforced by the concern or attention they are likely to elicit. GPM encourages patients with BPD to become more reliable and appealing partners in relationship to others and to stabilize their interpersonal hypersensitivity through promoting self-improvement and self-reliance over helplessness and dependency.

Case Example 2

Mariana dropped out of college and returned home to live in her parents' basement. She was asked to leave college because of failing grades; disruptive behavior in her dorm, including heated arguments with other students; and one mild overdose of acetaminophen, leading to a brief psychiatric hospitalization. Mariana was given a diagnosis of BPD by the first therapist she consulted while at school. This therapist also felt Mariana had elements of narcissistic personality disorder, but the therapist did not feel comfortable sharing this information with the patient. Mariana spent most of her time smoking marijuana and writing songs she hoped someday to sell, although she made no efforts to do so. Mariana began looking for a local therapist; she understood her treatment would be designed to help her gain "self-knowledge," with a focus on exploring what she considered to be the trauma of having parents who would not support her career in music.

When Mariana was referred to a local clinic, she met with a psychologist, Dr. Hong, who saw a number of patients with BPD and used GPM as an initial intervention for those patients, while reserving access to more intensive or specialized treatments for those patients who did not respond to a more flexible and less intensive intervention. Dr. Hong began her meetings with Mariana by explaining the need for discussion of her goals beyond just reduction of symptoms like her intense anger and intermittent impulsivity. Mariana found this request to be surprising. She had anticipated that treatment for her BPD would consist of something the therapist offered to supply her, not something linked to actual goals related to returning to school, finding work, or developing positive relationships.

This process of establishing realistic life goals at the outset of treatment allowed Dr. Hong to introduce the idea of Mariana's accountability as an integral part of the treatment. Mariana began to understand that she would be responsible for her behavior. Dr. Hong maintained this focus on Mariana's life outside of treatment in the initial sessions, reinforcing the value of structured activities (e.g., paid work, volunteer opportunities), as well as asking Mariana about the relationships she did have with friends and family.

Case Management

GPM's particular focus on case management suggests its emphasis on practicality. In this way GPM appreciates that some, maybe most, patients with BPD may not be appropriate candidates for intensive therapy, be it behavioral or psychodynamic. Gunderson stressed in his writings the limits of traditional psychoanalytic treatment for patients with BPD, noting well-described high dropout rates in this treatment (Gunderson 2009). Gunderson also believed that the 24-hours-per-day, 7-days-a-week skills coaching model of DBT could problematically breed increased dependency, rendering a treatment that an individual with BPD might not want to leave. The case management approach encourages clinicians to engage actively with patients, often with a goal of mobilizing patients who themselves may believe they are unable to accomplish basic life tasks (e.g., make doctors' appointments, apply for work). Clinicians are therefore expected to use time in sessions to accomplish concrete tasks that support the patient's mobilization and engagement. In general, GPM encourages clinicians to convey that they are interested and involved; the therapist's goal is to stay active in the treatment, and thus not fall into a pattern of being excessively or exclusively reactive to the patient's travails. By definition, GPM is an eclectic treatment intervention; it requires the clinician to integrate elements of different psychotherapies (psychodynamic, cognitive-behavioral, and supportive), while also using case management elements marked by action and practicality. It focuses on finding what works, rather than being dogmatic and rigid about technique. The GPM clinician will employ interventions determined by the patient's needs and the clinician's common sense; this might mean utilizing interventions that traditionally would fall outside of the boundaries of standard "talk therapy" or pharmacotherapy.

Case Example 3

Mrs. Jackson lives in a rural county with limited access to psychiatric treatment. She has to drive a considerable distance for her monthly meetings with Dr. Goldberg, a psychiatrist. Dr. Goldberg has a high-volume practice focused exclusively on prescribing medications; he does no psychotherapy, although he uses GPM-informed attitudes and interventions in his work.

Mrs. Jackson had been significantly symptomatic in her late teens and early 20s, requiring multiple hospitalizations for suicide gestures and attempts and metabolic instability related to bulimia nervosa. Now in her 30s, she is less overtly symptomatic, but she continues to have challenges with family relationships and with finding and maintaining steady employment. Dr. Goldberg has prescribed medications that have helped Mrs. Jackson in a limited way; she is aware that medications have an adjunctive use and work best when combined with her participation in an online DBT skills group.

Dr. Goldberg begins sessions by conducting a standard "medical model" of meeting with Mrs. Jackson, reviewing her ongoing target symptoms and her use of medications, and asking about medication side effects. He also employs supportive psychotherapy techniques when appropriate, including advice, guidance, and empathic listening. He also uses, when indicated, some of his time with Mrs. Jackson to focus on challenges she has with accessing appointments for her medical care and vocational rehabilitation resources. Mrs. Jackson can become easily overwhelmed or hopeless when negotiating bureaucracies of different kinds. Dr. Goldberg works with her to make important medical appointments and to help her fill out online applications for government services. Dr. Goldberg moves with ease between these different roles, acting as physician, supportive therapist, or case manager as determined by Mrs. Jackson's chief concerns and the most important barriers to her recovery.

Interpersonal Hypersensitivity

GPM's formulation of *interpersonal hypersensitivity* as a critical way to understand the behavior of individuals with BPD is the heart of the GPM approach (Figure 15–2). This theory provides clinicians and patients with a coherent way to understand the extreme shifts in the emotions, interpersonal reactions, and behavior that rapidly occur in BPD. Taking patients step-by-step through the different states described in the interpersonal hypersensitivity formulation, along with directly linking these states with the patient's experience of others, is a central task in the psychoeducation about BPD that any clinician can provide. The interpersonal hypersensitivity model identifies four key states frequently observed in patients with BPD: 1) connectedness, 2) feeling threatened, 3) aloneness, and 4) despair. The model also offers a theory about how the patient might move among these four BPD-related states and how those around the patient (clinicians, family) might intervene.

In the state of *connectedness*, the patient is anxious, receptive to help, and idealizing (e.g., of a romantic partner or the therapist) or dependent (on family, spouse, or treater). However, the patient remains in a precarious position, usually hypervigilant for signs of real or perceived abandonment or rejection. Inevitably, when signs of imminent rejection or separation are perceived, the connected state devolves into a *threatened* state, where the patient expresses intense anger, devalues others, and engages in self-harming behaviors to communicate distress. The reactions of others to patients in this state can vary. Some, including therapists, may be moved to increase involvement or try to "rescue" patients (thereby leading the patient back to a state of connectedness). Others may withdraw out of fear, futility, or frustration, leaving the patient with BPD truly alone.

In this state of *aloneness*, the patient with BPD will become dissociated, impulsive, and paranoid without the other person and relationship to ground, organize, and contain him or her. The states related to being alone are understandably riskier than the connected or threatened states described above. Without a holding environment, the patient with BPD becomes more truly *despairing* and suicidal. At this point, containment in a hospital allows the patient to reconnect and reconstitute with greater access to others, in either idealizing connected or hostile threatened ways.

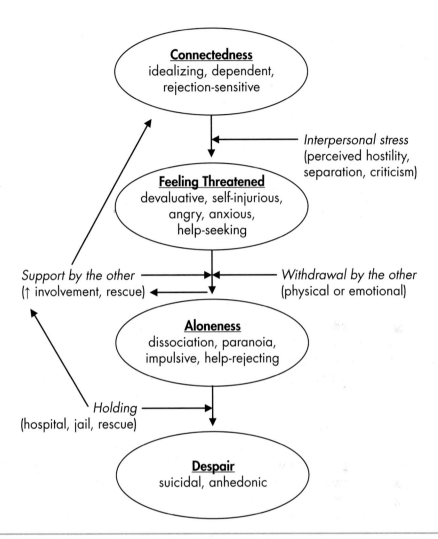

FIGURE 15–2. Borderline personality disorder interpersonal coherence model.

The *holding environment* refers to the calming influence of a relationship that the patient feels he or she can depend on. When others show concern, consistency, and responsiveness, the patient develops a belief that someone cares about him or her. When the patient is in a threatened state, aggressive behaviors may succeed in gaining attention from the desired caregiver. When the caregiver provides rescue or increased involvement, the patient calms down and goes back to a connected state. When the patient devolves into aloneness and despair, an external container (e.g., hospital or other settings where the patient can be reconnected with others) provides containment where the patient may encounter caregivers or sources of support that relieve his or her sense of loneliness.

Source. Reprinted from Gunderson JG, Links P: *Handbook of Good Psychiatric Management for Borderline Personality Disorder.* Washington, DC, American Psychiatric Publishing, 2014, p. 14. Copyright © 2014, American Psychiatric Association. Used with permission.

The GPM therapist familiar with this model will use the descriptions of the four oscillating states of BPD to convey to patients a sense that the patient's shifting affective states can be contextualized and predicted. For example, given the intense reactions patients with BPD experience in response to others, the GPM clinician will express doubt about the patient's dependency on exclusive relationships with anyone, including the clinician. At the same time, the GPM clinician will encourage the patient to widen his or her social network as a protective influence in light of the patient's intolerance of aloneness. (For example, use of 12-step groups, given their ubiquity and flexibility, can sometimes be of great use to patients with BPD, when indicated.) When the patient realizes that his or her hostile, devaluing, and self-injurious behaviors can scare or push others away, other strategies for managing and communicating distress are encouraged. These strategies might include connecting with members of a peer group program, using available 12-step meetings or contacts with a program sponsor, or reaching out to available resources on "hotlines" via phone, email, or text. Lastly, reasonable self-reliance is emphasized as a solution to the patient's tendency to decompensate when alone.

Patients often feel less alone and alienated knowing that these extreme shifts in their emotional and behavioral activity are indeed understandable and that there are strategies they can use to cope with their emotions. The GPM therapist will return repeatedly to the interpersonal hypersensitivity model as a framework for understanding BPD symptoms and educating the patient about what the therapist observes to be the patient's vulnerabilities and reflexive reactions. The overarching goal of this process is to have the patient develop his or her own capacity for self-awareness, so that he or she is aware of threats to stability and can take action accordingly.

Additionally, the GPM model of interpersonal hypersensitivity guides clinicians on points of intervention depending on the prevailing symptomatic presentation. Clinicians are taught to "lean in" rather than withdraw when the patient is in the transition between connected and threatened states. By making a point to engage rather than withdraw, the GPM therapist can take the opportunity to explore with the patient a conflicted, rather than either idealizing or devaluing, stance. While this intervention may seem counterintuitive, engaging when most others might naturally withdraw can contain the patient's distress and therefore restore the patient's receptivity to help from collaborators in challenging periods. At the same time, this model instructs clinicians that when a patient with BPD is in a paranoid, dissociated, or truly despairing suicidal state, containment in a hospital may be necessary to restore the patient's capacity to use clinical interactions more productively.

Case Example 4

Francesca sought counseling at a local clinic that specialized in treating patients in the lesbian, gay, bisexual, transgender, or queer/questioning (LGBTQ) community. She met with Ms. Roberts, a master's-level clinician. Francesca described to Ms. Roberts her history of tumultuous romantic relationships that often led to periods of impulsivity, isolation, and despair when she was reacting to a romantic breakup. Twice Francesca had been seen in a local emergency department when she failed to attend to her diabetic regimen during one of these crises, leading to serious medical consequences.

Francesca had searched the internet and identified BPD as her likely diagnosis, something she raised with Ms. Roberts, who agreed with Francesca about this conjecture after Ms. Roberts had conducted an initial interview and had spoken with Francesca's most recent therapist. Ms. Roberts used basic GPM interventions in her work with Francesca, focusing on the ways that Francesca's interpersonal hypersensitivity, mostly in the context of romantic relationships, would lead to a marked deterioration in her functioning and occasionally dangerous behavior, as in her impaired diabetes care.

Over time, Francesca developed an increased understanding about her pattern of behavior. She came to appreciate how she could easily become highly dependent on a new romantic partner when she felt that the new relationship would meet all of her needs. She came to recognize how she could easily come to feel threatened if a girlfriend did not immediately answer her calls or texts. Often Francesca would become anxious or needy, asking friends for reassurance during these episodes. Ms. Roberts reviewed with Francesca those episodes in the past when a breakup had led to a period of marked distress with associated impulsivity, such as when she had failed to administer her diabetes medications as was necessary. Francesca learned to recognize those dangerous periods when her despair would lead to suicidal impulses, a situation further compounded by her help-rejecting attitudes during those crises. Francesca would often review the familiar patterns outlined in the interpersonal model with Ms. Roberts using diary cards or chain analyses, which explore the vulnerabilities and prompting events that give rise to problem behaviors, as well as their consequences. For example, Francesca used the chain analysis intervention to more thoroughly examine the elements of a pattern familiar to her: perceived rejection would lead to isolation; in this isolated state Francesca would be more likely to turn off her phone, leading her to feel more lonely and despairing; when despairing, Francesca would become overwhelmed by her diabetes medication regimen, leading her to a state of intense futility and self-reproach. Doing chain analysis helped Francesca move from a pattern of feeling unable to control her moods and behaviors to one in which she felt some understanding of and therefore control over her reactions to her experiences with others.

Multimodality

The use of different treatment interventions either in sequence or together is a key aspect of GPM's flexibility. This approach is markedly different from the model of the closed treatment dyad of a generation ago; the GPM therapist is open to including whatever might be of use to the patient, including group treatment options (DBT skills groups, 12-step programs, family coaching, and psychoeducation), along with adjunctive pharmacotherapy. As noted, GPM itself borrows from various approaches to treatment; rather than considering concurrent treatment interventions as a liability or distraction, the GPM therapist remains open to whatever might be beneficial during the course of treatment. GPM has a specific and detailed approach to pharmacotherapy that has evolved since its early adherence to the APA practice guideline (American Psychiatric Association 2001); since that time, accruing evidence of the circumscribed benefits and concerning risks associated with medications used frequently with patients with BPD has informed the thinking about medication options. In addition, GPM has a well-considered algorithm for family involvement that reinforces a psychoeducation component and limits possibly unproductive family involvement.

Case Example 5

Mr. Sawada is a divorced man who is retired from his part-time work and living in an assisted living facility. Mr. Sawada had a history of multiple psychiatric hospitalizations in his youth, some lasting many months. Mr. Sawada had not been suicidal for many years, but continued to have interpersonal difficulties, including intense relationships with his nephews that often ended in dramatic relationship ruptures when Mr. Sawada felt ignored or mistreated in some way.

Mr. Sawada had been given a diagnosis of BPD by a therapist many years ago, but he only grudgingly accepted this diagnosis and felt it did not account for his prominent anxiety. Mr. Sawada had grown up with a mother who was addicted to alcohol, and he attributed many of his difficulties to his childhood. When he came to live at the assisted living facility, Mr. Sawada was referred to a team at a local geriatric psychiatry clinic. This clinic used GPM principles when treating individuals with personality disorder symptoms. His social worker at this clinic, Ms. Villa, broached with Mr. Sawada the possibility of using resources both in the clinic and in the local community as part of a treatment plan. Mr. Sawada was initially reluctant to follow this suggestion, as he had only been treated in the past by a psychiatrist who provided both counseling and medication management. Ms. Villa suggested that Mr. Sawada might benefit from seeing her individually in a flexible counseling modality while also seeing the clinic's psychiatrist for continued prescription of his medication for anxiety. Ms. Villa also suggested that Mr. Sawada consider participation in a local chapter of Adult Children of Alcoholics (ACOA), which held multiple meetings weekly at a convenient nearby location. Ms. Villa also offered to meet with Mr. Sawada and his nephews. Mr. Sawada wondered if this would constitute family therapy of some kind; Ms. Villa suggested that she would initially propose a meeting to provide information and psychoeducation for Mr. Sawada and his nephews, perhaps to be followed by some additional meetings focused on coaching should this be useful. This coaching could include advice for his nephews on managing Mr. Sawada's periods of perceived mistreatment: trying not to become defensive, "taking things slow," and setting limits in situations when Mr. Sawada might become verbally abusive.

Mr. Sawada found the ACOA meetings to be comforting. He often went to meetings when he was feeling isolated or alienated from the other residents at the residential facility. He especially appreciated the flexibility of the meetings, as he could drop in when he felt so inclined but did not feel an obligation to do so. Mr. Sawada also found that seeing a psychiatrist and a therapist separately allowed him to get different perspectives at times, particularly when he felt misunderstood or ignored by one of his treaters.

Duration and Intensity

GPM is distinguished by its relative flexibility with regard to the length of treatment recommended and the intensity of the treatment as reflected in frequency of visits. In this regard, GPM differs from the other empirically validated treatments that require a set number of visits weekly and/or an expected duration of treatment. GPM's flexibility therefore allows for treatment of patients with BPD symptoms with a range of severity of illness. This means that relatively stable patients who are not in crisis, for example, may be seen sporadically, while patients with prominent active difficulties can be seen more frequently as determined by the therapist. GPM's variable duration and intensity therefore allow individual clinicians to treat a larger number of patients, which is consistent with the treatment's overarching goal of serving a public health need by providing competent services to as many consumers as possible.

GPM's focus on therapist practicality informs the recommendation for variable treatment intensity and duration. In situations where treatment is offered to patients who may not have a set schedule, such as college students who are away for vacations or summer break, this flexibility can allow for good enough treatment. GPM should continue only if the patient and therapist feel that progress is being made. There is no "autopilot" setting for GPM, but rather the patient and therapist are always actively evaluating the benefit of the intervention. In addition, the GPM therapist will recommend a frequency usually of once weekly at the beginning of treatment, but even this recommendation is not set in stone. The therapist will adjust the number of sessions based on the clinical needs of the patients; again, this is markedly different from other evidence-based treatments that have a set frequency and duration. There will be cases when a patient may have no positive response to GPM, and in these cases the therapist may consider a referral for a different, more intensive treatment. There may be instances when the patient has benefited from the treatment but the patient prefers a different type of intervention to work more specifically on certain issues.

Case Example 6

Vy is a senior medical student who received her care through the counseling service offering treatment to graduate students and medical trainees at her university. Vy was treated for what she thought was a depressive disorder during her college years, but in her first year of medical school she concluded through her own research that the affective instability, recurrent thoughts of suicide, and binge eating she experienced might best be understood as reflecting a BPD diagnosis. This conjecture was affirmed by the psychologist, Dr. Wu, whom she saw at the counseling center. In the first weeks of Vy's treatment, Dr. Wu reviewed with her different treatment options available both through the counseling service and with clinicians in the community. Vy had strong feelings that she wanted to use her last year of medical school to travel, if she could; this made commitment to an extended treatment such as DBT, with its set commitment to a series of modules, somewhat impractical. Dr. Wu proposed that Vy meet with her using a GPM approach, meaning that they would begin with weekly treatment but would periodically revisit that schedule and assess what frequency of treatment worked best for the patient.

Vy met weekly with Dr. Wu during the months she remained local. They focused on understanding how Vy's experience of rejection by others was closely associated with her impulsive binge eating and her feelings of hopelessness; they repeatedly reviewed Vy's experience using a chain analysis exercise that helped Vy trace how these episodes evolved.

When Vy twice spent time out of state working in other medical facilities as part of her studies, she continued to work on these chain analysis exercises and used a trip back home to see Dr. Wu for a once-monthly meeting. Vy managed to complete her studies and to graduate from medical school. She had made a decision to choose a residency that would allow her more flexibility in her schedule than had been possible while in medical school. She continued to see Dr. Wu the following year, and together they decided that an adjunctive DBT skills group might be of help to Vy, as she had hoped to have some peer support for her challenges from her BPD. Vy and Dr. Wu continued to meet sporadically while Vy committed to the 6-month course of weekly evening DBT skills group. The opportunity to hear about others' challenges with BPD and to provide support in the group to her peers turned out to be a valuable and gratifying opportunity for Vy.

Clinician Attitude

The basic components of GPM listed in this chapter provide clinicians in any treatment setting with tools to structure their treatment of patients with BPD. Even in an emergency department setting or during brief inpatient hospitalization, GPM clinicians can make a diagnosis, provide basic psychoeducation, and utilize the interpersonal hypersensitivity model to understand BPD (Hong 2016, 2019). The clinical attitude of GPM involves all of the following: being flexible and pragmatic; anticipating the patient's presentation and needs; setting goals; avoiding unnecessary pharmacological interventions; expecting change through enhancing accountability; and treating the clinical relationship as both real and professional.

In GPM, the therapist is encouraged to do what works and what is most realistic. There is no set duration, intensity, or frequency of encounters. At the same time, the GPM clinician is firm in holding the patient accountable for what he or she says and does. Instead of reflexively trying to minimize the patient's feelings of guilt or shame, the clinician can validate the patient for having such feelings, which are preconditions for taking responsibility and eventual change.

Change is expected as part of the GPM treatment paradigm. This means that if the patient is not making progress, the clinician and patient both need to review the current treatment approach and make appropriate changes. This does not necessarily mean intensifying the treatment. Instead, it could mean stepping back from an approach that is not working. Patients should be informed that the course of BPD trends toward gradual improvement and that this improvement is dependent on the patient taking an active role. Although this level of accountability may feel threatening or abandoning, clinicians can demonstrate their engagement and investment by having a demeanor that is present and active, not reactive. An added element of the GPM stance is treating the clinical relationship as both real and professional. GPM encourages clinicians to express their humanity and acknowledge their own mistakes and limitations realistically and responsibly. Self-disclosure can be helpful when used judiciously, but keeping the relationship professional, consistent, and with boundaries is essential. (See Chapter 19, "Boundary Issues," in this volume for a detailed discussion of the importance of appropriate boundaries in the treatment of patients with personality pathology.)

The clinical attitude that is part of the GPM approach to patient care will automatically assist the clinician in avoiding various risk management pitfalls commonly associated with the treatment of patients with BPD (Gutheil 1985). The literature on risk management underscores the fact that, in general, psychiatry is a low-risk medical subspecialty, although it is notable that psychiatry ranks among the medical fields more frequently associated with patient complaints to state boards of medicine (Reich and Schatzberg 2014). That said, reviews of psychiatry malpractice emphasize that potential risks for legal action, such as suicide and suicide attempts, boundary violations, incorrect diagnosis, and inappropriate hospitalization, are all areas of concern for clinicians treating patients with BPD. The GPM Handbook stresses that increased liability in treating patients with BPD is usually associated with the following: 1) clinician inexperience; 2) "countertransference enactments," such as excessive availability, punitive hostility, or personal involvement; and 3) lack of ongoing consultation, when it is indicated. One overarching goal of GPM's approach is to enable clinicians to treat patients with BPD safely and confidently so that inordinate concerns about lawsuits or complaints do not cause them to avoid treating patients with BPD, thus exacerbating the already concerning shortage of services for this population.

Suicidality and Self-Harm Management

In the GPM model, suicidal and self-injurious symptoms are to be expected, prepared for, and understood in the context of the interpersonal hypersensitivity model described earlier. Both suicidal behavior and nonsuicidal self-harm are considered to be expressions of distress. First and foremost, it is critical for the GPM therapist to respond with an expression of concern. Using general principles for GPM regardless of diagnosis, clinicians are encouraged to evaluate the actual level of current risk, with the understanding that for most patients with BPD, the baseline risk for suicide is chronically elevated as compared with the general population. The generalist clinician responds with the knowledge that acute exacerbations of risk for any person can relate to comorbid mood disorders, substance use, withdrawal of support (such as recent hospital discharge), and negative interpersonal events.

The GPM therapist involves the patient as an active participant in creating a safety plan at the beginning of treatment rather than as a crisis is unfolding. The patient is asked to develop and use alternative ways to feel better, paying attention to managing interpersonal hypersensitivity practically. The patient is encouraged to recruit additional social support that will be available when he or she is feeling distressed or alone, and also, similarly, the patient is discouraged from engaging in relationships that are likely to be rejecting at points of crisis. In addition to promoting a sense of agency and autonomy, this collaborative approach provides another means of assessing risk—a patient who is readily engaged and can easily create a safety plan is at lower risk than one who cannot. Notably, GPM clinicians avoid asking the patient to passively agree to a "safety contract" that has been established by the provider alone.

The suicidal or self-injurious patient can understandably create high anxiety in the clinician. GPM strongly encourages clinicians to seek support, supervision, and consultation from colleagues, according to the adage that one should "never worry alone." It is also important for the GPM therapist to be open and clear about his or her limits. No therapist is omniscient, omnipresent, or omnipotent, and it is therefore unreasonable for a patient's safety to depend on the therapist's availability. (See Chapter 20, "Assessing and Managing Suicide Risk," in this volume for a further discussion.)

Conservative Psychopharmacology

Medications are considered to be adjunctive to psychosocial interventions for BPD. Medications can be helpful when they are targeted to specific symptoms (e.g., anger, paranoia) or comorbidity (e.g., major depressive episode), but no medication is uniformly or consistently helpful, nor has any medication been approved by the U.S. Food and Drug Administration for the treatment of BPD (American Psychiatric Association 2001; Ingenhoven 2015). The multiplication of different medications (i.e., polypharmacy) can increase the risk for side effects and promote dependency, and may send the message that the patient can passively expect to improve by taking medications, as opposed to mobilizing to build a life. Polypharmacy can have significant risks including obesity (from certain mood stabilizers, atypical antipsychotics, and antidepressant medications), sexual dysfunction (from antidepressants), and dependence (from stimulants and benzodiazepines). The recently described recommendation for "collaborative de-prescribing" for patients with BPD, or judiciously and deliberately engaging patients in tapering medications when they are not working or reducing doses when possible, is consistent with GPM's approach to medication management (Fineberg et al. 2019).

Given the lack of evidence that any agent or class of medications is more than adjunctive in the treatment of BPD, the GPM stance on prescribing promotes healthy skepticism about the use of medications in treatment (Gunderson and Choi-Kain 2018). Crawford and colleagues (2018) published a large long-term study on the effectiveness of lamotrigine in the treatment of BPD that challenged formerly held notions that lamotrigine was a reasonable drug of choice to treat a number of BPD symptoms. Their study outcomes showed significant clinical improvement in BPD symptoms in both lamotrigine and placebo conditions, suggesting that the common factors in the intervention arms—namely, diagnosis of BPD, monitoring of its symptoms, and regular predictable follow-up—could produce clinical improvement without pharmacotherapy. Lamotrigine, which carries its own rare but serious side-effect profile, did not show any superiority over placebo. Given the difficulty patients have with compliance, and the risk of life-threatening side effects such as Stevens-Johnson syndrome and hemophagocytic lymphohistiocytosis, clinicians and patients should evaluate carefully the risks and benefits of taking lamotrigine (or any psychotropic agent) as part of the treatment. This also incorporates patient accountability in making informed-consent decisions and being responsible for tracking their own response to medication to decide whether or not it is helping. (See Chapter 17, "Pharmacological Management," in this volume for more information on the adjunctive use of medications in patients with personality pathology.)

The fact that common factors led to improvements even in the placebo condition suggests that for some patients, even lower levels of care can help reduce symptomatology in the absence of other treatments. Depending on available resources, clinical severity, and responsiveness to various interventions, clinicians can consider increasing or decreasing treatment intensity to match the needs of their clients, as proposed by stepped care models.

Good Psychiatric Management and Stepped Care Models

Given their more straightforward training and practice requirements, GPM and other organized generalist approaches to BPD care could meaningfully address public health needs (Gunderson 2016) by providing an avenue to generic care that is "good enough" for most patients with BPD. However, as Gunderson notes in the GPM Handbook, the treatment is not meant to replace or compete with specialized brand-name evidence-based treatments such as DBT, MBT, or TFP that constitute the standard of care for BPD. Clinicians self-select to train in these intensive specialized approaches because of an interest and motivation to develop expertise in psychotherapeutic management. But specialists alone cannot bear the burden of treating all the patients with BPD who need treatment. Clinicians practicing DBT, MBT, or TFP adherently are not only few and far between but also restricted in the number of patients they can see, based on the frequency, length of sessions, and expected duration of treatment (Iliakis et al. 2019). A clinician working 40 hours weekly can at most see between 20 and 30 patients with BPD a year utilizing the specialist treatments as they have been studied in clinical trials.

Given this situation, a few experts in the treatment of BPD have proposed stepped care models based on different considerations. Joel Paris was the first to propose a stepped model (Paris 2013) and also has written a book dedicated to the topic (Paris 2017). His approach emphasizes brief treatment for most and an extended treatment only when patients fail to improve with a brief intervention and intermittent follow-up, or for those who relapse. This simple and pragmatic approach was tested naturalistically by Paris and his collaborators (Laporte et al. 2018). In their study, 681 patients with BPD initially evaluated were referred to either short-term treatment over 12 weeks (12 individual and 12 group therapy sessions) or extended treatment, which was offered in 6-month increments for a span of 6 months to 2 years. The majority of these patients (86%) were referred to short-term care, and the remainder of patients to extended care. In the short-term treatment, there was a 29% dropout rate, which is in the range published in other clinical trials of BPD, and of the remainder who completed the short-term course, only 12% either requested or were referred to more treatment because either they did not improve or they needed more at the discretion of the clinical team. The patients in short-term treatment showed significant decreases in self-reported measures of impulsivity, low self-esteem, depression, emotional dysregulation, impaired social adjustment, self-harm, and suicide attempts from pre- to post-treatment, but did not show statistically significant decreases in drug and alcohol use. The patients in extended treatment showed similar results, but also reported significant reduction of drug and alcohol use. In the latter group, no difference was observed between the changes in patients staying 6–12 months versus 18–24 months. While the study has limitations, these findings suggest that 1) most patients can improve with short-term or brief treatment, and 2) in the fraction of patients needing more treatment, longer treatment does not necessarily produce more change, except in outcomes related to substance use. Notably, no single evidence-based manualized model was used, but elements of a number of effective treatments were eclectically employed with a team-based approach directed by experienced and expert leadership.

Chanen, Berk, and Thompson have also proposed a model of stepped care based on clinical staging (Chanen and Thompson 2016; Chanen et al. 2016). Their stepped care model suggests the intensity of care should increase with clinical staging to allow for earlier intervention, reserving specialized and extended treatments for greater levels of clinical severity. The first step is to identify individuals at increased risk for mood disorders and BPD—that is, those with a family history of mood or personality disorder, childhood adversity, or substance abuse—before symptoms develop. For those at increased risk for mood or personality disorder, basic mental health literacy, defined as "knowledge and beliefs about mental disorders which aid their recognition, management, or prevention" (Jorm et al. 1997, p. 182), can be employed by health care staff of any discipline to increase awareness of psychiatric problems, availability of treatments, and general measures to promote mental health (e.g., sleep and avoidance of substances). Mental health literacy as a starting point could serve as good medical care for any patient, providing basic information about what psychiatric symptoms might look like and where to seek help. Next, with early mild or nonspecific symptoms, psychoeducation, problem-solving support, and general mental health counseling are indicated for risk reduction. Brief generalist care models are employed starting at a subthreshold level of symptoms and are enhanced when first episodes of BPD symptoms meeting diagnostic criteria occur, such that more intensive treatment is applied for more advanced clinical stages. Specialized treatments such as DBT are reserved for recurrent episodes of BPD symptoms meeting diagnostic criteria.

In 2016, we proposed a model of stepped care that extended Chanen, Berk, and Thompson's model (Choi-Kain et al. 2016). Like their model, our stepped care proposal starts with psychoeducation, supportive counseling, and problem solving at preclinical stages, but employs GPM as the basic approach to care at the first episode of full-criteria BPD, reserving specialist evidence-based treatments for those who do not improve or relapse with GPM (Choi-Kain et al. 2016). We also integrate a step-down, or taper, of intensive treatment resources in chronic cases when patient are unresponsive to them. Treatment of chronic cases can be focused on supportive therapy and case management, rather than intensive, demanding specialized therapies. This stepped care model integrates attention to clinical grading as well as responsiveness to treatment, balancing the need for more after less has been tried with suboptimal results with the need to de-intensify if the patient remains unresponsive to the gradation of steps of care applied. Importantly, at the most chronic stages, the door remains open to return to intensive treatment if motivation or other conditions in the patient's life change to facilitate more active use of treatment (i.e., sobriety or leaving an abusive relationship).

More recent developments have informed reconsideration of these models. Kramer et al. (2011, 2017) in Lausanne developed and studied the effectiveness of a 10-session variant of GPM, which yielded reductions in BPD symptoms, interpersonal problems, and distress. This 10-session variant of GPM serves as the gateway to any personality disorder psychotherapy treatment in the Lausanne clinic, which has specialists in a variety of empirically validated psychotherapies. In Australia, Brin Grenyer and colleagues implemented a brief stepped care approach to personality disorders, providing four weekly outpatient sessions of organized care immediately available as a step-down upon emergency department discharge, a time when the suicide rate is 200 times the global rate (Chung et al. 2017) and hazard ratios (HRs) for suicide are elevated (HR=3.0–8.9; Haglund et al. 2019). This study reported a reduction of demand on hospital services with shorter stays, fewer emergency visits, and an estimated cost savings of $2,720 per patient per year (Grenyer et al. 2018). In one clinic in this trial, it was found that at the conclusion of the intervention, less than 43% of patients needed referrals to psychiatric services, and only just under 14% needed to be stepped up to inpatient care (Huxley et al. 2019). Combining Paris's model of utilizing primarily brief treatments with a clinical staging model such as Chanen, Berk, and Thompson's approach, which advocates for early intervention, our current model of stepped care would propose brief psychoeducation and/or 10-session GPM as the entry point of treatment at the earliest possible point of intervention, when symptoms are subthreshold or reaching full criteria threshold at first episode. The key, as noted in the Grenyer et al. study, is for brief treatment to be readily available, rather than be so scarce as to generate waiting lists. Those responding to treatment could either step down to intermittent follow-up or continue for a longer course depending on motivation and availability of care.

Models such as GPM can be flexibly adapted to an infrequent schedule of monthly to yearly visits to provide psychiatric monitoring and primary care to patients with BPD who have remission of symptoms. Patients can start with 10 sessions of GPM or short-term GPM, depending on the resources available to the mental health care system adopting stepped care. This would ideally allow the majority of patients to receive standard, effective care, and only a minority might need more protracted, elaborated treatments, such as those the gold-standard manualized specialist BPD treatments provide. Regardless of the model, stepped care systems should incorporate resources to assist patients with BPD in vocational activities. Recent analysis of McMain's DBT versus GPM trial shows three types of patients: 1) rapid responders who sustain treatment gains, 2) slow responders who sustain gains, and 3) rapid responders who return to baseline postdischarge (McMain et al. 2018). The third group was distinguished by higher baseline depression, high utilization of health care, and unemployment. McMain and collaborators suggest this third group may need modifications to their treatment targeting these features. Specifically, they argue that occupational functioning may be a productive treatment focus to improve outcomes for this group. At any level of stepped care, GPM's emphasis on building a life outside treatment should be prioritized.

With respect to clinical staging, there is considerable consensus that "severity" is the most important aspect of personality pathology, predicting both current and prospective functioning and outcomes. Both the AMPD and the ICD-11 personality disorder classification have severity as the core component for this reason. One potential use of the severity rating of these classification systems would therefore be to quantify and assess outcomes in level of functioning via assessing severity using the Level of Personality Functioning Scale to help to determine the appropriate level of care, including step-ups and step-downs. Future research is needed to determine the effectiveness of incorporating these severity indexes more formally in the stepped care system, but these tools are already available to clinicians if they should want to use them. (See Chapter 3, "Articulating a Core Dimension of Personality Pathology," in this volume for a detailed discussion of the development and use of the DSM-5 Level of Personality Functioning Scale.)

Stepped care models encourage judicious allocation of resource-intensive treatments, in order to provide more accessible treatment. A meta-analysis of reducing costs for treating BPD showed that for every patient with BPD treated with an evidence-based treatment, there was an associated cost savings of around $2,988 per year (Meuldijk et al. 2017). This suggests that treating BPD more broadly and effectively would yield substantial cost savings broadly and would mitigate the unreasonably long wait-lists for more intensive psychotherapeutic follow-up. Allocating more care with less intensity and a shorter duration, and earlier in a patient's clinical trajectory, may lead to the best outcomes for patients, the clinicians who treat them, and the health care system at large. Further research is needed to test these claims. In the meantime, this preliminary evidence holds promise that we can do less for more and still achieve good enough outcomes.

Future Directions

The GPM approach can be adapted to diverse settings, for a wide array of practitioners, and in combination with different treatments. Guidelines have been developed for practitioners in inpatient units (Gunderson and Palmer 2019), emergency departments (Hong 2019), consultation-liaison services (Jenkins et al. 2019), outpatient practices (Price 2019), and college mental health services (Hersh and Finch 2019) that need a foundational understanding of how to treat patients with BPD in their respective settings. Different providers, such as social workers (Drozek 2019), primary care providers (Adler et al. 2019), psychopharmacologists (Mercer and Links 2019), and psychotherapy supervisors (Brickell and Gunderson 2019), can find specific guidance on how to implement GPM. There are also directives about how to integrate GPM with specialized treatments such as DBT (Mercer et al. 2019), MBT (Unruh et al. 2019), and TFP (Hersh 2019), either in sequence or simultaneously.

Two major adaptations of GPM have been developed. *Good Psychiatric Management and Dialectical Behavior Therapy: Integration and Stepped Care* outlines a pragmatic approach to integrating the basic principles of GPM with DBT skills training. It provides a practical guide in navigating the stepped care model, and it suggests ways in which components of each modality might be combined or sequenced in different clinical scenarios (e.g., a therapist deciding between GPM and DBT for a particular patient, a GPM therapist whose patient is also in a DBT skills group, a DBT therapist who would like to utilize GPM strategies in his or her work). The upcoming book can help clinicians deliberating between different levels of care within the stepped care models make well-informed decisions. Second, GPM for adolescents (GPM-A) is a new adaptation of GPM developed by BPD experts and child/adolescent psychiatrists to be specifically tailored for an emerging adult population. With a greater emphasis on family involvement and developmental concerns such as school, peer relationships, and autonomy, GPM-A is a promising generalist approach that may promote early diagnosis and intervention and help adolescents with BPD meet developmental milestones. Because of its focus on emerging personality disorder, and the general impairments in self-appraisal, self-regulation, and interpersonal functioning common to both personality disorders and adolescence, GPM-A incorporates more consideration of the more modern AMPD. (See Chapter 4, "The Alternative DSM-5 Model for Personality Disorders," in this volume for a detailed discussion of this new model.) *Handbook of Good Psychiatric Management for Borderline Personality Disorder in Adolescence* is expected to be published in 2021.

Conclusion

Specialized brand-name psychotherapies for BPD, such as DBT, MBT, and TFP, have revolutionized the field of BPD therapeutics by creating packages of care that survived the empirical test of randomized controlled trials. These trials showed the superiority of these specialist intensive therapies over relatively unstructured and uninformed "treatment as usual" in reducing the disorder's most fatal, destructive, and disabling features. From these packages of brand-name psychotherapeutics, we have been able to distill the essential ingredients of structured, informed general BPD management. It is these essential core ingredients that are embodied in generalist treatments we have reviewed here, including GPM primarily, but also other empirically supported models such as SCM and GCC, as well as GIT-PD in the Netherlands, which still requires formal empirical testing. We propose that these core ingredients, embodied in generalist treatments as a whole, can constitute a new generic market of effective and critical BPD care that can become more widely available and standard in every psychiatric setting, much as generic medications have expanded viability of broad care for other common psychiatric disorders not just nationally, but globally, including locales with more strained economic and health care resources. We provided an overview of GPM as a manualized but flexible clinical management approach to patients with BPD, based on the vast contributions and boiled-down pragmatic wisdom of the late John Gunderson, M.D. His hope and advocacy for ensuring that psychiatry better understands these patients and that patients receive more effective care live on in GPM. We have faith that GPM will be good enough for most, and those who need more or less can follow various stepped care pathways that can involve step-ups, or intensification of care to the brand-name psychotherapies where they are available, or a step-down, or taper-down, of care to limited or supportive approaches. Now we are fortunate to have many treatments that work, and we can organize them more effectively in pragmatic health care provision rather than in expert rarified care for the few that can access it.

References

Aalders H, Hengstmengel M: GIT-PD in Practice (in Dutch). Amsterdam, Hogrefe, 2019

Adler KA, Finch EF, Rodriguez-Villa AM, Choi-Kain LW: Primary care providers, in Applications of Good Psychiatric Management for Borderline Personality Disorder: A Practical Guide. Edited by Choi-Kain LW, Gunderson JG. Washington, DC, American Psychiatric Association Publishing, 2019, pp 169–186

American Psychiatric Association: Practice guideline for the treatment of patients with borderline personality disorder. Am J Psychiatry 158 (suppl 10):1–52, 2001

Bateman A, Fonagy P: Effectiveness of partial hospitalization in the treatment of borderline personality disorder: a randomized controlled trial. Am J Psychiatry 156:1563–1569, 1999

Bateman A, Fonagy P: Randomized controlled trial of outpatient mentalization-based treatment versus structured clinical management for borderline personality disorder. Am J Psychiatry 166:1355–1364, 2009

Bateman A, Fonagy P: Impact of clinical severity on outcomes of mentalisation-based treatment for borderline personality disorder. Br J Psychiatry 203:221–227, 2013

Bateman AW, Krawitz R: Borderline Personality Disorder: An Evidence-Based Guide for Generalist Mental Health Professionals. Oxford, UK, Oxford University Press, 2013

Brickell C, Gunderson JG: Psychotherapy supervisors, in Applications of Good Psychiatric Management for Borderline Personality Disorder: A Practical Guide. Edited by Choi-Kain LW, Gunderson JG. Washington, DC, American Psychiatric Association Publishing, 2019, pp 215–229

Caruana E, Cotton SM, Farhall J, et al: A comparison of vocational engagement among young people with psychosis, depression and borderline personality pathology. Community Ment Health J 54:831–841, 2018

Chanen AM, Thompson K: Borderline personality and mood disorders: risk factors, precursors, and early signs in childhood and youth, in Borderline Personality and Mood Disorders. Edited by Choi-Kain LW, Gunderson JG. New York, Springer, 2016, pp 155–174

Chanen AM, Jackson HJ, McCutcheon LK, et al: Early intervention for adolescents with borderline personality disorder using cognitive analytic therapy: randomized controlled trial. Br J Psychiatry 193:397–408, 2008

Chanen AM, Berk M, Thompson K: Integrating early intervention for borderline personality disorder and mood disorders. Harv Rev Psychiatry 24:330–341, 2016

Choi-Kain LW, Albert EB, Gunderson JG: Evidence-based treatments for borderline personality disorder: implementation, integration, and stepped care. Harv Rev Psychiatry 24:342–356, 2016

Choi-Kain LW, Finch EF, Masland SR, et al: What works in the treatment of borderline personality disorder. Curr Behav Neurosci Rep 4:21–30, 2017a

Choi-Kain LW, Glasserman EI, Finch EF: Borderline personality disorder: treatment resistance reconsidered. Psychiatric Times 34(11), Nov 27, 2017b

Chung DT, Ryan CJ, Hadzi-Pavlovic D, et al: Suicide rates after discharge from psychiatric facilities: a systematic review and meta-analysis. JAMA Psychiatry 74:694–702, 2017

Clarkin JF, Levy KN, Lenzenweger MF, et al: Evaluating three treatments for borderline personality disorder: a multiwave study. Am J Psychiatry 164:922–928, 2007

Colli A, Tanzilli A, Dimaggio G, et al: Patient personality and therapist response: an empirical investigation. Am J Psychiatry 171:102–108, 2014

Comtois KA, Fruhbauerova M: A dialectical tension in health services. Psychiatr Serv 70:749, 2019

Crawford MJ, Sanatinia R, Barrett B, et al: The clinical effectiveness and cost-effectiveness of lamotrigine in borderline personality disorder: a randomized placebo-controlled trial. Am J Psychiatry 175:756–764, 2018

Cristea IA, Gentili C, Cotet CD, et al: Efficacy of psychotherapies for borderline personality disorder: a systematic review and meta-analysis. JAMA Psychiatry 74:319–328, 2017

Drozek RP: Social workers, in Applications of Good Psychiatric Management for Borderline Personality Disorder: A Practical Guide. Edited by Choi-Kain LW, Gunderson JG. Washington, DC, American Psychiatric Association Publishing, 2019, pp 141–167

Fineberg SK, Gupta S, Leavitt J: Collaborative deprescribing in borderline personality disorder: a narrative review. Harv Rev Psychiatry 27:75–86, 2019

Fonagy P, Allison E: The role of mentalizing and epistemic trust in the therapeutic relationship. Psychotherapy (Chic) 51:372–380, 2014

Giesen-Bloo J, van Dyck R, Spinhoven P, et al: Outpatient psychotherapy for borderline personality disorder: randomized trial of schema-focused therapy vs transference-focused psychotherapy. Arch Gen Psychiatry 63:649–658, 2006

Greene JA: What's in a name? Generics and the persistence of the pharmaceutical brand in American medicine. J Hist Med Allied Sci 66:468–506, 2011

Greene JA, Kesselheim AS: Why do the same drugs look different? Pills, trade dress, and public health. New Engl J Med 365:83–89, 2011

Grenyer BFS, Lewis KL, Fanaian M, et al: Treatment of personality disorder using a whole of service stepped care approach: a cluster randomized controlled trial. PLoS One 13:e0206472, 2018

Gunderson JG: Borderline personality disorder: ontogeny of a diagnosis. Am J Psychiatry 166:530–539, 2009

Gunderson JG: The emergence of a generalist model to meet public health needs for patients with borderline personality disorder. Am J Psychiatry 173:452–458, 2016

Gunderson JG, Choi-Kain LW: Medication management for patients with borderline personality disorder. Am J Psychiatry 175:709–711, 2018

Gunderson JG, Links PS: Borderline Personality Disorder: A Clinical Guide, 2nd Edition. Arlington, VA, American Psychiatric Publishing, 2008

Gunderson JG, Links PS: Handbook of Good Psychiatric Management for Borderline Personality Disorder. Arlington, VA, American Psychiatric Publishing, 2014

Gunderson JG, Lyons-Ruth K: BPD's interpersonal hypersensitivity phenotype: a gene-environment-developmental model. J Pers Disord 22:22–41, 2008

Gunderson JG, Palmer BA: Inpatient psychiatric units, in Applications of Good Psychiatric Management for Borderline Personality Disorder: A Practical Guide. Edited by Choi-Kain LW, Gunderson JG. Washington, DC, American Psychiatric Association Publishing, 2019, pp 11–35

Gunderson JG, Fruzzetti A, Unruh B, et al: Competing theories of borderline personality disorder. J Pers Disord 32:148–167, 2018

Gutheil TG: Medicolegal pitfalls in the treatment of borderline patients. Am J Psychiatry 142:9–14, 1985

Haglund A, Lysell H, Larsson H, et al: Suicide immediately after discharge from psychiatric inpatient care: a cohort study of nearly 2.9 million discharges. J Clin Psychiatry 80:27–32, 2019

Hastrup LH, Jennum P, Ibsen R, et al: Societal costs of borderline personality disorders: a matched-controlled nationwide study of patients and spouses. Acta Psychiatr Scand 140:458–467, 2019

Hersh RG: Integration with transference-focused psychotherapy, in Applications of Good Psychiatric Management for Borderline Personality Disorder: A Practical Guide. Edited by Choi-Kain LW, Gunderson JG. Washington, DC, American Psychiatric Association Publishing, 2019, pp 327–351

Hersh RG, Finch EF: College mental health services, in Applications of Good Psychiatric Management for Borderline Personality Disorder: A Practical Guide. Edited by Choi-Kain LW, Gunderson JG. Washington, DC, American Psychiatric Association Publishing, 2019, pp 117–137

Hong V: Borderline personality disorder in the emergency department: good psychiatric management. Harv Rev Psychiatry 24:357–366, 2016

Hong V: Emergency departments, in Applications of Good Psychiatric Management for Borderline Personality Disorder: A Practical Guide. Edited by Choi-Kain LW, Gunderson JG. Washington, DC, American Psychiatric Association Publishing, 2019, pp 37–56

Hutsebaut J, Kaasenbrood A: Guideline-Informed Treatment for Personality Disorders: A Treatment Framework for Persons With a Personality Disorder (in Dutch). Utrecht, Netherlands, Kenniscentrum Persoonlijkheidsstoornissen, 2015

Huxley E, Lewis KL, Coates A, et al: Evaluation of a brief intervention within a stepped care whole of service model for personality disorder. BMC Psychiatry 19(1):341, 2019

Iliakis EA, Sonley AKI, Ilagan GS, et al: Treatment of borderline personality disorder: is supply adequate to meet public health needs? Psychiatr Serv 70:772–781, 2019

Ingenhoven T: Pharmacotherapy for borderline patients: business as usual or by default? J Clin Psychiatry 76:e522–e523, 2015

Jenkins J, Iliakis EA, Choi-Kain LW: Consultation-liaison service, in Applications of Good Psychiatric Management for Borderline Personality Disorder: A Practical Guide. Edited by Choi-Kain LW, Gunderson JG. Washington, DC, American Psychiatric Association Publishing, 2019, pp 57–83

Jorm A, Korten A, Jacomb P, et al: "Mental health literacy": a survey of the public's ability to recognize mental disorders and their beliefs about the effectiveness of treatment. Med J Aust 166:182–186, 1997

Keuroghlian AS, Palmer BA, Choi-Kain LW, et al: The effect of attending good psychiatric management (GPM) workshops on attitudes towards patients with borderline personality disorder. J Pers Disord 30:567–576, 2016

Kramer U, Berger T, Kolly S, et al: Effects of motive-oriented therapeutic relationship in early-phase treatment of borderline personality disorder: a pilot study of a randomized trial. J Nerv Ment Dis 199:244–250, 2011

Kramer U, Stulz N, Berthoud L, et al: The shorter the better? A follow-up analysis of 10-session psychiatric treatment including the motive-oriented psychotherapeutic relationship for borderline personality disorder. Psychother Res 27:362–370, 2017

Laporte L, Paris J, Bergevin T, et al: Clinical outcomes of a stepped care program for borderline personality disorder. Personal Ment Health 12:252–264, 2018

Linehan MM, Armstrong HE, Suarez A, et al: Cognitive-behavioral treatment of chronically parasuicidal borderline patients. Arch Gen Psychiatry 48:1060–1064, 1991

Masland SR, Price D, MacDonald J, et al: Enduring effects of one-day training in good psychiatric management on clinician attitudes about borderline personality disorder. J Nerv Ment Dis 206:865–869, 2018

McMain SF, Links PS, Gnam WH, et al: A randomized trial of dialectical behavior therapy versus general psychiatric management for borderline personality disorder. Am J Psychiatry 166:1365–1374, 2009

McMain SF, Guimond T, Streiner DL, et al: Dialectical behavior therapy compared with general psychiatric management for borderline personality disorder: clinical outcomes and functioning over a 2-year follow-up. Am J Psychiatry 169:650–661, 2012

McMain SF, Fitzpatrick S, Boritz T, et al: Outcome trajectories and prognostic factors for suicide and self-harm behaviors in patients with borderline personality disorder following one year of outpatient psychotherapy. J Pers Disord 32:497–512, 2018

Mercer D, Links PS: Psychopharmacologists, in Applications of Good Psychiatric Management for Borderline Personality Disorder: A Practical Guide. Edited by Choi-Kain LW, Gunderson JG. Washington, DC, American Psychiatric Association Publishing, 2019, pp 187–214

Mercer D, Links PS, Sonley AKI, et al: Integration with dialectical behavior therapy, in Applications of Good Psychiatric Management for Borderline Personality Disorder: A Practical Guide. Edited by Choi-Kain LW, Gunderson JG. Washington, DC, American Psychiatric Association Publishing, 2019, pp 281–305

Meuldijk D, McCarthy A, Bourke ME, et al: The value of psychological treatment for borderline personality disorder: systematic review and cost offset analysis of economic evaluations. PLoS One 12:e0171592, 2017

Ng FY, Bourke ME, Grenyer BF: Recovery from borderline personality disorder: a systematic review of the perspectives of consumers, clinicians, family and carers. PLoS One 11:e0160515, 2016

Ng FYY, Townsend ML, Miller CE, et al: The lived experience of recovery in borderline personality disorder: a qualitative study. Borderline Personal Disord Emot Dysregul 6:10, 2019

Oud M, Arntz A, Hermens MLM, et al: Specialized psychotherapies for adults with borderline personality disorder: a systematic review and meta-analysis. Aust NZ J Psychiatry 52:949–961, 2018

Paris J: Stepped care: an alternative to routine extended treatment for patients with borderline personality disorder. Psychiatr Serv 64:1035–1037, 2013

Paris J: Stepped Care for Borderline Personality Disorder: Making Treatment Brief, Effective, and Accessible. Cambridge, MA, Academic Press, 2017

Paris J, Zweig-Frank H: A 27-year follow-up of patients with borderline personality disorder. Compr Psychiatry 42:482–487, 2001

Price D: Generalist adult outpatient psychiatry practice, in Applications of Good Psychiatric Management for Borderline Personality Disorder: A Practical Guide. Edited by Choi-Kain LW, Gunderson JG. Washington, DC, American Psychiatric Association Publishing, 2019, pp 85–115

Reich J, Schatzberg A: An empirical data comparison of regulatory agency and malpractice legal problems for psychiatrists. Ann Clin Psychiatry 26:91–96, 2014

Ridolfi ME, Rossi R, Occhialini G, Gunderson JG: A clinical trial of a psychoeducation group intervention for patients with borderline personality disorder. J Clin Psychiatry 81:19m12753, 2019

Ryle A, Leighton T, Pollock P: Cognitive Analytic Therapy and Borderline Personality Disorder: The Model and the Method. Hoboken, NJ, Wiley, 1997

Soeteman DI, Verheul R, Busschbach JJ: The burden of disease in personality disorders: diagnosis-specific quality of life. J Pers Disord 22:259–268, 2008

Stoffers JM, Völlm BA, Rücker G, et al: Psychological therapies for people with borderline personality disorder. Cochrane Database Syst Rev (8):CD005652, 2012

Trull TJ, Jahng S, Tomko RL, et al: Revised NESARC personality disorder diagnoses: gender, prevalence, and comorbidity with substance dependence disorders. J Pers Disord 24:412–426, 2010

Unruh BT, Sonley AKI, Choi-Kain LW: Integration with mentalization-based treatment, in Applications of Good Psychiatric Management for Borderline Personality Disorder: A Practical Guide. Edited by Choi-Kain LW, Gunderson JG. Washington, DC, American Psychiatric Association Publishing, 2019, pp 307–326

Wnuk S, McMain S, Links PS, et al: Factors related to dropout from treatment in two outpatients treatments for borderline personality disorder. J Pers Disord 27:716–726, 2013

Zanarini MC, Frankenburg FR: A preliminary, randomized trial of psychoeducation for women with borderline personality disorder. J Pers Disord 22:284–290, 2008

Zanarini MC, Frankenburg FR, Reich DB, et al: The 10-year course of psychosocial functioning among patients with borderline personality disorder and axis II comparison subjects. Acta Psychiatr Scand 122:103–109, 2010

Zanarini MC, Frankenburg FR, Reich DB, et al: Attainment and stability of sustained symptomatic remission and recovery among patients with borderline personality disorder and axis II comparison subjects: a 16-year prospective follow-up study. Am J Psychiatry 169:476–483, 2012

Zanarini MC, Conkey LC, Temes CM, et al: Randomized controlled trial of web-based psychoeducation for women with borderline personality disorder. J Clin Psychiatry 79:16m11153, 2018

Zimmerman M, McGonigal P, Moon SS, et al: Does diagnosing a patient with borderline personality disorder negatively impact patient satisfaction with the initial diagnostic evaluation? Ann Clin Psychiatry 30:215–219, 2016

CHAPTER 16

Group, Family, and Couples Therapies

John S. Ogrodniczuk, Ph.D.
Amanda A. Uliaszek, Ph.D.
Jay L. Lebow, Ph.D.
David Kealy, Ph.D.

Although individual therapy has long been the mainstay of treatment for personality disorders (PDs), there is a growing appreciation for the place of multiperson therapies (group, family, couples) and the need for a multimodal approach when treating patients with PD. As Magnavita (1998) noted, "The dynamic interplay between our biological and intrapersonal organization interacts with the social systems and not only adds to the shaping of our personality, but also is crucial in the pathogenesis or maintenance of self-defeating patterns of behavior" (p. 8). Interpersonal dynamics help organize, shape, and consolidate individuals' self-perceptions and self-concepts and can be observed in the dynamics within family systems and other social groups. PDs and the clinical syndromes that they engender are not contained solely within the individual but are formed by early attachments, shaped by family dynamics, and consolidated by repetitive interactions and habitual patterns of communication and interaction (Magnavita 2000). As such, PDs are expressed relationally in various interpersonal configurations, evident in marriages and romantic partnerships, families, and other groups that are part of an individual's social system (Magnavita 2000). Indeed, the Alternative DSM-5 Model for Personality Disorders (AMPD) considers severity of interpersonal dysfunction as a defining feature of PD. Therapies that address personality functioning within an interpersonal milieu—involving interaction with others—are thus worthy treatment options for patients with PD.

This chapter focuses on multiperson therapies (group, family, couples) for PDs. These therapies may take many different forms based on their theoretical and technical orientations. Because of the presence of multiple patients, multiperson therapies have certain unique features that distinguish them from other types of therapy. These unique features may facilitate or complicate the treatment of PDs. Similarly, PDs have certain features that may facilitate or complicate their treatment with different types of multiperson therapies.

Considering each of these multiperson therapies (group, family, couples) separately, we discuss the facilitating and complicating features of these therapies and of PDs. For each of the three categories of multiperson therapies, we also review various forms, which differ in format, intensity, and objectives; discuss research support; and present case examples. Given its brevity, this chapter should be considered only as an abridged introduction to the use of group, family, and couples therapies for PD.

Group Therapy

Features of Group Therapy or PDs That Facilitate or Complicate Treatment of PDs

Features of Group Therapy That Facilitate Treatment

The AMPD emphasizes impairment in self functioning (with regard to identity and self-direction) and interpersonal relatedness (in the areas of empathy and intimacy) as defining PD, along with the presence of maladaptive personality traits (American Psychiatric Association 2013). Group therapy can be an effective approach for various combinations of maladaptive traits and self and interpersonal impairments that constitute different manifestations of PD. In group therapy, difficulties in the patient's capacity for self-regulation and relatedness with others are revealed through interactions with other group members. The intensive verbal and nonverbal interchanges within the group quickly unmask a patient's maladaptive personality traits, making repetitive dysfunctional patterns apparent. The other patients may recognize and identify with similar behavior patterns, provide feedback, and offer suggestions for change. The patient can subsequently practice adaptive behavior. This process is commonly referred to as *interpersonal learning*. Other patients may learn through observation and imitation. Simply recognizing that other patients share one's difficulties (universality) and helping other patients with their problems (altruism) can be therapeutic. A sense of "we-ness" or togetherness develops, providing patients with a feeling of belonging and cohesion with a caring group of others. These various processes (cohesion, interpersonal learning, imitation, universality, and altruism) are regarded as powerful unique therapeutic factors of group treatment (Yalom and Leszcz 2005). Moreover, the efforts of group members to empathize with and understand one another's behaviors—particularly in terms of underlying mental states, emotions, and motivations—may provide the patient with an adaptive model of self-regulatory functioning associated with mentalizing and epistemic trust (Fonagy et al. 2017). Such experience in group treatment may thus expand the patient's ability to self-reflect and utilize feedback from others beyond the termination of therapy.

Group treatments have other facilitative features as well. Paralyzing negative transference toward the therapist is less likely to occur in group therapy than in individual therapy because the situation is less intimate and because strong affects such as rage are diluted and expressed toward multiple targets. Similarly, feedback from the therapist in the individual therapy situation may be dismissed by the patient as biased, but this reaction is much less likely to occur in response to feedback from several peers in a therapy group. In addition, because of the variety of affects expressed by different patients, integration of positive and negative affects is facilitated.

Features of Group Therapy That Complicate Treatment

Group features may also produce complications in treatment of PDs. Some patients with PD resent sharing the therapist and feel neglected and deprived. In the group situation, regressive behaviors, such as emotional outbursts, aggressive actions, or suicidal threats, are more difficult to manage and contain than in individual therapy. Groups are prone to scapegoating; patients with PD provide many provocations. There are a number of concerns in the group situation, relative to individual therapy, that many patients with PD find troublesome, including loss of control, individuality, understanding, privacy, and safety. The therapist is subject to such concerns as well.

Features of PDs That Facilitate Group Therapy

The predominant feature of patients with PD that facilitates group treatment is their strong tendency to openly demonstrate interpersonal psychopathology through behavior in the group. Compared with patients without PD, patients with PD are more likely to demonstrate rather than describe their interpersonal problems. Although these problems are also demonstrated in individual therapy, the stimuli from multiple patients precipitate pathological interpersonal behavior more intensely and quickly in group therapy, allowing for the therapist to recognize it more clearly and address it immediately. A second facilitative feature of patients with some forms of PD (e.g., those with dependent or histrionic traits) is that they are "other seeking" and particularly oriented to valuing connections within the group.

Features of PDs That Complicate Group Therapy

Many of the behaviors that are characteristic of patients with PD can complicate group treatment. These behaviors can be offensive to other members of the group, thereby weakening cohesion and distracting members from working. Usually, such patients challenge the guidelines and norms that have been established in the group. Examples of antitherapeutic behaviors include stoic silence or, conversely, excessive disclosure; scapegoating; extragroup socializing; disregard for boundaries; and absenteeism.

When a patient's antitherapeutic behaviors persist in the group, the behaviors may be conceptualized as roles. The persons occupying the roles are commonly labeled as "difficult" patients in the group therapy literature (Bernard 1994). Patients who demonstrate these challenging behaviors are often those with PD. Examples of difficult roles and the DSM-5 PDs (American Psychiatric Association 2013) often associated with them are the silent or withdrawn role (schizoid, schizotypal, paranoid, avoidant); the monopolizing role (histrionic, borderline, narcissistic); the boring role (narcissistic, obsessive-compulsive); the therapist's helper role (histrionic, dependent); the challenger role (antisocial, borderline, obsessive-compulsive); and the help-rejecting complainer role (borderline, narcissistic, histrionic). Although these roles are occupied by individual persons, they often represent something shared by others in the group. The person occupying the role unwittingly serves a defensive function for the entire group, with the other members disavowing ownership of uncomfortable thoughts and feelings and projecting them onto particular members. In this way, the behavior of those fulfilling certain roles represents a wish or conflict that is shared by all members of the group. These roles can interfere with the work of the group by preventing the occupier of the role and the other group members who project onto that role from experiencing certain aspects of themselves. Therefore, when addressing "difficult" behavior represented by a particular patient role, the therapist must discern what aspect of the behavior is serving a defensive function for the group and what is an authentic reflection of the person's particular personality pathology. This task can be very difficult considering the complex and volatile nature of some PDs, such as borderline PD (Tuttman 1990). For that reason, a combination of group therapy and individual therapy is often recommended. Moreover, the membership composition of therapy groups, in terms of the mixture of different patients' personality tendencies, may need to be carefully considered in selecting patients with PD for a particular therapy group (Kealy et al. 2016).

Different Forms of Group Therapy

Group therapies differ in structure (format), intensity, and objectives. Four forms can be distinguished: short-term outpatient group therapy, long-term outpatient group therapy, day treatment, and inpatient or residential treatment.

Short-term outpatient group therapy often involves a single session per week for 20 or fewer weeks. Certain focal symptoms (e.g., depression) or behaviors (e.g., impaired affect expression or social skills) are targeted for change. These groups usually are not intensive in nature; they do not attempt to change the basic personality traits and personality structure that characterize PDs. An example of this type of group therapy is Systems Training for Emotional Predictability and Problem Solving (STEPPS), which was designed as an adjunctive treatment program for patients with borderline PD (Blum et al. 2008). Participants attend 2-hour weekly group seminars organized around learning specific emotional, cognitive, and behavioral self-management skills. STEPPS also involves a psychoeducation group for key members of the patients' support networks.

Long-term outpatient group therapy consists of one or two sessions per week for at least 1–2 years. It focuses on the interpersonal world of the patient, including the patient's sense of self and relatedness with others within a social context. Long-term group therapy is intensive in nature, involving exploration, confrontation, and interpretation of the patient's core conflicts, self-regulatory and defensive mechanisms, and maladaptive interpersonal patterns. In this way the core aspects of PD—impaired self and interpersonal functioning and maladaptive traits—are targeted within a social milieu that provides both support for the patient and exposition of dysfunctional patterns. This group approach assumes that over time the group comes to represent a social microcosm in which the interpersonal difficulties of the patients become vividly illustrated by the interpersonal behavior of the patients in the group. Examples of long-term group psychotherapy used with patients who have PDs are those of Jørgensen and colleagues (2014) and Lorentzen and colleagues (2015).

Day treatment is a form of partial hospitalization. It is designed for patients who do not require full-time hospitalization and who are unlikely to benefit a great deal from outpatient group therapy. Day treatment patients have often had an unsuccessful course of outpatient group therapy. Patients typically participate in a variety of therapy groups for several hours each day for 3–5 days per week. The therapy groups are often approached from different technical orientations. For example, behavioral and cognitive interventions can be used in structured, skills-oriented groups, whereas dynamic interventions can be used in unstructured, insight-oriented groups. Family and couples interventions may also be employed. This intensive, integrative form of treatment thus offers multiple potential mechanisms through which patients with PD can obtain symptom relief, modify dysfunctional personality traits, and improve social functioning.

Several other features contribute to making day treatment a powerful intervention. The first is the intensity of the group experience: patients participate in a number of different groups each day. Second, the groups vary in size, structure, objectives, and processes. This variety provides a comprehensive approach. Third, the different groups are integrated and synergistic. Patients are encouraged to think about the entire system. Fourth, patients benefit from working with multiple staff members and a large number of other patients. Fifth, day treatment capitalizes on the traditional characteristics of a therapeutic community (democratization, permissiveness, communalism, reality confrontation). These features strengthen cohesion, which helps patients endure difficult periods of treatment. The structure of day treatment programs encourages patients to be responsible, engenders mutual respect between patients and staff, and facilitates patients' participation in the treatment of their peers. Well-known approaches to day treatment programs are mentalization-based therapy (MBT), described by Bateman and Fonagy (2016), and time-limited day treatment, described by Piper et al. (1996).

As in day treatment, *hospital inpatient wards and residential treatment centers* commonly provide a variety of group treatment activities. Inpatient or residential treatment groups include admission groups, community groups, patient governance groups, insight groups, occupational therapy groups, support groups, and discharge groups. Although group sessions are a highly visible set of activities in acute treatment settings, they tend to be regarded as a minor part of the treatment regimen. Instead, psychotropic medications and problem solving regarding the acute crisis are viewed as the dominant interventions. An example of group-based inpatient treatment is described by Chiesa et al. (2003).

In North America, the lengths of stays in acute hospital settings have been decreasing significantly in response to escalating costs. Today, length of stay in such settings has come to represent short-term crisis management. Similarly, the cost of long-term care (i.e., lasting from several months to a year) in retreat settings that in the past provided powerful milieu therapies has become prohibitive, with many centers having closed down or greatly scaled back in size. Other centers have made accommodations to the changing health care environment but have preserved intensive hospital interdisciplinary treatment, carried out for an average length of stay of about 6 weeks (e.g., the Menninger Clinic). Conversely, in many European countries, most notably Germany, group-based, psychotherapeutically oriented, long-term inpatient treatment is common and supported by the national health care system.

Research Support for Group Therapy for PDs

Research on group therapy for PDs has been growing in recent years. However, because group therapy is often regarded as an adjunct to individual therapy for patients with PDs or as a component of comprehensive, multimodal treatment programs, relatively few studies have examined the effectiveness of group therapy as a stand-alone intervention for PDs. One example of such a study is that of Popolo and colleagues (2019), who compared metacognitive interpersonal group therapy (16 sessions) with treatment as usual (weekly individual consultations with a clinical psychologist) for 20 patients with mixed PDs. Patients in the metacognitive interpersonal group had symptomatic and functional improvements consistent with large effect sizes, along with similarly large effects for increased capacity to understand mental states and regulate social interactions using mentalistic knowledge. In a different type of study, Lorentzen and colleagues (2015) compared short- and long-term group analytic therapy for 167 patients, many of whom had a PD. Examining PD as a moderator of treatment outcome, the authors reported that patients with PD improved significantly more regarding all outcome variables in long-term group therapy (80 weekly sessions) than in short-term group therapy (20 weekly sessions). In another study of long-term treatment, Jørgensen and colleagues (2014) compared 2 years of stand-alone supportive group therapy (biweekly sessions) with combined individual and group mentalization-based treatment (twice-weekly sessions) for 58 patients with borderline PD. Reporting on treatment outcome 1.5 years after treatment completion, the authors noted that patients in both groups showed highly significant symptomatic and diagnostic remission during treatment, that were sustained over the follow-up period. There were no statistically significant differences between the two groups, though close to half (48%) of the patients who received 2 years of combined mentalization-based treatment met criteria for functional remission at 1.5-year follow-up, compared with less than a fifth (19%) of the patients who received supportive group therapy only.

More common are studies of treatment packages that include group therapy as one component. One of the more recognizable of such treatments is dialectical behavior therapy (DBT; Linehan 1993), which is a multimodal treatment for borderline PD. DBT uses a skills-training group (2.5 hours per week for the usual 1 year of treatment) that complements twice-weekly individual therapy and telephone coaching to address emotion regulation, distress tolerance, and interpersonal behavior. Several research studies support DBT as an effective treatment for the reduction of suicidal and self-injurious behaviors (Chapman 2006; McMain et al. 2012). It is important to note that these studies have examined a complete multimodal delivery of DBT; the effectiveness of any one singular component of DBT is unclear, though one study found that group skills training had benefits comparable to those of standard DBT (Linehan et al. 2015). Furthermore, DBT has not been established as superior to other structured treatments for borderline PD (Levy et al. 2018; McMain et al. 2012).

STEPPS was developed to supplement ongoing care for borderline PD with a 20-week course of cognitive-behavioral therapy and psychoeducation (Blum et al. 2008). STEPPS involves psychoeducation for the patient's family members and other health care providers so that the patient's support network can remain appropriately engaged and responsive. Patients also attend 2-hour seminars each week about cognitive-behavioral therapy and self-management skills. STEPPS is intended as an adjunct to the patient's regular treatment. Two randomized trials have shown that STEPPS plus treatment as usual is more effective than treatment as usual alone, leading to improvements in borderline PD symptoms, depressive symptoms, impulsiveness, and overall functioning

(Blum et al. 2008; Bos et al. 2011). The benefit of adding STEPPS to standard care is thus encouraging, given its relatively brief duration and its effect on affective symptoms, an area in which DBT has less impact.

Bateman and Fonagy (1999) developed MBT as a psychoanalytically oriented day treatment program that consists of a combination of group and individual therapies for 5 days per week for a maximum of 18 months. In a randomized controlled trial, they compared this program with a standard-care control condition, which consisted of infrequent meetings with a psychiatrist but no formal therapy, for a sample of 44 patients with borderline PD. Day treatment patients showed significant improvements that exceeded the minimal change for standard care on a variety of outcome variables, including suicide attempts and acts of self-mutilation and self-reports of depression, anxiety, general symptoms, interpersonal functioning, and social adjustment. Subsequent to discharge from day treatment, patients were provided with 18 months of psychoanalytically oriented outpatient group therapy. Five years following the completion of the outpatient group therapy, patients who had received day treatment and outpatient group therapy continued to have superior performance on a number of outcome indicators (Bateman and Fonagy 2008). The long time frame for the follow-up period in this study is unparalleled in contemporary psychotherapy research, and the impressive findings regarding the maintenance of gains (and continued improvement, in many ways) demonstrated by treated patients provide compelling evidence for the lasting effects of MBT for borderline PD, which have also been observed in a randomized trial of outpatient MBT (Bateman and Fonagy 2009).

Other randomized trials that have examined group therapy as an adjunct to individual therapy include those of Farrell and colleagues (2009) and Gratz and colleagues (2014). In Farrell and colleagues' study, schema-focused group therapy (30 weekly sessions), focused on emotional awareness training, psychoeducation, distress management training, and schema change, was investigated as an adjunct to individual supportive therapy (i.e., treatment as usual) for patients with borderline PD (N=32). The authors reported superior results for those patients who received the adjunctive schema group therapy relative to those in the treatment-as-usual condition. Gratz and colleagues (2014) more recently investigated emotion regulation group therapy as an adjunct to individual therapy for deliberate self-harm among 61 female patients with borderline PD. Findings from their study revealed significantly greater improvements in deliberate self-harm and other self-destructive behaviors, emotion dysregulation, borderline PD symptoms, depression and stress symptoms, and quality of life for patients who received emotion regulation group therapy relative to those patients in the wait-list control group.

Findings from a number of carefully conducted naturalistic outcome studies that focused on the group treatment of PDs also have been published. These investigations, which tend to be pre-post single-condition studies or studies with nonrandom assignment to conditions, involved group schema therapy (Fassbinder et al. 2016; Nenadic et al. 2017), mentalization-based group therapy (Bo et al. 2019; Edel et al. 2017), and acceptance and commitment group therapy (Chakhssi et al. 2015). In general, the findings from these naturalistic studies are consistent with those of randomized clinical trials in providing evidence of favorable outcomes for patients with PD, in particular those with borderline PD (McLaughlin et al. 2019).

Case Example 1

Debra, a 40-year-old associate professor at a prominent university, was diagnosed with narcissistic PD. While Debra was receiving long-term individual psychodynamic therapy, her therapist referred her to a long-term psychodynamic group because her therapist felt that a group experience could help with her entrenched interpersonal problems. Debra had sought psychological help for feelings of extreme loneliness, something she has felt for as long as she can remember, and for multiple physical complaints. Debra seemed unable or unwilling to recognize or accept her own contributions to her problems, and instead would blame others and show contempt and envy toward them. She considered her peers to be immature and inferior to her, but deep down inside, she felt the opposite.

Even though the group therapist managed to facilitate affective involvement of the group members and a strong sense of cohesion within the group, Debra remained aloof for a long time and missed a lot of sessions. She developed an erotic transference toward the group therapist—an older man who was a well-known figure in the medical community—but felt despised by him, as well as by the other group members. She was not ready to participate in the group work, which would mean disclosing emotionally charged experiences and exposing her vulnerability. To her, revealing intimate details about herself to others was too threatening and would lead to being humiliated and hurt. This was interpreted many times by the group therapist, but to no avail.

During one session, Debra carelessly made a condescending remark about the other group members. In line with the work ethic of the group to be relational and respectful, one member asked Debra if she realized the meaning and impact of what she had just said. Debra was taken off guard at being confronted with her contempt for others. She apologized and admitted tearfully how hard it was for her to deal with feeling miserable and inferior to others. The group's empathic response to her display of vulnerability shocked her, and this intense emotional experience seemed influential in shaping her subsequent attitudes toward the group and its members. Debra began to respond more respectfully to the other group members' emotional experiences. She started to attend the group regularly and slowly ventured into expressing and sharing her problems.

Family Therapy

Features of Family Therapy or PDs That Facilitate or Complicate Treatment of PDs

Features of Family Therapy That Facilitate Treatment

The unique features of family therapy make it well suited for the treatment of people with PDs. As described in DSM-5, a primary criterion for the diagnosis of a PD is the existence of considerable interpersonal dysfunction. Because significant interpersonal problems are found across PDs, treatments that target the entire family system may be necessary to achieve a full amelioration of PD symptoms. First, research shows that individual treatment rarely has a positive impact on unsatisfying family relationships (Gurman and Fraenkel 2002). Second, first-degree relatives of those with a PD are at increased risk of having their own psychopathology symptoms considering that they have shared genetic, personality, environmental, and biological vulnerabilities with the client (e.g., White et al. 2003). Family therapy can help family members cope and manage in the face of PD symptoms and promote relationship stability that is likely to be helpful for all members of the system. Other forms of therapy do not provide such direct help to family members.

An important component of family therapy is the assumption that families are systems in which individuals reciprocally influence one another (Lebow 2005). Recent advances in theory and research stress that the arcs of causal influence are not entirely equal in the circular pathways they follow, which leads to and maintains ongoing difficulties. In modern systems theory there is a place for acknowledging the power of individual behavior and individual psychopathology. From this viewpoint, family systems that include an individual with a PD tend to be dominated by that individual's problematic behavior in the family context; yet reciprocal patterns readily become established. For example, frequent rage episodes by someone with borderline PD might cause family members to walk on eggshells and give into demands, thus reinforcing the displays of emotion dysregulation. Family therapy is uniquely able to target this pattern by focusing not only on emotion regulation strategies for the person with the PD, but also on behavioral reinforcement and punishment strategies for the family members.

Finally, the stable holding environment provided by family members can mitigate some PD symptoms. Certain PDs are associated with high interpersonal sensitivity (e.g., borderline PD, avoidant PD). The family system can be a validating environment that reduces pain and distress. Family therapy can instruct family members in optimal ways of support and validation. The success of the family unit as a place of safety and support often ameliorates the impact of PD, whereas difficulty in relational systems promotes greater symptoms and problems. A mindful, supportive holding environment may be an essential ingredient to treatment success (Critchfield and Benjamin 2006).

Features of Family Therapy That Complicate Treatment

Although family therapy may be an appropriate setting to target the interpersonal dysfunction found in those with PDs, there are features of family therapy that may introduce problems when treating someone with a PD. First, family therapy may be contraindicated for certain people. This might include a person who is unable to speak in the presence of family members because of fear or anxiety. For example, a person with avoidant PD may feel overwhelming embarrassment and fears of criticism when discussing personal issues in front of family members, as per the diagnostic criteria for the disorder. In other cases, family members may be too afraid to participate in family therapy. Family members of someone with antisocial PD may fear retribution if they are open about feelings and behaviors in the home. Conjoint treatments with people with PDs are always works in progress—the perfect setting for the adage "first do no harm." Some people with PDs cannot manage the complex feelings that evolve in family settings, especially early in treatment. Therapists must always have at the ready an action plan for when sessions lose constructive value.

Second, families may seek treatment when the person with a PD does not want treatment (Friedlander et al. 2006). In this situation, family therapy may be overwhelmed by resistance and uncontrolled emotionality. When this is the case, considerable work must be done to enlist the cooperation and involvement of the person with the PD. If the person refuses to participate or if meetings within the context of family become the source of frequent dysregulation, one might recommend individual therapy for the patient and a psychoeducation group for the family.

Third, alliances in family therapy involving someone with a PD are likely to be complex; that is, different family members are likely to have different degrees of alliance with the therapist. This may cause split alliances whereby some family members have a strong alliance and some have a poor one. A split alliance is related to poor outcome (Friedlander et al. 2006); therefore, the strength of the alliance should be a target early in treatment, with an eye toward maintaining a positive alliance with all family members. (See Chapter 11, "Therapeutic Alliance," in this volume for a detailed discussion of forming and maintaining a therapeutic alliance with patients who have PDs.)

Fourth, although this chapter highlights the importance of interventions outside of individual psychotherapy, we consider a successful treatment plan to be one that combines family therapy with individual treatment. The nature of PDs makes them too pervasive a problem to be treated with a single treatment modality. Research has shown that for people with complex PD symptoms, treatments combining such diverse modalities as individual, family, couples, and group therapy are the most efficacious (e.g., Fruzzetti et al. 2007). Individual work promotes change in behavior, cognitions, and affect that may be largely inaccessible in family therapy. Without seeing immediate positive changes, families may lose their motivation to provide the support and nurturance that are essential to family therapy.

Finally, it is important to reiterate that first-degree relatives of individuals with PD are at increased risk of having their own psychopathology symptoms, considering that they have shared genetic, personality, environmental, and biological vulnerabilities with the client (e.g., White et al. 2003). Although the person with the PD might be the primary focus of the treatment plan, it is likely that other family members with their own complicated histories and current psychopathological symptoms could complicate the administration of family therapy.

Features of PDs That Facilitate Family Therapy

Many experiencing PDs have significant interpersonal problems within the family system and need help rectifying these issues. In addition, the family may be desperate for improved feelings of connectedness among members. The concurrent issues of high levels of distress and low levels of connectedness hopefully result in high levels of motivation among family members. The individual with the PD is likely motivated by the desire for closer and more stable relationships and/or by the necessity of cohabitation or financial support provided by family members.

Families that include a member with a PD often display interpersonal patterns and dynamics that are particularly well-treated by family therapy. One example of such a pattern involves expressed emotion, the extent to which a family member expresses critical, hostile, or emotionally overinvolved attitudes and behavior toward the family member with the disorder (Vaughn and Leff 1976). Expressed emotion is a strong predictor of poor outcome in a range of clinical disorders, including schizophrenia and bipolar disorder (e.g., Wearden et al. 2000). However, expressed emotion displays a unique pattern in families in which a family member has borderline PD. Some research suggests that emotional overinvolvement actually predicts positive outcomes, while the other aspects of expressed emotion (i.e., criticism, hostility) are unrelated to outcome (Hooley and Hoffman 1999). Hooley and Gotlib (2000) hypothesize that people with borderline PD are seemingly unaffected by high levels of hostility and criticism and respond well to emotional overinvolvement because they have a higher tolerance for affective stimulation within the family system and actually interpret it as a sign of care and nurturance. This view is based on data that show that people with borderline PD, when compared with control participants, exhibit less physiological arousal in response to emotional stimuli (see, e.g., Herpertz et al. 1999). Thus, those with borderline PD may be able to tolerate the stress of family therapy, without directly benefiting from having expressed emotion as a therapeutic target.

In addition to expressed emotion, family members of those with PDs often experience high levels of burden and distress regarding their caregiving roles. A systematic review of carers of those with PDs indicated that family members experience elevated objective and subjective burden, grief, and impaired empowerment (Bailey and Grenyer 2013). In addition, these family members are at greater risk for their own mental health problems, including depression and anxiety. Although this review primarily focused on borderline PD, it is likely that any family member in close contact with someone experiencing pervasive personality dysfunction will experience symptoms of burnout and may benefit from a family intervention. In fact, it is recommended that those in caregiving roles, specifically those caring for someone with borderline PD, seek out some form of support or mental health treatment (Lawn and McMahon 2015).

Features of PDs That Complicate Family Therapy

Although the interpersonal problems associated with many PDs are a prime treatment target in family therapy, there are some features of PDs that may cause complications. First, engagement may be difficult with someone with a PD; this supposition is justified by research demonstrating that empirically supported treatments for some clinical disorders tend to be less efficacious with individuals with comorbid PDs (see, e.g., Shea and Elkin 1996). Because family therapy may be more complex—involving, for example, coordinating schedules, turn-taking, and compromising on agenda items—it may be thwarted by the dysregulation evident in those with PD. In addition, it may be likely that, because of shared biology and environment, other family members display similar PD symptoms, thus compounding the difficulty in organizing and engaging in a family therapy session.

Second, PD patients and their families tend to have a high rate of therapy dropout (Strauss et al. 2006). Studies have found that early treatment dropout rates for individual treatment of PDs are as high as 38% to 57%, with the average estimate between 15% and 22% (Leichsenring and Leibing 2003). Research has found similar rates of dropout for family therapy, with rates between 15% and 55% (Boddington 1995). The combination of the presence of a PD and the complexities of family therapy make it likely that a family therapy intervention for PDs would result in a large loss of patients early in treatment.

Third, when dealing with patients who can be frustrating or challenging, a therapist can easily fall into the trap of blaming the patient or of assuming that the intended effect of the patient's behavior is to aggravate the therapist (e.g., Santisteban et al. 2003). In these cases, a therapist may become hopeless, disengaged, or hostile. These thoughts and emotions may have a negative direct effect on the therapy in terms of siding with other family members or avoidance of serious topics. Although these issues have been discussed almost exclusively in terms of borderline PD, they likely extend to all or most of the other PDs. Just as a person with borderline PD might tax the therapist with demands of immediate relief and late-night phone calls, a patient with avoidant PD might refuse to speak honestly because of judgement-related fears. A therapist must be aware of the urge to name an identified patient or to always believe the interpretation of the family members. It is important for the therapist to be open and compassionate to all participating members.

Finally, there is some evidence that those with certain PDs (namely borderline PD) have experienced neglect and/or abuse within the family context (e.g., Bornovalova et al. 2013). This includes childhood neglect as well as physical and sexual abuse. In these cases, it may be inappropriate to include named family members in treatment.

Forms of Family Therapy

We review here three primary types of family therapy: psychoeducation, cognitive-behavioral family therapy, and systemic therapy. These descriptions illustrate common ways that families are integrated and treated in the psychotherapy setting. However, other therapeutic orientations, including psychodynamic and experiential, often integrate the family into current practice.

Psychoeducational approaches to family therapy highlight educating the family on the etiology, course, presentation, and prognosis of the specific PD. This education also may include common behavioral patterns within the family, information about medication and treatment, ways for the family to cope with stress, and how to interact with the patient in order to best alleviate symptoms. These approaches are based on the assumption that certain mental disorders seriously impair day-to-day living and the education of the family can reduce bias, stigma, and family-induced exacerbation of symptoms. Psychoeducation is most commonly delivered in a group format without including the person with the mental disorder. These groups allow family members to gain support from others in similar situations. Treatments that target the psychoeducation of the family have been highly effective for individuals with severe mental illnesses, such as bipolar disorder and schizophrenia (see, e.g., Miklowitz et al. 2009).

Cognitive-behavioral approaches to family therapy begin with the assumption that the most efficacious pathway to change is to target dysfunctional thoughts and maladaptive behavioral patterns. One essential building block of cognitive-behavioral family therapy is the introduction of skills training. Techniques such as communication training and negotiating strategies are explained and practiced during therapy sessions through role-play and practiced at home through the implementation of homework. Social learning theory is a second essential building block for this approach, with social reinforcers assuming the greatest importance within the family. In this context, modeling becomes an important source of change. The family learns interpersonal skills by observing the therapist enacting them within the familial context. For example, a patient might learn how to be assertive with his mother by observing the therapist being assertive with the mother and then observing her positive reaction. In addition, parents learn the importance of modeling adaptive behaviors for their children.

Although all family therapies include attention to recursive patterns in families, the central focus of *systemic therapies* is on altering such patterns (Lebow 2005). The emphasis is on finding a place to interrupt dysfunctional sequences. Closely related, systemic therapies look to change dysfunctional aspects of family structure, such as disengagement or enmeshment. Efforts also extend into understanding whatever function the dysfunctional behavior may serve for the system and finding a more helpful way of accomplishing this function.

Research Support for Family Therapy for PDs

A sizable empirical literature exists on interpersonal difficulties and PDs, yet few studies have targeted these difficulties by examining family therapy interventions. There is growing evidence for family interventions for individuals with borderline PD (e.g., Fruzzetti et al. 2007; Grenyer et al. 2019), with little research regarding other PDs. Here we focus on the research relevant to borderline PD.

Psychoeducation approaches to the treatment of borderline PD have received some research support. One study found that family members of individuals with borderline PD knew very little about the disorder; however, those who reported having more information demonstrated heightened levels of criticism, hostility, and depression and less warmth (Hoffman et al. 2003). These findings stand in contrast to those from numerous studies that have demonstrated the positive use of psychoeducation in other disorders, ranging from depression to schizophrenia, and underscore the need for care in determining the content of the psychoeducation and the process for providing it. This study concluded that much of the family members' information was likely inaccurate and had been presented in a pessimistic style (possibly on the internet). A small amount of unedited knowledge can lead to pejorative use of labels and a profound sense of pessimism and hopelessness.

To respond to the perceived need for formalized psychoeducation for families of individuals with borderline PD, Hoffman and colleagues (2005) developed *Family Connections*, a 12-week multifamily manualized psychoeducation program. This program covers current information and research on borderline PD, its developmental course, available treatments, comorbidity, individual skills to promote patient well-being, family skills to improve familial interactions, instruction in validation, and problem-solving techniques. Families in the program decreased their level of burden and grief while increasing their level of mastery throughout the program and at a 3-month follow-up (Hoffman et al. 2005). A subsequent trial (not a randomized controlled trial) found that Family Connections improved burden and grief better than did an optimized treatment-as-usual family program (Flynn et al. 2017). This program has now been widely disseminated across the world (e.g., Krawitz et al. 2016).

Apart from Family Connections, other investigators have attempted to test similar structured group psychoeducation interventions for family members of people with borderline PD. One such group intervention focused on improving relationship patterns, education about the disorder, peer support, self-care, and skills to reduce burden (Grenyer et al. 2019). Compared with a wait-list control, this treatment improved adjustment, family empowerment, self-reported ability to play an active role in care, and expressed emotion. Notably, these gains were maintained after 12 months. Finally, a brief three-session group psychoeducation has been developed with promising initial research (Betts et al. 2018; Pearce et al. 2017). This group, *Making Sense of BPD*, is specifically aimed at supporting family members of youth with borderline PD. Initial results support its efficacy in improving burden, distress, and knowledge.

Dialectical behavior therapy is an efficacious treatment of borderline PD (Linehan 1993). An adaptation of this therapy for suicidal adolescents includes a family therapy component (Miller et al. 2007). This is a multifamily skills group where both the parents and the adolescents attend a weekly 2-hour group. This group is adapted from traditional DBT skills training (modules focused on mindfulness, interpersonal effectiveness, emotion regulation, and distress tolerance), but includes added components on behaviorism, validation, and dialectics. This group has been shown to be an effective addition to individual family therapy (Miller and Skerven 2017). In addition, this multifamily skills group has been shown to improve both caregiver-reported and clinician-assessed PD symptoms (borderline and antisocial PD, specifically) in youth as an add-on to individual therapy (Uliaszek et al. 2014).

Other researchers have explored an adaption of DBT for families (Fruzzetti et al. 2007; Miller et al. 2007; Santisteban et al. 2003). In this adaptation, the family members learn how to understand the other person, communicate that understanding genuinely, and reinforce the accurate expression of emotions. The emphasis on creating a validating environment for a person with borderline PD stems from a basic tenet of the biosocial model (Linehan 1993). This tenet states that an important cause of borderline PD is an inherent difficulty with emotion regulation, interacting with an invalidating childhood environment. In an invalidating environment, a person learns that only extreme emotional displays (often in the form of self-harm) succeed in garnering help (Linehan 1993). Emotion dysregulation is reinforced, and adaptive coping mechanisms are not formed. The process of validation within the family therapy context allows the person with borderline PD to trust his or her emotions and use more adaptive coping skills when feeling dysregulated.

Family-based DBT emphasizes the importance of mindfulness (Fruzzetti et al. 2007). In this activity, dubbed *relationship mindfulness*, a person is encouraged to transfer anger into more primary emotions and practice bringing attention to everyday interactions. These mindfulness skills have the potential to reduce the negative reactivity of a person with borderline PD to other members of the family system, thus reducing conflicts between family members. Mindfulness exercises have the added value of an established track record of impact on different types of PDs and could be implemented in family therapy for other PDs (Robins et al. 2004).

Finally, a recent study explores the efficacy of an MBT family treatment for those with borderline PD. MBT is a psychodynamically oriented treatment to help those with borderline PD better differentiate their own thoughts and feelings from the thoughts and feelings of those around them. Specifically, this supportive and skills-based group program, *Families and Carers Training Support* (MBT-FACTS), consists of five sessions delivered by family members, as in Family Connections. Research on this intervention demonstrated a significant reduction in adverse events compared to a wait-list control (Bateman and Fonagy 2019).

Case Example 2

Mary D, 28 years old and living with her parents, was diagnosed with borderline PD. In conjunction with her individual therapy and DBT skills group, Mary and her family participated in 6 months of weekly family therapy. The first set of sessions focused on helping the family understand borderline PD, which fit well with Mary's growing ability to label and monitor her own symptoms, a task important in individual therapy. Her family learned how to take a nonjudgmental stance in approaching Mary's symptoms and reduce using labels such as "manipulative" and "crazy." This helped Mary feel more supported, resulting in an improved ability to ask for help instead of using extreme displays of aggression or despair. Early in therapy, Mary and her family formed agreements regarding how to handle crises and moments of dysregulation. This included Mary's use of distress tolerance skills. When Mary needed to take a break, complete a self-soothing task, or engage in a distraction activity, her family gave her space and did not accuse her of being dramatic or high-maintenance. In addition, family members were able to use mindfulness to notice times when they were beginning to feel dysregulated and utilize some of the same skills that Mary was practicing. This fostered a mutually supportive environment and a reduction in Mary's sick role within the family. Building on these successes, the family sessions then moved to examine the family experience more broadly, including how the family could be helpful in relation to Mary's treatment plan, as well as discussing experiences in the family related to Mary's dysregulation. In addition, Mary and her mother spent considerable time processing their difficult relationship during Mary's childhood. The combined therapy ultimately helped improve Mary's emotion regulation strategies and increased feelings of connectedness among family members. Overall, conflict was reduced and positive affect among family members increased.

Couples Therapy

The following section outlines the intersection between couples therapy and the treatment of PDs. Many of the guiding principles, theories, and techniques used in common couples therapy are identical to those used in family therapy, as the two modalities often draw from the same pool of interventions. With the goal of reducing redundancy between this section and the previous section on family therapy, we only highlight the unique aspects of couples therapy that are relevant to the treatment of PDs.

Features of Couples Therapy or PDs That Facilitate or Complicate Treatment of PDs

Features of Couples Therapy That Facilitate Treatment

The primary aim of couples therapy is to aid the couple in the creation of an environment that is conducive to improving functioning and maintaining a soothing home environment. As outlined in the family therapy section, those with PDs have considerable interpersonal dysfunction. Individual therapy alone may not always have a positive effect on relationship satisfaction, even though relationship satisfaction has a direct association with overall functioning and symptom severity. Couples therapy is uniquely able to target problematic systemic patterns within a romantic relationship and aid both parties in making changes that affect PD symptoms. The success of the couple unit as a place of safety and support often ameliorates the impact of PD, whereas difficulty in relational systems exacerbates symptoms and problems.

Moreover, research demonstrates the beneficial effect of positive romantic relationships for those with PDs. Lewis (1998) reviewed a series of studies that examined the role of marriage in the adult consequences of childhood trauma. He found that a good marriage can have a healing effect on borderline PD characteristics in adulthood. In a longitudinal follow-up study of inpatients with borderline PD, marriage predicted a better clinical outcome and improved functioning. In addition, being in a stable marital relationship appeared to dampen levels of impulsivity (Links and Heslegrave 2000).

An additional benefit of couples therapy is that many topics related to individual functioning may come into focus only when raised by a concerned partner. These topics may include maladaptive behaviors that the individual with a PD lacks the insight or motivation to address. Examples may include medication compliance, frequent paranoid cognitions, or an increase in self-harm behavior. Furthermore, partners are often further along in the stages of change than the person with the PD. This motivation can help scaffold change in a person with PD, particularly when there is a feeling of safety in being with one's partner. This can spur the exploration of specific issues in patients who may have difficulty with the same issues in individual therapy.

Features of Couples Therapy That Complicate Treatment

In the family therapy section, we outlined four primary factors that could complicate family treatment of PDs: contraindication for certain patients, resistance, complex alliances, and the necessity of individual work. All four factors apply to couples therapy. A person with a PD may be experiencing strong emotions regarding a partner— urge to cheat, thoughts of divorce, the presence of domestic violence. In these cases, individual therapy focused on these issues may need to be done before couples therapy can commence. Again, complex alliances resulting in jealousy or resentment on the part of one member of the couple could compromise both the therapeutic relationship and the couple's relationship.

A special factor to consider in couples therapy is that a person with a PD may often choose a partner who is also experiencing psychopathology (see, e.g., Bouchard et al. 2009). In such instances, the expectation that the partner can assume a supportive, empathic position toward the individual with the PD is untenable. In this case, it may be beneficial for each partner to engage in individual therapy to stabilize symptoms and then reconnect at a later point for couples therapy. Furthermore, for those with a PD, the presence of a partner in session may be at times dysregulating and intolerable. Special plans for handling such circumstances should be discussed in early sessions.

Features of PDs That Facilitate Couples Therapy

The range of interpersonal problems evident in those with PDs increases the likelihood that romantic relationships will be affected (Fitzpatrick et al. 2019). For example, there is an increasing amount of research demonstrating the relationship between borderline PD and insecure attachment styles in adulthood (Agrawal et al. 2004). In a meta-analysis of 13 studies, borderline PD demonstrated a consistent inverse relationship with secure attachment styles; this was best characterized as fearfulness in romantic relationships. A second study examined the relationship between 10 PDs and attachment styles (Brennan and Shaver 1998). This study found that most PD symptoms corresponded to insecure and defensive attachment styles. Because of these difficulties, people with PDs may be specifically motivated to engage in couples therapy to address these issues.

In addition to problematic attachment styles, those with PDs have problematic romantic relationships. One study found that avoidant PD was associated with a lower likelihood of marriage. Avoidant, antisocial, and obsessive-compulsive PD were also associated with marital disruption, which included divorce and separation (Whisman et al. 2007). Another study found that among individuals with borderline PD,

29% of men and 52% of women were married at follow-up, compared with an average rate of marriage of their peers of 80%–90% (Stone 1990). A study examining heterosexual relationships in which the woman has borderline PD found a high risk of breakup during the 18 months of the study (Bouchard et al. 2009). This indicates that problems obtaining and maintaining long-term successful relationships may be an appropriate treatment target.

Specific attention has been paid to the difficulties of romantic partners of those with borderline PD. Similar to the family therapy treatments that focus on treating family members as caregivers of those with borderline PD, research on partners often sees them as carers as well. A systematic review of 22 studies focusing on the romantic partners of those with borderline PD revealed that partners noted significant emotional challenges, dual roles as both a partner and a therapeutic figure, and lack of control (Greer and Cohen 2018). The authors found a disconnect between psychoeducational and skills-based therapeutic programs that did little to address these specific needs. This disconnect, combined with research pointing to the dynamic bidirectional relationship between borderline PD and relational distress (see Fitzpatrick et al. 2019 for review), points to the potentially important role of couples therapies that emphasize partner-focused, relation-based skills as an avenue for improving the overall treatment of borderline PD.

Features of PDs That Complicate Couples Therapy

Earlier, in the family therapy section, we reviewed aspects of PDs that may complicate treatment; these included difficult engagement, high dropout rates, and interacting with persons that may increase frustration or burnout on the part of the therapist. These features also apply to couples therapy. Therapists should be aware of the importance of building a strong alliance within couples therapy in order to ensure treatment compliance and reduced hostility within sessions.

In addition, not only may persons with PDs have objectively more problems in relationships than persons without PDs, but they also perceive their relationships to be more difficult. For example, one study found that borderline PD patients perceived their relationships with families, partners, and children to be much more difficult than did a comparison group of depressed individuals (Gerull et al. 2008). This enhanced perception of relational difficulties may cause progress to feel slow or even intractable. The presence of easily hurt feelings, followed by angry outbursts, withdrawal, or total avoidance of feelings, may also complicate couples therapy.

A final complication, as in family therapy, is that the partner of a person with PD may be at an increased likelihood of also having a PD. Although the cause is different (obviously not due to shared genetics or environment as seen within families), some research has found that this may be particularly likely in borderline PD samples. For example, Bouchard and colleagues (2009) found that approximately 50% of the romantic partners of women with borderline PD met criteria for at least one PD.

Different Forms of Couples Therapy

In this section, we review three primary types of couples therapy: psychoeducation, cognitive-behavioral, and integrative therapy. The descriptions for some of these methods can be found in the family therapy section and will not be repeated here.

Psychoeducational approaches to couples therapy are nearly identical to what was described in the family therapy section. The main focus of these interventions is to educate the partner on facts about the PD and include helpful treatment and couple interaction information. Psychoeducation that specifically targets romantic partners may include information on intimacy, future-planning, and the sharing of household responsibilities.

Many aspects of *cognitive-behavioral approaches* to couples therapy are identical to those of family therapy—this includes social learning theory, skills training, and homework implementation. However, there are additional theoretical and technical aspects to cognitive-behavioral couples therapy. One is the importance of social exchange theory, which posits that individuals strive to increase their rewards and decrease their costs in social relationships. In other words, behavior from the partner is reciprocated to maintain a balance between partners: negative behavior is responded to with negative behavior and positive with positive. Often couples can be caught in mutually coercive behavioral patterns. In cognitive-behavioral couples therapy, there also is a focus on how to de-escalate arguments when one or both partners are emotionally dysregulated. Techniques include engaging in calming behaviors, slowing down, suggesting that affects have become too heated, and using other de-escalation techniques (e.g., breathing, taking a walk) until the conversation can be resumed.

Integrative treatments that blend acceptance and cognitive-behavioral strategies have proven highly effective in the treatment of couples (Jacobson and Christensen 1996). *Integrative behavioral couples therapy* focuses on changing what can be changed, building skills, changing cognitions, working with affects, and working with internal dynamics and object relations. This therapy retains a focus on acceptance by both the person with the PD and his or her partner; therapists and clients examine what cannot be changed and find ways to work within these constrictions.

One popular empirically supported integrative couples therapy, Gottman's *Sound Marital House* treatment (Gottman and Gottman 2008), emphasizes the positive effects of having a strong marital foundation made of friendship, fondness, admiration, and positive sentiment. According to this approach, resistance is common in therapy because people have a distorted working model of how relationships are supposed to function. This therapy works on increasing positive interactions between couples, de-escalating conflict, and developing a "love map" of shared future goals, memories, and hopes.

Research Support for Couples Therapy for PDs

There are few evidence-based couples therapies for PDs. Here we focus on treatments for borderline PD that have the potential for application to other PDs; this includes one adaptation of DBT and one case study that combines theories from DBT and Gottman's couples therapy.

DBT has been adapted for specific work with couples (Fruzzetti and Fruzzetti 2003). These researchers have adapted the dialectical dilemmas originally put forth by Linehan (1993) to better fit a couples therapy dynamic. The new dialectics for couples therapy include a) closeness versus conflict, b) partner acceptance versus change, c) one partner's needs and desires versus the other's, d) individual versus relationship satisfaction, and e) intimacy versus autonomy. From these central dialectics, they identify five functions that must be included in dialectical behavior couples therapy. The first of these functions, *skill acquisition or enhancement*, includes development of individual and relational skills that are taught and practiced in sessions. The second, *skill generalization*, refers to the transfer of skills from the therapeutic situation to life outside of therapy, and may combine outside planning and telephone coaching. The third function, *motivation/ behavior change*, involves collaboration between the therapist and clients to identify and change dysfunctional patterns. The fourth function, *therapist capability enhancement and motivation*, refers to the requirement that counselors who work from a DBT model acquire the necessary skills and maintain high levels of motivation. The final function is the *structuring of environment*. These modifications of DBT for couples in which one person has borderline PD can be adapted to fit couples when someone has a different PD.

Other researchers have begun to expand DBT to couples therapy by utilizing the work of Gottman and Gottman (2008). A case study presented by Oliver et al. (2008) demonstrates the positive effects of combining these theories. Again, this study focused on borderline PD but has the potential to be expanded to other PDs. DBT focuses on radical behaviorism, the balance between acceptance and change, and skill building, all with a foundation in mindfulness (Linehan 1993). Gottman's therapy focuses on the building of mutual appreciation and positive sentiment override through exercises and attention to positive exchanges. Gottman also targets what he calls the four horsemen of negative behaviors during conflict (i.e., criticism, defensiveness, contempt, and stonewalling), all behaviors likely to be manifested by those with PD.

Case Example 3

Jose and Susan presented for treatment after frequent fighting with complaints about difficulties morphing into violence. Susan demonstrated signs of borderline PD, including emotion sensitivity within the relationship; this included extreme reactivity to ambiguous responses from Jose and difficulty calming herself down after becoming upset. She had difficulties in interpersonal interactions that resulted in her alternating between passivity and aggressiveness. Susan would easily become inconsolable and cope with the extreme affect by taking substances or becoming violently aggressive. Jose presented as withdrawn and indifferent. He spent the majority of the day alone in his office, avoiding interactions with Susan and his children. He also showed signs of depression, including anhedonia and reduced motivation and concentration. When confronted with Susan's extreme affect, Jose would withdraw further. Eventually, he would try to remove himself from these conflicts, only to be met by physical confrontation from Susan. At this point, he would often lose control and respond with physical aggression. For example, a recent exchange involved Jose coming home late from work. Susan met him at the door, in tears, demanding to know what had kept him. Jose responded, "Traffic," and then went to his office to check his email. Susan followed him to his office and knocked his laptop to the floor while screaming accusations of cheating. Jose grabbed her roughly by the arms and shook her until she stopped screaming. At that point, they both retreated to separate areas in the home for the remainder of the night.

The treatment plan put a primary focus on de-escalating the emotion dysregulation and violence that surrounded many of the couple's arguments. This included practice in mindfulness, which emphasizes effective, nonjudgmental behavior, and self-soothing exercises, such as deep breathing and muscle relaxation. The treatment plan also focused on skill building. Jose and Susan and the therapist role-played adaptive communication patterns, and the therapist modeled validation techniques. The combination of acceptance (including de-escalation and self-soothing) and change (improvement of skills) gave balance to the treatment for such a high-conflict couple.

In approximately the eleventh session of couples therapy, the therapist began with an assessment of a recent event. An extremely volatile fight had resulted in the police being called. Susan had smashed Jose's hand with a hammer, and she was arrested for domestic battery. Susan almost immediately became flooded with affect. She raised her voice and began to cry uncontrollably. Jose angrily voiced his frustration, calling Susan "crazy" and saying that he should get a divorce. The therapist first paused the session so that each could tell his/her story separately, without using judgmental or blaming language (de-escalation of the argument). During that time, Susan was helped to engage in some self-soothing skills. The therapist focused on abdominal breathing and mindfulness practice so that Susan could calm herself and carry on the conversation further, and therapy continued, with the rule that it would pause again if the fight escalated. The therapist reframed the issue behind the fight (Susan wanted to go on a bike ride together, but Jose wanted to be left alone to do his work) as their struggling with how to be close with each other. This notion further calmed the fight and fostered empathy between the couple. The therapist then moved to contracting about how Susan and Jose could meet each of their needs when they wanted to do different things. This included assertiveness training for both, with Susan learning how to avoid insisting on time together in an aggressive way and Jose learning how to avoid being passive-aggressive when uninterested in spending time with Susan at that moment. As both Susan and Jose became more emotionally regulated, they were asked to look more directly at one another and see whether they could begin to find their better feelings for one another (promoting engagement and communication). The therapist also referred back to their discussions about what could be changed in their communication and engagement with each other and what could not: their core wants, desires, and personality (promoting a balance between acceptance and behavior change).

Conclusion

It could be argued that cultural bias toward individualism has led people to neglect the power of collectivity as a helping resource. The emphasis on individual psychotherapy puts out of reach the range of helping behaviors that are potentially available from parents, families, and other human groupings. Yet the scarcity of professional resources may force a return to more traditional (from a sociological sense) helping patterns and to the use of resources that exist within natural groups, such as the family and the community, or within groups developed by, or for, people with similar interests or problems.

The presence of many individuals in therapeutic settings, such as family, couples, or group therapy, also brings a greater variety of ways of intervening compared to individual psychotherapy. In individual therapy, a therapist does not usually directly observe the patient's interpersonal environment and may misinterpret the patient's experience, which is subjective and easily distorted by both parties, compared with the more objective interpersonal reality. Not observing the patient in an interpersonal setting limits the information gathered about the relational context in which the problem is embedded, even though this information is part of the patient's cognitive world. The patient may behave quite differently in different contexts, and individual therapy may not allow the therapist to observe the patient interacting with anyone other than the therapist. Some traits may not become readily apparent in individual treatment, whereas recapitulative interpersonal patterns are evoked automatically in group, family, or couples therapy.

A multiperson approach to treatment does not mean that the approach is simply interactional and ahistorical, based on overt behavior and not on content. Instead, a multiperson approach allows the clinician to take other levels of human functioning into consideration, because interactions and processes also instill content and affects, particularly the intersubjectivity that is present in any human interaction. Multiperson therapy often moves back and forth between process and content. How the content is discussed and how the members behave and react are observed in order to help them see how they may be ineffective in dealing with particular issues.

Clinicians who work with people who have PDs should be familiar with various treatment modalities, including individual, group, family, and couples therapies. Therapeutic flexibility is important, and the ability to shift or integrate modalities is likely crucial to a successful outcome. For example, when individual therapy seems stalled, couples therapy sessions may help address marital dynamics that may be perpetuating the patient's difficulties. That being said, a mix-and-match approach to treatment that utilizes techniques as and when the clinician deems appropriate is not ideal. Treatment decisions should be based on a coherent theory of the disorder, supported by an understanding of the mechanisms of change, which can be used to carefully craft a logically integrated therapeutic package. A team approach is likely necessary. In general, the more severe a person's problems are, the greater the need to include multiple components in the treatment. Using a diversity of approaches in a carefully considered, coherent, and well-structured manner helps keep clinicians from fulfilling the adage "If all you have is a hammer, everything looks like a nail."

References

Agrawal HR, Gunderson J, Holmes BM, et al: Attachment studies with borderline patients: a review. Harv Rev Psychiatry 12:94–104, 2004

American Psychiatric Association: Diagnostic and Statistical Manual of Mental Disorders, 5th Edition. Arlington, VA, American Psychiatric Association, 2013

Bailey RC, Grenyer BFS: Burden and support needs of carers of persons with borderline personality disorder: a systematic review. Harv Rev Psychiatry 21:248–258, 2013

Bateman A, Fonagy P: Effectiveness of partial hospitalization in the treatment of borderline personality disorder: a randomized controlled trial. Am J Psychiatry 156:1563–1569, 1999

Bateman A, Fonagy P: Eight-year follow-up of patients treated for borderline personality disorder: mentalization-based treatment versus treatment as usual. Am J Psychiatry 165:631–638, 2008

Bateman A, Fonagy P: Randomized controlled trial of outpatient mentalization-based treatment versus structured clinical management for borderline personality disorder. Am J Psychiatry166:1355–1364, 2009

Bateman A, Fonagy P: Mentalization-Based Treatment for Personality Disorders: A Practical Guide. New York, NY, Oxford University Press, 2016

Bateman A, Fonagy P: A randomized controlled trial of a mentalization-based intervention (MBT-FACTS) for families of people with borderline personality disorder. Personal Disord 10:70–79, 2019

Bernard HS: Difficult patients and challenging situations, in Basics of Group Psychotherapy. Edited by Bernard HS, MacKenzie KR. New York, Guilford, 1994, pp 123–156

Betts J, Pearce J, McKechnie B, et al: A psychoeducational group intervention for family and friends of youth with borderline personality disorder features: protocol for a randomised controlled trial. Borderline Personal Disord Emot Dysreg 5:13, 2018

Blum N, St John D, Pfohl B, et al: Systems Training for Emotional Predictability and Problem Solving (STEPPS) for outpatients with borderline personality disorder: a randomized controlled trial and 1-year follow-up. Am J Psychiatry 165:468–478, 2008

Bo S, Bateman A, Kongerslev MT: Mentalization-based group therapy for adolescents with avoidant personality disorder: adaptations and findings from a practice-based pilot evaluation. J Infant Child Adolesc Psychother 18:249–262, 2019

Boddington SJA: Factors associated with drop-out from a couples therapy clinic. Sex Relation Therapy 10:321–327, 1995

Bornovalova MA, Huibregtse BM, Hicks BM, et al: Tests of a direct effect of childhood abuse on adult borderline personality disorder traits: a longitudinal discordant twin design. J Abnorm Psychol 122:180–194, 2013

Bos EH, van Wel EB, Appelo MT, et al: Effectiveness of Systems Training for Emotional Predictability and Problem Solving (STEPPS) for borderline personality problems in a "real-world" sample: moderation by diagnosis or severity? Psychother Psychosom 80:173–181, 2011

Bouchard S, Sabourin S, Lussier Y, Villeneuve E : Relationship quality and stability in couples when one partner suffers from borderline personality disorder. J Marit Fam Therapy 35:446–455, 2009

Brennan KA, Shaver PR: Attachment styles and personality disorders: their connections to each other and to parental divorce, parental death, and perceptions of parental caregiving. J Pers 66:835–878, 1998

Chakhssi F, Janssen W, Pol SM, et al: Acceptance and commitment therapy group-treatment for non-responsive patients with personality disorders: an exploratory study. Personal Ment Health 9:345–356, 2015

Chapman AL: Dialectical behavior therapy: current indications and unique elements. Psychiatry 3:62–68, 2006

Chiesa M, Fonagy P, Holmes J: When less is more: an exploration of psychoanalytically oriented hospital-based treatment for severe personality disorder. Int J Psychoanal 84:637–650, 2003

Critchfield KL, Benjamin LS: Principles for psychosocial treatment of personality disorder: summary of the APA Division 12 Task Force/NASPR review. J Clin Psychol 62:661–674, 2006

Edel M, Raaff V, Dimaggio G, et al: Exploring the effectiveness of combined mentalization-based group therapy and dialectical behaviour therapy for inpatients with borderline personality disorder—a pilot study. Br J Clin Psychol 56:1–15, 2017

Farrell JM, Shaw IA, Webber MA: A schema-focussed approach to group psychotherapy for outpatients with borderline personality disorder: a randomized controlled trial. J Behav Ther Exp Psychiatry 40:317–328, 2009

Fassbinder E, Schuetze M, Kranich A, et al: Feasibility of group schema therapy for outpatients with severe borderline personality disorder in Germany: a pilot study with three year follow-up. Front Psychol 7:1851, 2016

Fitzpatrick S, Wagner AC, Monson CM: Optimizing borderline personality disorder treatment by incorporating significant others: a review and synthesis. Personal Disord 10:297–308, 2019

Flynn D, Kells M, Joyce M, et al: Standard 12 month dialectical behaviour therapy for adults with borderline personality disorder in a public community mental health setting. Borderline Personal Disord Emot Dysreg 4:19, 2017

Fonagy P, Campbell C, Bateman A: Mentalizing, attachment, and epistemic trust in group therapy. Int J Group Psychother 67:176–201, 2017

Friedlander ML, Escudero V, Heatherington L: Therapeutic Alliances in Couple and Family Therapy: An Empirically Informed Guide to Practice. Washington, DC, American Psychological Association, 2006

Fruzzetti AE, Fruzzetti AR: Borderline personality disorder, in Treating Difficult Couples: Helping Clients With Coexisting Mental and Relationship Disorders. Edited by Snyder DK, Whisman MA. New York, Guilford, 2003, pp 235–260

Fruzzetti AE, Stantisteban DA, Hoffman PD: Dialectical behavior therapy with families, in Dialectical Behavior Therapy in Clinical Practice: Applications Across Disorders and Settings. Edited by Dimeff LA, Koerner K. New York, Guilford, 2007, pp 222–244

Gerull F, Meares R, Stevenson J, et al: Beneficial effect on family life in treating borderline personality. Psychiatry 71:59–70, 2008

Gottman JM, Gottman JS: Gottman method couple therapy, in Clinical Handbook of Couple Therapy, 4th Edition. Edited by Gurman AS. New York, Guilford, 2008, pp 138–164

Gratz K, Tull M, Levy R: Randomized controlled trial and uncontrolled 9-month follow-up of an adjunctive emotion regulation group therapy for deliberate self-harm among women with borderline personality disorder. Psychol Med 44:2099–2112, 2014

Greer H, Cohen JN: Partners of individuals with borderline personality disorder: a systematic review of the literature examining their experiences and the supports available to them. Harv Rev Psychiatry 26:185–200, 2018

Grenyer BF, Bailey RC, Lewis KL, et al: A randomized controlled trial of group psychoeducation for carers of persons with borderline personality disorder. J Personal Disord 33:214–228, 2019

Gurman AS, Fraenkel P: The history of couple therapy: a millennial review. Fam Process 41:199–260, 2002

Herpertz SC, Kunert HJ, Schwenger UB, et al: Affective responsiveness in borderline personality disorder: a psychophysiological approach. Am J Psychiatry 156:1550–1556, 1999

Hoffman PD, Buteau E, Hooley JM, et al: Family members' knowledge about borderline personality disorder: correspondence with levels of depression, burden, distress, and expressed emotion. Fam Process 42:469–478, 2003

Hoffman PD, Fruzzetti AE, Buteau E, et al: Family connections: a program for relatives of persons with borderline personality disorder. Fam Process 44:217–225, 2005

Hooley JM, Gotlib IH: A diathesis-stress conceptualization of expressed emotion and clinical outcome. Appl Prev Psychol 9:135–151, 2000

Hooley JM, Hoffman PD: Expressed emotion and clinical outcome in borderline personality disorder. Am J Psychiatry 156:1557–1562, 1999

Jacobson NS, Christensen A: Integrative Couples Therapy: Promoting Acceptance and Change. New York, WW Norton, 1996

Jørgensen CR, Bøye R, Andersen D, et al: Eighteen months post-treatment naturalistic follow-up study of mentalization-based therapy and supportive group treatment of borderline personality disorder: clinical outcomes and functioning. Nord Psychol 66:254–273, 2014

Kealy D, Ogrodniczuk JS, Piper WE, Sierra-Hernandez CA: When it is not a good fit: clinical errors in patient selection and group composition in group psychotherapy. Psychotherapy (Chic) 53:308–313, 2016

Krawitz R, Reeve A, Hoffman P, Fruzzetti A: Family Connections in New Zealand and Australia: an evidence-based intervention for family members of people with borderline personality disorder. Journal of the New Zealand College of Clinical Psychologists 25:20–25, 2016

Lawn S, McMahon J: Experiences of family carers of people diagnosed with borderline personality disorder. J Psychiatr Ment Health Nurs 22:234–243, 2015

Lebow JL: Handbook of Clinical Family Therapy. Hoboken, NJ, Wiley, 2005

Leichsenring F, Leibing E: The effectiveness of psychodynamic therapy and cognitive behavior therapy in the treatment of personality disorders: a meta-analysis. Am J Psychiatry 160:1223–1232, 2003

Levy K, McMain S, Bateman A, et al: Treatment of borderline personality disorder. Psychiatr Clin North Am 41:711–728, 2018

Lewis JM: For better or worse: interpersonal relationships and individual outcome. Am J Psychiatry 155:582–589, 1998

Linehan MM: Cognitive Behavioral Treatment of Borderline Personality Disorder. New York, Guilford, 1993

Linehan MM, Korslund KE, Harned MS, et al: Dialectical behavior therapy for high suicide risk in individuals with borderline personality disorder: a randomized clinical trial and component analysis. JAMA Psychiatry 72:478–452, 2015

Links PS, Heslegrave RJ: Prospective studies of outcome: understanding the mechanisms of change in patients with borderline personality disorder. Psychiatr Clin North Am 23:137–150, 2000

Lorentzen S, Ruud T, Fjeldstad A, et al: Personality disorder moderates outcome in short- and long-term group analytic psychotherapy: a randomized clinical trial. Br J Clin Psychol 54:129–146, 2015

Magnavita JJ: Challenges in the treatment of personality disorders: when the disorder demands comprehensive integration. In Session: Psychotherapy in Practice 4:5–17, 1998

Magnavita JJ: Integrative relational therapy of complex clinical syndromes: ending the multi-generational transmission process. J Clin Psychol 56:1051–1064, 2000

McLaughlin SP, Barkowski S, Burlingame GM, et al: Group psychotherapy for borderline personality disorder: a meta-analysis of randomized-controlled trials. Psychotherapy (Chic) 56:260–273, 2019

McMain SF, Guimond T, Streiner DL, et al: Dialectical behavior therapy compared with general psychiatric management for borderline personality disorder: clinical outcomes and functioning over a 2-year follow-up. Am J Psychiatry169:650–661, 2012

Miklowitz DJ, Axelson DA, George EL, et al: Expressed emotion moderates the effects of family-focused treatment for bipolar adolescents. J Am Acad Child Adolesc Psychiatry 48:643–651, 2009

Miller AL, Rathus JH, Linehan MM: Dialectical Behavior Therapy With Suicidal Adolescents. New York, Guilford, 2007

Miller ML, Skerven K: Family skills: a naturalistic pilot study of a family-oriented dialectical behavior therapy program. Couple and Family Psychology: Research and Practice 6:79–93, 2017

Nenadic I, Lamberth S, Reiss N: Group schema therapy for personality disorders: a pilot study for implementation in acute psychiatric in-patient settings. Psychiatr Res 253:9–12, 2017

Oliver M, Perry S, Cade R: Couples therapy with borderline personality disordered individuals. The Family Journal 16:67–72, 2008

Pearce J, Jovev M, Hulbert C, et al: Evaluation of a psychoeducational group intervention for family and friends of youth with borderline personality disorder. Borderline Personal Disord Emot Dysreg 4:5, 2017

Piper WE, Rosie JS, Joyce AS, et al: Time Limited Day Treatment for Personality Disorders: Integration of Research and Practice in a Group Program. Washington, DC, American Psychological Association, 1996

Popolo R, MacBeth A, Canfora F, et al: Metacognitive Interpersonal Therapy in Group (MIT-G) for young adults with personality disorders: a pilot randomized controlled trial. Psychol Psychother 92:342–358, 2019

Robins CJ, Schmidt H, Linehan MM: Dialectical behavior therapy: synthesizing radical acceptance with skillful means, in Mindfulness and Acceptance: Expanding the Cognitive-Behavioral Tradition. Edited by Hayes SC, Follette VM, Linehan MM. New York, Guilford, 2004, pp 30–44

Santisteban DA, Muir JA, Mena MP, et al: Integrative borderline adolescent family therapy: meeting the challenges of treating adolescents with borderline personality disorder. Psychotherapy (Chic) 40:251–264, 2003

Shea M, Elkin I: The NIMH Treatment of Depression Collaborative Research Program, in Interpersonal Factors in the Origin and Course of Affective Disorders. Edited by Mundt C, Fiedler PL, Goldstein ML, et al. London, Gaskell/Royal College of Psychiatrists, 1996, pp 316–328

Stone MH: The Fate of Borderline Patients: Successful Outcome and Psychiatric Practice. New York, Guilford, 1990

Strauss JL, Hayes AM, Johnson SL, et al: Early alliance, alliance ruptures, and symptom change in a nonrandomized trial of cognitive therapy for avoidant and obsessive-compulsive disorders. J Consult Clin Psychol 74:337–345, 2006

Tuttman S: Principles of psychoanalytic group therapy applied to the treatment of borderline and narcissistic disorders, in The Difficult Patient in Group: Group Psychotherapy With Borderline and Narcissistic Disorders. Edited by Roth BE, Stone WN, Kibel HD. Madison, CT, International Universities Press, 1990, pp 7–29

Uliaszek AA, Wilson S, Mayberry M, et al: A pilot intervention of multifamily dialectical behavior group therapy in a treatment-seeking adolescent population: effects on teens and their family members. The Family Journal 22:206–215, 2014

Vaughn CE, Leff JP: The influence of family and social factors on the course of psychiatric illness. Br J Psychiatry 129:125–137, 1976

Wearden AJ, Tarrier N, Barrowclough C, et al: A review of expressed emotion research in health care. Clin Psychol Review 20:633–666, 2000

Whisman MA, Tolejko N, Chatav Y: Social consequences of personality disorders: probability and timing of marriage and probability of marital dysfunction. J Pers Disord 21:690–695, 2007

White CN, Gunderson JG, Zanarini MC, et al: Family studies of borderline personality disorder: a review. Harv Rev Psychiatry 11:8–19, 2003

Yalom ID, Leszcz M: The Theory and Practice of Group Psychotherapy, 5th Edition. New York, Basic Books, 2005

CHAPTER 17

Pharmacological Management

Katharine J. Nelson, M.D.
Sherab Tsheringla, M.D.

The emergence of the diagnostic category of personality disorder (PD) arose primarily from the field of psychoanalytic theory and practice. Therefore, the early treatment approaches tended to focus on psychodynamic and psychoanalytic therapies. The establishment of the DSM-III in 1980 as the manual for the categorization of objective diagnostic criteria for PDs (American Psychiatric Association 1980) opened the door for improved methodology and rate of completion of clinical trials of pharmacological agents. These efforts were aided by the development of structured diagnostic interviews, such as the Diagnostic Interview for Borderlines (Kolb and Gunderson 1980). At the same time, the field of psychiatry worked to expand its capacity to explore the neuroscientific basis of psychiatric illness, such as the theoretical relationships among specific neurotransmitters, neural pathways, and biological markers associated with specific symptoms. This neuroscientific approach led to an overall increase in clinical medication trials, with the goal of improving the outcomes of people living with difficult-to-treat psychiatric illnesses, such as borderline PD (BPD), schizotypal PD (STPD), and other symptoms classified in the realm of personality dysfunction.

Most of the literature on PDs is centered on the pathophysiology and treatment of BPD. BPD significantly impacts the lives of individuals living with the disorder, as well as their family, friends, and those participating in providing care in the medical treatment setting. The morbidity and mortality associated with BPD impacts the broader community, particularly because of the substantial rates of nonsuicidal self-injury,

---

Dr. S. Charles Schulz was an original contributor to this chapter in earlier editions of this volume.

suicidal behaviors, and suicide. People living with BPD suffer enormously with difficulties in emotion regulation and interpersonal functioning, resulting in disability and functional problems in multiple domains of living. Compared with the experience of living with other PDs, living with the symptoms of BPD is more likely to be experienced as disruptive and impairing. This prompts people living with BPD and their families to seek care from medical and mental health professionals. The other PDs tend to be experienced as more ego-syntonic, even when functioning is impaired. Thus, there are fewer opportunities for direct treatment and certainly fewer opportunities for enrollment in clinical trials for potential study participants meeting criteria for PDs other than BPD.

The second most studied PD is STPD, which is now described as being part of the continuum of schizophrenia spectrum disorders in DSM-5 (American Psychiatric Association 2013). This disorder is notable for the presence of ideas of reference, magical thinking, oddness, and eccentricity that significantly interfere with an individual's functioning but do not meet full criteria for a primary psychotic disorder, such as schizophrenia.

With the increase in clinical studies in the 1980s came the assessment of a number of first-generation antipsychotic and antidepressant medications for the treatment of PDs. Mood-stabilizing agents such as lithium were also tested based on the observation of rapidly changing mood in people who had disorders that met criteria for PDs. However, during the first decade of these medicines being tested, the positive results of studies were often outweighed by the side effects of the medications, such as movement disorders. During this same time, interest increased in the development and empirical substantiation of psychotherapeutic approaches such as dialectical behavior therapy (DBT; Linehan et al. 1991) and mentalization-based therapy (Bateman and Fonagy 2008).

The introduction of a number of second-generation medications—beginning with fluoxetine, which was followed by other selective serotonin reuptake inhibitors (SSRIs), and then second-generation/atypical antipsychotic medications and mood-stabilizing anticonvulsant medications such as divalproex—led to increased momentum and attention to medication treatment over the past three decades. The field has produced a number of positive medication studies for the treatment of people living with PDs, with fewer intolerable side effects observed compared with treatment with the first-generation medications. However, emerging controversy and diverging international opinion exist regarding the effect size of, and the generalizability of data and analysis arising from, these trials. Furthermore, because of the positive outcomes of structured therapies such as DBT, there has been considerable controversy and debate over the role of medications versus psychosocial therapies for the treatment of PDs. A challenge for medication management of PDs is rooted in comparisons of effect sizes when medications are matched against psychotherapies, concerns about potentially serious side effects, and other issues. However, it is worth noting that a gap exists between the academic conceptualization of evidence-based treatment approaches and "real-world" clinical practice. Not only are people living with PDs frequently prescribed medications, but the practice of polypharmacy is very common. Moeller and colleagues found that among 165 hospitalized participants, the participants with BPD were significantly more likely to be prescribed psychotropic medications than the group of participants diagnosed with major depressive disorder (Moeller et al. 2016). A global trend in similarly high psychotropic prescription for people diagnosed with BPD is reflected in Paton and colleagues' cross-sectional survey of United Kingdom mental health services, in which 92% of people receiving care for BPD were being treated with psychotropic medication (Paton et al. 2015).

Even with increasing clinical research on pharmacological treatment of PDs, as well as very interesting meta-analyses, psychotherapeutic approaches continue to be first-line treatments for PDs. Medications are widely prescribed for PDs, often with unclear evidence for use. We therefore review international guidelines whose consensus is that medications may have an adjunctive role in treating PDs but are not the primary treatment. In this chapter, we discuss pharmacotherapies for PDs, the medication classes used, indications for use, and clinical approaches to effective and compassionate treatment of people living with PDs. We also explore future directions for research.

Pharmacotherapies

Antipsychotic Medications

First-Generation Antipsychotics

Despite the fact that PDs were not officially described by diagnostic criteria until 1980, antipsychotic medications were historically tried for disorders that would now in retrospect be considered BPD and/or STPD. An initial description of people receiving what was termed "low-dose neuroleptic treatment" (Brinkley et al. 1979) led to a series of medication trials that were structured using protocols that were similar to those used in studies of psychotic illnesses, such as schizophrenia. The first placebo-controlled trial of low doses of first-generation antipsychotic medications for people diagnosed with BPD or STPD was conducted by Goldberg et al. (1986), who designed a double-blind, placebo-controlled trial of thiothixene given at a low dosage (8.7 mg/day) in participants recruited from the community. The research team noted statistically significant changes while evaluating outcome measures related to schizotypal symptoms. Of interest, however, was the fact that the group of participants receiving placebo had the same amount of global improvement as the group taking thiothixene. Soloff et al. (1989) designed a trial for participants with BPD comparing haloperidol at low dosages (4–16 mg/day) with amitriptyline at dosages typically used to treat depression (100–175 mg/day) and placebo. The participants were inpatients at the Western Psychiatric Institute and Clinic and therefore were clearly participants receiving care for severe symptoms rather than outpatient "symptomatic volunteers." In this study, haloperidol at low dosages was significantly superior to placebo and, compared with Goldberg et al.'s study, was better than placebo on essentially all outcome ratings. Haloperidol was superior to amitriptyline in this group.

Findings from two blinded and placebo-controlled trials were consistent with those of other studies in which two antipsychotic medications were compared with each other (Serban and Siegel 1984). These findings resulted in a significant interest in the use of antipsychotic medications for treating people living with BPD, mainly those with comorbid STPD.

Subsequent to these studies, Soloff et al. (1993) continued work examining haloperidol as a treatment for BPD and noted that in their second trial, haloperidol did not separate from placebo. As in the earlier trial, the design focused on the ability to compare the effects of an antipsychotic with an antidepressant. In this trial, the monoamine oxidase inhibitor (MAOI) phenelzine was included and was more effective than placebo. Other reports examined antipsychotic medications for people with symptoms meeting diagnostic criteria for STPD (Hymowitz et al. 1986) and reported some benefit, but also noted some difficulties with participants' management of side effects. Investigators noted that even if people did not have major movement disorders with the first-generation antipsychotic medications, they felt somewhat stultified or slowed and chose not to continue taking the medication.

In this same era, Cowdry and Gardner (1988) examined outpatients referred to their National Institute of Mental Health program in which they examined four classes of compounds in order to determine whether there was specificity for the complex illness of BPD. They studied the antipsychotic trifluoperazine, the benzodiazepine alprazolam, the anticonvulsive carbamazepine, and the antidepressant tranylcypromine. Many participants did not continue use of trifluoperazine beyond the first phase of the trial because of limited tolerability. There was no statistical difference in participant or staff symptom rating scale scores between the antipsychotic and placebo for the participants who did continue taking this medication. The authors noted that there may have been issues with the generalizability of this finding because the participants in this study tended to demonstrate symptoms that emphasized difficulties with affective and behavioral problems rather than transient psychotic states or schizotypy.

Second-Generation Antipsychotics

Clozapine was the first second-generation antipsychotic demonstrated to be effective for treatment-refractory schizophrenia in a large multicenter trial in the 1980s (Kane et al. 1988). Positive reports of efficacy and relative lack of movement disorder side effects led to substantial interest in its use for schizophrenia. Interestingly, clozapine was the first atypical antipsychotic medication to be studied for BPD. Frankenburg and Zanarini (1993) assessed the use of clozapine in significantly ill hospitalized participants with BPD and comorbid major psychiatric illness. The authors noted a significant decrease in the PD symptoms. This remains an excellent clinical contribution to the field, because most studies have examined outpatients. In further work using clozapine, researchers examined participants who had only a PD and no other psychiatric diagnoses. In one trial, 12 inpatients meeting diagnostic criteria for BPD and severe psychotic-like symptoms were treated with clozapine at dosages ranging from 25 to 100 mg/day. Participants in this small sample experienced overall improvement, specifically in impulsivity and affective instability (Benedetti et al. 1998). Over the years, several groups have made similar observations regarding the potential for clozapine to improve symptoms for people living with BPD. Frogley et al. (2013), in the United Kingdom, followed 22 female inpatient participants diagnosed with BPD who were receiving clozapine for 18 months and found significant reductions in symptom severity, and reductions in the need for one-to-one close observations for safety, the use of additional medication, and the number of aggressive incidents. Another group from the United Kingdom, Dickens et al. (2016), described 20 adult female participants with symptoms meeting diagnostic criteria for BPD in a secure inpatient facility, with many reporting profound subjective well-being on clozapine compared with past treatments. The increasing interest in clozapine appears to have been supported by at least some evidence for consideration for clinical use and further scientific inquiry.

In a Danish study from 2018, Rohde et al. examined the "real-world" effectiveness of clozapine in participants with BPD after a 2-year follow-up and found a significant reduction in psychiatric admissions, decreased psychiatric bed days by almost two-thirds, and a reduction in self-harm by almost half. Reduced self-injurious behavior in BPD with clozapine had previously been reported (Zarzar and McEvoy 2013), and systematic reviews (Zalsman et al. 2016) have shown that along with lithium, clozapine is considered effective in preventing suicide. Differences in clozapine's pharmacological profile, such as lower dopamine D_2 receptor affinity, rapid dissociation from receptors, D_4/D_2 receptor binding profile, and serotonin 5-HT_{2A} affinity, along with other unknown mechanisms, possibly explain the superior efficacy of clozapine in treatment-resistant schizophrenia and its potential to differentiate from other antipsychotics in treatment of PDs. The use of clozapine has been limited clinically by the need for initial assessment and monitoring of blood counts (specifically neutrophils) to assess for and minimize the risk of developing severe neutropenia, a life-threatening condition associated with use of this medication. Clozapine and all other second-generation antipsychotics are associated with metabolic risks, such as weight gain, diabetes, and elevated blood lipids. These conditions increase the risk of cardiovascular events such as coronary artery disease and myocardial infarction and present a higher incidence of stroke in older people. Movement side effects, such as dystonic reactions and tardive dyskinesia, have also been observed. Neuroleptic malignant syndrome, a rare but serious condition that could be life-threatening, can also occur with antipsychotic use.

Following the introduction of clozapine, other second-generation antipsychotics emerged. These medications are also referred to as *atypical* antipsychotics because they result in substantially decreased movement disorders compared with first-generation antipsychotics. Risperidone, the first second-generation antipsychotic approved for the treatment of schizophrenia, was tested in participants with BPD in an 8-week trial by Rocca et al. (2002). In this case series, there was a significant reduction in symptoms. Koenigsberg et al. (2003) examined the effect of risperidone on participants with STPD and found a statistically significant reduction in the symptoms of psychoticism in these participants with a low dosage of risperidone (starting dose of 0.25 mg, with the dosage titrated upward to 2 mg/day). The authors noted that two of the participants had received both STPD and BPD diagnoses, and these two participants also demonstrated improvement in outcome measures. Schulz et al. (1998) compared low doses of risperidone with placebo in symptomatic participants who qualified for the BPD diagnosis and were recruited through advertising media. This double-blind, placebo-controlled trial was conducted in an outpatient program in which the staff members were trained in DBT techniques and the participants were given education handouts and books and provided with 24-hour staff availability. In this report, the participants assigned to receive risperidone did have a significant reduction in symptoms on a number of rating scales; however, as the differences between the group treated with risperidone and the group treated with placebo were not statistically significant, risperidone did not separate from placebo. The investigators speculated that the substantial psychosocial support was of significant benefit for the participants with BPD in both the placebo and active medication groups.

The second atypical antipsychotic medication to be released in the United States was olanzapine. This medication was found, in comparisons with placebo, to reduce symptoms of schizophrenia, and was not observed to have as high a degree of movement disorder side effects compared with first-generation antipsychotic medications such as haloperidol (Tollefson et al. 1997). Initial assessments of olanzapine for BPD were open-label studies aimed at assessing the effect of the medication on standard rating scale symptoms (e.g., Hopkins Symptom Checklist–90 [SCL-90]; Derogatis et al. 1973) and examining potential side effects. The first trial by Schulz et al. (1998) assessed 11 participants taking olanzapine at a total daily dose of 7.5 mg, approximately half the dose used in people taking the medication for the treatment of schizophrenia. The results demonstrated a significant reduction in symptoms as assessed by the SCL-90, the Buss-Durkee Hostility Inventory, and the Barratt Impulsiveness Scale. The authors noted that 9 of the 11 participants who completed the 8-week study found the medication to be tolerable. In an open-label trial focusing on STPD, Keshavan et al. (2004) noticed improvement both in measures of psychoticism and in mood. This study, which took place over nearly 6 months, observed improvement in 8 of 11 participants and represented an important contribution to the field.

Following the initial open-label trials, other investigators designed placebo-controlled studies of olanzapine in participants with BPD. Zanarini and Frankenburg (2001) tested olanzapine in women and noted improvement compared with placebo. Of interest, the dosage of olanzapine in this study was low (average of 5.3 mg/day) compared with that used in the treatment of schizophrenia. A larger study compared olanzapine with placebo in 40 participants with BPD (Bogenschutz and Nurnberg 2004). This study was the first to use DSM-based criteria as an outcome measure. Of note, the severity of seven of the nine DSM-specified criteria for BPD was reduced in participants taking olanzapine compared with those receiving placebo.

Zanarini et al. (2004) compared olanzapine with fluoxetine and a combined olanzapine/fluoxetine compound. In this trial, the olanzapine/fluoxetine compound was most effective, but the gains were not statistically greater than those for olanzapine alone. Both the olanzapine/fluoxetine compound and olanzapine were superior to fluoxetine alone. This was of interest to the field because, at the time, there had previously been a number of successful fluoxetine case series.

An issue facing the field of treatment for people living with BPD has been the lack of information regarding medication treatment in the context of co-occurring structured psychosocial treatments. To address this issue, Soler et al. (2005) tested olanzapine by giving either the active medication or placebo to participants enrolled in DBT. The authors entered 60 participants in the study and found an advantage for olanzapine over placebo on depression and impulsivity rating scales. Linehan et al. (2008) similarly reported an advantage for olanzapine added to DBT compared with placebo added to DBT. Their results showed a reduction in anger during the study—an area of potential usefulness in engaging people in treatment.

To further address olanzapine's potential in the treatment of BPD, investigators conducted two large registration trials designed to test the medication versus placebo (Schulz et al. 2008; Zanarini et al. 2011). One aim of these industry-sponsored Phase III clinical trials was to provide evidence and data that could be used by the U.S. Food and Drug Administration (FDA) to decide whether to approve olanzapine for BPD. The design of these trials included participants with BPD, but to assess the specificity of the treatment, no participants with a comorbid PD were included. Also, comorbidities of other major psychiatric disorders were substantially limited. This design differs substantially from the design of a number of the earlier studies of antipsychotic medications in participants with comorbid BPD and STPD.

In the first published of these two large trials, Schulz et al. (2008) reported that olanzapine was not statistically significantly superior to placebo by the end of the 12-week study, and both the placebo and medication groups showed a reduction of symptoms over the course of the trial, as assessed by the Zanarini Rating Scale for Borderline Personality Disorder (ZAN-BPD). The authors also reported on the metabolic side effects in the two groups; the olanzapine group had significantly greater weight gain and a higher incidence of treatment-emergent abnormally high levels of prolactin. Later, in the largest BPD study performed to date, Zanarini et al. (2011) randomly assigned 451 outpatients ages 18–65 to receive a fixed low dose of olanzapine (2.5 mg), a higher dose of olanzapine (5–10 mg), or placebo. There was a significant reduction of ZAN-BPD symptoms in the 5- to 10-mg group, but the 2.5-mg group did not separate from the placebo group. As in the previous trial, the olanzapine groups showed significantly increased metabolic side effects. After completion of the two studies, the open-label continuation trial (Zanarini et al. 2012) showed that the participants who had been assigned to receive placebo in either of the two double-blind studies had a reduction in symptoms with open-label use of olanzapine. Also, participants who continued in the study after having taken olanzapine in an earlier study continued their improvement.

The third second-generation antipsychotic medication to be released in the United States for the treatment of schizophrenia was quetiapine. This antipsychotic medication was shown to reduce symptoms of schizophrenia relative to placebo (Small et al. 1997). The medication has since been assessed using an open trial methodology for both inpatients and outpatients with a BPD diagnosis (Adityanjee et al. 2008). Of interest is the wide range in dosing of quetiapine, with relatively high doses being assessed in the inpatient setting for people living with BPD. These open-label studies and case series frequently cite sedation as a side effect, as well as increased appetite, dry mouth, and weight gain (Adityanjee et al. 2008).

Aripiprazole is an antipsychotic medication with a unique activity in the brain: it is a partial agonist of dopamine receptors, in addition to having the usual dopaminergic antagonism effects of other antipsychotics. This medication was judged to have significant effectiveness in schizophrenia (Kane et al. 2002) and was tested by Nickel et al. (2006) for BPD. In this trial, 43 women and 9 men with DSM-III-defined BPD were randomly assigned to receive either 15 mg/day of aripiprazole (*n*=26) or placebo (*n*=26) for 8 weeks. The authors noted that symptoms of anxiety and depression, as well as anger, were broadly reduced. This study was extended to an 18-month follow-up to assess long-term use of the medication. The authors noted significant improvement on all outcome measures over this period (Nickel et al. 2007).

Since the approval of aripiprazole in 2002, there have been a few newer antipsychotics in the market that have received FDA approval for the treatment of schizophrenia. One open-label study comparing asenapine with olanzapine (51 outpatients in a 12-week trial) showed that asenapine was better than olanzapine for affective instability (Bozzatello et al. 2017). Oral paliperidone ER was studied in 18 outpatients with BPD, showing improvements in impulsive dyscontrol, anger, and cognitive-perceptual disturbances (Bellino et al. 2011).

Antipsychotic medications have the benefit of being available as long-acting injectable formulations, which can greatly support treatment adherence. The psychiatric literature contains reports of intramuscular long-acting injectable antipsychotics like paliperidone and risperidone for people receiving treatment for BPD, especially with comorbid psychosis, though further research on efficacy is required (Díaz-Marsá et al. 2008; Palomares et al. 2015).

With STPD now being conceptualized as part of the schizophrenia spectrum, there have been numerous trials of antipsychotics in this population. An early intervention trial in Denmark (Albert et al. 2017), the OPUS II study, with a follow-up 3.5 years later, showed that individuals with STPD may be an ultra-high-risk group, with 32% developing a psychotic disorder. In this study, low functioning at baseline was noted to be the strongest predictor of psychotic transition. The OPUS II study did not find any effect of specialized early intervention on this transition. Their findings are reflective of our current understanding of the uncertain efficacy of antipsychotics in treating at-risk or prodromal states of psychosis.

In summary, antipsychotic medications have been tested for BPD, BPD and STPD together, and STPD alone. Some, but not all, of the studies have shown symptom reductions in open-label trials. Antipsychotic medications have been superior to placebo in some, but not all, studies. Also, of note are the two studies in which an antipsychotic medication was delivered in the context of a structured psychosocial treatment (i.e., DBT), in which the combination demonstrated a statistical advantage. Because of the limiting nature of the side effects of this class of medications, clinicians and those receiving care must together carefully weigh the potential benefits of medication versus the side effects.

Antidepressant Medications

In the early stages of testing antidepressant medications in the treatment of BPD, Soloff et al. (1986) found that the tricyclic antidepressant (TCA) amitriptyline was no better than placebo, and also noted that approximately a quarter of the participants experienced deterioration in their behavior. This report, perhaps combined with some of the safety issues related to TCAs, such as the significant toxicity in the case of overdose, diminished interest in TCAs for the treatment of BPD. The group's next assessment of antidepressant medications examined the MAOI phenelzine at 60 mg/day (Soloff et al. 1993). This medication was selected on the basis of previous work demonstrating efficacy in people receiving care for anxiety disorders (Ravaris et al. 1976). In the Soloff et al. (1993) BPD treatment trial, phenelzine was superior to placebo. Despite the positive results of the study, issues related to side effects (including diet restriction of foods containing tyramine) discouraged significant use or further trials of MAOIs.

The MAOI tranylcypromine (40 mg/day) was tested by Cowdry and Gardner (1988) in a multiple medication study of 16 female outpatients. The authors noted that this MAOI was rated better than placebo by the participants and the physicians. They also commented on its potential usefulness in combination with the psychotherapy the participants were receiving. Examination of MAOI studies has shown dosing ranges similar to doses used in depression treatment. In this category of medication, the selegiline patch is a newer compound with less significant dietary side effects, but it appears to be underutilized even in treatment of depression (Asnis and Henderson 2014) and there are no studies of this compound in the treatment of BPD.

With the introduction in 1987 of fluoxetine, the first SSRI, investigators interested in BPD felt that fluoxetine might be useful in reducing symptoms of depression and anxiety. The first trials were open-label, and results on rating scales such as the SCL-90 indicated that the participants had a statistically significant reduction of symptoms. The first report, by Cornelius et al. (1990), noted improvements, mostly in depressive and impulsive symptoms, in five participants with BPD. In another early open-label trial, this time with 22 participants with BPD, Markovitz et al. (1991) noted decreased self-injury and SCL-90 scores. Additionally, Salzman et al. (1995) reported, in a 13-week double-blind, placebo-controlled study, the reduction of anger. In examining these latter two studies, it is interesting to note that the doses of fluoxetine appeared higher than those used in major depression. Dosages ranged from 20 to 80 mg/day in the study by Markovitz et al. (1991) and 20 to 60 mg/day in the study by Salzman et al. (1995). Markovitz and Wagner (1995) additionally examined venlafaxine, a serotonin-norepinephrine reuptake inhibitor (SNRI), in an open-label trial. In this study, participants who had not responded to SSRIs did show improvement with venlafaxine. At the time, the treatment of BPD symptoms with antidepressant medication was a significantly controversial topic.

The early investigations of medications for BPD focused on those participants whose personality functioning met the criteria for BPD on the basis of DSM-III criteria (American Psychiatric Association 1980) or the Diagnostic Interview for Borderline Patients (Gunderson et al. 1981). Of interest in the pharmacotherapeutic approach to BPD is examination of symptom or trait domains of the PDs, rather than the global DSM-based criteria. Coccaro and Kavoussi (1997) investigated impulsive/aggressive symptoms in participants who initially had PD characteristics. Coccaro and colleagues (Coccaro and Kavoussi 1991; Coccaro et al. 1997) examined the serotonergic underpinning of impulsive and aggressive disorders, using both behavioral and neuroscientific measures over the years preceding these studies. In a double-blind, placebo-controlled trial, fluoxetine, given at dosages of up to 60 mg/day, led to improvement in the early phase of the study that extended to the end of the trial (Coccaro et al. 1997). Thus, a combination of neuroscience and clinical trial studies indicated that fluoxetine could be useful in the domain of symptoms of impulsivity and aggression. In contrast to the previously reviewed studies, which assessed use of antidepressants alone in clinical trial format, Simpson et al. (2004) examined the addition of fluoxetine to DBT. In this study, in which all participants received DBT in combination with either fluoxetine or placebo, fluoxetine did not emerge as providing an advantage over placebo.

In summary, early studies of TCAs showed that this class of compounds did not lead to an improvement across participant groups and may have led to worsening of symptoms for inpatients with BPD (Soloff et al. 1986). The initial reports on SSRIs, based on open-label studies of fluoxetine, showed improvement in depressive and impulsive symptoms, and these open-label findings were confirmed in some, but not all, subsequent controlled studies. It is noteworthy that Markovitz and Wagner (1995) found that the SNRI venlafaxine may be useful in participants who have had a failed trial with an SSRI. With the emergence of PD studies examining trait domains rather than only DSM criteria, Coccaro and Kavoussi (1997) demonstrated the potential usefulness of fluoxetine in impulsive/aggressive participants. Also of note is the observation of the higher-than-usual dosage range of fluoxetine in the clinical treatment of BPD and the observed safety and tolerability. SSRIs may have limited evidence, but they continue to be the most commonly used medications in the treatment of people with BPD, especially in the first decade of treatment. Since 2011, the FDA has approved newer medications such as desvenlafaxine, vilazodone, levomilnacipran, and vortioxetine for treating depression. However, there are no studies yet on these medications for PDs. Similarly, even as ketamine treatments are being evaluated for depressive disorders, there is no evidence for these treatments in PDs or PDs with comorbid depression.

Anxiolytics

Anxiety is a prominent symptom for people living with BPD, who demonstrate difficulties in interpersonal relationships, sensitivity to rejection, and misperception of the intent of others. These challenges can lead to significant distress, and at times this may lead to highly consequential behaviors. Therefore, anxiolytic medications, such as benzodiazepines, appear to be a natural target for investigation. The highly creative study by Cowdry and Gardner (1988) examined four medications from different classes, including the benzodiazepine alprazolam (4.7 mg/day). The results of other parts of this study are presented elsewhere in the chapter (see "Antipsychotic Medications" and "Antidepressant Medications" above and "Anticonvulsants" below). Notably, in the alprazolam treatment arm of this study, participants experienced no improvement in symptoms, and their impulsivity and behavioral dyscontrol actually worsened, which led to the early discontinuation of this treatment arm (Gardner and Cowdry 1985). This carefully controlled study led to concern about using disinhibiting medications in this population, and further trials have not been pursued. Therefore, even though it might occur to a clinician to use benzodiazepines in treating symptoms of anxiety in people seeking and receiving care for BPD, there is no empirical evidence that this class of medications is useful, and these medications may in fact pose substantial risks. Of note are the emerging findings of functional imaging in participants with personality functioning meeting diagnostic criteria for BPD that are revealing a pattern of hypofrontal metabolism or blood flow that may be related to impulsive/aggressive behavior. In other words, the higher the rating of impulsive and aggressive behavior, the lower the frontal lobe activity (Goyer et al. 1996). Decreased neural mechanisms of self-control may be an underpinning of the observed disinhibition in people living with BPD and being treated with benzodiazepines. Comorbid BPD in high-dose benzodiazepine users has also been associated with a history of suicide attempt (Lekka et al. 2002). Clinicians should exert caution about benzodiazepine prescriptions, especially in this population with an elevated risk of suicide.

Lithium Carbonate

Lithium carbonate was approved by the FDA in the early 1970s for use in bipolar disorder. This medication had been found over the previous 20 years in other countries to be very effective in reducing mood dysregulation in people living with BPD. Furthermore, it did not have the side effects, such as sedation, movement disorders, or emotional flattening, that were associated with neuroleptic medication. In their pre-DSM-III study, Rifkin et al. (1972) described participants who would now be diagnosed with BPD as having "emotionally unstable character disorder." In this study of inpatient participants, lithium was substantially superior to placebo in the management of rapid mood swings. Dosages similar to those used for the treatment of bipolar disorder were used in this study. These results led to a continued interest in this compound, which was considered nonsedating and safe. In another study examining lithium carbonate in BPD, Links et al. (1990) noted some reduction in symptoms based on the therapists' rating scales, but participants' reports indicated no significant reduction in symptoms for lithium versus placebo. The authors noted that lithium reduced impulsive symptoms. Considering these reports on lithium carbonate and the observations of objective improvements in mood changes for people living BPD, the lack of further evidence is difficult to explain.

When lithium carbonate is used in people being treated for BPD, as when it is used to treat people living with mood disorders, assessment and monitoring of thyroid and kidney function are necessary. People taking lithium, and their families as well, need to know about side effects, such as tremor, thirst, and increased urination, as well as the potential for neurological complications in the setting of lithium toxicity. Lithium blood levels must be monitored. This medication may pose significant morbidity or mortality if taken in an overdose, which is a particular risk factor for people living with BPD, given the high risk of suicidal behavior. Some authors suggest that in people with a strong genetic link to bipolar affective disorder, mood stabilizers like lithium may be more effective (Stone 2019). There is also increasing evidence for the protective effects of lithium in suicide (Tondo and Baldessarini 2018), though such effects have yet to be established in comorbid depression and PDs (Rombold et al. 2014).

Anticonvulsants

During the 1970s, research emerged examining the impact of anticonvulsant medications on bipolar disorder. An early report from Japan noted a reduction in bipolar symptoms in participants treated with carbamazepine (Okuma 1983). This work was followed closely by reports examining the potential pathophysiology underpinning temporal lobe stimulation leading to an increased frequency of mood symptoms (Ballenger and Post 1978; Post et al. 1986). The first group of researchers to examine use of an anticonvulsant medication in BPD were Cowdry and Gardner (1988), drawing on their earlier work in bipolar disorder, in which carbamazepine was used in one of the arms of their four-medication treatment trial. The significantly useful outcome measure was a decrease in suicide attempts by this impulsive group. Interestingly, although there was no overall change in the participants' assessment of improvement in their own symptoms, an objective decrease in measured impulsivity and suicidality was considered meaningful. Unfortunately, there was also an increase in depressive symptoms in these participants during the anticonvulsant period of the trial. In a subsequent double-blind, placebo-controlled study, de la Fuente and Lotstra (1994) examined the use of carbamazepine in hospitalized patients with BPD. In this trial, there were no differences in symptomatic outcomes between participants given carbamazepine and those given placebo.

During the 1980s, there was a greater interest in assessing the utility of divalproex sodium for the treatment of bipolar disorder. Frankenburg and Zanarini (2002), in one of their studies of people with BPD, examined divalproex sodium in a group of participants with bipolar II disorder who also qualified for the diagnosis of BPD. This was a very useful study in light of the frequent comorbidity of these disorders. Interestingly, Frankenburg and Zanarini examined symptoms of impulsive aggression using a standardized rating scale and found a statistically significant reduction of symptoms with divalproex in this comorbid group. In a related trial of divalproex sodium in outpatients with BPD, Hollander et al. (2001) found a reduction of symptoms in the participants receiving divalproex sodium. However, there was a very significant dropout rate in the placebo group, which made interpretation of the results somewhat difficult. Hollander et al. (2005) later examined participants with impulsive and aggressive symptoms to look further into the borderline, narcissistic, antisocial, and histrionic PD groups. There was a reduction in symptoms in these diagnostic groups overall. When Hollander and colleagues then focused only on the participants with BPD, they noted a significant decrease in aggression and trait impulsiveness when divalproex was used. In these studies, the mean dosage was approximately 1,250 mg/day, similar to the dosages used for epilepsy and bipolar disorder. Because blood levels of divalproex can vary widely at a given dosage, assessment of blood levels is important. The monitoring of side effects, which include weight gain and sedation, is also warranted. Women with the potential to bear children should be counseled about the risk of birth defects, including neural tube abnormalities, especially following exposure to valproic acid in the first trimester.

Other anticonvulsant medications have been released since these early trials were begun, and medications such as oxcarbazepine and topiramate have been examined in the treatment of people living with PDs. Of note are studies by M.K. Nickel et al. (2004, 2005) and C. Nickel et al. (2005) examining topiramate. In this series of studies, topiramate was assessed in double-blind, placebo-controlled trials, first in women (Nickel et al. 2004) and then in men (M. K. Nickel et al. 2005). In both studies, the investigators used the State-Trait Anger Expression Inventory (STAXI; Spielberger et al. 1999) as an outcome measure and noted significant reductions in anger in both groups. The group given topiramate (at dosages up to 250 mg/day) interestingly lost more weight than the placebo group. This research group then used SCL-90 measures to assess the effects of topiramate and noted a significant decrease in scores on some of the scales, such as somatization, interpersonal sensitivity, anxiety, hostility, and phobic anxiety (Loew et al. 2006). In this study, the highest dosage was 200 mg/day. Of clinical note was the reduction in weight for participants taking topiramate, because weight gain has been a substantial clinical issue for second-generation antipsychotic medications and, to a lesser degree, other psychiatric medications, such as anticonvulsants and some antidepressants.

Topiramate has been studied in many areas of neurology and psychiatry, and observations have emerged indicating that it may have a negative impact on cognition. Loring et al. (2011) assessed this issue in a study of both participants with epilepsy and healthy volunteers. The authors noted a negative impact of topiramate on neuropsychological assessment and noted that it was dose-related, with the greatest impact for those given topiramate at the highest dosage (384 mg/day). The cognitive impact of topiramate related to its dose is important if the medication is used in the treatment of people living with PDs.

Oxcarbazepine at dosages of 1,200–1,500 mg/day has been evaluated in the outpatient setting by Bellino et al. (2005) in their study showing improvements in the BPD severity index domains of interpersonal relationships, impulsivity, affective instability, and outbursts of anger. Gabapentin is an anticonvulsant recognized as an increasingly used medication for multiple off-label indications. We found only one open-label study from Spain evaluating use of gabapentin in BPD (Peris et al. 2007). Off-label use of anticonvulsants for BPD requires further review.

Lamotrigine is another medication that has been explored for use in the treatment of people diagnosed with BPD. Some of this work was spawned from early studies of lamotrigine in bipolar disorder by Calabrese et al. (1999), who reported that lamotrigine had a positive impact on the depressive phase of bipolar disorder. These findings led to speculation about the potential usefulness of lamotrigine for depressive symptoms in people living with BPD. Pinto and Akiskal (1998) reported on an eight-participant case series in which three participants with BPD showed improvement in global functioning. Tritt et al. (2005) completed the first placebo-controlled study of lamotrigine in the treatment of participants with BPD, using the STAXI as the outcome tool, and they noted significant improvement and safety. Reich et al. (2009) assessed lamotrigine in participants with BPD in a double-blind trial using the ZAN-BPD and noted reductions in Affective Lability Scale scores and in the affective instability item. They also noted a reduction in impulsivity. Crawford et al. (2018), in a more recent study (Lamotrigine and Borderline Personality Disorder: Investigating Long-Term Effectiveness [LABILE]), reported results from a multicenter, double-blind, placebo-controlled randomized trial in the United Kingdom with 195 participants who were followed up for 52 weeks, using the ZAN-BPD as primary outcome measure. This study did not find that lamotrigine was clinically effective or cost-effective and also observed that only one-third of patients were taking this medication at 1-year follow-up. In an editorial from August 2018, Gunderson and Choi-Kain (2018) commented on this observation, emphasizing both the natural course of remission in BPD and significant placebo response in people with BPD, which has also been our clinical experience. The LABILE study was different from the previous positive trials in that it recruited from clinical referrals from inpatient and community care and not from advertisements as in previous trials, excluded participants with psychosis or mood disorder and those taking other mood stabilizers, had more men enrolled than previous studies, and possibly had lower-functioning participants (22% employed vs. 100% employed in Tritt et al.'s [2005] study). Regarding the clinical management of lamotrigine, it is worth noting the importance of using a slow titration of the medication as mandated by the manufacturer and monitoring for possible skin rash or lesions, to minimize the risk of potentially life-threatening development of Stevens-Johnson syndrome.

Other Pharmacological Treatments

Omega-3 Fatty Acids

Although much of the discussion of somatic treatments for PDs may focus on pharmaceuticals, omega-3 fatty acids have been the object of a double-blind, placebo-controlled trial for BPD (Zanarini and Frankenburg 2003). This study, in which participants were assigned to receive either omega-3 fatty acids (1 g/day) ($n=20$) or placebo ($n=10$), found a statistical advantage for the compound compared with placebo. The study's focus was on aggression and depressive symptoms. A 12-week randomized trial of combined therapy with omega-3 fatty acids and valproic acid showed improvement in impulsive-behavioral dyscontrol, outbursts of anger, and self-harm, with long-lasting effects even after discontinuation of omega-3 fatty acids with respect to anger control (Bellino et al. 2014).

NMDA Antagonists

Strategies that optimize the efficacy of medications used in the treatment of people with BPD have included medications like memantine, a glutamate N-methyl-D-aspartate (NMDA) receptor antagonist. NMDA has been implicated in BPD (Grosjean and Tsai 2007) by possibly mediating the vulnerability to environmental stress, while causing BPD symptoms through changes in neural plasticity, synaptic activity, sensory gating, or NMDA receptor function. Kulkarni et al. (2018) conducted an 8-week double-blind, placebo-controlled trial of adjunctive memantine. Both groups received treatment as usual, which included antidepressants, mood stabilizers, antipsychotics, psychotherapy, and psychosocial interventions. Seventeen participants diagnosed as having BPD received up to 20 mg/day of memantine and showed significant reductions in severity on the primary outcome measure, the ZAN-BPD.

Meta-analytic Studies of Medications in Personality Disorders

Personality Disorders Other Than BPD

Significant effort has been invested in reviewing the available literature to best advise practicing clinicians in the care of people with PDs. As described in this chapter, many clinical trials have been small, and the generalizability of individual studies is somewhat limited. The Cochrane Collaboration conducted a meta-analytic study of randomized controlled medication trials involving participants with antisocial PD (Khalifa et al. 2010). The existing evidence is sparse. Eight trials examining eight medications were identified, but data could be reviewed for only four of the trials. The quality of the studies was considered insufficient, and thus no conclusions could be drawn.

BPD and International Practice Guidelines

To address the significant need for evidence-based guidance on clinical management of BPD, researchers in several countries have developed practice guidelines based on meta-analytic reviews. A consistent theme among such efforts is the acknowledgment of methodological limitations due to the relatively limited number of clinical trials in the area of BPD treatment and to differences in study design, which challenge the pooling of data.

The first practice guideline for the treatment of people living with BPD was developed in the United States by the American Psychiatric Association (APA) in 2001, and it included a set of clinical algorithms for the adjunctive use of medications for BPD, based on the limited research available at the time. This guideline was developed prior to the majority of the research described earlier in this chapter and included only seven placebo-controlled clinical trials. The APA guideline suggested that clinicians consider symptom domains of BPD and pointed to antidepressant medications as a first-line treatment for affective symptoms. The guideline noted that the combination of psychotherapy and psychopharmacology is probably the most useful strategy in the overall management of BPD. The APA guideline is currently considered outdated because of the significant number of clinical medication and combined medication-psychotherapy trials that have been conducted since its development. Furthermore, the FDA has not approved any medication for use in the treatment of PDs. An APA steering committee is reviewing the practice guidelines, and a partial update of the BPD guideline is under development at the time of this writing.

The first European guidelines were released by the Swedish Psychiatric Society, which developed *Clinical Guidelines for Personality Disorders* in 2006 (updated in 2017) (Ekselius et al. 2017). These guidelines did not consider medications as the primary treatment for PDs, although they did address use of medications for co-occurring symptom disorders. A Cochrane Collaboration review conducted by German researchers serves to identify high-quality evidence that clinicians may use in making individualized practice decisions (Stoffers et al. 2010). The reviewers identified 28 qualifying studies for analysis of first- and second-generation antipsychotics, mood stabilizers, and antidepressants. Omega-3 fatty acids were also included. Outcome measures included treatment impact on BPD severity, amelioration of BPD core pathology (chronic feelings of emptiness, identity disturbance, and abandonment), changes in associated psychopathology (depression, anxiety, general psychiatric pathology, and overall mental health status), and participant attrition. In this comprehensive assessment, the reviewers noted some supporting evidence for medication therapy in the treatment of BPD—mostly for the second-generation antipsychotic medications, mood stabilizers, and omega-3 fatty acids. In the area of safety, the most prominent side effects were related to weight gain and metabolic abnormalities observed with olanzapine. Similar to the recommendations of the APA practice guideline, the reviewers in the Cochrane meta-analysis noted that medication treatment should be combined with psychotherapy, with close attention to the therapeutic relationship. On the basis of the limited long-term data on medication treatment, the authors recommended identification of clear treatment targets and discontinuation of treatment if improvement in these targets is not observed. The data suggested that SSRIs are possibly effective for the treatment of anxiety, depression, and affective instability symptoms. Evidence also suggested that atypical neuroleptics and mood stabilizers may possibly be effective for hostility, anger, impulsivity, aggression, and depression.

After examination of the individual medications, Stoffers et al. (2010) noted an important clinical point related to selection of treatment by clinicians—namely, that there were very few comparisons of medications (which are very useful in determining a treatment). The authors also noted that among the therapeutic effects of medications, changes in feelings of emptiness or abandonment were not reported. These symptoms are an important target of treatment and would be important to note in managing the expectations of clinicians and people seeking and receiving care. We note this important limitation in these medication trials because they fail to address the components of self and interpersonal psychopathology of BPD that manifest in these core symptoms.

In a subsequent Cochrane Collaboration review, Stoffers et al. (2012) carefully assessed psychological therapies for BPD, describing 28 studies that included psychological treatment modalities such as DBT, schema-focused therapy, mentalization-based therapy, group therapy, and Systems Training for Emotional Predictability and Problem Solving. Examination of the articles shows that in some studies, many of the participants were receiving medications on entry and throughout the studies. This observation highlights the fact that because many people being treated for BPD are being prescribed medications even if they are being referred to psychotherapy treatment, the evidence for the efficacy of psychotherapy is not necessarily derived in isolation from pharmacological treatment and effects. An updated Cochrane review is planned with data results from that study not published at this time.

In the Netherlands, Ingenhoven et al. (2010) conducted a meta-analysis of 21 BPD medication treatment studies, with the intent of identifying high-quality clinical evidence. This analysis focused specifically on BPD domains, which included cognitive-perceptual symptoms, impulsive-behavioral dyscontrol, affective regulation, and global functioning. The studies under consideration in the analysis used placebo-controlled trials that included participants with BPD and/or STPD. The authors reported a moderate to very large effect of mood stabilizers on impulsive-behavioral dyscontrol, anger, and anxiety, and a moderate effect on depression (Table 17–1). For antipsychotic medications, a moderate effect was seen on cognitive-perceptual disturbances and a moderate to large effect was seen on anger. For the antidepressants, there were small effects on anxiety and anger. The authors concluded that this analysis supports the use of medications to target specific symptom domains, a finding that is consistent with the American Psychiatric Association (2001) guideline, discussed at the beginning of this subsection. The Dutch have developed a clinical guideline that approaches BPD management through the use of hierarchical symptom-targeted treatment algorithms (Trimbos-Instituut 2008).

In the United Kingdom, the National Collaborating Centre for Mental Health (2009) issued its National Institute for Health and Clinical Excellence (NICE; now National Institute for Health and Care Excellence) guidelines for the treatment and management of BPD to equip clinicians practicing through the governmental health care system. The guidelines describe strategies for improved access to care, the importance of therapeutic relationships, patient autonomy and choice, and service planning in the community. The guidelines also clearly state, however, that the existing level of evidence for the use of medication in the treatment of BPD does not yet meet the standard needed in order to recommend use. The guidelines also nonempirically describe using sedating antihistamines, such as hydroxyzine, to assist in immediate crisis or insomnia. NICE has planned an exceptional surveillance review, due in 2021, to consider the potential impact on their guidelines of the implementation of ICD-11 and resulting changes in personality disorder classification.

The National Health and Medical Research Council (2012) of Australia guideline contained 63 recommendations for comprehensive patient care, including those related to diagnosis, treatment, management, and information for caregivers. The guideline stated that persons with BPD should be referred to structured psychotherapies designed for BPD and should be offered choices. Regarding medication treatment, the guideline noted that medication should not be used as a primary therapy for BPD because of effects that are modest, inconsistent, and not helpful for modifying the course of the disorder, although short-term use of medication as an adjunct to psychological therapy to manage specific symptoms may be considered. Similar to the NICE guidelines (National Collaborating Centre for Mental Health 2009), this guideline rec-

TABLE 17–1. Results of a meta-analysis of controlled trials of medications in the treatment of borderline personality disorder

Medication class	Target domains (effect size)	Medication (major trials)	Dosage range (mg/day)	Major side effects
Antipsychotics	Anger (moderate/large) Cognitive-perceptual (moderate)	Haloperidol Olanzapine Aripiprazole Risperidone	4–16 2.5–20 15 0.25–2	Weight gain, hyperlipidemia, diabetes mellitus, dystonia, tardive dyskinesia, neuroleptic malignant syndrome
Anticonvulsant mood stabilizers	Impulsive-behavioral dyscontrol (very large) Anger (very large) Anxiety (large) Depressed mood (moderate)	Valproate Lamotrigine Carbamazepine Topiramate	500 (or plasma level) 50–200 820 (or plasma level) 25–250	Dizziness, drowsiness, fatigue, tremor, weight gain, Stevens-Johnson syndrome, cognitive problems
Antidepressants	Anxiety (small) Depressed mood (small)	Phenelzine Fluoxetine Fluvoxamine Desipramine Tranylcypromine Amitriptyline	60–90 20–80 150 163 40 100–175	Nausea, constipation, dry mouth, agitation, irritability, loss of sexual desire and impairment in sexual functioning

Source. Adapted from Ingenhoven et al. 2010.

ommended that medications be used in acute crisis situations and discontinued after the crisis is resolved. The National Health and Medical Research Council guideline for management of borderline personality disorder stands rescinded at this time and is available only in the Australian government web archives.

The most recent guidelines from Europe are from 2018. The Swiss Association for Psychiatry and Psychotherapy Task Force issued guidelines, available in French and German, on management of PDs that mentioned the use of low-dose medications in critical situations and for a short time span, and also discussed a symptom-focused hierarchical organization of medication use. Lamotrigine and topiramate are advised for anger, aggression, and impulsivity. The task force also recommended quetiapine and aripiprazole for irritability and cognitive-perceptive symptoms. Of note is the strong recommendation to avoid benzodiazepines in the PD population (Euler et al. 2018)

Future Directions in Pharmacological Research in Personality Disorders

Even though the field of pharmacological treatment of PDs has advanced in many ways, with a significant number of clinical trials, specific and objective rating scales, and meta-analytic comparisons, myriad issues remain to be addressed. These include the following:

- In the study of PDs, there has been an emergence of the concept of *symptom domains* within the PDs, perhaps most frequently in BPD, and new analyses of clinical trials point to efficacy in specific symptom domains of PDs (e.g., affective instability) rather than in the treatment of the overall PD.
- With advances in neuroimaging and improving understanding of neural circuits, biological constructs are possible treatment targets. Perez et al. (2016) showed frontolimbic circuit changes and associated clinical improvement with transference-focused psychotherapy in BPD.
- For major psychiatric disorders, elaborate trials have been performed to examine the effects of medication alone versus medication plus specific therapies. Hogarty et al. (1986) showed that combined medication and therapy was better than medicine alone in the treatment of schizophrenia. However, at this point there is very little similar research for PDs.
- Very few new randomized controlled trials of pharmacotherapy for PDs have been conducted in the last decade, and several authors, including Ingenhoven (2015) and Paris (2015), have decried the overmedication of people receiving care for PDs. Good psychiatric management is strongly recommended, and there is growing evidence (Finch et al. 2019) that treatment as usual in the absence of specialized care can be a practical and effective option (see also Chapter 15, "Good Psychiatric Management: Generalist Treatments and Stepped Care for Borderline Personality Disorder," in this volume). Treatment as usual involves nonspecific interventions as opposed to manualized and standardized psychotherapies for BPD. With increasing knowledge about BPD among providers, the quality of nonspecific interventions has also improved. Separating treatment effects in that context, and with established strong placebo responses, will be challenging.

- For major psychiatric disorders, there has been continued exploration of the length of time to use medication treatment, yet in PDs there has been no similar empirical assessment.
- Although men and women are both affected by BPD, evidence suggests that the level of disability and psychopathology may be somewhat different. These differences have yet to be fully explored in the medication treatment literature.
- Clinical trials in BPD have tended to recruit *symptomatic volunteers*. There has been considerable controversy regarding potential differences in study outcome based on whether the participant was obtained through newspaper advertisements or recruited from clinics or inpatient units, as was also highlighted in the LABILE study (Crawford et al. 2018).
- Existing clinical trial methodology utilizes a variety of instruments to measure specific traits associated with PDs, and the field would benefit from agreed-on assessments to better compare trial data (Zanarini et al. 2010).
- DSM5 has retained the diagnostic criteria for PDs that appeared in DSM-IV (American Psychiatric Association 1994); however, DSM-5 Section III, "Emerging Measures and Models," contains proposed major changes to the criteria and categorization of PDs. (See Chapter 4, "The Alternative DSM-5 Model for Personality Disorders," in this volume.) The impact and application of existing research on this new model remain to be determined. Reconceptualization based on dimensional assessments of level of personality functioning in the aspects of identity, self-direction, empathy, and intimacy, along with trait measures of negative affect, detachment, antagonism, disinhibition, and psychoticism, as described in the alternative model, might change sample populations and also the target treatment outcomes.

Clinical Approaches

Although the various clinical practice guidelines may diverge on the subject of medication therapy indications and practices, all agree on the importance of skillful and effective treatment of people living with PDs. A careful psychiatric evaluation, which includes assessment of the presence of all psychiatric disorders, including comorbid PDs, will serve to inform management decisions and expectations. PDs are also often comorbid with other psychiatric disorders, including major depression, bipolar disorder, attention-deficit/hyperactivity disorder, and posttraumatic stress disorder. These comorbid disorders require identification and treatment; however, the presence of a PD has been noted to confer aspects of treatment resistance (Feske et al. 2004). This finding highlights the importance of identifying and treating comorbid personality and other disorders concurrently. It is of critical importance to correctly discriminate BPD from other types of mood disorders, such as major depression or bipolar disorder, or to identify the comorbid presence of both, because there are significant differences in treatment approaches and divergence in the weight placed on the role of pharmacotherapy.

Cultivation of healthy therapeutic relationships in which people are educated about their diagnoses and provided with autonomy and shared decision making will improve chances of recovery, based on clinical experience. People living with BPD benefit from diagnosis disclosure, which can often be facilitated through use of a symptom screening tool, such as the McLean Screening Instrument for Borderline Personality Disorder (Zanarini et al. 2003a). Symptoms can be followed over time with use of a continuous rating scale, such as the ZAN-BPD (Zanarini et al. 2003b). Zanarini and Frankenburg (2008) demonstrated a significant reduction in the core BPD symptoms of impulsivity and relationship conflict in participants provided with psychoeducation shortly after disclosure of the diagnosis compared with those on a wait-list, highlighting the critical role of informing and teaching people about their diagnosis.

People living with PDs have been known to present in acute distress or crisis. The level of affective intensity tends to prompt a pattern of adding or increasing medications, which may result in long medication lists that increase the risk of side effects, medication interactions, and expense, and that may negatively impact quality of life. Approaching people in a manner that is responsive and validates their distress while avoiding reactively adding or increasing a medication during a crisis has been noted clinically to stabilize the treatment course (Nelson and Schulz 2011). Iatrogenic harm has unfortunately played a role historically in well-meaning attempts to provide care for people living with PDs. A qualitative study of interviews with psychiatrists (Martean and Evans 2014) noted four main themes in the relational process of prescribing medications to people with BPD. Themes elaborated were 1) difficulty collaborating in emotionally charged consultations, 2) feelings of helplessness when the provider was unable to relieve suffering, 3) effects of discontinuity in the doctor-patient relationship, and 4) role of the drug as a facilitator in the doctor-patient relationship. These issues highlight the need for more support and training for psychiatrists in better understanding the dynamics of a medication management visit.

Many clinicians have noted that people being treated for BPD tend to be sensitive to side effects, and the general wisdom is to start at a low dose and titrate over time on the basis of tolerability of the medications. Even with the low doses of antipsychotic medication used for BPD, it is recommended to monitor movement disorder side effects and to assess and follow metabolic issues such as weight gain, diabetes mellitus, and other cardiovascular and metabolic side effects. Compliance and suicidal ideation are also necessary elements of care that require close monitoring and regular follow-up, ideally in a multidisciplinary manner through coordination with the primary care provider. Helping people receiving care for BPD to understand that medication will be used to target a problematic symptom domain, with the goal of facilitating recovery and emotional development, will help to set the stage for an understanding that future crises are to be expected and not necessarily representative of medication or psychotherapeutic treatment failure. Identifying the symptom domain that poses the most difficulty for a person experiencing symptoms can facilitate a discussion in which an evidence-based medication may be selected and titrated over time (Table 17–2). In patients with multiple symptom domains, we recommend identifying the domains associated with greatest functional impairment to guide treatment.

Case Example

Yvette is a 25-year-old college student referred to the psychiatry clinic by her primary care provider. She had been treated by her primary care provider for anxiety but wonders if she "might actually have bipolar disorder" and is seeking the opinion of a psy-

TABLE 17–2. Recommended medications for symptom domains in borderline personality disorder

Symptom domain	Effective medication class	Medication used	Dosage range (mg/day)	Treatment goals/comments
Cognitive-perceptual symptoms (e.g., hallucinations, paranoia, severe dissociation)	Antipsychotics	*Typical* Haloperidol *Atypical* Aripiprazole Risperidone Quetiapine Clozapine	 4–16 2.5 0.5–1 25–150 12.5–100	Start at low dose and continue as maintenance till therapeutic goals met. Taper in 6 months to 2 years. Chronic symptoms may need long-term medication.
Impulsive-behavioral dyscontrol (e.g., self-injury, aggression, risky behavior)	Mood stabilizers	Lithium	300–600	Response at lower doses. No target blood levels. Lithium possibly protective against suicide. Newer evidence less convincing for anticonvulsant use. No definitive evidence for antidepressant/anxiolytic medication.
Affective dysregulation (e.g., depressed mood, mood fluctuations, anger, anxiety, rejection sensitivity)	Mood stabilizers Antipsychotics	Lithium *Typical* Haloperidol *Atypical* Aripiprazole Risperidone Quetiapine Clozapine	300–600 4–16 2.5 0.5–1 25–150 12.5–100	Response at lower doses. No target blood levels. Start at low dose and continue as maintenance until therapeutic goals are met. Taper in 6 months to 2 years. Consider long-term risks of antipsychotic use.

chiatrist. She describes a long history of intense anxiety; she says, "I've always been this way." Her anxiety prompts mood swings, especially when she is talking with others on the phone or in person. She is frequently irritable and angry and has not been able to continue her part-time work in the same setting for more than 1 year. She has had frequent relationships with men that rarely last beyond 6 weeks. Yvette describes these relationships as becoming serious quickly and then ending suddenly without reason. She worries that her mental health and anxiety play a role in this pattern. She frequently stays up late wondering if people are angry with her and wondering what she has done wrong to lead to her multiple perceived failures. She has considered suicide, usually in the period following a breakup, and she has scars on her wrists and thighs from self-injury from early in college, but none from the past year. She avoids alcohol because her mother "was an alcoholic." She denies grandiosity or ever having a decreased need for sleep. When asked about elevated mood, she describes a period of elation lasting 3–4 hours, which occurred after she received a compliment. She has never experienced delusions, but she does describe frequent mistrust of others' intentions and worries that people will leave her based on her prior experiences. She also describes frequent periods of intense sadness prompted by interpersonal circumstances, which improve if others work to help her feel better. She states, "My moods are all over the place, and I can't live this way."

Her primary care provider had initiated citalopram 20 mg/day to help with anxiety and depression and recently prescribed lorazepam 1 mg three times daily as needed to offer additional treatment of anxiety symptoms, which had not improved after 6 weeks of treatment with citalopram. Yvette states that the citalopram causes nausea, has reduced her sex drive, and has not helped with her symptoms. She notes that the lorazepam is very helpful for 2–3 hours after taking the medication, but that she has had more angry outbursts and recently experienced increased urges toward self-injury. On the basis of these worsening symptoms, she observes that the lorazepam may need to be increased to better manage her anxiety.

As part of the diagnostic discussion, the psychiatrist offers Yvette a symptom screen for BPD. Yvette reads over the symptoms, looks up from the page, and states, "These symptoms perfectly describe me. What is this?" She is provided with education about the symptoms and hopeful prognosis of BPD. The psychiatrist has prepared a handout of reputable resources and websites for people to learn more about this disorder. Yvette is referred to psychotherapy and considers this option, but she is highly interested in pursuing medication treatment for her symptoms. The psychiatrist validates Yvette's response to lorazepam, acknowledging that this medication is helpful in temporarily relieving anxiety symptoms, but problems with its long-term use, such as tolerance, physiological dependency, disinhibitory effects, and impact on learning, indicate that it would seem reasonable to begin a slow taper of this medication. Yvette is initially reluctant but trusts this recommendation because of her strong agreement with the diagnosis. The psychiatrist provides coaching on breathing retraining to assist in the management of acute anxiety symptoms. Yvette identifies her primary problematic symptom as being affective instability. The risks and benefits of anticonvulsant mood-stabilizing medication are discussed, and Yvette opts to begin treatment with lamotrigine. The clinician gives Yvette the option of either continuing or discontinuing the citalopram, and Yvette decides to discontinue this medication. A follow-up session is scheduled for 2 weeks later. Yvette agrees to complete a symptom tracking card to monitor her symptoms and agrees to look into the feasibility of initiating a structured, evidence-based psychotherapy for the treatment of BPD.

Conclusion

Medications for the treatment of people living with PDs have been tried and evaluated for over 50 years. With the emergence of the Diagnostic Interview for Borderlines and DSM-III, clinical trials in PDs—mostly BPD and STPD—increased in pace. In this chapter, the results of studies using major classes of medications have been described and guidance regarding the practical management of medication treatment has been provided. Because the clinical trials mainly focused on diagnostic criteria and did not show large effect sizes, meta-analytic studies of trait and symptom domains have been reviewed, with results that may be very helpful in clinical decision making. Although more data and methods of analysis are available now than in the past, many issues remain that need to be addressed to lead to best treatments.

References

Adityanjee A, Romine A, Brown E, et al: Quetiapine in patients with borderline personality disorder: an open-label trial. Ann Clin Psychiatry 20:219–226, 2008

Albert N, Glenthøj LB, Melau M, et al: Course of illness in a sample of patients diagnosed with a schizotypal disorder and treated in a specialized early intervention setting: findings from the 3.5-year follow-up of the OPUS II study. Schizophr Res 182:24–30, 2017

American Psychiatric Association: Diagnostic and Statistical Manual of Mental Disorders, 3rd Edition. Washington, DC, American Psychiatric Association, 1980

American Psychiatric Association: Diagnostic and Statistical Manual of Mental Disorders, 4th Edition. Washington, DC, American Psychiatric Association, 1994

American Psychiatric Association: Practice guideline for the treatment of patients with borderline personality disorder. Am J Psychiatry 158 (10 suppl):1–52, 2001

American Psychiatric Association: Diagnostic and Statistical Manual of Mental Disorders, 5th Edition. Arlington, VA, American Psychiatric Association, 2013

Asnis GM, Henderson MA: EMSAM (deprenyl patch): how a promising antidepressant was underutilized. Neuropsychiatr Dis Treat 10:1911–1923, 2014

Ballenger JC, Post RM: Therapeutic effects of carbamazepine in affective illness: a preliminary report. Commun Psychopharmacol 2:159–175, 1978

Bateman A, Fonagy P: Eight-year follow-up of patients treated for borderline personality disorder: mentalization-based treatment versus treatment as usual. Am J Psychiatry 165:631–638, 2008

Bellino S, Paradiso E, Bogetto F: Oxcarbazepine in the treatment of borderline personality disorder: a pilot study. J Clin Psychiatry 66:1111–1115, 2005

Bellino S, Bozzatello P, Rinaldi C, Bogetto F: Paliperidone ER in the treatment of borderline personality disorder: a pilot study of efficacy and tolerability. Depress Res Treat 2011:680194, 2011

Bellino S, Bozzatello P, Rocca G, Bogetto F: Efficacy of omega-3 fatty acids in the treatment of borderline personality disorder: a study of the association with valproic acid. J Psychopharmacol 28:125–132, 2014

Benedetti F, Sforzini L, Colombo C, et al: Low-dose clozapine in acute and continuation treatment of severe borderline personality disorder. J Clin Psychiatry 59:103–107, 1998

Bogenschutz MP, Nurnberg HG: Olanzapine versus placebo in the treatment of borderline personality disorder. J Clin Psychiatry 65:104–109, 2004

Bozzatello P, Rocca P, Uscinska M, Bellino S: Efficacy and tolerability of asenapine compared with olanzapine in borderline personality disorder: an open-label randomized controlled trial. CNS Drugs 31:809–819, 2017

Brinkley JR, Beitman BD, Friedel RO: Low-dose neuroleptic regimens in the treatment of borderline patients. Arch Gen Psychiatry 36:319–326, 1979

Calabrese JR, Bowden CL, Sachs GS, et al: A double-blind placebo-controlled study of lamotrigine monotherapy in outpatients with bipolar I depression. Lamictal 602 Study Group. J Clin Psychiatry 60:79–88, 1999

Coccaro EF, Kavoussi RJ: Biological and pharmacological aspects of borderline personality disorder. Hosp Community Psychiatry 42:1029–1033, 1991

Coccaro EF, Kavoussi RJ: Fluoxetine and impulsive aggressive behavior in personality-disordered subjects. Arch Gen Psychiatry 54:1081–1088, 1997

Coccaro EF, Kavoussi RJ, Hauger RL: Serotonin function and antiaggressive response to fluoxetine: a pilot study. Biol Psychiatry 42:546–552, 1997

Cornelius JR, Soloff PH, Perel JM, et al: Fluoxetine trial in borderline personality disorder. Psychopharmacol Bull 26:151–154, 1990

Cowdry RW, Gardner DL: Pharmacotherapy of borderline personality disorder: alprazolam, carbamazepine, trifluoperazine, and tranylcypromine. Arch Gen Psychiatry 45:111–119, 1988

Crawford MJ, Sanatinia R, Barrett B, et al: The clinical effectiveness and cost-effectiveness of lamotrigine in borderline personality disorder: a randomized placebo-controlled trial. Am J Psychiatry 175:756–764, 2018

de la Fuente JM, Lotstra F: A trial of carbamazepine in borderline personality disorder. Eur Neuropsychopharmacol 4:479–486, 1994

Derogatis LR, Lipman RS, Covi L: The SCL-90: an outpatient psychiatric rating scale. Psychopharmacol Bull 9:13–28, 1973

Díaz-Marsá M, Galian M, Montes A, et al: Long-acting injectable risperidone in treatment resistant borderline personality disorder: a small series report (in Spanish). Actas Esp Psiquiatr 36:70–74, 2008

Dickens GL, Frogley C, Mason F, et al: Experiences of women in secure care who have been prescribed clozapine for borderline personality disorder. Borderline Personal Disord Emot Dysregul 3:12, 2016

Ekselius L, Herlofsson J, Palmstierna T, et al: Personlighetssyndrom: Kiniska Riktlinjer för Utredning Och Behandling. Stockholm, Gothia Förlag AB, 2017

Euler S, Dammann G, Endtner K, et al: Borderline-Störung: Behandlungsempfehlungen der SGPP. Psychiatr Psychother 169:135–143, 2018

Feske U, Mulsant BH, Pilkonis PA, et al: Clinical outcome of ECT in patients with major depression and comorbid borderline personality disorder. Am J Psychiatry 161:2073–2080, 2004

Finch EF, Iliakis EA, Masland SR, Choi-Kain LW: A meta-analysis of treatment as usual for borderline personality disorder. Personal Disord 10:491–499, 2019

Frankenburg FR, Zanarini MC: Clozapine treatment of borderline patients: a preliminary study. Compr Psychiatry 34:402–405, 1993

Frankenburg FR, Zanarini MC: Divalproex sodium treatment of women with borderline personality disorder and bipolar II disorder: a double-blind placebo-controlled pilot study. J Clin Psychiatry 63:442–446, 2002

Frogley C, Anagnostakis K, Mitchell S, et al: A case series of clozapine for borderline personality disorder. Ann Clin Psychiatry 25:125–134, 2013

Gardner DL, Cowdry RW: Alprazolam-induced dyscontrol in borderline personality disorder. Am J Psychiatry 142:98–100, 1985

Goldberg SC, Schulz SC, Schulz PM, et al: Borderline and schizotypal personality disorders treated with low-dose thiothixene vs placebo. Arch Gen Psychiatry 43:680–686, 1986

Goyer PF, Berridge MS, Morris ED, et al: PET measurement of neuroreceptor occupancy by typical and atypical neuroleptics. J Nucl Med 37:1122–1127, 1996

Grosjean B, Tsai GE: NMDA neurotransmission as a critical mediator of borderline personality disorder. J Psychiatry Neurosci 32:103–115, 2007

Gunderson JG, Choi-Kain LW: Medication management for patients with borderline personality disorder. Am J Psychiatry 175:709–711, 2018

Gunderson JG, Kolb JE, Austin V: The diagnostic interview for borderline patients. Am J Psychiatry 138:896–903, 1981

Hogarty GE, Anderson CM, Reiss DJ, et al: Family psychoeducation, social skills training, and maintenance chemotherapy in the aftercare treatment of schizophrenia, I: one-year effects of a controlled study on relapse and expressed emotion. Arch Gen Psychiatry 43:633–642, 1986

Hollander E, Allen A, Lopez RP, et al: A preliminary double-blind, placebo-controlled trial of divalproex sodium in borderline personality disorder. J Clin Psychiatry 62:199–203, 2001

Hollander E, Swann AC, Coccaro EF, et al: Impact of trait impulsivity and state aggression on divalproex versus placebo response in borderline personality disorder. Am J Psychiatry 162:621–624, 2005

Hymowitz P, Frances A, Jacobsberg LB, et al: Neuroleptic treatment of schizotypal personality disorders. Compr Psychiatry 27:267–271, 1986

Ingenhoven T: Pharmacotherapy for borderline patients: business as usual or by default? J Clin Psychiatry 76:e522–523, 2015

Ingenhoven T, Lafay P, Rinne T, et al: Effectiveness of pharmacotherapy for severe personality disorders: meta-analyses of randomized controlled trials. J Clin Psychiatry 71:14–25, 2010

Kane J, Honigfeld G, Singer J, et al: Clozapine for the treatment-resistant schizophrenic: a double-blind comparison with chlorpromazine. Arch Gen Psychiatry 45:789–796, 1988

Kane JM, Carson WH, Saha AR, et al: Efficacy and safety of aripiprazole and haloperidol versus placebo in patients with schizophrenia and schizoaffective disorder. J Clin Psychiatry 63:763–771, 2002

Keshavan M, Shad M, Soloff P, et al: Efficacy and tolerability of olanzapine in the treatment of schizotypal personality disorder. Schizophr Res 71:97–101, 2004

Khalifa N, Duggan C, Stoffers J, et al: Pharmacological interventions for antisocial personality disorder. Cochrane Database Syst Rev (8):CD007667, 2010

Koenigsberg HW, Reynolds D, Goodman M, et al: Risperidone in the treatment of schizotypal personality disorder. J Clin Psychiatry 64:628–634, 2003

Kolb JE, Gunderson JG: Diagnosing borderline patients with a semistructured interview. Arch Gen Psychiatry 37:37–41, 1980

Kulkarni J, Thomas N, Hudaib AR, et al: Effect of the glutamate NMDA receptor antagonist memantine as adjunctive treatment in borderline personality disorder: an exploratory, randomised, double-blind, placebo-controlled trial. CNS Drugs 32:179–187, 2018

Lekka NP, Paschalis C, Beratis S: Suicide attempts in high-dose benzodiazepine users. Compr Psychiatry 43:438–442, 2002

Linehan MM, Armstrong HE, Suarez A, et al: Cognitive-behavioral treatment of chronically parasuicidal borderline patients. Arch Gen Psychiatry 48:1060–1064, 1991

Linehan MM, McDavid JD, Brown MZ, et al: Olanzapine plus dialectical behavior therapy for women with high irritability who meet criteria for borderline personality disorder: a double-blind, placebo-controlled pilot study. J Clin Psychiatry 69:999–1005, 2008

Links PS, Mitton JE, Steiner M: Predicting outcome for borderline personality disorder. Compr Psychiatry 31:490–498, 1990

Loew TH, Nickel MK, Muehlbacher M, et al: Topiramate treatment for women with borderline personality disorder: a double-blind, placebo-controlled study. J Clin Psychopharmacol 26:61–66, 2006

Loring DW, Williamson DJ, Meador KJ, et al: Topiramate dose effects on cognition: a randomized double-blind study. Neurology 76:131–137, 2011

Markovitz PJ, Wagner SC: Venlafaxine in the treatment of borderline personality disorder. Psychopharmacol Bull 31:773–777, 1995

Markovitz PJ, Calabrese JR, Schulz SC, et al: Fluoxetine in the treatment of borderline and schizotypal personality disorders. Am J Psychiatry 148:1064–1067, 1991

Martean L, Evans C: Prescribing for personality disorder: qualitative study of interviews with general and forensic consultant psychiatrists. Psychiatr Bull 38:116–121, 2014

Moeller KE, Din A, Wolfe M, Holmes G: Psychotropic medication use in hospitalized patients with borderline personality disorder. Ment Health Clin 6:68–74, 2016

National Collaborating Centre for Mental Health: Borderline Personality Disorder: The NICE Guideline on Treatment and Management (National Clinical Practice Guideline No 78). London, RCPsych Publications, 2009

National Health and Medical Research Council: Clinical Practice Guideline for Management of Borderline Personality Disorder. Melbourne, Australia, National Health and Medical Research Council, 2012

Nelson KJ, Schulz SC: Pharmacotherapy for borderline personality disorder. Current Psychiatry 10:30–40, 2011

Nickel C, Lahmann C, Tritt K, et al: Topiramate in treatment of depressive and anger symptoms in female depressive patients: a randomized, double-blind, placebo-controlled study. J Affect Disord 87:243–252, 2005

Nickel MK, Nickel C, Mitterlehner FO, et al: Topiramate treatment of aggression in female borderline personality disorder patients: a double-blind, placebo-controlled study. J Clin Psychiatry 65:1515–1519, 2004

Nickel MK, Nickel C, Kaplan P, et al: Treatment of aggression with topiramate in male borderline patients: a double-blind, placebo-controlled study. Biol Psychiatry 57:495–499, 2005

Nickel MK, Muehlbacher M, Nickel C, et al: Aripiprazole in the treatment of patients with borderline personality disorder: a double-blind, placebo-controlled study. Am J Psychiatry 163:833–838, 2006

Nickel MK, Loew TH, Pedrosa Gil F: Aripiprazole in treatment of borderline patients, part II: an 18-month follow-up. Psychopharmacology (Berl) 191:1023–1026, 2007

Okuma T: Therapeutic and prophylactic effects of carbamazepine in bipolar disorders. Psychiatr Clin North Am 6:157–174, 1983

Palomares N, Montes A, Díaz-Marsá M, Carrasco JL: Effectiveness of long-acting paliperidone palmitate in borderline personality disorder. Int Clin Psychopharmacol 30:338–341, 2015

Paris J: Making psychotherapy for borderline personality disorder accessible. Ann Clin Psychiatry 27:297–301, 2015

Paton C, Crawford MJ, Bhatti SF, et al: The use of psychotropic medication in patients with emotionally unstable personality disorder under the care of UK mental health services. J Clin Psychiatry 76:e512–e518, 2015

Perez DL, Vago DR, Pan H, et al: Frontolimbic neural circuit changes in emotional processing and inhibitory control associated with clinical improvement following transference-focused psychotherapy in borderline personality disorder. Psychiatry Clin Neurosci 70:51–61, 2016

Peris L, Szerman N, Ruíz M: Efficacy and safety of gabapentin in borderline personality disorder: a six-month, open-label study (in Spanish). Vertex 18:418–422, 2007

Pinto OC, Akiskal HS: Lamotrigine as a promising approach to borderline personality: an open case series without concurrent DSM-IV major mood disorder. J Affect Disord 51:333–343, 1998

Post RM, Rubinow DR, Ballenger JC: Conditioning and sensitization in the longitudinal course of affective illness. Br J Psychiatry 149:191–201, 1986

Ravaris CL, Nies A, Robinson DS, et al: A multiple-dose, controlled study of phenelzine in depression-anxiety states. Arch Gen Psychiatry 33:347–350, 1976

Reich DB, Zanarini MC, Bieri KA: A preliminary study of lamotrigine in the treatment of affective instability in borderline personality disorder. Int Clin Psychopharmacol 24:270–275, 2009

Rifkin A, Quitkin F, Carrillo C, et al: Lithium carbonate in emotionally unstable character disorder. Arch Gen Psychiatry 27:519–523, 1972

Rocca P, Marchiaro L, Cocuzza E, et al: Treatment of borderline personality disorder with risperidone. J Clin Psychiatry 63:241–244, 2002

Rohde C, Polcwiartek C, Correll CU, Nielsen J: Real-world effectiveness of clozapine for borderline personality disorder: results from a 2-year mirror-image study. J Pers Disord 32:823–837, 2018

Rombold F, Lauterbach E, Felber W, et al: Adjunctive lithium treatment in the prevention of suicidal behavior in patients with depression and comorbid personality disorders. Int J Psychiatry Clin Pract 18:300–303, 2014

Salzman C, Wolfson AN, Schatzberg A, et al: Effect of fluoxetine on anger in symptomatic volunteers with borderline personality disorder. J Clin Psychopharmacol 15:23–29, 1995

Schulz SC, Camlin KL, Berry SA, et al: A double-blind study of risperidone for BPD (NR270), in 1998 New Research Program and Abstracts, American Psychiatric Association 151st Annual Meeting, Toronto, Ontario, Canada, May 30–June 4, 1998. Washington, DC, American Psychiatric Association, 1998

Schulz SC, Zanarini MC, Bateman A, et al: Olanzapine for the treatment of borderline personality disorder: variable dose 12-week randomised double-blind placebo-controlled study. Br J Psychiatry 193:485–492, 2008

Serban G, Siegel S: Response of borderline and schizotypal patients to small doses of thiothixene and haloperidol. Am J Psychiatry 141:1455–1458, 1984

Simpson EB, Yen S, Costello E, et al: Combined dialectical behavior therapy and fluoxetine in the treatment of borderline personality disorder. J Clin Psychiatry 65:379–385, 2004

Small JG, Hirsch SR, Arvanitis LA, et al: Quetiapine in patients with schizophrenia: a high- and low-dose double-blind comparison with placebo. Seroquel Study Group. Arch Gen Psychiatry 54:549–557, 1997

Soler J, Pascual JC, Campins J, et al: Double-blind, placebo-controlled study of dialectical behavior therapy plus olanzapine for borderline personality disorder. Am J Psychiatry 162:1221–1224, 2005

Soloff PH, George A, Nathan RS, et al: Paradoxical effects of amitriptyline on borderline patients. Am J Psychiatry 143:1603–1605, 1986

Soloff PH, George A, Nathan S, et al: Amitriptyline versus haloperidol in borderlines: final outcomes and predictors of response. J Clin Psychopharmacol 9:238–246, 1989

Soloff PH, Cornelius J, George A, et al: Efficacy of phenelzine and haloperidol in borderline personality disorder. Arch Gen Psychiatry 50:377–385, 1993

Spielberger CD, Sydeman SJ, Owen AE, et al (eds): Measuring anxiety and anger with the State-Trait Anxiety Inventory (STAI) and the State-Trait Anger Expression Inventory (STAXI), in The Use of Psychological Testing for Treatment Planning and Outcomes Assessment, 2nd Edition. Mahwah, NJ, Erlbaum, 1999, pp 993–1021

Stoffers JM, Völlm BA, Rücker G, et al: Pharmacological interventions for borderline personality disorder. Cochrane Database Syst Rev (6):CD005653, 2010

Stoffers JM, Völlm BA, Rücker G, et al: Psychological therapies for people with borderline personality disorder. Cochrane Database Syst Rev (8):CD005652, 2012

Stone MH: Borderline personality disorder: clinical guidelines for treatment. Psychodyn Psychiatry 47:5–26, 2019

Tollefson GD, Beasley CM Jr, Tran PV, et al: Olanzapine versus haloperidol in the treatment of schizophrenia and schizoaffective and schizophreniform disorders: results of an international collaborative trial. Am J Psychiatry 154:457–465, 1997

Tondo L, Baldessarini RJ: Antisuicidal effects in mood disorders: are they unique to lithium? Pharmacopsychiatry 51:177–188, 2018

Trimbos-Instituut: Practice Guideline on Diagnosis and Treatment of Adult Patients With a Personality Disorder (in Dutch). Utrecht, The Netherlands, Trimbos-Instituut, 2008

Tritt K, Nickel C, Lahmann C, et al: Lamotrigine treatment of aggression in female borderline-patients: a randomized, double-blind, placebo-controlled study. J Psychopharmacol 19:287–291, 2005

Zalsman G, Hawton K, Wasserman D, et al: Suicide prevention strategies revisited: 10-year systematic review. Lancet Psychiatry 3:646–659, 2016

Zanarini MC, Frankenburg FR: Olanzapine treatment of female borderline personality disorder patients: a double-blind, placebo-controlled pilot study. J Clin Psychiatry 62:849–854, 2001

Zanarini MC, Frankenburg FR: Omega-3 fatty acid treatment of women with borderline personality disorder: a double-blind, placebo-controlled pilot study. Am J Psychiatry 160:167–169, 2003

Zanarini MC, Frankenburg FR: A preliminary, randomized trial of psychoeducation for women with borderline personality disorder. J Pers Disord 22:284–290, 2008

Zanarini MC, Vujanovic AA, Parachini EA, et al: A screening measure for BPD: the McLean Screening Instrument for Borderline Personality Disorder (MSI-BPD). J Pers Disord 17:568–573, 2003a

Zanarini MC, Vujanovic AA, Parachini EA, et al: Zanarini Rating Scale for Borderline Personality Disorder (ZAN-BPD): a continuous measure of DSM-IV borderline psychopathology. J Pers Disord 17:233–242, 2003b

Zanarini MC, Frankenburg FR, Parachini EA: A preliminary, randomized trial of fluoxetine, olanzapine, and the olanzapine-fluoxetine combination in women with borderline personality disorder. J Clin Psychiatry 65:903–907, 2004

Zanarini MC, Stanley B, Black DW, et al: Methodological considerations treatment trials for persons with personality disorder. Ann Clin Psychiatry 22:75–83, 2010

Zanarini MC, Schulz SC, Detke HC, et al: A dose comparison of olanzapine for the treatment of borderline personality disorder: a 12-week randomized, double-blind, placebo-controlled study. J Clin Psychiatry 72:1353–1362, 2011

Zanarini MC, Schulz SC, Detke H, et al: Open-label treatment with olanzapine for patients with borderline personality disorder. J Clin Psychopharmacol 32:398–402, 2012

Zarzar T, McEvoy J: Clozapine for self-injurious behavior in individuals with borderline personality disorder. Ther Adv Psychopharmacol 3:272–274, 2013

CHAPTER 18

Collaborative Treatment

Victoria Winkeller, M.D.
Abigail B. Schlesinger, M.D.

Increasing interest in collaboration across providers, provider types, disciplines, and specialties has resulted in many definitions of collaborative treatment. In this chapter, *collaborative treatment* refers to the treatment relationship that occurs when two or more treatment modalities are provided by more than one mental health or medical professional. When two providers are working with a patient with no collaboration or integration, which could be viewed as the most troublesome of shared care situations, so-called split treatment can occur. We reserve the term *split treatment* for situations in which lack of communication and/or agreement between providers causes a potential impasse in treatment.

In the most common form of collaborative treatment, one clinician prescribes psychotropic medication (or somatic treatments) and another performs psychotherapy. In psychiatry, collaborative treatment often involves a psychiatrist prescribing psychiatric medication and another clinician (e.g., psychiatrist, psychologist, social worker, therapist, case manager) performing the therapy. Treatment can also be divided in many ways among the primary care provider physician, psychoanalysts, specialty medical doctors, psychiatrists, specialty psychiatrists, therapists, clinical nurse therapists, visiting nurses, physician assistants, case managers, different people and disciplines on an inpatient unit or in a partial hospital program, and many others. Increasingly, collaborative treatment has come to represent a situation in which a primary care provider prescribes psychotropic medication and a nonpsychiatric clinician conducts psychotherapy. Collaborative care models in which a psychiatrist provides consultation to a care manager, who along

Dr. Winkeller and Dr. Schlesinger would like to thank Dr. Kenneth Silk, who passed away April 18, 2016. He contributed to previous versions of this chapter. His commitment to helping patients struggling with mental health disorders was exceptional. He will be missed by his patients and by the many students and colleagues he mentored throughout the years.

with the primary care provider is systematically measuring the response of a patient to medication treatment, have gained increasing popularity in recent years because of evidence of their effectiveness (Gilbody et al. 2006) as well as the increasing necessity to meet the needs of more patients due to the Patient Protection and Affordable Care Act of 2010 (Donohue et al. 2010). The tenets described in this chapter should apply to these types of collaborative care models as well.

Use of the term *collaborative* highlights the need for treating clinicians to communicate and work together, because there are many legal, ethical, and treatment issues and pitfalls that can arise when more than one provider is involved in a person's treatment. Patients with personality disorders (PDs), especially those with emotional lability (Negative Affectivity), depressivity (Negative Affectivity), separation insecurity (Negative Affectivity), and hostility (Antagonism) (see Chapter 4, "The Alternative DSM-5 Model for Personality Disorders," in this volume), tend to "split" even without a "split" treatment relationship, and treaters must keep this propensity in mind when entering into a collaborative care model with another clinician for a patient with a PD. *Splitting*, in its most formal psychoanalytic sense, is a defensive process wherein a patient appears to attribute good characteristics almost exclusively to one person (or one provider of treatment) while attributing to the other person (treater) all bad or negative feelings. The patient appears to take the natural ambivalence one feels about almost all people and divide it into two packages—a positive package bestowed on one person and a negative package bestowed on another. Each package almost exclusively contains either good or bad attributes, rarely contaminated by the opposite attribute. In addition, the roles of "good" and "bad" treaters can shift back and forth over time, with the previously favored professional suddenly viewed negatively, and vice versa. Defensive splitting can be accompanied by *projective identification*, in which the patient projects disavowed aspects of himself or herself onto different treaters. The treaters, in turn, unconsciously identify with those projected characteristics and may experience pressure to respond accordingly (Gabbard 1989; Gabbard and Wilkinson 1994; Ogden 1982).

Case Example 1

Zia, a young woman diagnosed with borderline PD, was in psychotherapy with a psychologist and receiving medication from a psychiatrist. Zia had an extensive history of self-mutilating behavior. The psychologist was, even in his everyday interactions, quite restrained.

Zia was acutely aware of rejection, and she would call the psychiatrist to complain vociferously about her psychologist's lack of feeling or empathy. Every 6 or 9 months of this, she would try to convince the psychiatrist, whom she knew did psychodynamic psychotherapy, to take over all of her treatment. The psychiatrist always sent Zia back to discuss these issues with her psychologist, even though the psychiatrist was aware that many of the accusations made about the psychologist were, in some ways, not untrue.[1]

---

[1]This situation may occur frequently in collaborative treatment. The patient presents an observation about the collaborating psychotherapist that may be an astute and accurate perception of the psychotherapist. Despite the face validity of the observation, the psychiatrist must refrain from agreeing or disagreeing with the patient. Each patient brings his or her unique history and transference into play when making such observations, and a comment at this point might undermine that particular transferential process occurring in the psychotherapy.

As the therapy progressed, Zia's self-destructive behavior diminished and then eventually ceased as her interpersonal relationships grew more stable. Longer periods elapsed between her complaints about her psychologist, and eventually the complaints stopped. The treatment terminated successfully.

In this chapter, we discuss collaborative treatment in general and then collaborative treatment of patients with PDs. Much of what we address applies to any collaborative treatment, regardless of the patient's diagnosis, but the issues of collaboration are heightened when the patient has a diagnosis of a PD. Although the techniques, strategies, or issues presented are pertinent to many patients with PDs, they cannot be applied to all such patients because we often discuss treatments in which psychotherapy is conducted by one person and psychopharmacology is managed by another, and few data are available to support prescribing medications to patients with maladaptive personality functioning and traits.

Evidence for Effectiveness of Collaborative Care

Despite a lack of studies comparing behavioral health treatment delivered by more than one provider to that delivered by a sole provider (i.e., when a psychiatrist performs both therapy and medication management), the use of multiple providers in behavioral health treatment continues to increase. Although there are studies that compare the use of different pharmacological and nonpharmacological strategies (Greenblatt et al. 1965; Klerman 1990), either alone or in combination, none of them address the use of single versus multiple providers. In models in which a psychiatrist provides oversight of a care manager who is monitoring the response to a primarily pharmacological treatment, the "collaboration" is actually a typical consultative relationship. Patients who do not respond to the care manager intervention within a specified time often will be referred to a behavioral health provider, but the treatment results for the patients referred to the psychiatrist have not been well studied.

Collaborative care programs (CCPs) seek to improve the care of individuals with chronic and complicated illnesses, and nurses play a lead role in CCPs in their function as collaborative care managers. Stringer et al. (2015) developed a CCP as a treatment approach for individuals with severe PDs, specifically borderline PD or PD not otherwise specified, as an alternative to care as usual. This CCP was developed for patients no longer engaged in any form of psychotherapy. The components of the CCP included informing patients and their caregivers about the CCP and teaching the principles of autonomy and self-management. A team was formed that included the patient, caregiver(s), psychiatrist, and nurse(s). The patient described his or her treatment history, and a collaboration agreement was developed with the patient as the driver and the nurse the navigator. This approach allowed for shared decision making between the patient and the nurse and was designed to empower the patient to take the lead in the treatment. The treatment stage included early recognition of destructive behaviors, a relapse prevention plan, and problem solving, all part of a protocol that was taught to the nurses. The authors' preliminary results demonstrated a significant decrease in borderline symptoms within the CCP along with an increase in mental health utilization during the testing period (Stringer et al. 2015).

Angstman et al. (2017) did a retrospective review of patients in treatment with the collaborative care management (CCM) model within primary care practices and found that those with a personality disorder and major depressive disorder had worse CCM outcomes compared with those with only a depression diagnosis. The CCM model for depression treatment within primary care integrated a nurse care manager within the primary care practice; there was weekly psychiatry oversight, a depression registry and relapse prevention. Within the same institution, Solberg et al. (2018) examined the use of a CCM model for the treatment of patients with major depressive disorder with comorbid personality disorder compared with care as usual within primary care. The depression CCM model as designed by the authors' institution is based on the principle of shared decision making between patient and clinician. For patients with major depressive disorder and PD, clinical outcomes at 6 months were significantly improved when patients were treated with CCM; outcome was defined as remission of depressive symptoms or the presence of persistent depressive symptoms.

Many patients with PDs have complex biological and psychosocial issues and do not respond as well to medications as would patients with other primary diagnoses (except perhaps those with schizotypal PD [Duggan et al. 2008; Herpertz et al. 2007; Koenigsberg et al. 2003; Paris 2003; Soloff 1990, 1998]). Comorbidity is common in some personality disorders, though the presentations in these cases may be atypical. Treatment modalities beyond psychopharmacological treatment are necessary, and often each modality is provided by a different mental health professional. Thus, there are many clinical situations in which multimodal treatment implies and warrants collaboration between at least two mental health professionals.

Most current outcome studies in psychotherapy and psychopharmacology do not measure the effects of any treatment other than the one being studied. Surprisingly few studies—and even fewer randomized controlled trials—have compared psychotherapy alone, medication alone, and psychotherapy and medicine in combination to determine the differential efficacy or effectiveness (Browne et al. 2002). Studies of cognitive-behavioral therapy and nefazodone for depression (Keller et al. 2000) and cognitive-behavioral therapy and tricyclic antidepressants for panic disorder (Barlow et al. 2000) have yielded interesting findings about the course and continuation of response to specific interventions (Manber et al. 2003). de Jonghe et al. (2004) found equivalent results for groups of mildly to moderately depressed patients treated with psychotherapy (short-term psychodynamic supportive psychotherapy) or a combination of psychotherapy and psychopharmacology with antidepressants. More recently, per the 2010 American Psychiatric Association practice guideline for treatment of patients with major depressive disorder, the combination of psychotherapy and pharmacotherapy was found to be superior to either modality alone in several meta-analyses (American Psychiatric Association 2010).

Often patients with PDs are excluded from efficacy studies, or PDs are not assessed. Thus, for patients with PDs, no clear conclusions can be made concerning the effectiveness of medication versus psychotherapy. Furthermore, no conclusions about effectiveness or efficacy can be made if these treatments are combined. The exceptions are 1) the study by Kool et al. (2003), which found that patients with personality pathology and depression responded best to a combined approach of both psychopharmacology and psychotherapy, although personality pathology of patients with Cluster C diagnoses responded better than that of patients with Cluster B diagnoses;

2) the 12-week study by Soler et al. (2005), who found greater improvement in depression, anxiety, and impulsivity/aggression in patients assigned to dialectical behavior therapy (DBT) plus olanzapine than those assigned to DBT alone; and 3) the small study by Simpson et al. (2004), which randomly assigned patients to receive fluoxetine or placebo after completion of a course of DBT and found that those assigned to placebo had more positive pre/post treatment differences than those assigned to fluoxetine. None of these studies addressed the differential effectiveness of therapy and medication management performed by one provider versus two (or more) providers.

Importance of Collaborative Treatment in Current Personality Disorder Care

General Issues

A 1997 survey revealed that 38% of patients seen by a psychiatrist had been seen by another mental health professional in the prior 30 days (Pincus et al. 1999). Almost half of those patients seen by another mental health provider had received psychotherapy from that other provider. In more than two-thirds of the instances in which an additional mental health provider was caring for the patient, the psychiatrist indicated that he or she had discussed the diagnosis and/or treatment of the patient with this other provider. In an unpublished electronic survey conducted in 2010 by the American Psychiatric Association (involving 394 psychiatrists, representing a 14% response rate), 67% of the responding psychiatrists' patients received both psychotherapeutic and psychopharmacological treatment (West et al. 2012). Half of those patients received both modalities from the same psychiatrist. For almost half of the cases, the psychiatrist provided the pharmacological treatment while another clinician performed the therapy. In 2% of the cases, the psychiatrist was the therapist and another physician or psychiatrist managed the pharmacotherapy. Research suggests that about three-fourths of patients receive their antidepressants from their primary care physicians (up from 37.3% in 1987), and an increasing proportion of these prescriptions do not have a psychiatric diagnosis recorded in the medical record (Mojtabal and Olfson 2011).

Serotonin reuptake inhibitors are less complicated to prescribe, with fewer general side effects and less lethality, than tricyclic antidepressants (Healy 1997). Particularly with this class of medications, primary care physicians appear ready to provide the ongoing management of psychopharmacological medication in consultation with a psychiatrist. Although they do not always prescribe concurrent psychotherapy, a number of primary care physicians are collaborating with therapists of varying levels of training. An interesting triangular relationship can develop among a therapist, a primary care physician writing the prescriptions for psychotropic medication, and a psychiatrist for referral or collaboration. Smith (1989) noted, "In contemporary treatment situations that include a patient, a therapist, a pharmacotherapist, and a pill, the transference issues can become more complex than the landing patterns of airplanes at an overcrowded airport" (p. 80). Add a managed care utilization reviewer to the picture, and things really get complicated.

Managed care companies often believe that patients with PDs use too much or at least more than their share of treatment. One of the challenges associated with providing collaborative care for these patients is convincing utilization reviewers that more than one modality of care is needed. To avoid divergent reports that negatively affect the reimbursed care for the patient, it is best to designate one member of the team to report the progress of treatment and the treatment plan to the reviewer. In general, this designated "reporter" should be the psychiatrist.

Increasing Prescription of Antidepressants

Despite the lack of hard evidence for the benefits of psychopharmacology in PDs, the practice of prescribing antidepressants for a wide array of symptom complexes suggestive of depression continues to increase (Healy 1997). Although depression is prevalent among patients with PDs (Skodol et al. 1999), quite often the nature of the depression, especially among patients with Cluster B disorders, is not the classic psychophysiological presentation frequently seen in a major depressive episode (Silk 2010; Westen et al. 1992). There has been much debate about the type and nature of depression in patients with PDs. The effectiveness of antidepressants in treating depression in such patients is moderate at best, even as the number of patients given these medications is increasing (Paris 2003; Silk and Fuerino 2012). Many patients who may have been treated by psychotherapy alone in the past are now receiving psychopharmacological treatment as well. An emerging literature suggests that the use of antidepressants can be helpful in the treatment of specific symptom complexes, such as the use of selective serotonin reuptake inhibitors or mood stabilizers for impulsivity, affect lability, and aggression in patients with borderline PD, rather than the disorder itself (Coccaro and Kavoussi 1997; Coccaro et al. 1989; Cowdry and Gardner 1988; Fuerino and Silk 2011; Hollander et al. 2001, 2005; Loew et al. 2006; Markowitz 2001, 2004; Nickel et al. 2005; Rinne et al. 2002; Ripoll 2012; Salzman et al. 1995; Sheard et al. 1976; Silk and Fuerino 2012; Soloff 1998; Soloff et al. 1993; Tritt et al. 2005). The American Psychiatric Association's (2001) practice guideline for the treatment of patients with borderline PD recommends adjunctive treatment with selective serotonin reuptake inhibitors in a symptom-specific manner for patients with this disorder. This recommendation is based on evidence from several double-blind, placebo-controlled studies; a number of open studies; and clinical experience in conjunction with a relatively benign side-effect profile and risk of overdose (American Psychiatric Association 2001). Some strong evidence suggests that neuroleptics and atypical antipsychotics can be effective for patients with schizotypal and borderline PDs (Bogenschutz and Nurnberg 2004; Goldberg et al. 1986; Koenigsberg et al. 2003; Markowitz 2001, 2004; Nickel et al. 2006; Schulz and Camlin 1999; Soloff et al. 1986b, 1993; Zanarini and Frankenburg 2001). However, a more recent paper reviewed studies evaluating the use of second-generation antipsychotics in patients with a diagnosis of borderline PD and found that evidence supporting their use is lacking. That same article highlighted how this class of medication may be useful for targeting certain symptoms, such as depression or anger (Wasylyshen and Williams 2016).

Patients with PDs present with a complex admixture of symptoms and problems, some of which appear to arise from psychosocial issues and interpersonal events, whereas others appear more related to expressions of underlying traits such as baseline anxiety, emotional lability, and impulsivity (Livesley 2000; Livesley et al. 1998; Putnam and Silk 2005). When treatment is divided between two providers, the psychotherapist may believe that all problems arise from psychosocial issues and subtly demean, undermine, or dismiss the psychopharmacological treatment. Conversely, the psychopharmacologist may think that difficulties are due primarily to "trait expression" and that once the right combination of medications is discovered, all symptoms will be alleviated. The increasing use of polypharmacy in patients with PDs, despite limited to no evidence of effectiveness (Zanarini et al. 2003), can hopefully be abated with collaboration and communication among multiple providers (Silk 2011).

Strengths and Weaknesses of Collaborative Treatment

Collaborative treatment has many positive attributes, some of which have direct applicability to patients with personality pathology:

1. Collaborative treatment can provide the patient with both a clinician to idealize and a clinician to denigrate within one treatment relationship. Although this situation might at first appear to be problematic, it can be useful if both providers confer with each other and work to have the patient develop a more balanced view of each of them. For example, both treaters may have an opportunity to model more appropriate coping mechanisms for the patient, or the idealized provider might be able to work with the patient to modify or mollify the patient's denigration of the other treater and thus help keep the patient in treatment with the other provider being denigrated. The classic example is the patient with borderline PD, but patients with narcissistic PD also contemptuously devalue and criticize treaters who do not treat them the way they believe they are entitled to be treated. Feeling devalued can occur for the provider when faced with the moralistic, judgmental, and somewhat contemptuous attitude of the patient with obsessive-compulsive PD. In all of these instances, the "good" provider may be able to give support to the criticized, or "bad," provider. One way this support may occur is by the "good" provider coming up with examples of other situations in which he or she had the misfortune of owning and bearing the "bad" therapist label and describing how difficult it was to bear at the time but how useful it was to the eventual outcome of the treatment. The "good" provider may also try to minimize the negative countertransferential feelings the "bad" therapist is experiencing and may be able to ward off the "bad" therapist's wish to end treatment with the patient.
2. Collaborative treatment provides a basis for ongoing consultation between providers. It also provides the potential for multiple perspectives on complicated clinical and diagnostic situations. Such complex situations are not uncommon in patients with PDs, whose symptoms, behaviors, and interpersonal interactions can be so intertwined that it is difficult to unravel the trait biological functioning from the interpersonally and experientially learned behaviors and maneuvers (Cloninger et al. 1993; Livesley et al. 1998).
3. When collaboration is with a primary care physician, the mental health professional can confer with someone who may have a longitudinal relationship with and understanding of the patient. The primary care physician often is viewed as fairly neutral by the patient and may be more impervious to the distortions of transfer-

ence that appear frequently among patients with PDs. The primary care physician may be able to assist the patient in remaining medication compliant.

4. Patients with PDs can be very draining to treat. Patients with borderline PD can be demanding and threatening. Constant demands for attention from histrionic or narcissistic patients can become exhausting. The complaints of histrionic patients can be very difficult to listen to and to take seriously. Patients with dependent traits can be draining and pulling, whereas the chronic anger and distrustfulness of patients with paranoid pathology can be quite difficult to tolerate. Therefore, therapists and psychiatrists working as a team to provide overall patient management can support and confer with one another to reduce burnout.

Collaborative treatment can readily turn into a split treatment when the collaborators fail to collaborate. There can be many causes for this failure. Some patients with PDs have a tendency, as explained earlier, to split by attributing all good to one person and all bad to another. Although this splitting is most blatant among patients with borderline PD, it occurs in more subtle forms among patients with schizotypal, narcissistic, antisocial, and obsessive-compulsive PDs. Failure to collaborate in the treatment of these patients can lead to serious problems in the treatment. Table 18–1 presents specific issues that need to be considered in collaborative treatment for each of the DSM-5 Section II PDs.

Failure to collaborate or the end of collaboration can develop when the treaters identify with the projections of the patient. In this situation, each of the treaters begins to lose respect for the other treater as each begins to identify and psychologically "own" some of the patient's negative projections (Gabbard 1989; Ogden 1982). Such events or situations are not uncommon on inpatient units, where the split is often between the attending or resident psychiatrist and a member or members of the nursing staff, although they can occur between nurses as well (see Gabbard 1989; Gunderson 1984; Main 1957; Stanton and Schwartz 1954).

Case Example 2

A ward staff member suddenly accused another staff member of deliberately trying to jeopardize the treatment of a specific patient, while each staff member believed that he or she alone really knew best. The director of the ward, who had frequently encountered such sudden disagreements, had decided to deal with these types of difficulties by bringing together the "warring parties" and wondering out loud with them why each had suddenly begun to despise his or her other colleague on the unit. The director emphasized that prior to the disagreement, each person had appeared to have great respect for and to enjoy working with the other person. The director moved to a discussion of the patient and tried to show the parties how each was really only seeing a part of the patient, from which they each had constructed the idea that they alone knew how best to treat the patient.

Collaboration in divided treatment is essential but does not always occur easily or frequently; a concerted effort must be made. Regularly scheduled phone calls or e-mail exchanges may be the best way to sustain the collaboration, even when there is skepticism as to its value or a belief that another provider is causing difficulty.

TABLE 18–1. Specific issues to address in collaborative treatment with classic personality disorder features

Personality disorder	Classic personality features	Tips for providers of collaborative treatment
Paranoid	Distrust, suspiciousness	Be clear about frequency of contact among providers and be sure to inform patient whenever a contact between any providers has occurred. Regularly remind patient about sources of specific information and be sure that each treater knows whether information he or she has about the patient comes from the patient or other sources (providers).
Schizoid	Detachment from emotional relationships	Work among providers to minimize redundancy of visits so that patient can visit providers as infrequently as possible. Coordinate treatment visits so patient can visit all providers on same day.
Schizotypal	Discomfort with close relationships, cognitive or perceptual distortions, eccentricities of behavior	Be prepared to contact other providers when increased distortions arise in sessions. Work together to minimize redundancy of visits (see schizoid above).
Antisocial	Disregard for rights of others	Convey clearly that all members of the treatment team will communicate regularly. Be prepared for misrepresentations of facts. Be prepared to verify information with providers. If different providers are getting very different facts from the patient, a designated provider needs to discuss discrepancies with the patient.
Borderline	Instability in mood and interpersonal relationships, impulsivity	Provide support for patient without becoming caught up in splitting among providers. Discuss strong countertransference feelings with other providers. Have a clear plan about roles and responses of all providers to emotional outbursts, threats, increased suicidality, other crises, and medication changes. Be careful that repeated crises or turmoil is not reinforced by increased attention from providers.
Histrionic	Excessive emotionality, attention seeking	Have a clear plan among providers as to how to handle emotional outbursts. Be prepared to contact other providers at periods of increasing physical symptoms and/or increasing attention-seeking behavior.

TABLE 18–1. Specific issues to address in collaborative treatment with classic personality disorder features *(continued)*

Personality disorder	Classic personality features	Tips for providers of collaborative treatment
Narcissistic	Grandiosity, lack of empathy	Be prepared to contact other providers when overt or covert signs of increasing contempt toward a treater occur. Have a clear plan among providers regarding how to handle contemptuous behavior so that one provider addresses the issue even if patient is expressing contempt toward only one treater.
Avoidant	Social inhibition, feelings of inadequacy, hypersensitivity to negative evaluation	Work among providers to encourage consistent treatment relationships and attitudes in all treatments involved in the collaboration. Be prepared to communicate with other providers whenever patient misses appointments with any provider. Coordinate treatment visits so patient can visit all providers on same day.
Dependent	Submissive behavior, a need to be taken care of	Work with patient to minimize appointments and avoid overutilization of services. Work together to anticipate how to handle patient needs during vacations. Plan to ensure that increasing distress does not lead to an increasing number of appointments.
Obsessive-compulsive	Preoccupation with order, cleanliness, control	Ensure that consistent recommendations are made by each provider. Be prepared to communicate with other providers when patient is having difficulty adhering to recommendations. Have a clear plan regarding how to confront a patient who constantly obsesses and complains about lack of consistency or thoroughness of treatment when, in this situation, obsessing is a sign of disdain toward other people.

Note. Because many patients' presentations meet criteria for more than one personality disorder, features of multiple disorders may need to be considered in treatment. In addition, when personality disorders have no clear indication or no data to support the use of medications, collaborative treatment might arise because there is psychopharmacological treatment of a comorbid symptom disorder. This table provides tips with respect to how the patient might be dealt with in collaborative treatment even if the medication is being administered for reasons other than the patient's personality disorder diagnosis.

Collaborative Treatment and Personality Disorders

Treatment with combined psychopharmacology and psychotherapy is more common now in the treatment of all PDs than it has ever been. A number of factors are probably involved, including the following:

1. Use of psychopharmacological agents among all psychiatric patients has increased, reflecting the general ascendancy of biological psychiatry (Siever and Davis 1991; Siever et al. 2002; Silk 1998; Skodol et al. 2002).
2. Since the early 1990s, there has been an expansion of specific types of psychotherapy for patients with PDs; these therapies include DBT (Linehan et al. 1993), transference-focused psychotherapy (Clarkin et al. 1999; Kernberg et al. 2000), mentalization-based therapy based on dynamic therapy (Bateman and Fonagy 1999, 2001), interpersonal reconstructive psychotherapy (Benjamin 2003), cognitive-behavioral therapy (Beck and Freeman 1990; Davidson et al. 2006), and schema-focused cognitive-behavioral therapy (Young et al. 2003). None of these therapies oppose the concurrent use of psychopharmacological agents. (See other chapters in Part III ["Treatment"] of this volume for more detailed discussions of effective psychotherapies for patients with personality pathology.)
3. Psychopharmacological agents are more commonly used in psychiatric treatment today, and the medications used are generally safer and have more tolerable side-effect profiles than in the past (Healy 2002). Safety is especially important among a subgroup of PD patients, particularly patients with borderline PD, who have very high suicide rates (Paris 2002; Stone 1990).
4. Managed care companies play a significant role in types of treatment. They are reluctant to approve treatment sessions with seriously ill patients (including a significant number of patients with PDs) who are not receiving medication.
5. There is a growing appreciation of the role of biological and constitutional factors in the etiology of PD symptoms. The nature-nurture dichotomy has been replaced by consideration of the subtle role played by biological predisposition, resulting in traits that are expressed through behavior that is affected by experiential and environmental factors (both shared and nonshared) (Rutter 2002). Such a theory of interaction between biological predispositions and life experience supports a multimodal treatment approach (Paris 1994).
6. The comorbidity of PDs and other disorders more amenable to psychopharmacological intervention has received increased consideration. If one prefers to treat personality problems with psychotherapy, one must still consider and treat comorbid conditions so as not to worsen the clinical manifestation of the PD (Yen et al. 2003; Zanarini et al. 1998). Comorbid mental health diagnoses may respond to pharmacological agents, and even in the absence of a clear comorbid diagnosis, the patient with PD may have pharmacologically responsive symptom clusters that are reminiscent of other comorbid conditions (such as mood and anxiety disorders) and should be treated as such. (See Chapter 17, "Pharmacological Management," for a complete and up-to-date discussion of the use of medications in the treatment of personality pathology.)

Specific Situations in Which Collaborative Treatment Might Occur

Although *collaborative treatment* usually refers to the arrangement in which a nonmedical psychotherapist performs psychotherapy and a psychiatrist or other medical doctor prescribes medication, variations on that arrangement still qualify as collaborative treatment. Some such variations occur regardless of the diagnosis, but others are more prone to occur in the treatment of patients with personality pathology.

Comorbid Substance Abuse Treatment

Collaboration should occur when the patient is undergoing both treatment for substance abuse and treatment with a psychiatrist for PD issues. Continuous use of substances can exacerbate PD psychopathology, and in these instances, it is very important that the substance abuse counselor and/or psychotherapist and the treating psychiatrist immediately confer (Casillas and Clark 2002; de Groot et al. 2003). If an increase in substance use or a resumption of substance use after a period of abstinence should occur, the counselor or psychotherapist needs to initiate contact with the psychiatrist. Sometimes, a patient will feel embarrassed about resuming use of substances after a period of sobriety and may ask the counselor or psychotherapist not to inform the psychiatrist. Obviously, this wish cannot be granted, because there would be 1) collusion between the counselor or psychotherapist and the patient to keep the psychiatrist in the dark and 2) a splitting between the counselor or psychotherapist and the psychiatrist. (See Chapter 21, "Substance Use Disorders," for a detailed discussion of substance use by patients with personality pathology.)

Case Example 3

An engineer in his mid-50s, Sam was referred for substance abuse treatment after his second citation for driving while intoxicated. The substance abuse counselor referred Sam to a psychiatrist for treatment of narcissistic PD. Whenever Sam increased his alcohol use, he would miss his appointments with the psychiatrist because he was embarrassed, although he *would* attend his substance abuse sessions. The psychiatrist called the substance abuse counselor whenever Sam missed an appointment, and the counselor always convinced Sam to return to and continue with the psychiatrist. The psychiatrist eventually concluded that Sam's shame about his substance abuse behavior related more to avoidance than narcissism in interpersonal functioning, and this information allowed the substance abuse counselor to modify his approach to Sam.

Somatic Complaints, the Primary Care Physician, and the Psychiatrist

Patients with PDs, particularly those with Cluster B and Cluster C PDs, have a tendency to be somatically preoccupied (Benjamin et al. 1989; Frankenburg and Zanarini 2006). Although the treating psychiatrist may suspect mere somatic preoccupation, he or she cannot make the mistake of not taking the complaint seriously. If complaints persist or if different somatic concerns frequently appear, it is important for the psychiatrist to share his or her concern with the physician who is working up the somatic issues. Together, the two physicians can decide how much physical exploration of somatic concerns should occur and coordinate a consistent therapeutic response to persisting somatic issues (Williams and Silk 1997). (See Chapter 23, "Personality Disorders in the Medical Setting," for a discussion of the presentation and management of patients with personality pathology and physical symptoms or disorders.)

Seven Principles to Follow in Collaborative Treatment

A number of principles can apply to any collaborative treatment, but they have special application in the treatment of patients with PDs. Adherence to these principles can lead to a smoother and more synergistic approach to collaborative treatment (Silk 1995).

Understanding and Clarifying the Relationship Between Therapist and Prescriber

The relationship that includes the patient, the psychotherapist, and the pharmacotherapist (or "prescriber") has been described as the "pharmacotherapy-psychotherapy triangle" (Beitman et al. 1984). In managed care, psychiatrists may be expected to provide medical backup for therapists whose work they do not know, whose approach they may not agree with, or whom they do not respect (Goldberg et al. 1991). Conversely, the psychotherapist may have to deal with a psychiatrist whom he or she does not know or agree with. In the best of worlds, neither the psychiatrist nor the psychotherapist would feel obligated to collaborate with a provider whom he or she does not respect.

Patients with PDs are quite sensitive to disagreements among members of the treatment team (Main 1957; Stanton and Schwartz 1954). When there is a lack of communication and sharing of knowledge among treaters and other professionals involved in the case, the patient can become caught in the middle of a disagreement (Stanton and Schwartz 1954). Each treater should respect what the other is trying to accomplish. This respect for the treatment modality should be separated from personal feelings (although it is always easier if there is mutual regard). Each provider should be free to conduct open communication with the other so that treatment collaboration and coordination can occur (Koenigsberg 1993).

Ideally, the prescriber and the therapist will know each other or at least know something about each other's practice and practice reputation. The prescriber should have an appreciation for the basic psychological issues involved in treatment and a general understanding of how they may manifest in psychopharmacological treatment. The prescribing psychiatrist needs to be clear with the therapist as to his or her beliefs in the putative efficacy of psychotherapy for the PD in general as well as for each patient specifically. Psychotherapy will not proceed constructively if the prescriber does not believe in the usefulness of psychotherapy, particularly with patients with PDs (especially those with Cluster B PDs). Maintenance of therapeutic boundaries between treaters is crucial in working with patients with PDs and must be clarified (Woodward et al. 1993). Some questions to consider follow:

- Should between-session phone calls be permitted in the pharmacological treatment if they are not permitted or are frowned upon in the psychotherapy?
- In what quantities will pills be prescribed, and what course should the therapist take if there is a sudden increase in the suicidality of the patient?
- When the patient requests a change or an increase in dosage, will the prescriber contact the therapist beforehand to understand better what issues might be coming up in the psychotherapy?
- How frequently will discussions between the prescriber and the therapist take place?
- How will issues that belong primarily in the psychotherapy be dealt with if they are brought up with the prescriber?
- Will the psychopharmacologist notify the patient or therapist that he or she has directed some issue back to the therapist?

The psychotherapist also needs to have respect for the prescriber and for the intervention of psychopharmacology (Koenigsberg 1993). Although there is probably little need for nonmedical therapists to be experts in psychotropic drug usage, nonmedical psychotherapists should understand the general indications for pharmacotherapy and be aware of the specificity as well as the limitations of the psychopharmacological treatment. The therapist should have some rudimentary knowledge of both the expected therapeutic effects and the possible side effects of at least the broader classes of psychotropic medications. In the course of the psychotherapy, the therapist should be willing to discuss, albeit on a limited basis, the patient's experience (both positive and negative) of taking the medication(s). Additionally, the therapist needs to have some knowledge of medications so that he or she can have some appreciation of what might be subjective versus objective reactions of the patient to taking the medications.

As stated earlier, no psychotherapist or psychopharmacologist should feel obligated to work with a collaborative partner whom he or she does not agree with or respect. Each treater must respect the roles and competence of the other. In this atmosphere of mutual respect, both the prescriber and the therapist need to appreciate the perceived efficacy as well as limitations of each of the interventions. Both need to be able to tolerate treatment situations in which progress is often slow, punctuated by periods of improvement and regression, and in which the long-range prognosis is often guarded but not necessarily negative. Appreciating the other's difficulties and those of the patient in the treatment may help each treater avoid blaming the other (or the patient) during difficult periods.

Appelbaum suggested that, to address clarity of treatment and treatment expectations, as well as medicolegal issues, the therapist and prescriber should draw up a formal contract that delineates their respective roles as well as the expected frequency and range of, or limitations on, their communication (Appelbaum 1991). Such a contract works well when the two people share responsibility for a number of patients (Smith 1989). These ideas about contracts are merely suggestions, and contracts certainly may not be necessary or useful when the two collaborators work in the same clinic or the same health system.

Much of what is diagnosed as PD reflects a group of patients with chronic maladaptive interpersonal functioning across a wide range of settings. The Alternative DSM-5 Model for Personality Disorders (AMPD) (see Chapter 4 in this volume), which is included in Section III of DSM-5, defines any personality disorder as moderate or greater impairment in personality functioning (related to a sense of self and reflected in interpersonal relationships) and the presence of pathological personality traits (Oldham 2015). Though the AMPD does not replace traditional PD diagnoses, including it in DSM-5 highlights a way of thinking about PDs in terms of dimensions of personality pathology, rather than set categories (Oldham 2015). Interpersonal dysfunction cannot and should not be ignored, dismissed, or denied, and whenever and wherever it occurs in the therapeutic endeavor, it should be discussed not only between the two providers but among the treaters *and* the patient. Transference is not solely reserved for transference-oriented psychotherapy (Beck and Freeman 1990; Goldhamer 1984), and "pharmacotherapy is [also] an interpersonal transaction" (Beitman 1993, p. 538).

Understanding What the Medication Means to Both Therapist and Prescriber

Medications may play both positive and negative roles in treatment. The therapist and the prescriber need to be attuned to what the initiation of medication means to each of them.

In Section III, "Emerging Measures and Models," of DSM-5 (American Psychiatric Association 2013), an alternative model to the categorical approach to PD diagnosis has been published. In clinical practice, patients with PDs defy easy classification and do not always fit neatly into any DSM categories (Westen and Arkowitz-Westen 1998). In addition, no medications have yet been indicated as the primary treatment for any specific PD. Although there are algorithms with respect to the pharmacological treatment of PDs (particularly borderline PD [American Psychiatric Association 2001; Soloff 1998]), there are no clear-cut rules as to when or what medication should be used in any given personality disorder. In circumstances of prescriber self-doubt, ambivalence, and uncertainty about either the diagnosis or, more probably, the chosen pharmacological agent, a defensive and authoritarian posture might be assumed by the prescriber in an attempt to assure that the pharmacological decision was correct. The prescriber and/or the therapist may deny ambivalence about the medication, become intolerant of the patient's (or the other provider's) questions and concerns, and present the possible therapeutic effects of the medication in a more positive light than the evidence would imply. This idealization of the medication, similar to the patient's periodic idealization of the treatment, will usually be short-lived, however.

Pessimism about progress in the therapy was given as a reason to consider prescribing medications by 65% of the respondent psychotherapists in a study by Waldinger and Frank (1989). Given that some patients with PDs, particularly borderline PD, seem especially attuned to feelings, a treater's pessimism or frustration with the course of therapy may be inadvertently and unconsciously conveyed to the patient. Conversely, a referral to a psychopharmacologist could be viewed as an opportunity for consultation and a second opinion (Chiles et al. 1991).

When there is little apparent therapeutic progress, treaters can easily develop anger and rage at patients with PDs, particularly patients with substantial borderline, narcissistic, and paranoid personality characteristics (Gabbard and Wilkinson 1994). At these times, one treater may try to pull back from the treatment or, conversely, try to take over control of the entire treatment. The best way to handle these feelings is not to isolate oneself but to approach the other provider and be willing to share one's frustrations. More often than not, the first provider will discover that the other provider shares similar frustrations. This shared frustration will lead not only to less tension in each provider and in the therapy but also, at times, to a discussion and a review of the treatment.

When medication is being considered in a collaborative treatment, the following questions may be asked:

- Where is the impetus for the medication coming from?
- Does the therapist think the medication will affect or change the therapeutic relationship?

In turn, the prescriber should be able to let the therapist know if he or she feels that the therapist's expectations for the medication are unrealistic and what might be a reasonable expected response.

Understanding What the Medication Means to the Patient

Beginning pharmacotherapy or changing medication may not always be seen as favorable by patients, and a negative reaction to the idea of medication needs to be anticipated. A propensity to put the most negative spin on interpersonal encounters or perceived intentions may cause patients with PDs to experience the introduction of medication as a failure of their role in treatment or as the psychotherapist giving up on them. Patients might also, albeit rarely, experience the introduction of medication as a hopeful sign, as an additional modality that might help speed the progress of the treatment (Gunderson 1984, 2001; Waldinger and Frank 1989). Whatever the patient's reaction, both therapist and prescriber need to understand what the medication means to the patient and how the patient understands the use of medication within the context of the therapy as well as in the context of his or her own life experience (Metzl and Riba 2003).

Understanding the patient's reaction to the introduction of medication can be important not only for the patient's cooperation and compliance but also for transferential issues. The patient may take medication in a spirit of collaboration with the therapist and the prescriber. The patient may disagree with the decision but cooperate out of a strong need to please. A patient's reactions will depend on whether the therapist and prescriber are truly collaborating or at odds.

The introduction of medication into any therapy, even if by a conferring psychiatrist, has repercussions on the transference (Goldhamer 1984). If the idea of medication is introduced early in the treatment process, the potential negative transferential reaction to the introduction of medications later may be minimized. It is important that the therapist and the prescriber be on the same page as to "how" medication will be chosen, introduced, continued, discontinued, and so on. Discussions at the beginning of treatment can model the ethos of an open forum for exchange of information about medications and other feelings.

Case Example 4

Charles, a 50-year-old man with histrionic PD and panic disorder, was referred to an anxiety disorder clinic after several emergency department visits because of uncomfortable arousal symptoms precipitated by an antidepressant (Soloff et al. 1986a). He received cognitive-behavioral therapy and responded well, although he had trouble starting an antidepressant without having his panic symptoms increase. He did tolerate a low-dose benzodiazepine but was fearful of becoming "addicted" to the medication and would intermittently reduce his dosage despite his therapist's attempts to discourage his doing so. When Charles's insurance ran out, he stopped seeing his therapist because he was "doing so well," and he also stopped his medication. He began to have emotional outbursts and increased panic attacks and called the psychiatric emergency room inquiring about rehabilitation for drug abuse. Therapy was reinitiated after both the therapist and the psychiatrist discussed Charles's concerns about medication and considered how these concerns were affecting his life. The providers developed clear plans as to whom Charles would call for "medication questions," whom for "exposure questions," and how they would respond to emotional upheavals.

Both therapist and prescriber should be aware that patients may use medications as transitional objects (particularly patients with borderline, histrionic, and perhaps severely dependent personality pathology [Cardasis et al. 1997; Gunderson et al. 1985; Winnicott 1953]). In this context, the patient's attachment and/or resistance to changing or altering medications may seem out of proportion to the actual therapeutic benefit derived from the medication (Adelman 1985). It may also explain why the patient who has repeatedly complained about the medications is unwilling to change them even when there has been little clear evidence that the medications have been effective.

Understanding That the Medication Will Probably Have Limited Effectiveness

Therapists and prescribers need to appreciate the therapeutic benefits and limitations of medications. Therapists should inquire about a patient's medications at moments of calm, not during periods of crisis. Perhaps the most instructive and useful time for discussion about or change of medication is when things are actually going well and treatment does not seem bleak or hopeless.

The prescriber should describe what features of a specific medication may or may not be useful for this specific patient at this particular time. The prescriber should tell the therapist what unusual idiosyncratic reactions to the medication might occur (Gardner and Cowdry 1985; Soloff et al. 1986a), especially because these paradoxical reactions or tendencies toward dependency may not always be listed in the package insert or in the *Physician's Desk Reference*.

With effective therapist-prescriber collaboration, medication decisions will not be solely in the hands of the prescriber. A dialogue between therapist and prescriber should take place as to how each particular type or category of medication might work for the particular patient.

Case Example 5

After moving to a new city, Diane was referred by a psychiatrist from out of town for treatment of anxiety and depression. Diane had a long history of major depressive episodes. At the time of the evaluation, she was taking five medications: two mood stabilizers, a low-dose atypical antipsychotic, an antidepressant, and a benzodiazepine. She insisted that this combination was the correct regimen for her and that the new psychiatrist not tamper with her medications. She said it took many months and finally a referral to the most prominent psychopharmacologist in her region before the right combination was found. She also stated that she was going to remain in psychotherapy with her old therapist through weekly long-distance phone contacts.

The new psychiatrist, after seeing Diane five or six times, began to feel that Diane primarily had a narcissistic PD and that her depressions were brought about by her extreme sensitivity to anything that could remotely represent a narcissistic injury. The psychiatrist called Diane's therapist, who acknowledged that although Diane did have some narcissistic issues, she really had experienced a number of major depressive episodes during their treatment together.

After a few months, Diane grew more depressed, but her depression was marked primarily by lethargy, absenteeism from work, and an inability to concentrate. She was, however, able to date and had no loss of libido or appetite. Instead of feelings of guilt or worthlessness, she had feelings of grandiosity and entitlement. Diane requested a psychostimulant to help with her concentration and lethargy. The psychiatrist balked and tried to address some of the ways in which he felt her depression was atypical. He pointed out that she seemed more invested in wanting the psychiatrist to figure out what pills would make her better than in exploring events in her life that might be leading to what she thought was depression. She stormed out of the office. Later that week, Diane called the psychiatrist to say that her therapist also believed that she could benefit from a psychostimulant, and she was going to find a psychiatrist who was an expert in depression and more up-to-date about treatment. Calls the psychiatrist made to Diane's long-distance therapist went unanswered.

Understanding How the Medication Fits Into the Patient's Overall Treatment

If a psychotherapist considers using medications at some time during the course of treatment, ideally, he or she already has an ongoing arrangement or relationship with a prescriber. It is never wise to begin searching for a prescriber during a time of pressing need for medications.

The goal of treatment for a patient with personality pathology cannot be cure. A decision to use or change medications should not imply that one is "going for the cure." The goal of treatment should be to try to improve the ways in which patients cope, to help them develop increased awareness of their cognitive rigidity and distortions, to assist them in becoming somewhat less impulsive and less affectively labile, and to try to both increase the distance between and reduce the amplitude of their interpersonal crises (Koenigsberg 1993). These goals are attributable to both the psychotherapy and psychopharmacology and need to be appreciated by both the therapist and the prescriber. A prescriber who conveys a powerful belief in finding the "right" medication will promote an unrealistic and difficult situation.

Any therapy for patients with character disorders must have realistic and limited goals set early in the therapy, lest any of the players begin to idealize another player or another modality. Such idealization can only lead to disappointment and the multiple repercussions that occur in the treatment as a result.

Understanding the Potential and Actual Lethality of the Medication

Many psychotropic medications can be lethal, particularly tricyclic antidepressants, lithium, and mood stabilizers/anticonvulsants. Monoamine oxidase inhibitors and benzodiazepines also have significant morbidity and mortality associated with over-dose, especially when combined with other agents. Suicide potential needs to be con-tinually assessed, and when it increases, a plan should be enacted that takes into account when the therapist will contact the prescriber, whether the prescriber is going to limit the size of the prescription, which of the treating professionals might hold onto the medications if a decision is made to limit their administration, and so on. At a minimum, if the therapist believes there is an increase in suicide potential, then the prescriber should be notified. If the therapist is fearful that the patient may overdose, this issue should be discussed openly with the prescriber.

Patients with PDs, particularly borderline PD, are potentially volatile and can act out when they feel that relationships are threatened (Gunderson 1984). The therapist-patient relationship is one that, when complicated by transference, can increase the possibility of a patient's acting out in ways that include suicidal and other self-destructive behaviors; the prescriber-patient relationship is another that holds the po-tential for these types of dangers. Mutual respect and communication between thera-pist and prescriber are indispensable to ensuring that a crisis is defused.

Understanding That Interpersonal Crises and Affective Storms Cannot Be Relieved Simply Through Initiation or Modification of Medication

Introducing medication into the treatment of a patient with PD should not be a spur-of-the-moment decision. It should be done in a controlled manner with forethought and not in the midst of an interpersonal or transferential crisis. Patients' lives and af-fects do not follow well-designed courses or even respond to well-designed plans. Even if careful plans are made, the interpersonal crises and affective storms that occur in treatment, combined with the interpersonal demandingness and/or helplessness and passivity of the patient, put enormous pressure on the therapist to do something, to change something, to make the pain go away. There is a tendency to promise much more than can be accomplished, ultimately leading to idealization, disappointment, and subsequent devaluation. If a collaborative relationship exists, and it is very good and mutually supportive, then neither treater should deal with the patient's attacks and demands alone. The two can collaborate to think through and resolve the crisis.

Collaboration During a Crisis

In a crisis, all seven points just described come into play. The therapist and prescriber need to consider various questions:

- How well has there been open collaboration between the psychotherapist and the prescriber?
- How well do they work together, and can they trust each other and each other's judgment?
- How does each of them, as well as the patient, understand the role of medication in the treatment and the medication's benefits and symbolic meaning?
- How well does each person understand the limits of the medication, and is one of the treaters overreacting, merely prescribing or wanting a prescription written for med-ication to feel that a crisis is being defused?

- What has been said about medications in the treatment in the past, and how and when have medications been used in the treatment?
- Have medications been employed successfully, and have they been used safely by the patient?

Contraindications to Collaborative Treatment

Before concluding, we need to make mention of situations in which collaborative treatment may be contraindicated. First, however, we must point out that when a patient needs both medication and psychotherapeutic treatment, it is very common that both treatments are provided by a single psychiatrist. We continue to urge treatment by one individual psychiatrist whenever possible if the psychiatrist feels capable of and competent in providing both the medication and the specific form of psychotherapy most useful to the patient.

In some situations, collaborative treatment is contraindicated. The first situation would be when the patient is extremely paranoid or psychotic. These types of patients may not agree to having people "talk about them" and thus would not sign a release of information for such exchanges to occur. Also, paranoid persons often think that all or most other people are talking about them, and the therapist may not wish to reinforce this idea by means of an arrangement wherein people are talking about the patient.

There may also be instances in which patients have an admixture of serious medical and psychiatric problems. The medical problems may directly affect the patient's psychological problems and presentation, as well as the patient's cognitive processes and ability to comprehend. A physician who understands the impact of medical conditions on psychological presentation and functioning and who can conduct the psychotherapy as well as manage the medications would be most helpful in these cases, especially if the medical condition or related psychological problems wax and wane. In this instance, drug-drug interactions may have a direct impact on psychological and medical well-being, and changes in a medical condition may warrant repeated reevaluation of psychotropic drug regimens.

In other instances, practical reality issues may lead to treatment by a single provider rather than collaborative treatment. If a patient has a severe limit on the number of sessions of psychological or psychiatric treatment because of third-party payer restrictions, then the psychiatrist must consider how to use those sessions most efficiently and cost-effectively for the patient. In this instance, being able to manage medications and conduct psychotherapy in a single session may be important. A similar situation can occur when the patient has severely restricted financial resources or lives so far away that a trip to the psychotherapist and/or psychiatrist involves a significant expenditure of time or money. In this case, if both psychotherapy and psychopharmacology can be accomplished in a single trip or visit, then this approach should be seriously considered.

Conclusion

Collaborative treatment is increasing for a number of reasons, including economic, medical (i.e., advances in neuroscience and pharmacology), and structural (i.e., managed care and the way health care in the United States is delivered). The various combinations and permutations of collaborative treatment are growing beyond the standard combination of one person writing prescriptions for psychiatric medications while another person provides the psychotherapy. Psychiatrists, psychologists, primary care physicians, social workers, case managers, physician assistants, and visiting nurses are just some of the players involved in a collaborative treatment.

Advances in neuroscience and trends toward using psychotropic medications more regularly for patients with PDs have led to more of these patients receiving collaborative treatment. Managed care puts pressure on psychiatrists to use medications for a "quicker" response, and patients, bolstered by direct-to-consumer advertising, assume that a medication is available for every ailment. Given the co-occurrence of many disorders with PDs, it is not uncommon to find one provider managing medications while another directs or conducts psychodynamic, cognitive-behavioral, or interpersonal psychotherapy.

Patients with PDs have major difficulties in interpersonal relationships, and every visit with a psychopharmacologist or a psychotherapist is an interpersonal encounter. These interpersonal encounters must be managed carefully, and when there are two or more providers of treatment, the providers must communicate with each other on a regular basis. This communication is not only a hallmark of good psychiatric care but also a method whereby two or more providers can coordinate their treatment approach and collaborate on decision making so that the experience can be a synergistic rather than a divisive one.

Collaborative treatment at its best occurs in an atmosphere of respect and results in open and free communication with fellow providers. An opportunity for collaborators to consult and learn from one another exists, and this collaboration has the potential to result in more comprehensive and thoughtful care for difficult-to-treat groups of patients.

References

Adelman SA: Pills as transitional objects: a dynamic understanding of the use of medication in psychotherapy. Psychiatry 48:246–253, 1985

American Psychiatric Association: Practice guideline for the treatment of patients with borderline personality disorder. Am J Psychiatry 158 (10 suppl):1–52, 2001

American Psychiatric Association: Practice Guideline for the Treatment of Patients With Major Depressive Disorder, 3rd Edition. Arlington, VA, American Psychiatric Association, 2010

American Psychiatric Association: Diagnostic and Statistical Manual of Mental Disorders, 5th Edition. Arlington, VA, American Psychiatric Association, 2013

Angstman KB, Seshadri A, Marcelin A, et al: Personality disorders in primary care: impact on depression outcomes within collaborative care. J Prim Care Community Health 8:233–238, 2017

Appelbaum PS: General guidelines for psychiatrists who prescribe medications for patients treated by nonmedical psychotherapists. Hosp Community Psychiatry 42:281–282, 1991

Barlow DH, Gorman JM, Shear MK, et al: Cognitive-behavioral therapy, imipramine, or their combination for panic disorder: a randomized controlled trial. JAMA 28:2529–2539, 2000

Bateman A, Fonagy P: Effectiveness of partial hospitalization in the treatment of borderline personality disorder: a randomized controlled trial. Am J Psychiatry 156:1563–1569, 1999

Bateman A, Fonagy P: Treatment of borderline personality disorder with psychoanalytically oriented partial hospitalization: an 18-month follow-up. Am J Psychiatry 158:36–42, 2001

Beck A, Freeman A: Cognitive Therapy of Personality Disorders. New York, Guilford, 1990

Beitman BD: Pharmacotherapy and the stages of psychotherapeutic change, in American Psychiatric Press Review of Psychiatry, Vol 12. Edited by Oldham JM, Riba MB, Tasman A. Washington, DC, American Psychiatric Press, 1993, pp 521–539

Beitman BD, Chiles J, Carlin A: The pharmacotherapy-psychotherapy triangle: psychiatrist, non-medical psychotherapist, and patient. J Clin Psychiatry 45:458–459, 1984

Benjamin J, Silk KR, Lohr NE, et al: The relationship between borderline personality disorder and anxiety disorders. Am J Orthopsychiatry 59:461–467, 1989

Benjamin LS: Interpersonal Reconstructive Therapy. New York, Guilford, 2003

Bogenschutz MP, Nurnberg GH: Olanzapine versus placebo in the treatment of borderline personality disorder. J Clin Psychiatry 65:104–109, 2004

Browne G, Steiner M, Roberts J, et al: Sertraline and/or interpersonal psychotherapy for patients with dysthymic disorder in primary care: 6-month comparison with longitudinal 2-year follow-up of effectiveness and costs. J Affect Disord 68:317–330, 2002

Cardasis W, Hochman JA, Silk KR: Transitional objects and borderline personality disorder. Am J Psychiatry 154:250–255, 1997

Casillas A, Clark LA: Dependency, impulsivity, and self-harm: traits hypothesized to underlie the association between cluster B personality and substance use disorders. J Pers Disord 16:424–436, 2002

Chiles JA, Carlin AS, Benjamin GAH, et al: A physician, a nonmedical psychotherapist, and a patient: the pharmacotherapy-psychotherapy triangle, in Integrating Pharmacotherapy and Psychotherapy. Edited by Beitman BD, Klerman GL. Washington DC, American Psychiatric Press, 1991, pp 105–118

Clarkin JF, Yeomans FE, Kernberg OF: Psychotherapy for Borderline Personality. New York, Wiley, 1999

Cloninger CR, Svrakic DM, Przybeck TR: A psychobiological model of temperament and character. Arch Gen Psychiatry 50:975–990, 1993

Coccaro EF, Kavoussi RJ: Fluoxetine and impulsive aggressive behavior in personality-disordered subjects. Arch Gen Psychiatry 54:1081–1088, 1997

Coccaro EF, Siever L, Klar HM, et al: Serotonergic studies in patients with affective and personality disorders. Arch Gen Psychiatry 46:587–599, 1989

Cowdry RW, Gardner DL: Pharmacotherapy of borderline personality disorder: alprazolam, carbamazepine, trifluoperazine, and tranylcypromine. Arch Gen Psychiatry 45:111–119, 1988

Davidson K, Norrie J, Tyrer P, et al: The effectiveness of cognitive behavior therapy for borderline personality disorder: results from the Borderline Personality Disorder Study of Cognitive Therapy (BOSCOT) trial. J Pers Disord 20:450–465, 2006

de Groot MH, Franken IH, van der Meer CW, et al: Stability and change in dimensional ratings of personality disorders in drug abuse patients during treatment. J Subst Abuse Treat 24:115–120, 2003

de Jonghe F, Hendricksen M, van Aalst G, et al: Psychotherapy alone and combined with pharmacotherapy in the treatment of depression. Br J Psychiatry 185:37–45, 2004

Donohue J, Garfield R, Lave J: The Impact of Expanded Health Insurance Coverage on Individuals With Mental Illnesses and Substance Use Disorders. Washington, DC, U.S. Department of Health and Human Services, 2010

Duggan C, Huband N, Smailagic N, et al: The use of pharmacological treatments for people with personality disorder: a systematic review of randomized controlled trials. Personality and Mental Health 2:119–170, 2008

Frankenburg FR, Zanarini MC: Personality disorders and medical comorbidity. Curr Opin Psychiatry 19:428–431, 2006

Fuerino L III, Silk KR: State of the art in the pharmacologic treatment of borderline personality disorder. Curr Psychiatry Rep 13:69–75, 2011

Gabbard GO: Splitting in hospital treatment. Am J Psychiatry 146:444–451, 1989

Gabbard GO, Wilkinson SM: Management of Countertransference With Borderline Patients. Washington, DC, American Psychiatric Press, 1994

Gardner DL, Cowdry RW: Alprazolam-induced dyscontrol in borderline personality disorder. Am J Psychiatry 142:98–100, 1985

Gilbody S, Bower P, Fletcher J, et al: Collaborative care for depression: a cumulative meta-analysis and review of longer-term outcomes. Arch Intern Med 166:2314–2321, 2006

Goldberg RS, Riba M, Tasman A: Psychiatrists' attitudes toward prescribing medication for patients treated by nonmedical psychotherapists. Hosp Community Psychiatry 42:276–280, 1991

Goldberg SC, Schulz SC, Schulz PM, et al: Borderline and schizotypal personality disorders treated with low-dose thiothixene vs. placebo. Arch Gen Psychiatry 43:680–686, 1986

Goldhamer PM: Psychotherapy and pharmacotherapy: the challenge of integration. Can J Psychiatry 38:173–177, 1984

Greenblatt M, Solomon MH, Evans A, et al (eds): Drug and Social Therapy in Chronic Schizophrenia. Springfield, IL, Charles C Thomas, 1965

Gunderson JG: Borderline Personality Disorder. Washington, DC, American Psychiatric Press, 1984

Gunderson JG: Borderline Personality Disorder: A Clinical Guide. Washington, DC, American Psychiatric Publishing, 2001

Gunderson JG, Morris H, Zanarini MC: Transitional objects and borderline patients, in The Borderline: Current Empirical Research. Edited by McGlashan TH. Washington, DC, American Psychiatric Association, 1985, pp 43–60

Healy D: The Antidepressant Era. Cambridge, MA, Harvard University Press, 1997

Healy D: The Creation of Psychopharmacology. Cambridge, MA, Harvard University Press, 2002

Herpertz SC, Zanarini M, Schulz CS, et al: World Federation of Societies of Biological Psychiatry (WFSBP) guidelines for biological treatment of personality disorders. World J Biol Psychiatry 8:212–244, 2007

Hollander E, Allen A, Lopez RP, et al: A preliminary double-blind, placebo-controlled trial of divalproex sodium in borderline personality disorder. J Clin Psychiatry 62:199–203, 2001

Hollander E, Swann AC, Coccaro EF, et al: Impact of trait impulsivity and state aggression on divalproex versus placebo response in borderline personality disorder. Am J Psychiatry 162:621–624, 2005

Keller MB, McCullough JP, Klein DN, et al: A comparison of nefazodone, the cognitive behavioral-analysis system of psychotherapy, and their combination for the treatment of chronic depression. N Engl J Med 342:1642–1670, 2000

Kernberg O, Koenigsberg H, Stone M, et al: Borderline Patients: Extending the Limits of Treatability. New York, Basic Books, 2000

Klerman GL: The psychiatric patient's right to effective treatment: implications of Osheroff vs. Chestnut Lodge. Am J Psychiatry 147:409–418, 1990

Koenigsberg HW: Combining psychotherapy and pharmacotherapy in the treatment of borderline patients, in American Psychiatric Press Review of Psychiatry, Vol 12. Edited by Oldham JM, Riba MB, Tasman A. Washington, DC, American Psychiatric Press, 1993, pp 541–563

Koenigsberg HW, Reynolds D, Goodman M, et al: Risperidone in the treatment of schizotypal personality disorder. J Clin Psychiatry 64:628–634, 2003

Kool S, Dekker J, Duijsens IJ, et al: Changes in personality pathology after pharmacotherapy and combined therapy for depressed patients. J Pers Disord 17:60–72, 2003

Linehan MM, Heard HL, Armstrong HE: Naturalistic follow-up of a behavioral treatment for chronically parasuicidal borderline patients. Arch Gen Psychiatry 50:971–974, 1993

Livesley WJ: A practical approach to the treatment of patients with borderline personality disorder. Psychiatr Clin North Am 23:211–232, 2000

Livesley WJ, Jang KL, Vernon PA: Phenotypic and genetic structure of traits delineating personality disorder. Arch Gen Psychiatry 55:941–948, 1998

Loew TH, Nickel MK, Muehlbacher M, et al: Topiramate treatment for women with borderline personality disorder: a double-blind, placebo-controlled study. J Clin Psychopharmacol 26:61–66, 2006

Main TF: The ailment. Br J Med Psychol 30:129–145, 1957

Manber R, Arnow B, Blasey C, et al: Patient's therapeutic skill acquisition and response to psychotherapy, alone or in combination with medication. Psychol Med 33:693–702, 2003

Markowitz P: Pharmacotherapy, in Handbook of Personality Disorders: Theory, Research, and Treatment. Edited by Livesley WJ. New York, Guilford, 2001, pp 475–493

Markowitz PJ: Recent trends in the pharmacotherapy of personality disorders. J Pers Disord 18:90–101, 2004

Metzl JM, Riba M: Understanding the symbolic value of medications: a brief review. Prim Psychiatry 10:45–48, 2003

Mojtabal R, Olfson M: Proportions of antidepressants prescribed without a psychiatric diagnosis. Health Aff (Millwood) 30:1434–1439, 2011

Nickel MK, Nickel C, Kaplan P, et al: Treatment of aggression with topiramate in male borderline patients: a double-blind, placebo-controlled study. Biol Psychiatry 57:495–499, 2005

Nickel MK, Muehlbacher M, Nickel C, et al: Aripiprazole in the treatment of patients with borderline personality disorder: a double-blind, placebo-controlled study. Am J Psychiatry 163:833–838, 2006

Ogden TH: Projective Identification and Psychotherapeutic Technique. New York, Jason Aronson, 1982

Oldham JM: The alternative DSM-5 model for personality disorders. World Psychiatry 14:234–236, 2015

Paris J: Borderline Personality Disorder: A Multidimensional Approach. Washington, DC, American Psychiatric Press, 1994

Paris J: Chronic suicidality among patients with borderline personality disorder. Psychiatr Serv 53:738–742, 2002

Paris J: Personality Disorders Over Time: Precursors, Course, and Outcome. Washington, DC, American Psychiatric Publishing, 2003

Pincus AH, Zarin DA, Tanielian MA, et al: Psychiatric patients and treatments in 1997: findings from the American Psychiatric Practice Research Network. Arch Gen Psychiatry 56:441–449, 1999

Putnam KM, Silk KR: Emotion dysregulation and the development of borderline personality disorder. Dev Psychopathol 17:899–925, 2005

Rinne T, van de Brink W, Wouters I, et al: SSRI treatment of borderline personality disorder: a randomized, placebo-controlled clinical trial for female patients with borderline personality disorder. Am J Psychiatry 159:2048–2054, 2002

Ripoll LH: Clinical psychopharmacology of borderline personality disorder: an update on the available evidence in light of the Diagnostic and Statistical Manual of Mental Disorders. Curr Opin Psychiatry 25:52–58, 2012

Rutter M: The interplay of nature, nurture, and developmental influences: the challenge ahead for mental health. Arch Gen Psychiatry 59:996–1000, 2002

Salzman C, Wolfson AN, Schatzberg A, et al: Effect of fluoxetine on anger in symptomatic volunteers with borderline personality disorder. J Clin Psychopharmacol 15:23–29, 1995

Schulz SC, Camlin KL: Treatment of borderline personality disorder: potential of the new antipsychotic medications. Journal of Practical Psychiatry and Behavioral Health 5:247–255, 1999

Sheard M, Marini J, Bridges C, et al: The effect of lithium on impulsive aggressive behavior in man. Am J Psychiatry 133:1409–1413, 1976

Siever LJ, Davis KL: A psychobiological perspective on the personality disorders. Am J Psychiatry 148:1647–1658, 1991

Siever LJ, Torgersen S, Gunderson JG, et al: The borderline diagnosis III: identifying endophenotypes for genetic studies. Biol Psychiatry 51:964–968, 2002

Silk KR: Rational pharmacotherapy for patients with personality disorders, in Clinical Assessment and Management of Severe Personality Disorders. Edited by Links P. Washington, DC, American Psychiatric Press, 1995, pp 109–142

Silk KR (ed): Biology of Personality Disorders. Washington, DC, American Psychiatric Press, 1998

Silk KR: The quality of depression in borderline personality disorder and the diagnostic process. J Pers Disord 24:25–37, 2010

Silk KR: The process of managing medications in patients with borderline personality disorder. J Psychiatr Pract 17:311–319, 2011

Silk KR, Fuerino L III: Psychopharmacology of personality disorders, in The Oxford Handbook of Personality Disorders. Edited by Widiger TA. Oxford, UK, Oxford University Press, 2012, pp 713–724

Simpson EB, Yen S, Costello E, et al: Combined dialectical behavior therapy and fluoxetine in the treatment of borderline personality disorder. J Clin Psychiatry 65:379–385, 2004

Skodol AE, Stout RL, McGlashan TH, et al: Co-occurrence of mood and personality disorders: a report from the Collaborative Longitudinal Personality Disorders Study (CLPS). Depress Anxiety 10:175–182, 1999

Skodol AE, Siever LJ, Livesley WJ, et al: The borderline diagnosis II: biology, genetics, and clinical course. Biol Psychiatry 51:951–963, 2002

Smith JM: Some dimensions of transference in combined treatment, in The Psychotherapist's Guide to Pharmacotherapy. Edited by Ellison JM. Chicago, IL, Year Book Medical, 1989, pp 79–94

Solberg JJ, Deyo-Svendsen ME, Nylander KR, et al: Collaborative care management associated with improved depression outcomes in patients with personality disorders, compared to usual primary care. J Prim Care Community Health 9:2150132718773266, 2018

Soler J, Pascual JC, Campins J, et al: Double-blind, placebo-controlled study of dialectical behavior therapy plus olanzapine for borderline personality disorder. Am J Psychiatry 162:1221–1224, 2005

Soloff PH: What's new in personality disorders? An update on pharmacologic treatment. J Pers Disord 4:233–243, 1990

Soloff PH: Algorithms for pharmacological treatment of personality dimensions: symptom-specific treatments for cognitive-perceptual, affective, and impulsive-behavioral dysregulation. Bull Menninger Clin 62:195–214, 1998

Soloff PH, George A, Nathan RS, et al: Paradoxical effects of amitriptyline in borderline patients. Am J Psychiatry 143:1603–1605, 1986a

Soloff PH, George A, Nathan RS, et al: Progress in pharmacotherapy of borderline disorders: a double-blind study of amitriptyline, haloperidol, and placebo. Arch Gen Psychiatry 43:691–697, 1986b

Soloff PH, Cornelius J, George A, et al: Efficacy of phenelzine and haloperidol in borderline personality disorder. Arch Gen Psychiatry 50:377–385, 1993

Stanton AH, Schwartz MS: The Mental Hospital: A Study of Institutional Participation in Psychiatric Illness and Treatment. London, Tavistock, 1954

Stone MH: The Fate of Borderline Patients: Successful Outcome and Psychiatric Practice. New York, Guilford, 1990

Stringer B, van Meijel B, Karman P, et al: Collaborative care for patients with severe personality disorders: preliminary results and active ingredients from a pilot study (Part I). Perspect Psychiatr Care 51:180–189, 2015

Tritt K, Nickel C, Lahmann C, et al: Lamotrigine treatment of aggression in female borderline patients: a randomized, double-blind, placebo-controlled study. J Psychopharmacol 19:287–291, 2005

Waldinger RS, Frank AF: Clinicians' experiences in combining medication and -psychotherapy in the treatment of borderline patients. Hosp Community Psychiatry 40:712–718, 1989

Wasylyshen A, Williams AM: Second-generation antipsychotic use in borderline personality disorder: what are we targeting? Ment Health Clin 6:82–88, 2016

West JC, Perry JC, Plakun E, et al: Psychotherapy practices of psychiatrists in the US: patterns, trends, and barriers to psychotherapy. Presentation at the 165th Annual Meeting of the American Psychiatric Association, May 2012, Philadelphia, PA, and the Institute on Psychiatric Services, New York, New York, October 2012

Westen D, Arkowitz-Westen L: Limitations of Axis II in diagnosing personality pathology in clinical practice. Am J Psychiatry 155:1767–1771, 1998

Westen D, Moses M, Silk KR, et al: Quality of depressive experience in borderline personality disorder and major depression: when depression is not just depression. J Pers Disord 6:382–393, 1992

Williams BC, Silk KR: "Difficult" patients, in Primary Care Psychiatry. Edited by Knesper DJ, Riba MB, Schwenk TL. Philadelphia, PA, WB Saunders, 1997, pp 61–75

Winnicott D: Transitional objects and transitional phenomena. Int J Psychoanal 34:89–97, 1953

Woodward B, Duckworth KS, Gutheil TG: The pharmacotherapist-psychotherapist collaboration, in American Psychiatric Press Review of Psychiatry, Vol 12. Edited by Oldham JM, Riba MB, Tasman A. Washington, DC, American Psychiatric Press, 1993, pp 631–649

Yen S, Shea MT, Pagano M, et al: Axis I and Axis II disorders as predictors of prospective suicide attempts: findings from the collaborative longitudinal personality disorders study. J Abnorm Psychol 112:375–381, 2003

Young JE, Klosko JS, Weishaar ME: Schema Therapy: A Practitioner's Guide. New York, Guilford, 2003

Zanarini MC, Frankenburg FR: Olanzapine treatment of female borderline personality disorder patients: a double-blind, placebo-controlled pilot study. J Clin Psychiatry 62:849–854, 2001

Zanarini MC, Frankenburg FR, Dubo ED, et al: Axis I comorbidity of borderline personality disorder. Am J Psychiatry 155:1733–1739, 1998

Zanarini MC, Frankenburg FR, Hennen J, et al: The longitudinal course of borderline psychopathology: 6-year prospective follow-up of the phenomenology of borderline personality disorder. Am J Psychiatry 160:274–283, 2003

CHAPTER 19

Boundary Issues

Thomas G. Gutheil, M.D.

Experience teaches that any discussion of boundary issues—boundary crossings and violations—must begin with certain caveats, best delivered in the form of three axioms. First, only the professional member of the treatment dyad has a professional code to honor or to violate; thus, only the professional is responsible for setting and maintaining professional boundaries. Second, patients, having no professional code, may transgress or attempt to transgress professional boundaries; if they are competent adults, they are responsible or accountable for their *behavior*. However, per axiom 1 above, it is the professional who must hold the line. Third, exploring the dynamics of interaction between therapist and patient is not intended to "blame the victim" (i.e., the patient) or to exonerate the professional from responsibility for the boundaries.

Boundary issues in the treatment of psychiatric patients are universal, as are concerns about these issues. Therefore, by discussing boundary issues in relation to patients with personality disorders (PDs), I do not imply that *all* patients with PDs or that *only* patients with PDs experience or pose boundary problems. Instead, the purpose of this chapter is to examine a subset of the wider universe of boundary-related potential problem areas.

The profession as a whole has had its consciousness raised by the emergence of careful study of trauma victims, many of whom had become highly sensitive to boundary transgressions by their treaters; indeed, boundary issues within the nuclear families of these individuals may have constituted, or been a component of, the trauma. The frequent association of boundary problems as precursors to actual sexual misconduct also focused attention on the subject. Nevertheless, the cases continue to appear (Brooks et al. 2012).

It is critically important to retain nonjudgmental clarity in this important area, especially because the consequences of confusion about this topic may be serious. This chapter aims at alleviating some of this confusion. Before turning attention to PDs and their implications for boundary theory, I review the basic elements of this theory.

Basic Elements of Boundary Theory

What exactly is a boundary? The following serves as a working definition: a boundary is the edge of appropriate, professional conduct. It is highly context dependent. The relevant contexts might be the treater's ideology, the stage of the therapy, the patient's condition or diagnosis, the geographical setting, the cultural milieu, and others. Another dimension of context, quite relevant for PDs, is the clinical versus the forensic setting (Faulkner and Regehr 2011; Zwirn and Owens 2011). Context is a critical and determinative factor.

Unfortunately, a number of boards of registration and some attorneys ignore the matter of context, to the detriment of fair decision making. Boards may draw from case law and complaints and resort to a "list of forbidden acts," ignoring context entirely (Gutheil and Brodsky 2008), as discussed in the following section.

Besides the data derived from complaint procedures and their aftermath, data about boundary issues come from consultations, supervision and training settings, the literature, professional meetings, informal remarks by colleagues, and formal studies. These data permit empirical examination of the varieties of boundary phenomena, the criteria for boundary assessment, and the clinical or forensic contexts in which problems arise. An extensive literature has grown up around this subject in recent decades, and the reader is directed to it for additional discussion beyond the narrower focus of this chapter (Baca et al. 2017; Epstein and Simon 1990; Gabbard 1999; Gabbard and Lester 2003; Gutheil and Gabbard 1993, 1998; Gutheil and Simon 2000, 2002; Ingram 1991; Langs 1976; Pope and Keith-Spiegel 2008; Simon 1989, 1992; Smith 1977; Spruiell 1983; Zur 2018). In sum, boundary problems may emerge from role issues, time, place and space, money, gifts and services, clothing, language, and physical or sexual contact (Gutheil and Gabbard 1993).

A special type of boundary problem is what has been called in a number of professional codes a "dual relationship" and has been warned against. This term applies to conflicted treatment relationships that also have a nonclinical dimension, such as a business, sexual, academic, or supervisory relationship.

Boundary Crossings and Boundary Violations

In an earlier publication Gabbard and I (Gutheil and Gabbard 1993) proposed a distinction that has proven important in both theory and litigation related to boundaries: the difference between boundary crossings and boundary violations. *Boundary crossings* are defined as transient, nonexploitative deviations from classical therapeutic or general clinical practice in which the treater steps out to a minor degree from strict verbal psychotherapy. These crossings do not hurt the therapy and may even promote or facilitate it. Examples might include offering a crying patient a tissue, helping a fallen patient up from the floor, helping an elderly patient to put on a coat, giving a fragile patient a home telephone number for emergencies, giving a patient on foot a lift in a car during a blizzard, writing a patient cards during a long absence, making home visits based on the patient's medical needs, answering selected personal questions, disclosing selected personal information, and the like. None of these actions is psychotherapy in its pure "talking" form—they constitute instead a mixture of manners, helpfulness, support, or social amity—yet no one could reasonably claim they are exploitative of the patient or the patient's needs. Depending on the context, the appropriate response to such actions is for the therapist to explore their impact to maximize their therapeutic utility and to detect and neutralize any difficulties the patient may have as a result; even the therapist's well-mannered gesture of putting out a hand for a handshake may be experienced by a patient with a horrendous trauma history as an attack or threat.

An important point about boundary crossings is that when they occur, the therapist should review the matter with the patient on the next available occasion and fully document the rationale, the discussion with the patient, and the description of the patient's response. This advice may be summarized as the "3 Ds": demeanor (remaining professional at all times), debriefing (with the patient at the next session), and documentation (of both the crossing event and its rationale).

Boundary violations, in contrast, constitute essentially harmful deviations from the normal parameters of treatment—deviations that *do* harm the patient, usually by some sort of exploitation that breaks the rule "first, do no harm"; usually, it is the therapist's needs that are gratified by taking advantage of the patient in some manner. In the case of violations, the therapy is not advanced and may even be destroyed. Examples might include taking advantage of the patient financially; using the patient to gratify the therapist's narcissistic or dependency needs; using the patient for menial services (cleaning the office, getting lunch, running errands); or engaging in sexual or sexualized relations with the patient. A useful test that may distinguish a boundary crossing from a violation is whether the event is discussable in the therapy (Gutheil and Gabbard 1993); an even better test might be whether the behavior in question would be discussable (hence, admissible) with a colleague, because many violators admit that they did not seek a consultation because they knew the consultant would tell them to stop the behavior. In any case, the only proper response to boundary violations is not to do them in the first place.

It is characteristic of boundary violations that they develop incrementally; that is, almost never does the dyad go from therapy to bed, as it were. Rather, more and more informality and increasing loss of therapeutic focus on the patient's needs develop during the treatment encounter. This may represent a "slippery slope" on the way to misconduct, because of inexperience, lack of knowledge, or inadequate supervision of the treater or other factors. Unfortunately, this process may have a more venal aspect called "grooming"; an exploitative treater may successively make greater boundary incursions while attempting to gauge what he or she can get away with.

As discussed in the next subsection, the difference between crossings and violations is highly context dependent. However, forensic experience demonstrates that some agencies, such as the more punitive state boards of registration, tend to view all boundaries from a rigid "checklist" perspective that does violence to clinical flexibility and the essential relevance of context, as in this real-life example.

In a hearing before the board of registration, one complaint was that the therapist, who was treating the wife in a couple, had been given a book by the husband in appreciation for the therapist's work. In some contexts, gift giving to therapists may be a boundary problem. The therapist's expert was on the stand.

BOARD'S PROSECUTING ATTORNEY (*forcefully and accusingly*): Now, Dr. Expert, are you aware that the husband *gave the therapist a book*?
EXPERT: Yes, and I cannot wait to hear how you believe that that exploited the wife.

The attorney moved directly to the next topic.

Context Dependence

In a conceptual and contextual vacuum, it may be impossible to make a clear distinction between a boundary crossing and a boundary violation. A therapist, say, who sends a dependent patient a reassuring postcard from his vacation is merely crossing the boundary; however, if the postcard is highly erotized, contains inappropriate content, and is part of an extended sexual seduction, the same gesture carries an entirely different weight.

Another element of context is the type and goal of the therapy. A favorite example is this: for an analyst doing classical psychoanalysis, no justification would exist for accompanying an adult patient into the bathroom; however, in the behaviorist treatment of paruresis (fear of urinating in public rest rooms), the last step in a behavioral paradigm of treatment might well be the therapist accompanying the patient there (Goisman and Gutheil 1992). This example also implies that the context may be affected by issues such as informed consent to the type of therapy, the nature and content of the therapeutic contract, the patient's expectations, and so on.

Power Asymmetry and Fiduciary Duty

The concepts of power asymmetry and fiduciary duty play an important theoretical role in analyzing boundary problems and are frequently used in discussing the consequences of boundary breaches. *Power asymmetry* refers to the unequal distribution of power between the two parties in the therapeutic dyad: the therapist has greater social and legal power than the patient. Part of this power derives from the fact that the therapist often has detailed knowledge of the patient, including, theoretically, the patient's weaknesses and vulnerabilities—knowledge that may be used for good or ill. With this power comes the greater responsibility for directing and containing the therapeutic envelope. The occasional plaint "It's not my fault—the patient seduced me" carries little weight under this formulation.

A *fiduciary duty* is a duty that is based on trust and obligation. The doctor, as a fiduciary, owes a duty to the patient to place the latter's interests first; primarily, the doctor does what the patient needs, not what the doctor wants to do. Exploitative boundary violations, therefore, are viewed as breaches of the doctor's fiduciary duty to the patient: the treater has placed his or her own gratification ahead of the patient's needs.

Consequences of Boundary Problems

The consequences of boundary problems may be divided into those *intrinsic* to the therapy and those *extrinsic* to the therapy. As discussed in the previous section, "Basic Elements of Boundary Theory," a serious and exploitative boundary violation may doom the therapy and cause the patient to feel (accurately) betrayed and used. The clinical consequences of boundary violations, including sexual misconduct, may encompass the entire spectrum of emotional harms from mild and transient distress to suicide. Intrinsic harms may include loss of good therapy, provision of harmful therapy, and loss of a window of opportunity for healing. One survivor commented, "I gave up my adolescence for that guy."

The *extrinsic* harms fall into three major categories: civil lawsuits (in some jurisdictions, criminal charges for overtly sexual activity); complaints to the state's board of registration, the licensing agency; and ethics complaints to the professional society (e.g., the district branch of the American Psychiatric Association), usually directed to the ethics committee of the relevant organization.

Civil Litigation

A civil lawsuit for boundary problems is based on the concept that the treater's deviation(s) from the appropriate standard of care constitute professional negligence and the patient consequently sustained some form of damages (Gutheil and Appelbaum 2020). This blunt legal analysis scants the commonly encountered clinical complexity of these claims. Although lawsuits for clinician sexual misconduct were a serious problem in past decades, observers have noted an increase in what might be termed "pure" boundary cases—that is, cases in which actual sexual intercourse has not occurred, but the patient is claiming harm from boundary violations short of that extreme.

Other factors may come into play in the litigation arena. The growing awareness of both boundary issues and their common precursor role in actual sexual misconduct has led some disgruntled patients to use a boundary claim as a means of taking revenge against a disliked clinician. A current joke holds that with the advent of managed care and the severe restrictions placed on length of treatment, no therapy will continue long enough for the patient to develop erotic transferences for the doctor.

Although most malpractice suits against the clinician will be defended and—in case of a loss—paid for by the malpractice insurer, many insurance policies contain exclusionary language that avoids coverage for the more sexualized forms of boundary violation; some insurers will pay only for the defense, and if the doctor loses the suit, the cost may be levied out of pocket.

Board of Registration Complaints

A board of registration complaint is the most serious because it challenges the physician's fitness to practice, which is supposedly rendered questionable by the boundary problem at issue. There are three serious problems with this form of complaint. First, registration boards in some areas are extremely punitive, seeking to meet quotas of delicensed practitioners and ignoring both context and evidence. Second, unlike in a malpractice case, a loss in a board of registration case may cost the clinician his or her license and, hence, livelihood. Finally, because this complaint is not a malpractice issue, one's insurance policy will often not fund the defense, leaving the doctor with out-of-pocket legal expenses. One implication of this grim scenario is that board complaints should be taken very seriously and must include legal assistance, no matter how bizarre, overreactive, and trivial the complaint may seem. Some companies offer "administrative" insurance that may provide legal coverage for board and ethics complaints (see below).

Ethics Complaints

The field of ethics has produced a vast wealth of philosophical opinion and literature as to what does and does not constitute ethical conduct, but an ethics complaint to one's professional society has an extremely concrete denotation; for example, it could assert that a specific section of the American Psychiatric Association's (2009) code of ethics has been violated by the boundary issue in question. What is ethical is what is in the "book." The outcome of a formal ethics complaint (informal ones are not accepted) ranges from censure and warning (not reportable to the National Practitioner Data Bank) to suspension or expulsion from the professional society (both of which are reportable). Such reportage may plague every subsequent job application and will usually also reach the relevant board.

Summary

The three types of complaints discussed in this section constitute the most common forms of negative consequence from boundary problems. Alas for fairness, attorneys, boards, and ethics committees may not be sufficiently sophisticated to distinguish between boundary crossings and violations. Thus, any boundary issues should be clearly described in the records, together with their rationales, as well as readily discussed and explored in the therapy itself.

Some Personality Types Encountered in Clinical Practice

I turn now to boundary issues that come up in relation to various PDs. As discussed in the introduction to this chapter, our study of the clinical correlation of boundary problems with a patient with a PD neither blames the victim nor exonerates the treater, nor does it remove from the treater the burdens of setting and maintaining boundaries. Indeed, it takes two to generate a true boundary problem. Thus, the following discussion addresses the interactions between patients with PDs and the clinicians attempting to treat them.

As might be inferred from earlier sections of this chapter, no particular therapist, patient, or PD should be considered immune from actual or potential boundary problems (Norris et al. 2003). Indeed, both members of the dyad may present risk factors that increase the likelihood of boundary problems. Therapist issues may include life crises; transitions in a career; illness; loneliness, and the impulse to confide in someone; idealization of a "special patient"; pride, shame, and envy; problems with limit setting; denial; and issues peculiar to being in a small-town environment where interaction with patients outside the office is unavoidable. Patient issues that increase vulnerability may include enmeshment with the therapist; retraumatization from earlier childhood abuse and felt helplessness from that earlier event; the repetition compulsion; shame and self-blame; feelings that the transference is "true love"; dependency; narcissism; and masochism (Norris et al. 2003).

Empirically, boundary issues are less likely to occur in the Cluster A group of PDs, which are marked by a tendency toward detachment, than in the other two clusters;

however, individuals in the group with very poor social skills and poor perspective-taking of others may cross boundaries more out of social ineptness than other dynamics.

Histrionic and Dependent Personality Disorders

Note that these examples refer to the DSM-IV/DSM-5 Section II model, but similar situations and dynamics would apply to patients diagnosed with Personality Disorder—Trait Specified according to the Alternative DSM-5 Model for Personality Disorders (AMPD) in Section III for patients with pathological trait patterns resembling these Section II diagnoses.

Consultative experience demonstrates that two symptoms manifested by patients with either histrionic or dependent PD tend to play roles in boundary excursions: neediness and drama. A patient's intense need for contact, self-esteem or approval, or relief from any anxiety or tension may pressure clinicians into hasty actions that cross boundaries. Other relevant histrionic traits according to the DSM 5 AMPD might include attention seeking, emotional lability, and manipulativeness; dependent traits might include submissiveness, separation insecurity, and anxiousness. These traits may inspire or lead to boundary problems.

A dependent patient who had been out drinking for an evening called her therapist in a panic and begged him to pick her up at the bar and drive her home. Feeling somewhat trapped and choiceless, the therapist did so. The situation, though presented by the patient as an emotional emergency, was clearly one merely of "urgency."

Although probably harmless, such an event may well be used by a board of registration as evidence of boundary problems in the treater. Appropriate responses may have included calling a cab, recommending public transportation if available, or making a call to family or friends.

Dramatic behavior may "trigger" a boundary problem because of the clinician's wish to "turn down the volume."

> A patient with histrionic PD, who was distraught after a session over a therapist's just-announced vacation plan, seated herself on the floor just outside the therapist's door and moaned loudly for a prolonged interval. The therapist, embarrassed by this scene taking place in full view of the clinic waiting room in front of other patients and staff, brought the patient back into the office and conducted an impulsive, prolonged session, intruding into other patients' appointments.

Although patients are free to cross boundaries, the limits must be set by the clinician. The therapist in this example might have told the patient that the behavior was inappropriate and should be discussed at the next appointment; should the patient refuse to leave, security might be called, and the matter explored at the next session. It appears likely that the dynamic operating in the vignette was the therapist's countertransference-based inability to deal with his or her own sadistic feelings about both planning a vacation (and thus causing abandonment feelings in the patient) and being able to turn the patient away when the latter was behaving inappropriately. Conflicts about sadism are a common source of boundary difficulties, especially in younger therapists; the issue of countertransference is further addressed in the section "Countertransference Issues" below.

One of the earliest and most famous examples of histrionic (it would then have been called "hysterical") behavior was the hysterical pregnancy and pseudo-childbirth of

Anna O., who was in the throes of an erotic transference to Joseph Breuer, as described in the "Studies on Hysteria" (Breuer and Freud 1893–1895/1955). Although Breuer is not recorded as violating any boundaries, the point can be made that patient reactions in this disorder may operate independently of the clinician's actual behavior, a fact leading to confusion among decision-making bodies.

Antisocial Personality Disorder

Individuals with antisocial personality disorder (ASPD) may strain the boundary envelope with the intent of furthering manipulation of either the therapist or, through the therapist, others in the environment. That environment may be clinical or forensic (Faulkner and Regehr 2011; Zwirn and Owens 2011). Examples might include getting the therapist to advocate for the patient at work, at school, and in other areas where the therapist is induced to step out of the limits of the clinical role to abet the patient's purposes.

A mentor of mine made the point that the differential diagnosis of ASPD includes "normal," because of the ability of such patients to blend in and to simulate normal responses (L. Havens, personal communication, 1981); this ability may disguise the underlying psychopathy for some time. Consultative experience reveals that yet another pitfall in diagnosis of such patients is the tendency of frontline clinicians to view patients with ASPD who endorse mood swings as actually bipolar; in some trainees that appears to represent an attempt to make a treatable diagnosis stand in for one regarded as far less treatable.

Another boundary issue seen with patients in this category is excessive familiarity and pseudo-closeness designed to get the therapist to perform uncharacteristic actions that transgress boundaries.

> DOCTOR (*on first meeting*): How do you do, I am Dr. Thomas Gutheil.
> PATIENT (*with warm handclasp*): Very glad to meet you, Thomas.
> DOCTOR (*slightly nonplused*): Um, well, Thomas *is* my given name, but I go by "Doctor Gutheil."
> PATIENT (*affably*): Whatever you say, Tommy.

As illustrated, the patient may shift on first acquaintance to a first-name or nickname basis to establish an artificial rapport designed to persuade the therapist to alter the rules of proper conduct. The therapist may feel silly or stuffy about correcting this undue familiarity or even bringing it up at all, but the effort should probably be made, in concert with attempts to explore the meaning of the behavior.

Some common goals of this tendency toward pseudo-closeness are obtaining excusing or exculpatory letters sent to nonclinical recipients; obtaining prescription of inappropriate or inappropriately large amounts of controlled substances; and intervention in the patient's extratherapeutic reality ("I need you to meet with my parole officer to go easier on me; you know how ill I am").

From the patient's viewpoint, the boundaries, even if recognized, may be ignored in a goal-directed manner. From the clinician's viewpoint, the boundary transgressions may lead to trouble, especially if the patient's actions encompass illegal behavior (e.g., selling of prescriptions) into which the doctor is drawn by association.

An unfortunately common clinically observed constellation of boundary problems is the following: a female psychotherapist is treating a male patient with antisocial PD but misses the antisocial elements in the patient, seeing the latter as a needy infant who requires loving care to "get better." In the course of this rescue operation, boundary incursions occur and increase (Gabbard and Lester 2003). In a "ladies love outlaws" paradigm, a female therapist may occasionally interpret her role as "taming a wild [male] psychopath." Such an effort may lead to enmeshment and blurred boundaries.

Borderline Personality Disorder

Like patients with ASPD, patients with borderline personality disorder (BPD) may manifest conscious or unconscious manipulative tendencies for a number of reasons. Some scholars assert that these patients manipulate because their low self-esteem leaves them feeling unentitled to ask directly to have their needs met. It is a clinical truism that unentitlement may be masked by an overt attitude of entitlement; the patient operates from the position that he or she is special and deserving of extra attention. This assertion of specialness can lead therapists to grant favors that transgress boundaries with these patients.[1]

> A patient with BPD in a subsequent psychotherapy commented out of the blue that she really felt her previous therapist should not have charged her a fee but should in fact have paid her, because her case was so interesting.

The surprising power of the manipulation to slip under the clinician's radar, as it were, is one of the more striking findings in the boundary realm. "I sensed that I was doing something that was outside my usual practice and, in fact, outside the pale," the therapist will lament to the consultant, "but somehow I just found myself making an exception with this patient and doing it anyway."

In an earlier article (Gutheil 1989), I described my experience with therapists seeking consultation, who would begin their narratives by saying, "I don't ordinarily do this with my patients, but in this case I...[insert a broad spectrum of inappropriate behaviors here]." The patient's sense of entitlement and of being "special" may infect the therapist with the same view of their specialness, such that even inappropriate exceptions are made. Clearly, a therapist who realizes that an exception to usual practice is about to be made should view this impulse as a "red flag" signaling the need for reflection and consultation.

The patient's own boundary problems—both in the ego boundary sense (Gabbard and Lester 2003) and in the interpersonal space—may evoke comparable boundary blindness in the therapist:

> A therapist noted that a patient with very primitive BPD would slide out of the office along the wall in a puzzling manner that seemed to convey a fearful state. On exploration the patient revealed that she was struggling with the fantasy that—if she passed too close to the therapist—she might accidentally fall forward and sink into the therapist's chest and be absorbed as though into quicksand. (D. Buie, personal communication, 1969)

---

[1]Because BPD empirically poses the greatest boundary difficulties, the reader may wish to review the axioms given at the outset of this chapter in order to maintain a properly nonjudgmental perspective.

Although the reader may detect the unconscious wishes for fusion hidden under this fear, the point of the anecdote is that for some patients, the boundary even of the physical self may be extremely tenuous. Indeed, wishes for fusion in both patient and therapist may provide the stimulus to boundary transgressions.

> A female therapist treating a female patient exhibited a number of interactions that revealed a wish for fusion. When the patient went to the office bathroom after a session, the therapist would take the adjoining stall and attempt to continue the session through the wall. When the relationship had progressed to the therapist sleeping over at the patient's home, and lying in her arms discussing problems, the therapist wore the patient's clothing to work the next day.

The patient with BPD may manifest impulsivity—"I need you to do this now, right now!"—that presses the therapist to act precipitously without forethought. The patient may demand an immediate appointment, an immediate telephone contact, an immediate home visit, an immediate ride home, an extended session, a medication refill, or a fee adjustment. Note, of course, that any or all of these may be clinically indicated but may also constitute or lead to boundary problems.

Research data indicate that patients with BPD often have a trauma history; that is, they were at one time victims (J. Herman, personal communication, 1980; cited in Gutheil and Gabbard 1993). Some of these patients adopt a posture of victimization (an element of entitlement distinguishable from narcissistic entitlement). This posture may mobilize rescue feelings, fantasies, or attempts in the therapist that lead him or her to "bend the rules" to achieve the rescue and thus to transgress boundaries (Gabbard 2003; Gutheil 2005). Indeed, consultative experience leads to the conclusion that a number of cases of sexual misconduct spring ultimately from claimed attempts to rescue the patient, to prevent suicide, to elevate the patient's self-esteem, or to provide a "good" relationship in an effort to counter a string of bad ones that the patient has experienced.

Borderline rage is also a factor leading to boundary problems, often through its power to intimidate.

> A 6-foot 7-inch former college linebacker, now a therapist, was asked in consultation why he went along with a boundary violation that he knew was inappropriate but that was demanded by the patient. When asked why he did not simply refuse, he looked down from his height and stated, "I just didn't dare."

As I have noted elsewhere, this rage may leave therapists feeling pressured into inappropriate self-disclosure, conceding to inappropriate requests, and manifesting other signs of being "moved through fear" (Gutheil 1989, p. 598).

Disappointed in many past relationships, the patient with BPD may contrive to "test the therapist's care or devotion" in boundary-transgressing ways that often represent reenactments of earlier developmental stages. For example, a patient may perceive that therapy offers some form of promise—such as inclusion in the therapist's idealized family (Gutheil 1989; Smith 1977). The patient may demand to sit on the therapist's lap or to be held or hugged, arguing that without this demonstration of caring, there can be no trust in the therapy. J. Herman (personal communication, 1980; cited in Gutheil and Gabbard 1993, p. 598) pointed out that because so many patients with

BPD have histories of sexual abuse, they may have been conditioned to interact with significant others on whom they depend in eroticized or seductive ways.

Forensic experience reveals the sad truth of how often these primitive maneuvers to obtain inappropriate closeness or contact actually succeed, to the detriment of the therapy and often to the censure of the therapist. As might well be expected, the wellspring of these deviations is commonly the countertransference in the dyad, my next topic.

Countertransference Issues

The patient's need for help and the treater's membership in a helping profession ordinarily provide a salutary and symmetrical reciprocity, but one that is not immune to distortion or miscarriage. The basic wish to help and heal, unfortunately, may inspire efforts that—no matter how well intended—transgress professional boundaries in problematic ways. The patient's transferential neediness and dependency may evoke a countertransferential need in the therapist to rescue, save, or heal the patient at any cost. Wishes to save the patient from anxiety, depression, or suicide are common stimuli to boundary violations in the name of rescue.

An example of this problem is what I call the "brute force" attempt at a cure. Frustrated by the difficulty of working with the patient and disappointed at the latter's lack of progress, the therapist sees the patient more and more often each week, for longer and longer session times; weekends, holidays, even vacations are no exception to this relentless crescendo. Therapists in this situation are being held hostage by the patient's insatiable need and are setting themselves the wholly unrealistic goal of meeting that need by "giving more" (Gutheil and Brodsky 2008).

In a related manner, such patients' suicide risk may lead the therapist to try desperate measures to prevent this outcome at all costs, including the cost of violating boundaries to achieve this rescue. Gabbard (1999) described this phenomenon in detail as the therapist's masochistic surrender, a dynamic issue closely linked to boundary problems.

The therapist's frustration may rise to the level of overt anger, in which the therapist acts out countertransference hostility by violating boundaries such as confidentiality; the therapist who angrily and inappropriately calls the patient's partner at home and rails at him or her to protest some action involving the patient has lost the compass that would keep one in bounds.

In a useful discussion, Smith (1977) defined the "golden fantasy" entertained by some patients with BPD and others; the golden fantasy is the belief that all needs—relational, supportive, nurturant, dependent, *and* therapeutic—will be met by the treater. As the patient loses track of what constitutes the therapeutic aspect of the work, the therapist, too, may begin to lose track of the actual parameters within which the treatment should take place.

The "Practice Guideline for the Treatment of Patients with Borderline Personality Disorder" (American Psychiatric Association 2001) stresses four basic points relating to patients with BPD and boundaries. The therapist should 1) monitor countertransference carefully, 2) be alert to deviations from usual practice ("red flags"), 3) always avoid boundary violations, and 4) obtain consultation for "striking deviations from the usual manner of practice" (American Psychiatric Association 2001, p. 24). These points are fully congruent with the material in this chapter.

In sum, because of their own difficulties with boundaries, their capacity to evoke powerful countertransference reactions, and the particular elements of their interpersonal style, patients with BPD pose some of the most noteworthy examples of boundary problems and challenges to clinicians to maintain proper limits.

Some Cross-Cultural Observations

Culture, of course, is itself a context; although some forms of boundary issues might be expected in all cultures, the majority of litigation and theoretical discussion seems to occur in the United States (e.g., Stone 1976). A cross-cultural study (Commons et al. 2006), however, comparing boundary matters in the United States and in Rio de Janeiro, Brazil, turned up some interesting findings. The U.S. sample and the Brazilian sample agreed at the extremes; that is, in both countries overt sexual misconduct at one end of the spectrum was seen as proscribed, and trivial deviations at the other end were seen as harmless. In the middle ranges, divergence was revealed. For example, subjects in the U.S. sample believed hugging a patient was suspect and kissing was surely wrong, but it was fully acceptable to display licenses, certificates, and some honors on the wall. In contrast, the Brazilian cohort found kissing the cheek in greeting to be universally acceptable and an accepted manner of greeting patients, but display of certificates was considered a deviation.

Risk Management Principles and Recommendations

Clearly, a rigid formalism and an icy demeanor are not the solution to boundary problems when dealing with patients with PDs; patients so treated will simply leave treatment. Rather, some basic guidelines may prove helpful to the clinician desirous of staying out of trouble while preserving the therapeutic effect of the work.

1. Clinicians of any ideological stripe must obtain some basic understanding of the dynamic issues relating to transference and countertransference. Training programs that foolishly boast of having transcended "that Freudian stuff" do a serious disservice to their graduates. A patient with BPD in the idealizing phase of treatment may worship the therapist, but a therapist who is untrained in the vagaries of transference may be left to assume that his or her own natural gifts of person have evoked this reaction—a dangerous view indeed.

2. Treaters of patients with PDs must keep in mind the latter's capacity to distort or overreact. A therapist who writes to such a patient and signs the letter, "Love, Dr. Smith," may intend *agape* (nonerotic love), but the patient may interpret *eros* and expect treatment consistent with that emotion. Even if the patient initially understands the meaning, the regulatory agencies may interpret that salutation as a sign that the clinician has lost objectivity and may assume boundaries have been vio-

lated (note that this sequence of events is not speculative but empirical). Therapists should, of course, take responsibility for their actions, but these patients can evoke strong feelings of guilt that distort the clinician's perception of what happened and who is responsible. Some basic and broad guidelines may be helpful (Gutheil 2011). In a board of registration complaint, a patient claimed to have been hurt by some action of a doctor. Instead of writing, "I am sorry you feel hurt," the doctor wrote, "I am sorry I hurt you." This ill-chosen expression of inappropriate self-blame made it almost impossible to convince the board that the doctor had remained within proper boundaries. The learning point here: When in doubt, obtain forensic or legal consultation.

3. The therapist should develop a "red flag" warning response when finding himself or herself doing what he or she would not usually do—that is, making an exception to customary practice. The exception in question may be an act of laudable creativity in treatment, but it may also be a boundary problem. Self-scrutiny and consultation may be most useful under the circumstances.

4. Simon and I (Gutheil and Simon 1995) observed that the neutral space and time when both parties rise from their chairs and move toward the door at the end of a session represents an occasion when both parties may feel that the rules do not really apply, because the session is theoretically over. We recommended that therapists pay attention to their experiences and the events and communications occurring during this "window"; a tendency toward crossing or even violating boundaries may emerge in embryonic form during this period, allowing the therapist to open the subject for exploration in the following session and, one hopes, to deflate its problematic nature.

5. When in doubt, a therapist should seek consultation; this honors my favorite maxim, "Never worry alone." Although getting consultation before taking a step that might present boundary ambiguities is an excellent idea, the therapist should also begin presenting the case to a colleague or supervisor when boundary problems begin to appear on the horizon or when the transference becomes erotized. Such consultation will aid in keeping perspective and in ensuring that the standard of care is being met.

6. Any potential boundary excursion of uncertain meaning should be marked by three critical steps: maintenance of professional behavior, discussion with the patient, and documentation. Under some circumstances a tactful apology to the patient for misreading a situation may also be in order. Failure to perform these steps casts the therapist in the light of one who wants to conceal wrongdoing. The "3 Ds" noted earlier (see subsection "Boundary Crossings and Boundary Violations") should be invoked, as in this example:

> Driving home from a late last appointment, a therapist sees his patient slogging wearily homeward on foot through the 2-foot-high drifts that a recent blizzard has deposited on the area. To prevent the patient from dying of exposure in the subfreezing weather, he offers her a ride home in his Jeep. In the car he continues to behave in a formal, professional manner, despite the odd circumstances. Next day at the office he records a careful note outlining his reasoning and the risk-benefit analysis of the incident. At the patient's next appointment, the therapist inquires how the incident felt to the patient, and its therapeutic significance is explored.

7. Therapists can avert the majority of boundary difficulties by taking this approach: "Explore before acting." Impulsive responses to patient demands are likely to go astray, as well as to inappropriately model impulsivity. Boundary issues pose special challenges for therapists; adherence to the basic principles described in this chapter may aid in protecting both therapists and patients.

References

American Psychiatric Association: Practice guideline for the treatment of patients with borderline personality disorder. Am J Psychiatry 158 (10 suppl):1–52, 2001

American Psychiatric Association: The Principles of Medical Ethics with Annotations Especially Applicable to Psychiatry, 2009 Edition, Revised. Arlington, VA, American Psychiatric Association, 2009

Baca C, Drogin EY], Gutheil TG: Sexual misconduct by mental health professionals, in The SAGE Encyclopedia of Abnormal and Clinical Psychology. Edited by Wenzel A. Thousand Oaks, CA, Sage, 2017, pp 3133–3134

Breuer J, Freud S: Studies on hysteria (1893–1895), in The Standard Edition of the Complete Psychological Works of Sigmund Freud, Vol 2. Translated and edited by Strachey J. London, Hogarth Press, 1955, pp 1–319

Brooks E, Gendel MH, Early SR, et al: Physician boundary violations in a physicians' health program: a 19-year review. J Am Acad Psychiatry Law 40:590–566, 2012

Commons ML, Miller PM, Gutheil TG: Cross-cultural aspects of boundaries: Brazil and the United States. J Am Acad Psychiatry Law 34:33–42, 2006

Epstein RS, Simon RI: The exploitation index: an early warning indicator of boundary violations in psychotherapy. Bull Menninger Clin 54:450–465, 1990

Faulkner C, Regehr C: Sexual boundary violations committed by female forensic workers. J Am Acad Psychiatry Law 39:154–163, 2011

Gabbard GO: Boundary violations, in Psychiatric Ethics, 3rd Edition. Edited by Bloch S, Chodoff P, Green SA. Oxford, UK, Oxford University Press, 1999, pp 141–160

Gabbard GO: Miscarriages of psychoanalytic treatment with suicidal patients. Int J Psychoanal 84:249–261, 2003

Gabbard GO, Lester EP: Boundaries and Boundary Violations in Psychoanalysis, 2nd Edition. Washington, DC, American Psychiatric Press, 2003

Goisman RM, Gutheil TG: Risk management in the practice of behavior therapy: boundaries and behavior. Am J Psychotherapy 46:532–543, 1992

Gutheil TG: Borderline personality disorder, boundary violations, and patient-therapist sex: medicolegal pitfalls. Am J Psychiatry 146:597–602, 1989

Gutheil TG: Boundaries, blackmail and double binds: a pattern observed in malpractice consultation. J Am Acad Psychiatry Law 33:476-481, 2005

Gutheil TG: A "pocket guide" to avoiding the commonest boundary pitfalls. Psychiatric Times February 2011, p 15

Gutheil TG, Appelbaum PS: Clinical Handbook of Psychiatry and the Law, 5th Edition. Philadelphia, PA, Wolters Kluwer, 2020

Gutheil TG, Brodsky A: Preventing Boundary Violations in Clinical Practice. New York, Guilford, 2008

Gutheil TG, Gabbard GO: The concept of boundaries in clinical practice: theoretical and risk management dimensions. Am J Psychiatry 150:188–196, 1993

Gutheil TG, Gabbard GO: Misuses and misunderstandings of boundary theory in clinical and regulatory settings. Am J Psychiatry 155:409–414, 1998

Gutheil TG, Simon RI: Between the chair and the door: boundary issues in the therapeutic "transition zone." Harv Rev Psychiatry 2:336–340, 1995

Gutheil TG, Simon RI: Non-sexual boundary crossings and boundary violations: the ethical dimension. Psychiatr Clin North Am 25:585–592, 2000

Gutheil TG, Simon RI: Non-sexual boundary crossings and boundary violations: the ethical dimension. Psychiatr Clin North Am 25:585–592, 2002

Ingram DH: Intimacy in the psychoanalytic relationship: a preliminary sketch. Am J Psychoanal 51:403–411, 1991

Langs R: The Bipersonal Field. New York, Jason Aronson, 1976

Norris DM, Gutheil TG, Strasburger LH: This couldn't happen to me: boundary problems and sexual misconduct in the psychotherapeutic relationship. Psychiatr Serv 54:517–522, 2003

Pope KS, Keith-Spiegel P: A practical approach to boundaries in psychotherapy: making decisions, bypassing blunders and mending fences. J Clin Psychol 64:638–652, 2008

Simon RI: Sexual exploitation of patients: how it begins before it happens. Psychiatr Ann 19:104–122, 1989

Simon RI: Treatment boundary violations: clinical, legal and ethical considerations. J Am Acad Psychiatry Law 20:269–288, 1992

Smith S: The golden fantasy: a regressive reaction to separation anxiety. Int J Psychoanal 58:311–324, 1977

Spruiell V: The rules and frames of the psychoanalytic situation. Psychoanal Q 52:1–33, 1983

Stone MH: Boundary violations between therapist and patient. Psychiatric Annals 6:670–677, 1976

Zur O: To cross or not to cross: do boundaries in therapy protect or harm? Psychother Bull 39:27–32, 2018

Zwirn I, Owens H: Commentary: boundary violations in the correctional versus therapeutic setting: are the standards the same? J Am Acad Psychiatry Law 39:164–165, 2011

PART IV

Special Problems, Populations, and Settings

CHAPTER 20

Assessing and Managing Suicide Risk

Paul S. Links, M.D., FRCPC

Philippe Boursiquot, M.D., FRCPC

Madison Links, M.D.

Personality disorders (PDs) are highly prevalent disorders that impart significant morbidity and mortality. In the National Comorbidity Survey Replication, the prevalence of PDs was found to be approximately 9% in the general population (Lenzenweger et al. 2007). Borderline personality disorder (BPD), in particular, is a disabling condition affecting approximately 2% of the general population, 10% of psychiatric outpatients, and 20% of psychiatric inpatients (Lieb et al. 2004). Individuals with BPD are significant users of health services (Zanarini et al. 2004), and their lifetime risk of suicide ranges between 3% and 10% (Paris and Zweig-Frank 2001). As a result of the risk of suicide and repeated suicidal behavior (referring to behaviors with some level of intent to die), the illnesses of these patients are often considered difficult to treat, and these patients are actively avoided by clinicians. However, recent research indicates that appropriate psychiatric care can reduce the risk of future suicidal behavior in patients with BPD and thus is highly indicated. This chapter provides an understanding of the associations among PDs, suicidal behavior, nonsuicidal self-injury (NSSI), and suicide and also a discussion of the nonmodifiable and potentially modifiable risk factors for suicide and suicidal behavior. The final sections of the chapter discuss proposed causal pathways to NSSI and suicidal behavior and an approach to assessing acute suicide risk in patients with PDs.

Much of this chapter focuses on patients with BPD, which is the only PD in DSM-IV and DSM-5 (American Psychiatric Association 1994, 2013) to have recurrent suicidal or self-injurious behavior as one of the diagnostic criteria. In Section III of DSM-5, the proposed revision to BPD in the Alternative DSM-5 Model for Personality Disorders includes "self-harming behavior under emotional distress" as a defining feature of the disorder (American Psychiatric Association 2013, p. 767). Although suicidal behaviors are associated with other PDs, our emphasis on BPD in this review results from the clinical importance of this disorder and the fact that much of the research and progress over the last three decades has been focused on BPD.

We have organized our discussion of the assessment of suicide risk in patients with PDs based on the model of an "acute-on-chronic" risk (i.e., the acute risk that occurs over and above the ongoing chronic risk). *Chronic risk for suicide* relates to factors that have existed for many months or years and generally are not modifiable. In contrast, *acute risk for suicide* relates to factors that have existed for days, weeks, or months and are often modified by clinical interventions. The acute-on-chronic risk model is presented as a way of assessing and communicating the suicidal risk of patients with BPD, and in particular those patients with histories of repeated suicidal behaviors. This model should be differentiated from other models of suicide, suicidal behavior, and NSSI, such as the stress-diathesis model (Mann et al. 1999), which is a proposed causal model of suicidal behavior. Several of the most prominent models of causal pathways to suicidal behavior are discussed later in the chapter.

Literature Search

We completed a literature search to determine relevant literature to update and revise our previously published work. In our literature search using the McMaster University Health Sciences Library online catalogue search tool, our search parameters involved sources limited to peer-reviewed journal articles published between January 1, 2013, and May 1, 2019. In addition, we used the university's Health Sciences Library website, which has a health-related article database. The databases we used to search for articles included Ovid Medline, PubMed, ClinicalKey, Cochrane Library, DynaMed Plus, and PsycINFO. The key words and phrases we used for the literature search included the following: antisocial, obsessive-compulsive, schizotypal, borderline, avoidant, and narcissistic PDs; suicide; suicidal behavior; nonsuicidal self-injurious behavior; clinical studies; epidemiology; risk factors; and longitudinal course. We reviewed only English language papers. Articles were omitted if they were review chapters, review articles, treatment studies, studies not specific to PDs, and studies addressing related concepts (e.g., reward processing in BPD) but not specifically suicide, suicidal behavior, or NSSI.

Epidemiology

PDs are associated with a significant burden of illness and a relatively high prevalence of suicidal behavior and death by suicide. In one psychological autopsy study of 163 suicide decedents diagnosed using semi-structured diagnostic interviews with informants, 72.3% of men and 66.7% of women had features that met the criteria for at least one PD, and 42.6% of men and 30.8% of women had features that met the criteria in multiple PD clusters (Schneider et al. 2006). Another autopsy study of 229 suicide victims diagnosed by two pairs of psychiatrists found that 29.3% of their sample had features that met the criteria for at least one PD (Isometsa et al. 1996).

In Schneider et al.'s (2006) psychological autopsy study of deaths by suicide, 20% of men and 17.9% of women had features that met the criteria for paranoid PD, 10.8% of men and 12.8% of women met the criteria for schizoid PD, and 6.5% of men and 5.1% of women met the criteria for schizotypal PD. Isometsa et al. (1996) found a much lower rate, with 0.4% of suicide victims ($n=1$) having features that met the criteria for paranoid PD; in no cases were the criteria for other Cluster A PDs met.

In a retrospective study of patients with schizotypal PD followed for an average of 19 years, 3% died by suicide, 24% attempted suicide, and 45% expressed suicidal ideation (Fenton et al. 1997). Using data from the National Epidemiological Survey on Alcohol and Related Conditions, Lentz et al. (2010) reported that individuals with schizotypal PD ($n=307$) were 1.51 times more likely to have attempted suicide than individuals in the general population. In a study of inpatients with a primary diagnosis of PD, Ahrens and Haug (1996) found that 44% of individuals with schizoid PD and 47% of individuals with paranoid PD displayed "suicidal tendencies."

Jahn et al. (2016), in a sample of undergraduate students, tested whether the association between interpersonal schizotypy and suicidal ideation or suicide attempts was explained by psychological mediators, namely depressive symptoms, self-esteem, intimate disclosure in peer relationships, and social anxiety. The study found that depressive symptoms and low self-esteem explained the relationship between interpersonal schizotypy and lifetime worst-point suicidal ideation. In general, the authors suggested that schizotypy had an indirect rather than direct relationship to suicide risk.

Levi-Belz et al. (2019) researched whether schizotypal personality symptoms contributed to suicidal behavior, and particularly more-lethal suicide attempts. Comparing across four groups that included medically serious suicide attempters, medically nonserious suicide attempters, and psychiatric and healthy controls, the authors found that schizotypal personality symptoms were common to all suicide attempters; however, interpersonal difficulties and emotional detachment were important characteristics of those who engaged in highly lethal versus nonserious suicide attempts.

In the Isometsa et al. (1996) study of suicides mentioned previously, the prevalence of Cluster C PDs in the total sample was 10%. Of the suicide victims who met criteria for PDs, 7% had features that met the criteria for dependent PD, 6% for avoidant PD, and 3% for obsessive-compulsive PD. In the Schneider et al. (2006) study, also introduced above, 21.3% of men and 15.4% of women had features that met the criteria for avoidant PD, 6.2% of men and 5.1% of women met the criteria for dependent PD, and 23.1% of men and 17.9% of women met the criteria for obsessive-compulsive PD.

A cross-sectional study of psychiatric inpatients examined for Cluster C PDs found that 35% of patients with dependent PD, 18% of patients with avoidant PD, and 14% of patients with obsessive-compulsive PD had made a suicide attempt in the past (Chioqueta and Stiles 2004). In a study of 31 patients with depression and comorbid obsessive-compulsive PD, 52% had made a suicide attempt and 37.5% had made multiple attempts (Diaconu and Turecki 2009).

The estimated rates of suicide among individuals with BPD have ranged from 0% to 10%, depending on the setting, patient characteristics, and method of study. In their 27-year follow-up study of patients previously hospitalized with a diagnosis of BPD, Paris and Zweig-Frank (2001) reported a suicide rate of 10%, and a similar Japanese long-term follow-up study reported a suicide rate of 6.9% (Paris 2004; Yoshida et al.

2006). Several prospective studies, however, have found lower rates of suicide. In a 10-year prospective study by Zanarini et al. (2006), the rate of death by suicide was 4%. This same cohort at 24 years of prospective follow-up demonstrated a 5.9% rate of death by suicide (Temes et al. 2019). In a study of patients with BPD recruited at the Austen Riggs Center, a voluntary residential treatment facility, and followed in treatment for 7 years, Perry et al. (2009) found no deaths by suicide. Links et al. (2013), in a prospective follow-up study of BPD patients who received 1 year of BPD-indicated treatment, found that none died by suicide during 1 year of treatment and 2 years of follow-up. These results suggest that patients receiving regular outpatient treatment may be at significantly lower risk compared to an untreated or undertreated population of patients with BPD.

In patients with BPD, the rate of attempted suicide is much higher than the rate of suicide, and it is estimated that around 85% of patients have a history of attempted suicide (Paris 2004). In one cohort of previous suicide attempters, the rate of medically significant suicide attempts was 27.8% by year 6 of follow-up (Soloff and Chiappetta 2012). In another cohort recruited from an inpatient setting, 79.3% had made an attempt at baseline and 32% made an attempt within the first 2 years of follow-up (Wedig et al. 2012). Neither of these studies controlled for the amount or type of treatment received. In the prospective study of treated patients, Links et al. (2013) reported that 81.1% of patients had made a suicide attempt in the past, 26% of participants made a suicide attempt during the 1-year treatment phase, and 16.7% made an attempt during the 2-year follow-up period.

Patients with antisocial PD are also considered to be at elevated risk for suicide. One 5-year follow-up study found that 5.7% of subjects died of suicide within the follow-up period (Maddocks 1970). A Finnish psychological autopsy study of adolescents ages 13–19 years found that 17% had features that met the criteria for conduct disorder or antisocial PD (Marttunen et al. 1991). Cleckley (1976) considered that persons with psychopathy that often characterizes antisocial PD had "a disinclination" toward suicide. The psychopathic factors of emotional detachment, superficial charm, manipulativeness, callousness, and lack of empathy (the so-called Factor 1 features) have been found by some investigators to have a negative relationship to suicide attempts (Harrop et al. 2017; Verona et al. 2005); however, these findings are mixed, and further research is needed (Harrop et al. 2017).

Data on narcissistic PD and suicide risk are limited but growing. Apter et al. (1993) studied 43 consecutive suicides by Israeli males ages 18–21 that occurred during their compulsory military service. Psychological autopsies were carried out using pre-induction assessment information, service records, and extensive postmortem interviews. The most common PDs were schizoid personality in 16 of 43 (37.2%) and narcissistic personality in 10 of 43 (23.3%).

Stone's (1990) extensive follow-up study of 550 patients admitted to the general clinical research service of the New York State Psychiatric Institute provided some information on suicide for individuals hospitalized with the diagnosis of narcissistic PD. According to the 15-year follow-up, patients with the disorder or narcissistic traits were significantly more likely to have died by suicide compared with patients without the disorder or traits (14% vs. 5%; $P<0.02$). One report suggested that narcissistic personality was a risk factor for suicidal ideation in elderly patients with depression (Heisel et al. 2007). Blasco-Fontecilla et al. (2009b) compared suicide attempts among patients with various Cluster B PDs. In contrast to suicide attempters with other Cluster B PDs, those with narcissistic PD were less impulsive in their attempts, suggesting that they were more intentional in their suicidal behavior. Attempters with narcissistic PD also reported significantly higher expected lethality from their attempt compared to suicide attempters without narcissistic PD. The authors concluded that suicide attempters with narcissistic PD may be different from other Cluster B PD attempters in that their suicidal behavior is more intentional and less impulsive.

Some evidence has suggested that narcissistic pathology may be negatively associated with the risk for suicide. Svindseth et al. (2008) examined the relationship between scores on the Narcissistic Personality Inventory–21 item version (NPI-21) and violence, suicidality, and other psychopathology among patients admitted to acute psychiatric wards. In their sample, male gender, involuntary admission, severe violence, and high self-esteem were significantly associated with a high level of narcissism. However, the level of suicidality as measured by the Brief Psychiatric Rating Scale was significantly associated with low levels of narcissism. Anxiety, depression, and withdrawal/retardation were also associated with low levels of narcissism. These results may be a function of the particular qualities of the NPI-21, which is considered to capture aspects of "adaptive expressions" of the narcissistic concept; therefore, these concepts are likely to be inversely related to psychological distress and risk of suicide (Pincus and Lukowitsky 2010). Jaksic et al. (2017) studied a sample of 250 psychiatric outpatients and demonstrated that narcissistic vulnerability had unique significant positive associations with acute suicidal ideation, whereas narcissistic grandiosity was not significantly related to acute suicidal ideation. The researchers found that certain dimensions of shame-proneness mediated the relationship between narcissistic vulnerability and suicidal ideation.

Bolton and Robinson (2010) found in a general population cross-sectional survey that, after controlling for other diagnoses, narcissistic PD respondents versus those without narcissistic PD were 1.7 times less likely to report a suicide attempt. Giner et al. (2013) compared 636 adult suicide attempters and suicide decedents on various characteristics and from their multivariate analyses found that suicide decedents were 20 times more likely than attempters to be diagnosed with narcissistic PD and to have health problems. Coleman et al. (2017) studied a sample of 657 mood disorder patients and determined that narcissistic PD patients were 2.4 times less likely to have a suicide attempt history and that narcissistic PD was not related to either clinician- or self-rated lethality of suicide attempts.

Nonsuicidal self-injury is defined as the purposeful destruction of one's bodily tissue that is without cultural significance or lethal intent (Klonsky et al. 2014). In patients with BPD, self-poisonings should also be included, although self-poisonings are more commonly engaged in with suicidal intent (Andover and Gibb 2010). Although NSSI has been differentiated from suicidal behavior (based on some intent to die), many experts posit that these behaviors exist on a continuum and should be conceptualized as belonging to the same family of behaviors (Klonsky et al. 2014).

NSSI is common. Although approximately 15%–38% of college students engage in NSSI, most do not meet full criteria for a diagnosis of BPD (Brickman et al. 2014). Approximately 65%–80% of individuals with BPD report NSSI (Brickman et al. 2014), and NSSI is still one of the best predictors of an accurate diagnosis of BPD, both at baseline (Grilo et al. 2001) and at 2-year follow-up (Grilo et al. 2007). Studies of individuals with BPD and NSSI, compared to individuals with NSSI without BPD, demonstrated that BPD is associated with greater NSSI severity (e.g., cutting, burning, swallowing dangerous objects), greater likelihood of repetitive NSSI, and greater diversity of methods of NSSI (Vega et al. 2017). Research has observed that individuals with BPD have a peak in the prevalence of NSSI during early and middle adolescence and a decline into adulthood (Klonsky et al. 2014).

In summary, although research evidence shows a meaningful association between PD diagnoses and death by suicide, the strongest association seems to be between BPD and death by suicide. BPD is also related to frequent, repetitive, and severe suicidal behavior and NSSI. Narcissistic PD may have a very unique relationship to suicide; individuals demonstrating grandiose characteristics may be protected against suicidality, whereas those with vulnerable characteristics have increased risk. Narcissistic PD also may confer a risk more related to death by suicide than suicide attempts, because patients with narcissistic PD may carry out very lethal attempts but hold various motives for their actions (e.g., wanting death before dishonor) and have no conscious intention to die (Ronningstam and Maltsberger 1998).

Risk Factors

Using the acute-on-chronic risk model, the ongoing risk of suicide is determined by chronic risk factors (typically nonmodifiable risk factors), whereas discrete periods of increased risk arise from acute risk factors (Zaheer et al. 2008). Most empirical work on chronic risk factors in PDs has been done in BPD. The limited data related to the other PDs will be presented separately in indicated subsections of this section.

Chronic or Nonmodifiable Risk Factors

Demographics

The literature on BPD has reported little association between age, race, or sex and suicide attempter or high-lethality status (Links et al. 2013; Sher et al. 2019; Soloff 2005; Wedig et al. 2012). However, older patients with BPD with a chronic course of illness may be at increased risk for suicide as discussed later in this chapter (see the section "Course of Suicidal Behavior").

Personality Disorder Features

Three subcategories of BPD symptoms have been investigated with respect to suicide risk: impulsivity, affective instability, and dissociation. Impulsivity has been considered a risk factor for suicide (Wedig et al. 2012). Some research, however, has called this finding into question. Comparing individuals with BPD with Cluster B comorbidity who completed suicide, individuals with BPD without Cluster B comorbidity who completed suicide, and individuals living with BPD, McGirr et al. (2007) found a gradient of psychopathology across the groups, particularly for substance-dependent disorders and impulsive aggressiveness, with the highest levels of psychopathology being found in those individuals with BPD and Cluster B comorbidity. With respect to attempter status, Wedig et al. (2012) similarly found that impulsivity did not predict attempter status when self-harm and substance use disorder (SUD) were not incorporated into the measurement. These findings suggest that these specific components of impulsivity may be the true predictors of risk (Wedig et al. 2012) and that more precise clinical definitions of impulsivity as it relates to suicide risk are needed.

Affective instability and dissociation were associated with attempter status in Wedig et al.'s (2012) longitudinal follow-up study. In an experience sampling study, Links et al. (2008) found that negative mood intensity and mood amplitude were the facets of affective instability most associated with a history of suicidal behavior. Affective instability was correlated with the variability of suicidal ideation in patients with BPD and a history of suicide attempts (Rizk et al. 2019). Although emotional dysregulation has been thought to be associated with parasuicide and suicide attempts in patients with BPD (Gratz and Gunderson 2006; Hasking et al. 2010; Zanarini et al. 1998), a study examining the impact of emotional dysregulation (as measured by the Difficulties in Emotion Regulation Scale) on lifetime suicide attempts in a transdiagnostic sample showed no such association; however, BPD itself was associated with lifetime suicide attempts (Harris et al. 2018). By contrast, Mou et al. (2018) found that when experiencing negative affective states, such as feeling abandoned or humiliated, patients with BPD were more likely to experience suicidal thoughts.

Both affective instability and dissociative symptoms were protective against death by suicide in McGirr et al.'s (2009) study. These findings may suggest two distinct trajectories of suicidal behavior in BPD, one involving multiple low-lethality behaviors and another involving high-lethality and potentially fatal behaviors (Soloff and Chiappetta 2012). In a 1-year prospective study of NSSI, borderline personality features other than the suicide/self-injury criterion were identified as predictors, along with history of NSSI (Glenn and Klonsky 2011).

In an adolescent psychiatric inpatient sample, Glenn et al. (2013) also found that, compared with other BPD features, affective instability was uniquely related to suicidal thoughts and behaviors and uniquely differentiated suicide attempters among suicide ideators over and above general negative emotionality. Sadeh et al. (2014) tested whether specific features of BPD were related to NSSI functions in a small sample of adolescents and youth attending a psychotherapy clinic. They found that affective dysregulation BPD features were related to the intrapersonal functions of NSSI (e.g., regulating affect, punishing oneself), whereas the interpersonal dysfunction BPD features were related to interpersonal functions of NSSI (e.g., bonding with peers, establishing autonomy).

National Epidemiologic Survey on Alcohol and Related Conditions–III (NESARC-III) examined the covariates of self-directed, other-directed, and combined (self- and other-directed) violence (Harford et al. 2018). Survey participants with BPD showed higher odds for combined violence relative to participants with only self- or other-directed violence.

Psychosocial Functioning and Treatment History

Markers of impaired function, such as low socioeconomic status, poor global functioning, and preexisting treatment history, represent significant risk factors for suicidal behavior in patients with BPD over the longer term (Soloff and Chiappetta 2012, 2017, 2019). Over the 10-year follow-up, Soloff and Chiappetta (2019) continued to find that nonspecific measures of illness severity and baseline social, vocational, and psychosocial functioning were the most robust predictors of suicide attempts over the follow-up period.

Childhood Abuse

Childhood abuse and its aftereffects are a nonmodifiable risk factor for suicide attempts that may persist in spite of treatment (Links et al. 2013). Most research has focused on sexual abuse, but childhood abuse of any type can be a risk factor (Zaheer et al. 2008). Childhood emotional neglect was found to predict self-harm behavior as well as suicide attempts via separate pathways in patients with BPD (Blasczyk-Schiep et al. 2018, discussed below).

In Wedig et al.'s (2012) naturalistic follow-up of patients with BPD, posttraumatic stress disorder (PTSD) was an independent predictor of attempter status, whereas childhood abuse was not. Conversely, in a treated sample of individuals with BPD, severity of childhood sexual abuse emerged as a continuing risk factor, whereas PTSD did not (Links et al. 2013). Ferraz et al. (2013) examined the relationship of impulsiveness-related traits and the history of childhood sexual abuse to suicidal behavior in patients with BPD. They found that hostility and a history of childhood sexual abuse, but not impulsiveness and other temperament traits, were related to the presence, number, and severity of previous suicide attempts in patients with BPD. The authors suggested that hostility may be associated with the impulsive-aggression dimension and that future research must consider the composite nature of impulsivity. These findings suggest that certain shared factors may explain the association between trauma and the risk for suicide. Potential mediators of this risk between impulsive-related traits and history of childhood sexual abuse to suicidal behavior include the Cluster A traits, impulsive aggression and poor social adjustment, as well as neurobiological changes (Soloff et al. 2008). Blasczyk-Schiep et al. (2018) proposed explanatory models in which failure of state orientation (primarily ruminative vs. primarily pertaining to decision making) plays a mediating role between emotional neglect and the outcomes of suicide attempts and self-harm in patients with BPD. Rumination was posited to lead to depression, loss of reasons to live, and suicide attempts, whereas impaired decision making was linked to an inability to improve low positive affect in the face of stress, thereby leading to self-harm.

Chronic Risk Factors: Other Personality Disorders

Limited information is available about chronic risk factors for suicide in PDs other than BPD. The Collaborative Longitudinal Personality Disorders Study (CLPS), in which the sample included patients with schizotypal, avoidant, and obsessive-compulsive PDs as well as BPD, found no association between attempter status and age, gender, race, occupation, or education level (Yen et al. 2005).

Some evidence indicates an association between suicide risk and treatment history, burden of illness, and PD features. In Ahrens and Haug's (1996) sample of inpatients with any PD, the number of previous attempts was associated with "suicidal tendencies"; hospitalizations and other exposures to psychiatric treatment were not investigated. In a study by Blasco-Fontecilla et al. (2009a), "diffuse" PD (PD comorbidity across multiple PD clusters) was associated with number of suicide attempts but not lethality. Similarly, in a psychological autopsy, multiple-cluster pathology was associated with an increased odds ratio of 16.13 in men and 20.43 in women for death by suicide (Schneider et al. 2006). In NESARC-III, both schizotypal and antisocial PDs, similar to BPD, were associated with a higher odds of combined violence compared with no violence. Antisocial PD was also associated with a higher odds of combined violence compared to self-directed violence (Harford et al. 2018). Lastly, in a sample of patients with Cluster B PDs, all suicide attempters except those with narcissistic PD had significantly higher impulsivity than non-attempters, suggesting that impulsivity may be important in histrionic PD and antisocial PD (Blasco-Fontecilla et al. 2009b).

Collectively, these data suggest that some of the chronic risk factors that apply to BPD, including burden of illness and extensive treatment history, may also apply to the other PDs. More research is necessary to fully explore this area.

Acute or Modifiable Risk Factors

Comorbidities

The role of psychiatric comorbidity in suicide attempter status and in lethality of attempts in patients with BPD has been investigated extensively, particularly with respect to PTSD, major depressive disorder (MDD), SUD, and antisocial PD; however, the results have been inconsistent (McGirr et al. 2007; Soloff 2005; Zaheer et al. 2008). Wedig et al. (2012) found that MDD, SUD, and PTSD were all significantly associated with attempter status during 16 years of naturalistic follow-up. Mellesdal et al. (2015) found that PTSD—directly as well as through mediation of emotional dysregulation—was associated with hospital admission for self-harm. Conversely, in the prospective follow-up of a treated sample, Links et al. (2013) found that none of these diagnoses predicted attempter status. One way to interpret this discrepancy is to view comorbid conditions as modifiable risk factors and treatment status as an important consideration in evaluating the evidence (Links et al. 2013).

Sher et al. (2016) compared patients with BPD and a history of suicide attempts, BPD patients without a history of attempts, and healthy volunteers. Patients with a history of suicide attempts had higher levels of affective lability, aggression, depression, anxiety, and NSSI than patients with BPD but no history of suicide attempts. In addition, patients with a history of suicide attempts were more likely than those without to have comorbid MDD and BPD but less likely to be diagnosed with comorbid narcissistic PD.

Predictors of high-lethality status have been similarly inconsistent. Zaheer et al. (2008) identified the presence of specific phobias, lifetime PTSD, and schizotypal traits as risk factors for increased lethality, whereas Soloff et al. (2005) found an association only with antisocial PD. In a study of nonclinical participants, Chabrol and Raynal (2018) reported higher suicidal ideation in individuals with the co-occurrence of high borderline and autistic traits than in participants with low traits of both conditions or in participants with autistic or borderline traits alone.

The heterogeneity of studied populations, of the measurement tools used, and of the definitions of high lethality employed across studies may explain the variable findings (Zaheer et al. 2008). Another explanation is that comorbid conditions may act nonspecifically by increasing the burden of illness experienced by an individual; this burden of illness may lead to an increased risk of suicide (Zaheer et al. 2008). Comorbid psychopathologies, in general, are frequently reported among individuals with suicidal behavior, regardless of diagnosis. There is a substantial elevation in the risk of suicidal behavior for individuals with two or more psychiatric disorders. Nock et al. (2015) reported that among a sample of new soldiers, the odds ratio for suicidal ideation increased from 3.1 for those with one disorder to 11.7 for those with seven or more disorders. A similar pattern was seen for suicide attempts, with the odds ratio increasing from 4.1 to 39.8.

Finally, it is possible that comorbid conditions are surrogates for more specific risk factors included among their symptoms (Zaheer et al. 2008). For example, a subgroup of patients with PTSD could experience perceptual/dissociative symptoms that put them at higher suicide risk independent of the overall diagnosis (Zaheer et al. 2008). In another study with a nonclinical sample, BPD traits were associated with suicide risk, an effect that was mediated by insomnia but not nightmares (DeShong and Tucker 2019).

Stressful Life Events

Stressful life events present significant obstacles to patients with BPD, whose pathology often renders them unable to cope effectively. In addition, patients' BPD features may be responsible for causing stressful life events to occur.

Acute interpersonal stress is especially pertinent to the evaluation of suicide risk in patients with BPD. In a study by Brodsky et al. (2006), patients with BPD were more likely to report interpersonal triggers for both initial and subsequent suicide attempts. Interpersonal triggers may be characteristic stressors for patients with BPD, but other kinds of loss and transitions may also be relevant. For example, recent hospital discharge and the associated loss of supportive structures can be a risk factor for patients with BPD (Kolla et al. 2008). Shame surrounding an interpersonal stressor has been suggested as an intermediate risk factor between interpersonal events and suicidal behavior (Brown et al. 2009).

In the McLean Study of Adult Development, a 16-year follow-up study, Wedig et al. (2013) found that predictors of suicide threats included feeling abandoned and hopeless, as well as being demanding and manipulative, all emotions connected with interpersonal relationships. From the same study, Zanarini et al. (2013) noted that in addition to interpersonal reasons for engaging in self-harm, participants with more extensive self-harm reported internally directed reasons (e.g., to control emotional pain, to punish self, to prevent being hurt in a worse way) to a greater extent.

Other Personal Risk Factors

In Glenn and Klonsky's (2011) prospective study, participants' behavioral forecast of their future engagement in NSSI was a predictor of NSSI over the 1-year follow-up, as were past NSSI and borderline personality features, both chronic risk factors. In preliminary results from a study of hospitalized adolescents ages 11–17 years admitted with a suicide attempt, those with BPD engaged in nonproductive coping, mostly avoidant strategies, more than did those without BPD (Knafo et al. 2014). In a cross-sectional study of 80 patients with BPD, meaning in life has been shown to negatively correlate with suicide risk (García-Alandete et al. 2014).

Acute Risk Factors: Other Personality Disorders

Yen et al. (2005) found a relationship between negative life events and suicide attempts in the CLPS sample of individuals with mixed PDs. Specifically, negative events pertaining to love/marriage and crime/legal matters (both as victim and as perpetrator) were significant predictors of suicide attempts in the next month after their occurrence.

It remains to be determined whether some life events are as pertinent to suicide risk in patients with other PDs as interpersonal events are to risk in patients with BPD. Blasco-Fontecilla et al. (2010) explored this question in a mixed sample of patients from all three clusters of PDs. Only in patients with Cluster B disorders were suicide attempts found to be associated with specific stressors independent of Axis I diagnosis. Attempts by individuals with antisocial PD were associated with jail terms, minor violations of the law, and spousal death, whereas attempts by individuals with narcissistic PD were associated with marital arguments, personal injury/illness, and mortgage foreclosure. Although confounded by the presence of Axis I pathology, some relationships were also identified between specific event categories and Cluster A and Cluster C disorders.

Summary

This review suggests that stressful life events and some comorbid psychiatric disorders might be modifiable risk factors for reducing an acute-on-chronic exacerbation of suicide risk in patients with PDs (see the section "Assessing Suicide Risk in Patients with Personality Disorders" later in this chapter). Over the longer course of the disorder, markers of impaired function such as low socioeconomic status, poor global functioning, and preexisting treatment history represent significant risk factors for suicidal behavior. Early and sustained outpatient treatment directed at enhancing family, social, and vocational functioning might decrease long-term suicide risk in patients with BPD. Current treatment modalities for BPD (e.g., dialectical behavior therapy [DBT; Linehan 1993], pharmacotherapy) are focused on symptomatic relief. Efforts to increase overall psychosocial functioning might be more relevant to long-term prognosis. A rehabilitation model of treatment (as in the treatment of schizophrenia) might be required to optimize outcome in BPD (Links 1993).

Course of Suicidal Behavior

Despite a fatal outcome in a minority of PD patients (e.g., 3%-10% for BPD [Paris and Zweig-Frank 2001]), the vast majority can expect significant symptom relief over time. Recent prospective longitudinal studies of BPD patients report remission in both symptoms and diagnosis over the course of 10 or more years follow-up (Gunderson et al. 2011; Shea et al. 2002, 2009; Zanarini et al. 2010). In spite of symptom improvement, functional impairment in social relationships changed little over both the short term and at 10 years follow-up in BPD patients (Gunderson et al. 2011; Skodol et al. 2005). The McLean Study found that half of BPD subjects failed to achieve social and vocational recovery at 10 years follow-up despite symptomatic remission of BPD diagnostic criteria in 93% (Zanarini et al. 2010).

In terms of suicidal behavior, suicide attempts, which were found in 56.4% of subjects at the 2-year follow-up, were only reported in 4.3% by the 10th year (Zanarini et al. 2010). In the prospective study by Soloff and colleagues, suicide attempts occurred most frequently in the first two years of follow-up (e.g., 19% of 137 subjects in the first 12 months, 24.8% of 133 subjects by the second year) (Soloff and Fabio 2008). Thereafter, the number of new attempts decreased rapidly with time (Soloff and Chiappetta 2012). Death by suicide has been noted to occur at various points in the course of the disorder, as early as 30 months after the first suicidal communication or attempt (Runeson et al. 1996) or as late as the 10-year follow-up (Paris and Zweig-Frank 2001). In their 27-year follow-up study, Paris and Zweig-Frank (2001) reported that suicide occurred at an average age of 37 years. Temes et al. (2019) found the steepest increases in suicide occurred in younger individuals in their study cohort of former inpatients with BPD. Conceivably, younger patients with BPD tended to make frequent lower-lethality attempts while older patients after years of illness died by suicide.

Research evidence indicates that prospective predictors of suicide attempts changed dramatically over time. The CLPS found that 20.5% of treatment-seeking BPD patients attempted suicide during the first 2 years of study (Yen et al. 2003). Over the first 2 years, worsening of MDD predicted suicide attempts in the following month in the CLPS sample of four PDs, as did the occurrence of negative life events (Yen et al. 2005). In the shortest follow-up interval (12 months), Soloff and Chiappetta (2012) found attempts were predicted by comorbidity with MDD. Thereafter, no acute clinical stressors predicted interval attempts. Soloff and Chiappetta (2012) found that suicide attempts over a 6-year interval were best predicted by poor psychosocial functioning at baseline, a family history of suicide, and the absence of any outpatient treatment (prior to any attempt). Good psychosocial functioning at baseline was a protective variable that decreased risk. It is noteworthy that any outpatient treatment in the 12-month interval diminished the suicide risk. Importantly, absence of outpatient treatment remained a predictor of suicide risk to the 6-year follow-up. Similarly, at 10-year follow-up, Soloff and Chiappetta (2019) continued to find illness severity and poor baseline social, vocational, and psychosocial functioning to be the strongest predictors of suicide attempts over the follow-up interval.

Ansell et al. (2015), using data from the CLPS study, examined personality pathology predictors of suicide attempts over a 10-year follow-up of their cohort of 431 participants. BPD pathology uniquely predicted ever attempting suicide over other PD severity, and that observation indicates that BPD pathology may capture a general factor of psychopathology that creates the risk for suicidal behavior (Caspi et al. 2014). However, Ansell et al. (2015) found that narcissistic PD pathology was the unique predictor of an increasing number of suicide attempts over the follow-up period. The authors conjectured that shame proneness, which has been used to explain the link between narcissistic PD pathology and suicide-related outcomes, might explain the finding of multiple suicide attempts over time.

Across many studies, poor psychosocial functioning (defined by socioeconomic status, social relationships, and educational and vocational achievement) is a predictor of suicide attempt behavior independent of diagnoses. In one study, community subjects with PDs who died by suicide and complained of loneliness had suffered more interpersonal loss and conflicts compared with similar subjects with no PD diagnoses who died by suicide (Heikkinen et al. 1997).

Who dies by suicide? Are there clinical characteristics that predict attempts of higher lethality over time? In one prospective longitudinal study of attempters with BPD, Soloff and Chiappetta (2012) defined clinical characteristics of 91 repeat attempters who made increasingly lethal attempts over time. The time from the first attempt to the attempt of maximum lethality was long and extremely variable. Among attempters with up to five lifetime attempts, the time to maximum medical lethality was 8.94 years, with a median of 6.81 years and a range of 8 weeks to 37.1 years. High-lethality attempts (defined operationally by a Medical Lethality Scale score greater than or equal to 4) were best predicted by older age and a history of prior hospitalizations, suggesting that chronicity and illness severity play critical roles in the vulnerability to high-lethality behavior over time. A trajectory analysis separated two groups of attempters, one with increasingly greater Medical Lethality Scale scores over time (the high-lethality group) and another with recurrent attempts of low lethality. High-lethality subjects were predominantly recruited from inpatient units and had poorer psychosocial functioning at baseline compared to the low-lethality group. High-lethality subjects were characterized by poor relationships in the immediate family and a poor work history. The low-lethality group endorsed more negativism (on the Buss-Durkee Hostility Inventory), lifetime SUD, and comorbidity with Cluster B histrionic and/or narcissistic PD. This group is more likely to include patients whose suicidal acts are "communicative gestures" indicating extreme emotional distress and attempting to elicit caring responses from others.

Pathways to Nonsuicidal Self-Injury and Suicidal Behavior

Although more is being learned about the causal pathways leading to NSSI and suicidal behavior in patients with PD, many questions remain. Klonsky et al. (2014) concluded that NSSI in general most commonly serves to (temporarily) alleviate overwhelming negative emotion, thereby having *intrapersonal functions* (e.g., regulating affect). Of course, this mechanism of regulating affect has been applied to NSSI in patients with BPD and has led to therapies such as DBT (Linehan 1993) and emotion regulation group therapy (Gratz et al. 2014). However, NSSI may serve other purposes; for example, self-injury may be driven by a need for self-punishment or self-criticism or by interpersonal needs, and thereby have *interpersonal functions* (e.g., seeking support or revenge). Sadeh et al. (2014) suggested that knowing the function of NSSI can help in formulating an appropriate intervention. For example, for patients with problems with emotional dysregulation, clinicians might first teach distress tolerance and emotion regulation skills. In work with patients who have interpersonal functions of NSSI, clinicians should prioritize enhancing social and communication skills, social support, and boundary setting. NSSI is known to be an important risk factor for suicidal behavior, and Klonsky et al. (2014) suggested that NSSI might be more important than depression, anxiety, impulsivity, and BPD. However, the role of NSSI in the pathway to suicidal behavior remains to be explicated.

The causes of suicidal behavior are not well understood; however, the behavior clearly results from complex interactions of different factors. The stress-diathesis model by Mann et al. (1999) integrates neurobiology and psychopathology and suggests that the negative results of preexisting vulnerability factors such as emotion dysregulation or impulsive aggression are especially pronounced when activated by stress.

Extending the escape theory of suicide by Baumeister (1990) provides a foundation for understanding how self-punishment or shame-driven emotion might lead to NSSI and/or suicidal behavior in patients with narcissistic personality pathology.

Baumeister's theory suggests that when individuals perceive they have failed to live up to their rigid self-strivings, a causal chain of events is triggered: 1) the person falls short of personal standards or expectations; 2) these failures lead to attributions to the self; 3) high self-awareness then generates negative affect; 4) the person tries to escape from the negative affect and heightened self-awareness; 5) the person's escape through cognitive deconstruction leads to disinhibition; and 6) the consequences of deconstruction may include suicidal ideation and behavior. According to Tracy and Robins (2004), self-conscious emotions such as shame and hubristic pride are differentiated from basic emotions because they are evoked by self-reflection and self-evaluation. Shame is known to be an "acutely painful emotion," more intense than guilt, and is accompanied by a sense of worthlessness and powerlessness (Tangney and Tracy 2012). Shame impairs the individual's ability to maintain the dimensions of self, and the self becomes weakened or lost (Wilson et al. 2006). In this state of mind with decreased self-agency, rational, safe action will not be available to the patient and disinhibited, impulsive actions (e.g., NSSI, suicidal behavior, suicide) are more likely to occur.

More recently, the interpersonal theory of suicide (Van Orden et al. 2010) has focused much more attention on those factors that move an individual from desiring suicide to acting on this desire. This theory endorses a hypothesis that an acquired capability for suicidal behavior, involving an increased fearlessness about death and pain tolerance, may move a person from suicidal ideation to action. Repetitive NSSI and/or suicide attempts by an individual with BPD may create greater fearlessness about death. Nock et al. (2010) found that some factors, such as anxiety disorders, may elevate suicide risk by intensifying the desire for death or suicide, whereas the disorders characterized by impulsivity and poor conduct control may increase the risk of suicide by heightening the likelihood of individuals acting on their suicidal ideation. In patients with BPD, the desire for death may be activated by factors such as hopelessness (Perez et al. 2014) or shame, and impulsivity may interact with emotion dysregulation and lead to suicide and suicidal behavior (Terzi et al. 2017). Understanding the exact pathways to suicidal behavior beyond suicidal ideation will greatly enhance clinicians' ability to develop effective intervention strategies.

The neurobiology of BPD is under active investigation, and several reviews have summarized the current status of this research (Bani-Fatemi et al. 2018; Gunderson et al. 2018; Perez-Rodriguez et al. 2018; Ruocco and Carcone 2016). Certain proposed biological models may be most relevant to understanding the risk for suicidal behavior that characterizes BPD but also likely have transdiagnostic relevance for other PDs and psychiatric disorders. Affective instability has been associated with suicidality, and brain imaging studies find reduced top-down regulatory prefrontal cortex activity (orbitofrontal cortex, anterior cingulate cortex) and enhanced amygdala and insula activity when patients with BPD are viewing emotional stimuli (Perez-Rodriguez et al. 2018; Ruocco and Carcone 2016). In addition, patients with BPD may have emotional hypersensitivity (e.g., may be overly attentive to negative stimuli) and/or fail to habituate to repeated negative stimuli and fail to recruit adaptive affect regulation strategies to process emotions (Gunderson et al. 2018; Perez-Rodriguez et al. 2018). The interpersonal hypersensitivity model proposed by Gunderson (Gunderson and Links 2014) indicates that patients with BPD are hypersensitive to rejection, and research suggests that common neural substrates regulate both physical pain and the pain of social rejection (Perez-Rodriguez et al. 2018). Interpersonal rejection and the associated emotional pain can be proximal triggers for suicidal behavior. Neuropeptide research has studied whether patients with BPD have dysfunction of the opiate system that may modulate intrapsychic pain and whether NSSI may be the patient's response to increased internal opioid levels. Dysregulation of oxytocin is also being researched in patients with BPD because oxytocin abnormalities may lead to misreading social cues or to increased difficulties with forming trusting relationships (Perez-Rodriguez et al. 2018). Impulsivity or behavioral dysregulation may also be associated with increased suicidal behavior. Impairments in delay discounting (ability to delay a smaller immediate reward for a larger non-immediate reward), high emotional interference in cognitive functioning, and a reduction in response inhibition in the context of emotional stress have been reported in patients with BPD (Gunderson et al. 2018). Soloff et al. (2012) carried out one of the few imaging studies of subjects with PDs done specifically to ascertain potential causes of suicidal behavior. A voxel-based morphometry study of suicidal behavior in BPD found that specific structural abnormalities discriminate high- from low-lethality attempters (Soloff et al. 2012). High-lethality attempters differed from low-lethality attempters in that the former had significant decreases in gray matter concentrations in areas of orbitofrontal, temporal, insular, and paralimbic cortex—areas broadly involved in emotion regulation, behavioral control, executive cognitive function, and adaptive responses to social situations (Soloff et al. 2012).

Assessing Suicide Risk in Patients With Personality Disorders

Although empirical evidence is limited, the assessment and management of an acute risk of suicide might vary depending on the patient's predominant PD pathology. Treating patients with BPD can be challenging because of the potential for these patients to present in suicidal crises. These patients frequently have a history of previous suicidal behavior. Clinicians may avoid accepting such patients in their practice because they feel unskilled to manage these crises; however, recent evidence-based therapies, such as good psychiatric management (Gunderson and Links 2014), have demonstrated that outpatient management can be effective in preventing future suicidal behavior and in reducing the medical risk of future suicide attempts (McMain et al. 2009). (See Chapter 15, "Good Psychiatric Management: Generalist Treatments and Stepped Care for Borderline Personality Disorder," in this volume for a more detailed discussion of patient management.)

The clinical assessment of BPD patients in crisis is complicated. These patients often have made multiple suicide attempts, and it is unclear whether a short-term admission will have any impact on the ongoing risk of suicidal behavior. In patients with BPD, the acute-on-chronic level of risk is related to several factors. Patients with BPD typically are at a chronically elevated risk of suicide, much higher than that of the general population. This risk exists primarily because of a history of multiple previous attempts, although in some studies the patients' history of nonsuicidal self-injurious behavior has been shown to also increase the risk for suicide (Linehan 1993; Stanley et al. 2001). The patient's level of chronic risk can be estimated by taking a careful history of the previous suicidal behavior and focusing on the times when the patient may have demonstrated attempts with the greatest subjective intent, objective planning, and medical lethality. By studying the patient's most serious suicide attempts, one can estimate the severity of the patient's ongoing chronic risk for suicide, particularly as the method of previous attempts tends to predict the seriousness of suicide vulnerability (Modai et al. 2004). Some of the important factors that contribute to an acute risk of suicide for patients with BPD have been reviewed in this chapter and are discussed below; however, for a full discussion of suicide risk factors and suicide risk assessment in psychiatric patients, we recommend other resources such as the American Psychiatric Association's (2003) "Practice Guideline for the Assessment and Treatment of Patients With Suicidal Behaviors," the Zero Suicide Toolkit (Suicide Prevention Resource Center 2020), and the Veterans Affairs/Department of Defense's "Assessment and Management of Patients at Risk for Suicide" (U.S. Department of Veterans Affairs 2019).

An acute-on-chronic risk will be present if the patient has comorbid major depression or is demonstrating high levels of hopelessness or depressive symptoms. Also, patients with BPD are known to be at risk for suicide around times of hospitalization and discharge. The recently discharged patient is potentially at an acute-on-chronic risk, and the assessment cannot be truncated because of the recent discharge. Proximal substance abuse also can increase the suicide risk in a patient with BPD. Additionally, the risk is acutely elevated in patients who have less immediate family support, those who have lost or perceive the loss of an important relationship, or those who have suffered recent stressful events including contacts with the criminal justice system (Yen et al. 2005).

Using the acute-on-chronic model can be very effective for communicating the decisions regarding interventions in the health record. For example, if a patient is felt to be at a chronic but not acute-on-chronic risk for suicide, one can document and communicate that a short-term hospital admission will have little or no impact on a chronic risk that has been present for months and years. However, an inpatient admission of a patient demonstrating an acute-on-chronic risk might well be indicated. In this latter circumstance, a short-term admission may allow the level of risk to return to chronic preadmission levels.

When patients with BPD present in a suicidal crisis, they can pose a challenge even to experienced clinicians. Bergmans et al. (2007) discussed the fact that health care providers responsible for treating patients with BPD in the emergency department (ED) faced emotions including anxiety, anger, a lack of empathy, and frustration over repetitive behavior, as well as a perception that patients are not appropriately using the ED. Patients with BPD who present in crisis are often experiencing intense and dysregulated emotions; as a result, they have difficulty articulating how they are feeling, and their problem-solving abilities are compromised. Clinicians can help de-escalate patients by validating their emotional distress, confirming that seeking help was a good decision, and treating the patient with respect, dignity, and empathy. When the patient has de-escalated, the clinician and the patient can begin the process of problem solving and establishing a safety plan.

Patients with BPD who present in crisis with significant emotional dysregulation or extreme agitation can be difficult to assess and de-escalate. For the ED staff, these patients can be likened to patients who present with a bleeding wound; the first task with patients in a suicidal crisis is to stop the "emotional bleeding." The staff needs to recognize that these patients cannot participate in constructive problem solving until their emotional intensity has been de-escalated. The staff can use simple strategies such as monitoring the patients' breathing, distraction techniques such as having patients name items in the room, or soothing strategies such as recommending that patients listen to their smartphone resources or use appropriate apps. The staff can point out examples of how patients have made positive choices to be safer, such as choosing to come to the ED before making a suicide attempt.

Despite some inconsistent findings regarding the effectiveness of low-dose antipsychotics for affective dysregulation, depression, anger, and impulsivity in patients with BPD, antipsychotics may acutely temper the core symptoms of BPD. For example, in one randomized controlled trial, aripiprazole (15 mg/day) was found after 8 weeks to be more effective than placebo for symptoms of depression, anxiety, and aggressiveness/hostility in patients with BPD; however, no significant reductions in self-injurious behavior were observed (Nickel et al. 2006). Antipsychotic medications can be helpful in reducing a patient's anxiety, anger, hostility, and agitation in the ED, facilitating assessment, de-escalation of the patient, and development of a treatment plan.

Patients with a known diagnosis of BPD often have access to clinicians and support in the community. A patient frequently has a treatment plan with his or her primary caregiver that recommends going to the ED if the patient feels unsafe or is in crisis. In the ED, it is important for staff to connect with a patient's health care team to inform them of the situation, arrange appropriate follow-up for the patient if admission is not indicated, and coordinate ongoing care with other professionals on the team. Patients may benefit from family involvement in a crisis situation. A clinician can ask the patient which family members are helpful in times of crisis or can develop specific crisis interventions to avoid the interpersonal conflicts that may have precipitated the original suicidal crisis. Educating family members about restricting access to means should be incorporated into the care of all mental health patients presenting in crisis (Links et al. 2019).

One of the most critical issues is differentiating suicidal from nonsuicidal intentions. Too often, cutting oneself or other self-harm behaviors are assumed to be suicidal, although these behaviors also can be deliberate acts by the patient—intended for self-soothing and dealing with overwhelming emotional distress. To avoid misinterpretation, the clinician and patient should develop a method to differentiate nonlethal self-harm behavior, in which the patient's intent is to seek a reduction in emotional distress, from "true" suicidal intention, in which the patient's intent is to end his or her life. The clinician must attend to the risk of suicidal behavior when the risk moves toward true suicidal intention yet must avoid being therapeutically constrained by concerns about the patient's chronic suicidality. An important strategy is for the patient to develop a method of scaling his or her severity of suicidal thinking. For example, the patient can be asked to consider the question, "How intense are your suicidal thoughts today?" and to rate the intensity (from 1, *very low intensity*, to 10, *extreme intensity*). In addition, the patient can be asked to rate his or her intent to act on these thoughts: "In the next 24 hours, how likely do you think it is that you will act on your suicidal thoughts?" (rating the likelihood from 1, *very unlikely*, to 10, *almost certain*). These methods of scaling should be undertaken in a collaborative manner, with the patient joining the clinician in the responsibility of monitoring the level of risk over time (Craven et al. 2011). In light of the increased odds of combined violence in BPD patients—compared with individuals without BPD with no history of violence, a history of self-directed violence, or a history of other-directed violence—the assessment of suicidal ideation should address violent and homicidal ideation as well (Harford et al. 2018).

The clinician should work with the patient to develop a safety plan. Stanley and Brown (2012) have developed a very useful tool for such a purpose. The following vignette demonstrates use of that tool to develop a safety plan with a patient with BPD who presented to an ED.

Case Example

Ms. A was a 53-year-old single female with a diagnosis of BPD as well as a history of previous major depressive episodes and current social phobia. She came to the attention of psychiatry at a somewhat older age, having relatively minor self-harm behaviors and, in more recent years, some low-lethality overdose attempts. The clinician had seen Ms. A several times for her presentations to the ED after overdosing on small amounts of medication. The self-harm behaviors were often precipitated by arguments with her adult daughter. After completing an assessment of the patient's risk for suicide following her current overdose attempt, the clinician discussed creating a safety plan with the patient. Working through the six steps listed below, Ms. A came up with a safety plan for herself:

Step 1: What are your warning signs that you are going into a crisis?

- *Feeling panicky; can't breathe; wanting to get out; wanting to take pills or drink*

Step 2: What coping strategies such as distraction or soothing techniques have you used successfully in the past?

- *Petting my dog*

Step 3: What social situations and/or people can help distract you when you are in crisis?

- *Two girlfriends can be helpful to distract me*

Step 4: Who can you ask for help when you are in crisis (or who is unhelpful when you are in crisis)?

- *Do not ask my mother for help during a crisis*

Step 5: What professionals or agencies can you contact during a crisis?

- *Crisis phone line; therapist; family doctor*

Step 6: What can you do to make your home environment safer?

- *Lock up my medications so they are not readily available*[1]

In addition, patients should be educated to be better consumers of the ED. They should prepare for the next crisis by developing a safety plan similar to Ms. A's above. The clinician should encourage patients to recognize their personal early warning signs and to prepare a crisis kit to take with them to the ED. This kit would include a list of their medications, physicians' contact information, and important personal supports. The kit should include recommended distraction and soothing strategies that

---

[1]Steps adapted from Stanley B, Brown GK: "Safety Planning Intervention: A Brief Intervention to Mitigate Suicide Risk." *Cognitive and Behavioral Practice* 19:256–264, 2012.

could be used in the ED. The clinician should also rehearse with patients how the ED staff experiences their presentations to the ED. This preparation helps patients understand the multiple demands faced by the ED staff and recognize that clear repeated attempts at communication are likely the best way to have patients' needs heard in such a chaotic setting.

For patients with narcissistic personality pathology, the outpatient clinician can take the following steps to assess and manage the risk of suicide and suicide-related behavior. The clinician should routinely monitor the patient for evidence of coexisting major depression or, even when not depressed, for an acute episode of lowered self-esteem resulting from a felt narcissistic injury. When narcissistic persons feel ashamed, they hide their emotions and withdraw from the therapist. To avoid being exposed, the narcissistic patient may be deceitful by acts of omission rather than outright lying. Therefore, the therapist has to be sensitive to signs of withdrawal, missed sessions, sudden guardedness, or defensive anger. The therapist will likely have to directly inquire about suicidal thoughts, planning, and intent. A patient who has suffered a serious narcissistic injury has to experience a sense of safety within the therapeutic relationship in order to address these issues.

When working with a suicidal patient with narcissistic pathology, the therapist should anticipate that during crises, the patient will become isolated from family and be less communicative. From the outset of therapy with such patients, the therapist should contract to have permission to speak with the patient's significant supports. Following this initial consent, the patient's family and other significant supports should be made aware of the patient's risk for suicide and for the potential for an acute onset of suicidal feelings. The family must be informed about how to access help should a crisis arise and advised to remove access to lethal means if that becomes necessary.

Because suicide-related behavior in narcissistic individuals tends to arise abruptly, the risk can be lessened by preventing the patient from having access to a means of suicide. Specific inquiries should be made about access to guns, availability of large quantities of pills, and proximity to high venues. If guns or large quantities of pills are accessible in the home, the therapist should enlist a responsible family member or support person to remove the items in question. In addition, the therapist should receive firsthand evidence from the enlisted family member that the means of suicide have been removed and safely secured away from the patient.

The creation of a stable therapeutic relationship seems to be an important factor that can lessen the risk of suicide for patients with pathological narcissism and should be recommended in the ongoing management of suicidal patients with narcissistic pathology. Kohut (1972) suggested that narcissistic patients may be at less risk of acting out suicidal behavior once they have established a stable transference within a therapeutic relationship and the therapist has established some empathic closeness to the patient's fragmented self.

Finally, in some instances, patients with narcissistic pathology are thrown into a suicidal crisis when an intimate relationship is threatened. When a suicidal crisis is driven by a rupture or perceived rupture in the narcissistic patient's intimate relationship, couples therapy should be considered both to lessen the immediate crisis and to address the underlying relationship issues (Links and Stockwell 2002).

In working with patients with antisocial personality pathology, the clinician should carefully assess for active comorbid disorders (e.g., anxiety disorders, MDD, SUDs) that may be contributing to an acute risk of suicidal behavior. The clinician should also assess these patients for psychopathic features, such as "emotional detachment" manifesting as superficial charm, manipulativeness, callousness, and lack of empathy. Before considering a hospital admission, the clinician must consider that patients with these psychopathic attributes may be more of a risk to others than themselves, and this will be an important consideration given the existence of many vulnerable individuals on inpatient units.

Conclusion

Clinicians need to assess patients with PDs for evidence of both nonmodifiable (chronic) and modifiable (acute) risk factors for suicide. Although BPD diagnosis, for example, is associated with the risk for suicide, suicidal behavior, and NSSI, psychotherapeutic interventions and outpatient psychiatric care appear to be very effective in reducing the short- and long-term risk of recurrent suicidal behavior in patients with BPD. When they have the appropriate knowledge and skills, clinicians will find that working collaboratively with patients with PDs can be effective and rewarding.

References

Ahrens B, Haug HJ: Suicidality in hospitalized patients with a primary diagnosis of personality disorder. Crisis 17:59–63, 1996

American Psychiatric Association: Diagnostic and Statistical Manual of Mental Disorders, 4th Edition. Arlington, VA, American Psychiatric Association, 1994

American Psychiatric Association: Practice Guideline for the Assessment and Treatment of Patients With Suicidal Behaviors. Arlington, VA, American Psychiatric Association, 2003

American Psychiatric Association: Diagnostic and Statistical Manual of Mental Disorders, 5th Edition. Arlington, VA, American Psychiatric Association, 2013

Andover MS, Gibb BE: Non-suicidal self-injury, attempted suicide and suicidal intent among psychiatric inpatients. Psychiatry Res 178:101–105, 2010

Ansell EB, Wright AGC, Markowitz JC, et al: Personality disorder risk factors for suicide attempts over 10 years of follow-up. Personal Disord 6:161–167, 2015

Apter A, Bleich A, King RA, et al: Death without warning? A clinical postmortem study of suicide in 43 Israeli adolescent males. Arch Gen Psychiatry 50:138–142, 1993

Bani-Fatemi A, Tasmin S, Graff-Guerrero A, et al: Structural and functional alterations of the suicidal brain: an updated review of neuroimaging studies. Psychiatry Res Neuroimaging 278:77–91, 2018

Baumeister RF: Suicide as escape from self. Psychol Rev 97:90–113, 1990

Bergmans Y, Brown A, Carruthers A: Advances in crisis management of the suicidal patient: perspectives from patients. Curr Psychiatry Rep 9:74–80, 2007

Blasco-Fontecilla H, Baca-Garcia E, Dervic K, et al: Severity of personality disorders and suicide attempt. Acta Psychiatr Scand 119:149–155, 2009a

Blasco-Fontecilla H, Baca-Garcia E, Dervic K, et al: Specific features of suicidal behavior in patients with narcissistic personality disorder. J Clin Psychiatry 70:1583–1587, 2009b

Blasco-Fontecilla H, Baca-Garcia E, Duberstein P, et al: An exploratory study of the relationship between diverse life events and specific personality disorders in a sample of suicide attempters. J Pers Disord 24:773–784, 2010

Blasczyk-Schiep S, Kazen M, Jaworska-Andryszewska P, et al: Volitional determinants of self-harm behaviour and suicidal risk in persons with borderline personality disorder. Eur J Psychiatry 3:77–86, 2018

Bolton JM, Robinson J: Population attributable fractions of Axis I and II mental disorders for suicide attempts: findings from a representative sample of the adult, noninstitutionalized U.S. population. Am J Public Health 100:2473–2480, 2010

Brickman LB, Ammerman BA, Look AE, et al: The relationship between non-suicidal self-injury and borderline personality disorder symptoms in a college sample. Borderline Personal Disord Emot Dysregul 1:14, 2014

Brodsky BS, Groves SA, Oquendo MA, et al: Interpersonal precipitants and suicide attempts in borderline personality disorder. Suicide Life Threat Behav 36:313–322, 2006

Brown MZ, Linehan MM, Comtois KA, et al: Shame as a prospective predictor of self-inflicted injury in borderline personality disorder: a multi-modal analysis. Behav Res Ther 47:815–822, 2009

Caspi A, Houts RM, Belsky DW, et al: The p factor: one general psychopathology factor in the structure of psychiatric disorders? Clin Psychol Sci 2:119–137, 2014

Chabrol H, Raynal P: The co-occurrence of autistic traits and borderline personality disorder traits is associated to increased suicidal ideation in nonclinical young adults. Compr Psychiatry 82:141–143, 2018

Chioqueta AP, Stiles TC: Assessing suicide risk in cluster C personality disorders. Crisis 25:128–133, 2004

Cleckley H: The Mask of Sanity, 5th Edition. St Louis, MO, Mosby Medical Library, 1976

Coleman D, Lawrence R, Parekh A, et al: Narcissistic personality disorder and suicidal behavior in mood disorders. J Psychiatr Res 85:24–28, 2017

Craven MA, Links PS, Novak G: Assessment and management of suicide risk, in Psychiatry in Primary Care: A Concise Canadian Pocket Guide. Edited by Goldbloom DS, Davine J. Toronto, ON, Canada, Centre for Addiction and Mental Health, 2011, pp 237–248

DeShong HL, Tucker RP: Borderline personality disorder traits and suicide risk: the mediating role of insomnia and nightmares. J Affect Disord 244:85–91, 2019

Diaconu G, Turecki G: Obsessive-compulsive personality disorder and suicidal behavior: evidence for a positive association in a sample of depressed patients. J Clin Psychiatry 70:1551–1556, 2009

Fenton WS, McGlashan TH, Victor BJ, et al: Symptoms, subtype, and suicidality in patients with schizophrenia spectrum disorders. Am J Psychiatry 154:199–204, 1997

Ferraz L, Portella MJ, Vallez M, et al: Hostility and child sexual abuse as predictors of suicidal behavior in borderline personality disorder. Psychiatry Res 210:980–985, 2013

García-Alandete J, Salvador JHM, Rodriguez SR: Predicting role of the meaning in life on depression, hopelessness, and suicide risk among borderline personality disorder patients. Universitas Psychologica 13:1545–1555, 2014

Giner L, Blasco-Fontecilla H, Perez-Rodriguez M, et al: Personality disorders and health problems distinguish suicide attempters and completers in a direct comparison. J Affect Disord 151:474–483, 2013

Glenn CR, Klonsky ED: Prospective prediction of nonsuicidal self-injury: a 1-year longitudinal study in young adults. Behav Ther 42:751–762, 2011

Glenn CR, Bagge CL, Osman A: Unique association between borderline personality disorder features and suicide attempts and ideation in adolescents. J Pers Disord 25:604–616, 2013

Gratz KL, Gunderson JG: Preliminary data on an acceptance-based emotion regulation group intervention for deliberate self-harm among women with borderline personality disorder. Behav Ther 37:25–35, 2006

Gratz KL, Tull MT, Levy R: Randomized controlled trial and uncontrolled 9-month follow-up of an adjunctive emotion regulation group therapy for deliberate self-harm among women with borderline personality disorder. Psychol Med 44:2099–2112, 2014

Grilo CM, McGlashan TH, Morey LC, et al: Internal consistency, intercriterion overlap, and diagnostic efficiency of criteria sets for DSM-IV schizotypal, borderline, avoidant, and obsessive-compulsive personality disorders. Acta Psychiatr Scand 104:264–272, 2001

Grilo CM, Sanislow CA, Skodol AE, et al: Longitudinal diagnostic efficiency of DSM-IV criteria for borderline personality disorder: a two-year prospective study. Can J Psychiatry 6:357–361, 2007

Gunderson JG, Links PS: Handbook of Good Psychiatric Management of Borderline Personality Disorder. Arlington, VA, American Psychiatric Publishing, 2014

Gunderson JG, Stout RL, McGlashan TH, et al: Ten-year course of borderline personality disorder: psychopathology and function from the Collaborative Longitudinal Personality Disorders Study. Arch Gen Psychiatry 68:827–837, 2011

Gunderson JG, Herpertz SC, Skodol AE, et al: Borderline personality disorder. Nat Rev Dis Primers 4:18029, 2018

Harford TC, Chen CM, Kerridge BT, Grant BF: Self- and other-directed forms of violence and their relationship with lifetime DSM-5 psychiatric disorders: results from the National Epidemiologic Survey on Alcohol Related Conditions–III (NESARC-III). Psychiatry Res 262:384–392, 2018

Harris L, Chelminski I, Dalrymple K, et al: Suicide attempts and emotion regulation in psychiatric outpatients. J Affect Disord 232:300–304, 2018

Harrop TM, Preston OC, Khazem LR, et al: Dark traits and suicide: associations between psychopathy, narcissism, and components of the interpersonal-psychological theory of suicide. J Abnorm Psychol 126:928–938, 2017

Hasking PA, Coric SJ, Swannell S, et al: Brief report: emotion regulation and coping as moderators in the relationship between personality and self-injury. J Adolesc 33:767–773, 2010

Heikkinen ME, Isometsa ET, Henriksson MM, et al: Psychosocial factors and completed suicide in personality disorders. Acta Psychiatr Scand 95:49–57, 1997

Heisel MJ, Links PS, Conn D, et al: Narcissistic personality and vulnerability to late-life suicidality. Am J Geriatr Psychiatry 15:734–741, 2007

Isometsa ET, Henriksson MM, Heikkinen ME, et al: Suicide among subjects with personality disorders. Am J Psychiatry 153:667–673, 1996

Jahn DR, DeVylder JE, Hilimire MR: Explanatory risk factors in the relations between schizotypy and indicators of suicide risk. Psychiatr Res 238:68–73, 2016

Jaksic N, Marcinko D, Hanzek MS, et al: Experience of shame mediates the relationship between pathological narcissism and suicidal ideation in psychiatric outpatients. J Clin Psychol 73:1670–1681, 2017

Klonsky ED, Victor SE, Saffer BY: Nonsuicidal self-injury: what we know, and what we need to know. Can J Psychiatry 59:565–568, 2014

Knafo A, Labelle R, Guilé J-M, et al: Coping, suicidalité et trouble de personnalité limite à l'adolescence. Neuropsychiatr Enfance Adolesc 62:431–436, 2014

Kohut H: Thoughts on narcissism and narcissistic rage. Psychoanal Study Child 27:360–400, 1972

Kolla NJ, Eisenberg H, Links PS: Epidemiology, risk factors, and psychopharmacological management of suicidal behavior in borderline personality disorder. Arch Suicide Res 12:1–19, 2008

Lentz V, Robinson J, Bolton JM: Childhood adversity, mental disorder comorbidity, and suicidal behavior in schizotypal personality disorder. J Nerv Ment Dis 198:795–801, 2010

Lenzenweger MF, Lane MC, Loranger AW, et al: DSM-IV personality disorders in the National Comorbidity Survey Replication. Biol Psychiatry 62:553–564, 2007

Levi-Belz Y, Gvion Y, Levi U, et al: Beyond the mental pain: a case-control study on the contribution of schizoid personality disorder symptoms to medically serious suicide attempts. Compr Psychiatry 90:102–109, 2019

Lieb K, Zanarini MC, Schmahl C, et al: Borderline personality disorder. Lancet 364:453–461, 2004

Linehan MM: Cognitive-Behavioral Treatment of Borderline Personality Disorder. New York, Guilford, 1993

Links PS: Psychiatric rehabilitation model for borderline personality disorder. Can J Psychiatry 38 (suppl 1):535–538, 1993

Links PS, Stockwell M: The role of couple therapy in the treatment of narcissistic personality disorder. Am J Psychother 56:522–538, 2002

Links PS, Eynan R, Heisel MJ, Nisenbaum R: Elements of affective instability associated with suicidal behaviour in patients with borderline personality disorder. Can J Psychiatry 53:112–116, 2008

Links PS, Kolla NJ, Guimond T, McMain S: Prospective risk factors for suicide attempts in a treated sample of patients with borderline personality disorder. Can J Psychiatry 58:99–106, 2013

Links PS, Eynan R, Shah R: Are new standards for assessing and managing suicidal patients needed in Canada? Can J Psychiatry 64:400–404, 2019

Maddocks PD: A five-year follow-up of untreated psychopaths. Br J Psychiatry 116:511–515, 1970

Mann JJ, Waternaux C, Haas GL, Malone KM: Toward a clinical model of suicide behavior in psychiatric patients. Amer J Psychiatry 156:181–189, 1999

Marttunen MJ, Aro HM, Henriksson MM, et al: Mental disorders in adolescent suicide: DSM-III-R Axes I and II diagnoses in suicides among 13- to 19-year-olds in Finland. Arch Gen Psychiatry 48:834–839, 1991

McGirr A, Paris J, Lesage A, et al: Risk factors for suicide completion in borderline personality disorder: a case-control study of cluster B comorbidity and impulsive aggression. J Clin Psychiatry 68:721–729, 2007

McGirr A, Paris J, Lesage A, et al: An examination of DSM-IV borderline personality disorder symptoms and risk for death by suicide: a psychological autopsy study. Can J Psychiatry 54:87–92, 2009

McMain SF, Links PS, Gnam WH, et al: A randomized trial of dialectical behavior therapy versus general psychiatric management for borderline personality disorder. Am J Psychiatry 166:1365–1374, 2009

Mellesdal L, Gjestad R, Johnsen E, et al: Borderline personality disorder and posttraumatic stress disorder at psychiatric discharge predict general hospital admission for self-harm. J Trauma Stress 28:556–562, 2015

Modai I, Kuperman J, Goldberg I, et al: Suicide risk factors and suicide vulnerability in various psychiatric disorders. Med Inform Internet Med 29:65–74, 2004

Mou D, Kleiman EM, Fedor S, et al: Negative affect is more strongly associated with suicidal thinking among suicidal patients with borderline personality disorder than those without. J Psychiatr Res 104:198–201, 2018

Nickel MK, Muehlbacher M, Nickel C, et al: Aripiprazole in the treatment of patients with borderline personality disorder: a double-blind placebo-controlled study. Am J Psychiatry 163:833–838, 2006

Nock MK, Hwang I, Sampson NA, Kessler RC: Mental disorders, comorbidity and suicidal behavior: results from the National Comorbidity Survey Replication. Mol Psychiatry 15:868–876, 2010

Nock MK, Ursano RJ, Heeringa SG, et al: Mental disorders, comorbidity, and pre-enlistment suicidal behavior among new soldiers in the U.S. Army: results from the Army Study to Assess Risk and Resilience in Servicemembers (Army STARRS). Suicide Life Threat Behav 45:588–599, 2015

Paris J: Half in love with easeful death: the meaning of chronic suicidality in borderline personality disorder. Harv Rev Psychiatry 12:42–48, 2004

Paris J, Zweig-Frank H: A 27-year follow-up of patients with borderline personality disorder. Compr Psychiatry 42:482–487, 2001

Perez S, Marco JH, Garcia-Alandete J: Comparison of clinical and demographic characteristics among borderline personality disorder patients with and without suicidal attempts and non-suicidal self-injury behaviors. Psychiatric Res 220:935–940, 2014

Perez-Rodriguez MM, Bulbena-Cabre A, Bassir A, et al: The neurobiology of borderline personality disorder. Psychiatr Clin North Am 41:633–650, 2018

Perry JC, Fowler JC, Bailey A, et al: Improvement and recovery from suicidal and self-destructive phenomena in treatment-refractory disorders. J Nerv Ment Dis 197:28–34, 2009

Pincus AL, Lukowitsky MR: Pathological narcissism and narcissistic personality disorder. Annu Rev Clin Psychol 6:421–446, 2010

Rizk MM, Choo T-H, Galfalvy H, et al: Variability in suicidal ideation is associated with affective instability in suicide attempters with borderline personality disorder. Psychiatry (Chic) 82:173–178, 2019

Ronningstam EF, Maltsberger JT: Pathological narcissism and sudden suicide-related collapse. Suicide Life Threat Behav 28:261–271, 1998

Runeson BS, Beskow J, Waern M: The suicidal process in suicides among young people. Acta Psychiatr Scand 93:35–42, 1996

Ruocco AC, Carcone D: A neurobiological model of borderline personality disorder. Systematic and integrative review. Harv Rev Psychiatry 24:311–329, 2016

Sadeh N, Londahl-Shaller EA, Piatigorsky A, et al: Functions of non-suicidal self-injury in adolescents and young adults with borderline personality disorder symptoms. Psychiatry Res 216:217–222, 2014

Schneider B, Wetterling T, Sargk D, et al: Axis I disorders and personality disorders as risk factors for suicide. Eur Arch Psychiatry Clin Neurosci 256:17–27, 2006

Shea MT, Stout R, Gunderson J, et al: Short-term diagnostic stability of schizotypal, borderline, avoidant, and obsessive-compulsive personality disorders. Am J Psychiatry 159:2036–204, 2002

Shea MT, Edelen MO, Pinto A, et al: Improvement in borderline personality disorder in relation to age. Acta Psychiatr Scand 119:143–148, 2009

Sher L, Fisher AM, Kelliher CH, et al: Clinical features and psychiatric comorbidities of borderline personality disorder patients with versus without a suicide attempt. Psychiatry Res 246:261–266, 2016

Sher L, Rutter SB, New AS, et al: Gender differences and similarities in aggression, suicidal behaviour, and psychiatric comorbidity in borderline personality disorder. Acta Psychiatr Scand 139:145–153, 2019

Skodol AE, Pagano ME, Bender DS, et al: Stability of functional impairment in patients with schizotypal, borderline, avoidant, or obsessive-compulsive personality disorder over two years. Psychol Med 35:443–451, 2005

Soloff PH: Risk factors for suicidal behavior in borderline personality disorder: a review and update, in Borderline Personality Disorder. Edited by Zanarini MC. Boca Raton, FL, Taylor & Francis, 2005, pp 333–365

Soloff PH, Chiappetta L: Prospective predictors of suicidal behavior in borderline personality disorder at 6-year follow-up. Am J Psychiatry 169:484–490, 2012

Soloff PH, Chiappetta L: Suicidal behavior and psychosocial outcome in borderline personality disorder at 8-year follow-up. J Pers Disord 31:774–789, 2017

Soloff PH, Chiappetta L: 10-year outcome of suicidal behavior in borderline personality disorder. J Per Disord 33:82–100, 2019

Soloff PH, Fabio A: Prospective predictors of suicide attempts in borderline personality disorder at one, two, and two-to-five year follow-up. J Per Disord 22:123–134, 2008

Soloff PH, Fabio A, Kelly TM, et al: High-lethality status in patients with borderline personality disorder. J Pers Disord 19:386–399, 2005

Soloff PH, Feske U, Fabio A: Mediators of the relationship between childhood sexual abuse and suicidal behavior in borderline personality disorder. J Per Disord 22:221–232, 2008

Soloff PH, Pruitt P, Sharma M, et al: Structural brain abnormalities and suicidal behavior in borderline personality disorder. J Psychiatr Res 46:516–525, 2012

Stanley B, Brown GK: Safety planning intervention: a brief intervention to mitigate suicide risk. Cogn Behav Pract 19:256–264, 2012

Stanley B, Gameroff MJ, Michalsen V, Mann JJ: Are suicide attempters who self-mutilate a unique population? Am J Psychiatry 158:427–432, 2001

Stone MH: The Fate of Borderline Patients. New York, Guilford, 1990

Suicide Prevention Resource Center: Zero Suicide Toolkit. Education Development Center. 2015–2018. Available from: https://zerosuicide.edc.org/toolkit/zero-suicide-toolkit. Accessed August 29, 2020.

Svindseth MF, Nottestad JA, Wallin J, et al: Narcissism in patients admitted to psychiatric acute wards: its relation to violence, suicidality and other psychopathology. BMC Psychiatry 8:13, 2008

Tangney JP, Tracy JL: Self-conscious emotions, in Handbook of Self and Identity, 2nd Edition. Edited by Leary M, Tangney JP. New York, Guilford, 2012, pp 446–478

Temes CM, Frankenburg FR, Fitzmaurice GM, Zanarini MC: Deaths by suicide and other causes among patients with borderline personality disorder and personality-disordered comparison subjects over 24 years of prospective follow-up. J Clin Psychiatry 80:30–36, 2019

Terzi L, Martino F, Berardi D, et al: Aggressive behavior and self-harm in borderline personality disorder: the role of impulsivity and emotion dysregulation in a sample of outpatients. Psychiatry Res 249:321–326, 2017

Tracy JL, Robins RW: Putting the self into self-conscious emotions: a theoretical model. Psychological Inquiry 15:103–125, 2004

U.S. Department of Veterans Affairs: VA/DoD Clinical Practice Guideline for the Assessment and Management of Patients at Risk for Suicide, Version 2.0. Washington, DC, U.S. Department of Veterans Affairs, 2019. Available at: https://www.healthquality.va.gov/guidelines/mh/srb/index.asp. Accessed December 14, 2019.

Van Orden KA, Witte TK, Cukrowicz KC, et al: The interpersonal theory of suicide. Psychol Rev 117:575–600, 2010

Vega D, Torrubia R, Soto A, et al: Exploring the relationship between non-suicidal self-injury and borderline traits in young adults. Psychiatry Res 256:403–411, 2017

Verona E, Hicks BM, Patrick CJ: Psychopathy and suicidality in female offenders: mediating influences of personality and abuse. J Consult Clin Psychol 73:1065–1073, 2005

Wedig MM, Silverman MH, Frankenburg FR, et al: Predictors of suicide attempts in patients with borderline personality disorder over 16 years of prospective follow-up. Psychol Med 42:2395–2404, 2012

Wedig MM, Frankenburg FR, Reich DB, et al: Predictors of suicide threats in patients with borderline personality disorder over 16 years of prospective follow-up. Psychiatry Res 208:252–256, 2013

Wilson JP, Drozdek B, Turkovic S: Posttraumatic shame and guilt. Trauma Violence Abuse 7:122–141, 2006

Yen S, Shea T, Pagano M, et al: Axis I and Axis II disorders as predictors of prospective suicide attempts: Findings from the Collaborative Longitudinal Personality Disorders Study. J Abnorm Psychol 112:375–381, 2003

Yen S, Pagano ME, Shea MT, et al: Recent life events preceding suicide attempts in a personality disorder sample: findings from the collaborative longitudinal personality disorders study. J Consult Clin Psychol 73:99–105, 2005

Yoshida K, Tonai E, Nagai H, et al: Long-term follow-up study of borderline patients in Japan: a preliminary study. Compr Psychiatry 47:426–432, 2006

Zaheer J, Links PS, Liu E: Assessment and emergency management of suicidality in personality disorders. Psychiatr Clin North Am 31:527–543, 2008

Zanarini MC, Frankenburg FR, DeLuca CJ, et al: The pain of being borderline: dysphoric states specific to borderline personality disorder. Harv Rev Psychiatry 6:201–207, 1998

Zanarini MC, Frankenburg FR, Hennen J, Silk KR: Mental health service utilization by borderline personality disorder patients and Axis II comparison subjects followed prospectively for 6 years. J Clin Psychiatry 65:28–36, 2004

Zanarini MC, Frankenburg FR, Hennen J, et al: Prediction of the 10-year course of borderline personality disorder. Am J Psychiatry 163:827–832, 2006

Zanarini MC, Frankenburg FR, Reich DB, Fitzmaurice G: Time to attainment of recovery from borderline personality disorder and stability of recovery: a 10-year prospective follow-up study. Am J Psychiatry 167:663–667, 2010

Zanarini MC, Laudate CS, Frankenburg FR, et al: Reasons for self-mutilation reported by borderline patients over 16 years of prospective follow-up. J Pers Disord 27:783–794, 2013

CHAPTER 21

Co-occurring Substance Use Disorders

Lauren R. Gorfinkel, M.P.H.

Seth J. Prins, Ph.D., M.P.H.

Jennifer C. Elliott, Ph.D.

Jacquelyn L. Meyers, Ph.D.

Deborah S. Hasin, Ph.D.

Since the introduction of DSM-III in 1980 (American Psychiatric Association 1980), interest has grown in the study of personality disorder (PD) comorbidity among individuals with substance use disorders (SUDs). The driving force behind this interest is the high comorbidity of these disorders and the complex clinical management of dual-diagnosis patients. Although the evaluation of co-occurring PDs has been the subject of many studies by substance use researchers, PD researchers have paid less attention to the co-occurrence of SUDs. This lack of attention may be because the field of PD research started relatively recently, in the 1980s, whereas the field of substance use has long recognized the interconnection with personality dysfunction, in part due to the fact that the first two editions of DSM placed alcohol and drug addiction under the larger heading of sociopathy (American Psychiatric Association 1952, 1968). Historically, a large proportion of PD studies have actually been conducted with samples of patients referred for treatment of other mental disorders, including SUDs. Some exceptions to this come from forensic or criminological research that addresses substance use issues among individuals with PDs (e.g., Ogloff et al. 2015; Skeem and Cooke 2010; Skeem et al. 2011; Wetterborg et al. 2015).

One consequence of this research history is that much of this chapter is based on studies focusing on the occurrence and implications of PDs in individuals with SUDs. In addition, evidence from the literature on (normative) personality traits will be included whenever informative. We focus in this chapter on the epidemiology of co-occurring PDs and SUDs, diagnostic issues, causal pathways and treatment, and the latest genetic research on these disorders.

Epidemiology

In this section, we review the epidemiology of co-occurring SUDs and PDs in the U.S. general population, first examining SUDs among individuals with PDs, and then examining PDs among individuals with SUDs. Much of the research on this subject comes from the National Epidemiologic Survey on Alcohol and Related Conditions Wave 1 (NESARC Wave 1; Grant et al. 2004), NESARC Wave 2 (Grant et al. 2004), and NESARC-III (Grant et al. 2015a), nationally representative community samples of approximately 43,000 U.S. adults. These three surveys, conducted in 2001–2002, 2004–2005, and 2012–2013, respectively, remain the only nationally representative studies to assess both PDs and SUDs in the general population. The NESARC Waves 1 and 2 sampled the same individuals, whereas the NESARC-III sampled new individuals. All surveys used a diagnostic interview designed for use by lay interviewers, with fair to excellent reliability for specific PDs and SUDs (Grant et al. 2003; Grant et al. 2015b; Ruan et al. 2008; for some criticism of NESARC PD diagnoses, see Trull et al. 2010).

Within the general population, SUDs are highly prevalent among individuals with PDs. The prevalence of 12-month SUD was estimated to be 44.1% among individuals with schizotypal PD (Pulay et al. 2009), 50.7% among individuals with borderline PD (BPD) (Grant et al. 2008), 40.6% among individuals with narcissistic PD (Stinson et al. 2008), and 60.1% among individuals with antisocial PD (Goldstein et al. 2017). Overall, individuals with antisocial, borderline, and schizotypal PDs had significantly higher odds than individuals with other PDs of lifetime SUDs involving alcohol, tobacco, cannabis, heroin/opioids, and other drugs (Harford et al. 2018; Hasin et al. 2016). SUDs among PD clusters have also been examined. For example, Blanco et al. (2018) found that Cluster A PDs were associated with greater likelihood of nicotine use, Cluster C PDs with greater likelihood of alcohol use, and Cluster B PDs with greater likelihood of nicotine, alcohol, cannabis, and cocaine use. Another study by Pulay et al. (2008) used a dimensional categorization of PDs and found that the 12-month prevalence of alcohol dependence was 4.48% for individuals with subthreshold PD, 8.28% for those with simple PD, and 14.27% for those with complex PD (i.e., at least two PDs). For 12-month drug dependence, prevalence was 0.54%, 1.98%, and 5.03% across those three PD categories, respectively (Pulay et al. 2008).

The prevalence of PDs is also high among individuals with SUDs. Again, numerous findings are available from studies based on the NESARC surveys. Among individuals with 12-month SUD, 8.2% had schizotypal PD (Pulay et al. 2009), 14.1% had BPD (Grant et al. 2008), and 11.8% had narcissistic PD (Stinson et al. 2008). The prevalence of specifically antisocial PD was 18.3% among respondents with lifetime drug use disorders, and 9.1% among respondents with lifetime alcohol use disorder (AUD) (Goldstein et al. 2007a, 2007b). After controlling for sociodemographic characteristics, Grant et al. (2015a) reported odds ratios for 12-month AUD and lifetime antisocial, borderline, and schizotypal PDs of 2.7, 3.1, and 2.3, respectively. However, odds ratios for 12-month AUD and avoidant, dependent, obsessive-compulsive, paranoid, histrionic, and schizoid PDs were not statistically significant (Grant et al. 2015a; Hasin et al. 2007). Again, some research has examined the prevalence of PD clusters, rather than individual PDs. For example, among individuals with 12-month nicotine dependence, the lifetime prevalence rates of Cluster A, B, and C PDs were 19.04%, 28.59%, and 14.84%, respectively (Pulay et al. 2010). Table 21–1 summarizes prevalence estimates and odds ratios for co-occurring PDs and SUDs in the general population, including alcohol and drug use disorders. Only PDs with published prevalence estimates are included.

Studies of patient populations have also demonstrated a high co-occurrence of SUDs and PDs. For example, in a clinical sample of nearly 700 treatment-seeking individuals with DSM-IV (American Psychiatric Association 1994) PDs, the prevalence of AUD was 40.9% and the prevalence of drug use disorders was 37.3% (McGlashan et al. 2000). Zanarini et al. (2011a) examined psychiatric inpatients with BPD and found the prevalence of 12-month SUD to be 62%. Rounsaville et al. (1998) examined 370 patients in treatment for SUD, finding a prevalence of antisocial PD of 27.0%, BPD of 18.4%, narcissistic PD of 9.5%, schizotypal PD of 4.6%, and any PD of 57%, when excluding substance-related symptoms. Casadio et al. (2014) similarly found that the prevalence of PDs among outpatients in addiction services was 62.2%, whereas the prevalence of two or more comorbid PDs was 27.2%. By cluster, the prevalence of Cluster A PDs was 8%, Cluster B PDs 33%, and Cluster C PDs 14%.

Overall, compared with those without SUDs, individuals with SUDs experience higher prevalence rates of antisocial, borderline, narcissistic, and schizotypal PDs, and compared to those without PDs, individuals with PDs experience higher prevalence rates of alcohol and drug use disorders. This high comorbidity is found consistently in both general population and clinical samples. However, interpretation of this comorbidity remains unclear, because the extent to which it is attributable to conceptually overlapping diagnostic criteria and measurement issues, such as state-trait artifacts, is unknown.

An important development in the study of personality psychopathology is the substantial evidence for a "metastructure" of psychopathology (Krueger 1999). This metastructure, represented by two latent dimensions—"internalizing" (e.g., unipolar mood and anxiety disorders) and "externalizing" (e.g., disinhibitory disorders)—may help explain patterns of psychiatric comorbidity (Keyes et al. 2013). For instance, using NESARC data, the externalizing dimension was shown to include antisocial PD and SUDs, whereas avoidant, schizoid, schizotypal, and paranoid PDs may be components of a "thought disorder" subdimension of the internalizing dimension (Keyes et al. 2013). BPD, in contrast, may straddle the internalizing and externalizing dimensions (Eaton et al. 2011). This ongoing line of research has significant implications for optimizing the treatment of individuals with PDs, in that treatment can be guided by shared underlying pathopsychological structures, rather than distinct diagnostic categories (Keyes et al. 2013).

Assessment and Diagnosis

In this section, we review the literature on the assessment and diagnosis of comorbid PDs and SUDs. In 2001, Ball et al. used semi-structured interviews and self-report questionnaires to examine DSM-IV PDs among substance-dependent inpatients,

TABLE 21–1. Summary of NESARC findings on the prevalence and odds ratios of substarnc use disorders and personality disorders

PD	Prevalence (%)		OR of lifetime PD and:							
	PD among SUD	SUD among PD	12-month SUD	12-month AUD	12-month DUD	Lifetime AUD	Lifetime TUD	Lifetime CUD	Lifetime OUD
Antisocial	18.3 (DUD)	64.1	5.0[a]	2.7[a]	11.3[d]	5.3[c]	5.1[c]	4.7[a]	8.1[c]
Borderline	14.1	50.7	3.4[b]	3.1[a]	5.6[b]	4.2[c]	3.8[c]	4.5[a]	7.1[c]
Narcissistic	11.8	40.6	2.4[b]	2.2[b]	3.7[b]	1.9[b]	1.9[b]	—	—
Schizotypal	5.9	44.1	2.5[b]	2.3[a]	4.7[b]	3.1[c]	2.9[c]	4.0[a]	6.2[c]

Note.   AUD=alcohol use disorder; CUD=cannabis use disorder; DUD=drug use disorder; NESARC=National Epidemiologic Survey on Alcohol and Related Conditions; OR=odds ratio; OUD=opioid/heroin use disorder; PD=personality disorder; SUD=substance use disorder; TUD=tobacco use disorder.
[a]OR significant at $\alpha=0.05$, and adjustment made for sociodemographic characteristics.
[b]OR significant at $\alpha=0.01$, and adjustment made for sociodemographic characteristics.
[c]OR significant at $\alpha=0.01$.
[d]OR significant at $\alpha=0.05$.
Source.   Data from NESARC studies as described in text.

finding reliability comparable to other diagnoses when standardized procedures were used. In a study of veterans in treatment for substance use, DeMarce et al. (2013) found evidence for the concurrent validity of DSM-IV antisocial PD diagnoses when using both clinical interviews and computerized surveys.

Instruments based on self-report, however, may result in overdiagnosis of PDs (Zimmerman and Coryell 1990); this may be even more of a concern with patients who have SUDs, because these instruments do not ask respondents to differentiate personality traits from the effects of substance use or other prolonged changes in mental status (van den Bosch and Verheul 2012). Diagnostic interviews may have greater specificity because clarifications can be made about whether a symptom is chronic and pervasive, more situation specific, or related to substance use (van den Bosch and Verheul 2012). An interview also allows for behavioral observations of the patient's interpersonal style, which may inform clinical judgment (Zimmerman 1994). Some studies have shown promising findings in favor of the validity of PD diagnoses in individuals with SUDs obtained using a semi-structured interview schedule. For example, Skodol et al. (1999) reported similar prevalence rates of PDs among patients with a current SUD and patients with a lifetime SUD. Also, in a sample of 273 patients with SUDs, remission of the disorder was not significantly associated with remission of personality pathology, suggesting that the two conditions follow independent courses (Verheul et al. 2000).

Part of the issue regarding reliability and validity of PD diagnosis in patients with SUDs centers on whether to include or exclude PD symptoms that seem to be substance related (i.e., behaviors directly related to intoxication and/or withdrawal or other behaviors required to maintain an addiction). The magnitude of the effect of exclusion on the prevalence estimate seems partly attributable to the strategy used for exclusion. Measures with more stringent criteria exclude any symptom that has ever been linked to substance use and yield significantly reduced rates. Measures that exclude symptoms only if they were completely absent before substance use or during periods of extended abstinence show minimal effects on rates. The more stringent strategy will likely exclude all secondary personality pathology and possibly primary personality pathology. The less stringent strategy is meant to exclude behaviors and/or symptoms that do not persist beyond periods of substance use and do not qualify for a PD diagnosis. Consequently, the less stringent approach will probably not exclude primary personality pathology and will have only a limited impact on the diagnosis of secondary PD.

Intuitively, one might suggest that excluding substance-related symptoms (at least following the less stringent strategy) would result in more valid diagnoses. Diagnosing PDs independent of SUDs is consistent with guidelines suggested in DSM-IV and carried over to DSM-5 Section II, "Diagnostic Criteria and Codes" (American Psychiatric Association 2013). However, the task of differentiating substance-related symptoms from personality traits is not easy for patients or clinical interviewers and therefore may not be reliable. This task becomes more difficult when substance use is chronic. Furthermore, although most patients with SUDs can distinguish behaviors that are only related to substance intoxication or withdrawal, they have greater difficulty making the same distinction for other activities, such as lying or breaking the law, which may be related to obtaining substances. In other words, there is a difference between symptoms of intoxication or withdrawal and symptoms that may be viewed as drug-seeking behaviors. Such a distinction requires a high level of introspection and cognitive competence in making the judgment necessary to differentiate a trait from a situation or state. It also requires self-awareness and accountability (Zimmerman 1994). Furthermore, PD criteria in DSM-IV and in DSM-5 Section II are a mix of symptoms, traits, behaviors, and consequences, making such distinctions even more difficult in practice.

Patients with SUDs may be particularly impaired in the skills necessary to make these distinctions. Rounsaville et al. (1998) found that excluding substance-related symptoms reduced the reliability of antisocial PD diagnoses but not of BPD diagnoses. Furthermore, the authors found that patients with independent PD diagnoses and patients with substance-related diagnoses had rather similar clinical profiles, thereby calling into question the feasibility and clinical utility of exclusion.

If one chooses to exclude substance-related symptoms from the measurement of any PD, several considerations are in order:

- Symptoms should be eliminated as being substance related on an item-by-item basis.
- Unless there are behavioral indicators of a trait present that are not substance related, criteria in which substance use is an inherent component should be scored as due to substance use.
- The interviewer should remind patients that questions refer to the way the patients usually are—that is, when they are not symptomatic with either substance abuse or other disorders (e.g., when sober at work, when with friends who do not use substances).

Causal Pathways

High comorbidity that cannot be explained by chance or measurement artifacts suggests that the co-occurrence of SUDs and PDs reflects some type of causal link. Causal models of comorbidity have often been organized under "primary SUD," "primary PD," and "common factor" categories, although it is unclear whether these distinctions remain relevant, for reasons discussed below. The behavioral disinhibition pathway, stress reduction pathway, reward sensitivity pathway, and common factor model (with an emphasis on genetics) are also summarized in this section.

"Primary" Disorder Models

The primary SUD model postulates that SUDs contribute to the development of PDs. For example, one study of adolescent inpatients in alcohol and drug treatment facilities found that drug use predicted the progression of conduct disorder to antisocial PD (Myers et al. 1998). Overall, however, evidence for the primary SUD model is scarce. Bernstein and Handelsman (1995) pointed out that it is unclear to what extent the effects of substance use can "overwrite" or interact with preexisting personality patterns to form new personality configurations. Furthermore, distinguishing new enduring personality patterns from temporary patterns that disappear with reductions of substance use is a methodological challenge in need of robust measurement and long-term prospective studies. As discussed in the "Assessment and Diagnosis" section above, according to DSM-5, only when PD symptomatology cannot be attributed to the physiological effects of a substance should these symptoms be considered personality pathology.

The primary PD model postulates that pathological personality traits contribute to the development of SUD. This model has empirical support. For example, a study by Cohen et al. (2007) found that individuals diagnosed with schizotypal, borderline, narcissistic, or passive-aggressive PD or with conduct disorder by age 13 years had significantly elevated rates of SUDs between early adolescence and young adulthood, independent of correlated family risks, participant sex, and other disorders. Bahlmann et al. (2002) found that among psychiatric inpatients, the onset of antisocial PD characteristics preceded that of alcohol dependence by approximately 4 years. However, the primary versus secondary distinction may not be an accurate one, given that both types of disorders may be equally severe, have shared genetic origin, and be of indeterminate temporality.

Behavioral Disinhibition Pathway

The behavioral disinhibition pathway to SUDs hypothesizes that individuals with antisocial and impulsive traits and low constraint or conscientiousness have lower thresholds for behaviors such as alcohol and drug use. Although these personality traits are not necessarily pathological in and of themselves, several longitudinal studies have shown that teachers' ratings of low constraint, low harm avoidance, lack of social conformity, unconventionality, antisociality, and aggression in children, particularly boys, predicted alcohol and drug use in adolescence and young adulthood (Caspi et al. 1997; Cloninger et al. 1988; Krueger et al. 1996; Masse and Tremblay 1997; Trucco et al. 2016; Vincent et al. 2017). The same pattern was observed in university students (Kaiser et al. 2016; Sher et al. 2000).

The relationship between behavioral disinhibition and early-onset substance use behaviors may be mediated by problems with socialization, academic achievement, family conflict, and affiliation with peers who also engage in problem behaviors (Elam et al. 2016; Sher and Trull 1994; Tarter and Vanyukov 1994; Wills et al. 1998). The behavioral disinhibition pathway is associated with earlier onset of drinking, more rapid development of alcohol dependence once drinking begins, and more severe symptoms among individuals with antisocial PD than among those without the disorder (Verheul et al. 1998).

In experimental settings, impulsivity is measured with several standardized tasks, including Delayed Reward Discounting, the Go/No-Go Task, the Iowa Gambling Task, the Stop-Signal test, and other paradigms (Grant and Chamberlain 2014). Some evidence suggests that higher scores on these measures underlie both SUDs (Grant and Chamberlain 2014; MacKillop et al. 2011) and Cluster B PDs (Barker et al. 2015; Bazanis et al. 2002). For example, the Iowa Gambling Task was used to compare impulsivity in individuals with AUD and comorbid Cluster B PDs, individuals with comorbid AUD and Cluster A or C PDs, individuals with AUD alone, and non-SUD controls (Dom et al. 2006). Those with AUD and Cluster B PDs had the highest impulsivity scores, followed by AUD alone, AUD and Cluster A or C PDs, and controls. Another study by Rubio et al. (2007) similarly found individuals with AUD and comorbid Cluster B PDs to score higher on a variety of impulsivity paradigms compared to individuals with AUD alone and a non-substance-using comparison group. It is therefore possible that the relationship between PDs and SUDs is due, in part, to a shared association with behavioral and/or trait impulsivity.

Stress Reduction Pathway

The stress reduction pathway regards substance use as self-medication for the anxiety and mood instability that individuals with PDs may exhibit in response to stressful life events. In longitudinal studies, teacher ratings of negative emotionality, stress reactivity, and low harm avoidance in children predicted substance use in adolescence and young adulthood (Caspi et al. 1997; Cloninger et al. 1988; Wills et al. 1998). Coping and fear dampening—as motives for drinking alcohol—are also more pronounced among men scoring high on anxiety sensitivity (Conrod et al. 1998). Cackowski et al. (2014) found that under stressful conditions, response inhibition among women with BPD was impaired compared to being in nonstressful conditions and to non-BPD controls, suggesting that stress response is worsened among individuals with BPD; however, this finding has not been consistent when using all measures of response inhibition (Cackowski et al. 2014; Lawrence et al. 2010). Early life stresses, including physical, sexual, and emotional abuse, have been associated with both SUDs and PDs in adults (Carr et al. 2013). It is therefore plausible that life stress, and particularly early life stress, plays a role in the comorbidity between SUD and PDs in later life.

Reward Sensitivity Pathway

The reward sensitivity pathway regards the positive, reinforcing properties of substance use as the motivating factor among individuals scoring high on traits such as novelty seeking, reward seeking, extraversion, and gregariousness—traits also common to some PDs. Again, although these traits are not necessarily pathological, longitudinal studies have shown that novelty seeking in childhood and adolescence predicts later substance use problems (Cloninger et al. 1988; Foulds et al. 2017; Jensen et al. 2017; Masse and Tremblay 1997; Wills et al. 1998), as well as BPD (van Dijk et al. 2012). Some evidence suggests that students' extraversion predicts alcohol dependence at age 30 among students without a family history of alcoholism (Schuckit et al. 1994). Hyperresponsiveness or hypersensitivity to the positive reinforcing effects of substances might develop most strongly among individuals with a more general sensitivity to positive reinforcement (Zuckerman 1999). Delayed Reward Discounting, a measure that characterizes the desire for smaller immediate rewards over larger delayed rewards, is heightened among individuals with SUDs (MacKillop et al. 2011; Petry 2002) and Cluster B PDs (Barker et al. 2015; Bazanis et al. 2002) compared with non-SUD or non-PD controls. It has therefore been suggested that the higher reward sensitivity associated with certain PDs may account for the high comorbidity between PDs and SUDs (Verheul 2001).

Common Factor Model

The common factor model holds that PDs and SUDs share a common cause. This model is consistent with a psychobiological perspective of some PDs that suggests they are phenomenologically, genetically, and/or biologically related to impulse disorders such as substance abuse (Siever and Davis 1991; Zanarini 1993). This model is also consistent with findings from psychiatric epidemiology (see section "Epidemiology" above) that explore the metastructure of psychopathology, and is reflected in the structure of DSM-5, wherein at least some "externalizing" disorders are grouped together. In this section, we explore the common factor model from the perspectives of genetic epidemiology, molecular genetics, and biological markers. However, this focus is not intended to downplay or deprioritize common factors originating in developmental, environmental, and social experiences and exposures.

Genetic Epidemiological Studies

Epidemiological studies find that individuals rarely abuse a single substance (Swendsen et al. 2012). Instead, polysubstance abuse and dependence are normative, with high rates of comorbidity across various drug classes (Swendsen et al. 2012). Twin studies, in which the relationships between monozygotic (identical) and dizygotic (fraternal) twins are used to differentiate genetic and nongenetic (social environmental) sources of variance in a given trait, suggest that this comorbidity is due at least in part to a shared genetic etiology. Several twin and family studies have found evidence of a shared underlying genetic susceptibility to substance use and other psychopathologies, including antisocial PD (Cloninger et al. 1988; Goldman et al. 2005; Roysamb et al. 2011) and BPD (Bornovalova et al. 2013; Gillespie et al. 2018; Kendler et al. 2011; Long et al. 2017). Furthermore, this shared genetic factor appears to be more heritable than the individual disorders themselves (Goldman et al. 2005). Data from Few et al. (2014) suggest that genetic correlations between BPD and SUDs may result from shared personality traits, including neuroticism and affective instability.

Molecular Genetic Studies

Since the completion of the Human Genome Project in 2003, technological advances have enabled researchers to identify specific genetic variants influencing human behavior and disorder. Psychiatric disorders are complex behavioral traits, influenced by a multitude of genetic variants of subtle effect, which act in conjunction with each other (gene-gene interaction) and the individual's social context (gene-environment interaction). Because of the challenges of gene discovery for disorders with complex genetic architecture—for example, that extremely large study populations are required to detect the subtle effects of individual genetic loci—researchers have only begun to identify specific genetic risk factors for psychiatric disorders, including SUDs and PDs.

In the last few years, several large psychiatric genetic consortia/biobanks have formed (e.g., Psychiatric Genomics Consortium [Walters et al. 2018], GSCAN [Genome-Wide Association Studies and Sequencing Consortium of Alcohol and Nicotine Use] [Liu et al. 2019], UK Biobank [Clarke et al. 2017], 23andMe [Sanchez-Roige et al. 2019], Million Veterans Project [Kranzler et al. 2019]) and published landmark studies in SUDs, with efforts under way for PDs. For example, a recent publication from the Million Veterans Project (Kranzler et al. 2019) examined AUD in 274,424 individuals and identified 18 genome-wide significant loci, including several known candidate genes (e.g., *ADH1B*, *ADH4*, *DRD2*, *KLB*, *GCKR*, *SCL39A8*) and several novel variants for follow-up. Preliminary molecular genetic studies also further support the premise that shared genetic factors influence both SUDs and PDs. For example, data on Han Chinese males demonstrate that individuals with genetic risk factors previously associated with alcohol dependence—that is, dopamine receptor 2 (*DRD2*) and alde-hyde dehydrogenase 2 (*ALDH2*)—were at a 5.39 times greater risk for antisocial PD than were those without the genetic risk (Lu et al. 2012). Furthermore, data from the Collaborative Study on the Genetics of Alcoholism (Aliev et al. 2015) found that several genetic risk factors for alcohol dependence were also associated with antisocial PD, including genes in the alcohol dehydrogenase cluster (e.g., *ALDH2, ADH1C, ADH4*), cholinergic nicotinic receptors (e.g., *CHRNA3, CHRNA5*), and γ-aminobutyric acid receptors (*GABRG1, GABRP, GABRR2*), as well as notable candidate genes (*NRNX1* and *PTPRG*). As larger genetic studies of individual PDs begin to emerge, evaluation of genomic risk factors shared among SUDs and PDs will be an important next step toward understanding one aspect of shared liability for these disorders, as well as increasing understanding of genomic factors unique to each disorder.

Biological Markers

A final piece of evidence suggesting a shared genetic liability across externalizing psychopathology comes from the electrophysiological literature. Electrophysiological endophenotypes, which are thought to index genetic vulnerability to psychiatric phenotypes, are also shared across SUDs and comorbid psychiatric disorders (Iacono et al. 1999; Porjesz et al. 2005). A classic endophenotype in the SUD literature is a reduced P3 event-related potential amplitude, which has consistently been found in individuals with SUDs (Polich et al. 1994; Porjesz and Begleiter 1985) as well as in their at-risk family members. This was particularly salient when it was first observed in at-risk adolescents (offspring of individuals with SUDs) who had not yet initiated substance use, suggesting that this measure may indicate risk for SUDs rather than representing a consequence of substance use (Begleiter et al. 1984). Importantly, reduced P3 amplitudes are also observed among individuals with antisocial PD (Gilmore et al. 2010; Iacono et al. 2002), providing additional evidence of shared neural risk factors among SUDs and antisocial PD.

Treatment Outcome

Many clinicians believe PDs to be associated with poor treatment response in patients with SUDs. This is consistent with findings from some studies showing that individuals with PDs (usually antisocial PD) have worse substance use treatment outcomes (Galen et al. 2000; Grella et al. 2003; Haro et al. 2004; Krampe et al. 2006). Furthermore, several PDs (including antisocial [Daughters et al. 2008], histrionic [Fernandez-Montalvo and Lopez-Goni 2010], and borderline [Samuel et al. 2011; Tull and Gratz 2012]) have been linked to lower retention in substance use treatment. Large nationally representative samples also show more chronic SUDs in individuals with PDs (Fenton et al. 2012; Hasin et al. 2011). However, these findings contrast with more optimistic studies about the outcome for these individuals. Several studies suggest that although personality pathology may be associated with individuals' SUD severity, it may not predict how much they improve in response to SUD treatment (e.g., Cacciola et al. 1995; Verheul et al. 1999). Other studies show that PD comorbidity (again often focusing on antisocial PD) does not predict SUD treatment outcomes (Easton et al. 2012; Gill et al. 1992; Longabaugh et al. 1994; Messina et al. 2002; Ouimette et al. 1999; Ralevski et al. 2007) or premature dropout (Easton et al. 2012; Gill et al. 1992; Marlowe et al. 1997). These conflicting results do not allow for firm conclusions about the prognosis of SUD patients with comorbid PDs. However, some studies show that PDs predict a shorter time to relapse after discharge (Mather 1987; Thomas et al. 1999), even after controlling for baseline severity of substance use (Verheul et al. 1998). Therefore, although SUDs in patients with PDs may improve with treatment, these patients may be more susceptible to relapse following treatment, dictating increased caution and monitoring.

In contrast to the extensive literature on the effects of PDs on substance use treatment outcomes, less research has been done on the impact of SUDs on PD outcomes. This is likely because the literature on the efficacy of PD interventions in general is underdeveloped (with the possible exception of interventions for BPD) (Bateman et al. 2015). The lack of research may also reflect the exclusion of dual-diagnosis patients from treatment systems and research studies, illustrating the limitations of mental health systems and research policies oriented toward the treatment of single rather than multiple disorders (Ridgely et al. 1990). Whereas one study showed that recovery from SUDs did not relate to recovery from PDs (Verheul et al. 2000), other studies have found improvement in pathological personality traits following treatment for SUDs (Borman et al. 2006) and higher dropout rates from psychiatric treatment among substance users (Karterud et al. 2009), suggesting a potential impact of active substance use on success of PD treatment. More research is needed that specifically addresses whether SUD status affects outcome of PD treatment.

Outcomes of Dual Focus Treatments

Therapy protocols have been developed for comorbid PDs and SUDs. Dual Focus Schema Therapy (DFST) and Dialectical Behavior Therapy for Substance Abusers (DBT-S) have been the focus of ongoing study and are described below. Dynamic deconstructive psychotherapy (Goldman and Gregory 2010; Gregory et al. 2008) has received some support in multiple follow-ups of a single trial. Integrated dual disorder treatment, generally used for individuals with severe mental illness and comorbid SUDs, has also been argued to be adaptable for individuals with comorbid PDs and SUDs (van Wamel et al. 2010). However, more research is needed on these treatments.

Dual Focus Schema Therapy

DFST, developed by Ball and Young (Ball 1998; Ball and Young 2000), is a treatment designed to address both substance use problems and PD symptomatology. DFST is a manual-guided program that incorporates relapse prevention, coping skills, and discussion of maladaptive schemas. It proposes a core set of strategies that are meant to be adaptable for any PD, and targets reducing symptomatology in lieu of complete elimination of personality pathology (Ball 1998). Most studies of DFST have been conducted in small samples. In 2005, Ball et al. evaluated DFST among 52 individuals with PDs who abused substances and were receiving services at a drop-in center for the homeless. Participants were randomly assigned to receive either DFST or standard drug counseling group sessions for 24 weeks, both delivered on-site as enhancements to case management services. Results indicated more overall utilization of DFST, but patients with more severe Cluster A and C symptomatology preferred drug counseling. In 2007, Ball tested DFST against 12-Step Facilitation Therapy (TSFT) with 30 methadone maintenance patients. Treatment retention and utilization were similar for the two treatments; however, DFST patients evidenced a quicker decrease in substance use and stronger therapeutic alliance, whereas TSFT patients reported more improvement in dysphoric symptoms. In a third study, Ball et al. (2011) compared DFST with individual drug counseling in 105 patients receiving residential treatment. Their results suggested similar retention for the two groups, with more sustained changes among severe patients in the individual drug counseling group. In addition to these evaluations of DFST, Nielsen et al. (2007) found Personality-Guided Treatment for Alcohol Dependence (which was largely inspired by DFST) to be associated with increased abstinence from alcohol but found no difference in binge quantity or time to relapse. Firm conclusions about efficacy cannot be made from these small studies of DFST that have conflicting results. However, at best, efficacy for DFST thus far seems comparable to that of existing treatments such as drug counseling or TSFT.

Case Example 1

Andrew was a 36-year-old divorced male whose primary PD diagnosis was obsessive-compulsive PD. In addition to having symptoms of depression, obsessive thoughts, compulsive behavior, and paranoid ideation, he had interpersonal problems related to being exploitative and aggressive in response to even minor irritation. He began using substances at age 14 and had occasionally sold drugs or stolen property to fund his use. Andrew had had several prior substance abuse treatments and had been taking methadone for 1 year before starting individual therapy. His heroin dependence was in remission, and his primary drug abuse problem was cocaine, with more sporadic use of a high-potency solvent to which his job gave him ready accessibility. Andrew also met criteria for antisocial PD. This diagnosis does not frequently co-occur with obsessive-compulsive PD; however, it was difficult to determine whether the antisocial PD diagnosis was independent of substance abuse given, the very early age at onset and his persistent use of multiple substances during adolescence and adulthood.

Andrew was treated for 6 months as part of a research protocol evaluating DFST. His core early maladaptive schema was unrelenting standards/hypercriticalness (i.e., perfectionism, rigid rules, and preoccupation with time and efficiency), which appeared to originate from parental perfectionism (with physical or emotional abuse for Andrew's "failures" as a child). Andrew put a great deal of pressure on himself, and any minor deviation in his striving for perfection triggered an impulsive return to substance use, missing work or appointments, and antisocial acting out. He engaged in maladaptive coping behaviors that perpetuated this schema, including expecting too much of himself and others. At other times, he sought relief from the pressures of these standards and would avoid occupational or social commitments, develop somatic symptoms, procrastinate, or give up on himself and use drugs when he could not get things to be perfect. These avoidance strategies actually reinforced his high standards even more because he would subsequently have to redouble his efforts to get desired outcomes.

Andrew began therapy in a loud, challenging manner, wanting to know for sure that therapy was going to help him and that he was going to get as much out of it as the researchers would get out of him as a research participant. Because he continued to abuse cocaine and inhalants for the first 3 months, therapy necessarily remained more focused on relapse prevention while he struggled to grasp cognitively any of the schema-focused psychoeducational material. By month 4, he had achieved complete abstinence from solvents and was using cocaine much less frequently. This change had a significant positive effect on his personality (more agreeable and sociable, less depressed and agitated); however, his unrelenting standards/hypercriticalness schema was expressed even more strongly.

Cognitively oriented interventions included cost-benefit analyses of his unrelenting standards and reducing the perceived risks of imperfection. A core cognitive distortion targeted for dispute was "When I don't accomplish or get what I want, I should get enraged, give up, use drugs, and be dejected." Experiential techniques involved imagery dialogues with his parents about how they always made mistakes seem like catastrophes. Behavioral techniques included learning to accept "good enough" work from himself and others, accepting directions from people he did not respect, and redeveloping old leisure interests. Therapeutic relationship interventions included the therapist modeling acceptance of his own mistakes, processing homework noncompliance due to self-imposed rigid standards, and confronting Andrew's dichotomous views of the therapist. Much of the work in Andrew's outside relationships and in therapy involved helping him change his dichotomous view of other people and of his own recovery (i.e., all good/sober vs. all bad/relapsed).

Despite a rather turbulent course of treatment, Andrew appeared genuinely interested in improving himself and made some significant changes. In addition to his reduced substance abuse, he also experienced significant reductions in psychiatric symptoms and negative affect.

Dialectical Behavior Therapy for People Who Use Substances

Standard DBT has been shown to be associated with more reduction of substance use than has treatment as usual in some studies of patients with PDs (Harned et al. 2008) but not others (van den Bosch et al. 2002). However, DBT-S, a modified version of DBT, was developed specifically for individuals with comorbid BPD and SUDs (Linehan and Dimeff 1997). DBT-S includes individual and group treatment components similar to standard DBT, but also tailors DBT skills to substance use issues. Several small studies have assessed the efficacy of DBT-S in individuals with co-occurring SUDs and BPD. Linehan et al. (1999) tested DBT-S in 28 patients with BPD and various SUDs. They found that patients treated with DBT-S had greater reductions in substance use and greater gains in adjustment than did individuals referred for psychotherapy in the community. Dimeff et al. (2000) found DBT-S to be useful in increasing drug abstinence in three methamphetamine-dependent patients with BPD. Linehan et al. (2002) compared DBT-S and a comprehensive validation therapy (including 12-step facilitation) in 23 BPD patients with heroin dependence. Both groups showed improvements in opiate use and psychopathology. Although the comprehensive validation therapy group showed better retention, it also demonstrated slightly increased opiate use at the end of treatment compared with patients receiving DBT-S. Rizvi et al. (2011) found that even a smartphone adaptation of DBT-S was useful in decreasing distress and substance craving among 22 individuals with co-occurring BPD and SUD. Axelrod et al. (2011) examined the effects of DBT among 27 women with BPD and SUD; these patients reduced substance use and experienced improved mood. Finally, Beckstead et al. (2015) examined the effects of DBT-S adapted for American Indian/Alaska Native youth. Their sample of 229 evidenced significant decreases in distress over the course of treatment. In addition to its use in targeting BPD alone, or samples with comorbid BPD and SUD, DBT has also been studied in primarily SUD samples (with PD rates ~50%) (Cavicchioli et al. 2019; Maffei et al. 2018). Although most studies of DBT-S to date have utilized small samples and/or pretest-posttest designs, they suggest some support among patients with BPD and comorbid SUD. However, DBT-S has not been studied for PDs other than BPD. Encouraging results from patients with BPD should not be extrapolated to other PDs, especially because antisocial PD has been described as a possible contraindication for DBT (Linehan and Korslund 2006).

Case Example 2

Belinda was a 27-year-old patient with BPD. Her first suicide attempt was at age 12; alcohol abuse began at age 16, followed by abuse of cannabis, cocaine, and heroin. Her first admission into a psychiatric hospital was at age 12, and she had had a criminal record since age 16. In addition to her abuse of heroin, cocaine, cannabis, and alcohol, she had interpersonal problems, anger outbursts, parasuicidal behaviors, and aggressive impulsiveness. Previously, she had been in psychiatric and addiction treatments as both an outpatient and an inpatient. Among her typical therapy-interfering behaviors was attempting to invite the therapist into a very close and sometimes intimate relationship. She usually dropped out each time she failed to seduce a therapist. At the time of admission to the DBT program, she was in an addiction-oriented day hospital program.

Soon after Belinda started therapy, a basic behavior pattern became clear to the therapist: After work on Friday evening, Belinda would start to feel lonely. The thought "I need to comfort myself" would pop up. She would close the curtains, drink a glass of wine, and smoke cannabis while listening to music. Around 10 P.M. she would become restless, followed by feeling angry because she deserved "some company." Then she would dress up in sexy clothes and go out for a drink. In the pub, she would often meet familiar drug dealers. After a few drinks together, the drug dealers would offer her cocaine. Because Belinda could not afford to buy it, she would agree to have sex with them. Feelings of guilt would lead to more substance abuse, and finally she would lose contact with reality. The next morning, she would awake next to a stranger and would become self-destructive, usually making a series of cuts on her arm.

This behavior pattern was targeted for treatment. Because of its threshold-lowering capacities for impulsive and self-destructive behavior, the alcohol abuse was given high priority early in treatment. Telephone consultation was of utmost importance in this stage. After 3 months, Belinda succeeded for the first time in not acting on the impulse to go to the bars late at night. Her contact with her father, mother, and sisters was gradually restored, and she resumed contact with a network of old friends who were not involved in substance abuse. Reinforcement contingencies were thus introduced such that she would have enjoyable interactions with her friends and family when she chose to contact them instead of going to the bar by herself.

Despite Belinda's verbalized commitment to stop using all drugs, cannabis use was the most change-resistant behavior. The therapist introduced the concept of mindfulness, which allowed Belinda to practice being more aware of her cravings and more intentional in her response to them. After 8 months she was clean and was able to "surf the craving" (i.e., be fully aware of—but resist—the urge to use cannabis). Then, finally, her attachment problems were targeted in treatment. Belinda's efforts to become more intimate with the therapist failed, as did all her efforts to make the therapist reject her (e.g., stalking by telephone, anger outbursts). The therapist was able to validate Belinda's behavior as fear of abandonment, and she finally recognized that she was more afraid of saying good-bye than of being rejected. After 54 sessions Belinda left the program and the therapist by mutual agreement; she left a bouquet of flowers, along with a note that read, "This relationship is the most horrible thing that has ever happened to me in my life. Thanks so much."

Comment on Treatment Outcome

In summary, we have discussed that 1) personality pathology may affect response to treatment of SUDs, although the effect is not found as consistently as might have been anticipated; 2) more research is needed on the effect of SUD on response to PD treatment; and 3) some treatments with a dual focus exist (with greatest support for DBT-S), but more empirical evidence is needed. Together, these data emphasize the importance of and need for effective treatment approaches that pay simultaneous attention to substance and personality problems. Attention to the feasibility of these treatments is also required, because DFST and DBT-S require additional clinical training and supervision, and both treatments can be time intensive. The development of integrated, multitargeted treatment programs, rather than separate symptom-specific programs, could offer great benefit to patients with comorbid conditions. Relatedly, therapist training should incorporate training on working with individuals with comorbid disorders.

Treatment Guidelines

Patients with PDs are often treated with psychotherapy, and pharmacotherapy is used to address specific symptoms as needed. We see no reason to deviate substantially from this general protocol in dual-diagnosis patients, although effective treatment of these patients often requires modifications to traditional programs and methods. We provide some clinical recommendations for psychotherapy and pharmacotherapy, respectively.

Psychotherapy

Dual Focus

Dual focus does not necessarily mean that attention to both foci should always take place simultaneously. During the earlier sessions, it is often best to place the greatest emphasis on the establishment and maintenance of abstinence but with a secondary focus on identification of and psychoeducation about maladaptive personality traits. During later sessions, once a strong therapeutic relationship is established and substance-related concerns have become less pressing, a greater emphasis can be placed on confronting and changing maladaptive traits, cognitive-affective processes, or interpersonal relationships.

Clinical Setting

Psychotherapy with patients with both SUD and PD is often insufficient as a standalone treatment. Psychotherapy is likely to be most useful if it is offered as part of a comprehensive program incorporating varied treatment modalities (individual and group therapy, pharmacotherapy if needed) and external resources (e.g., Alcoholics Anonymous or Narcotics Anonymous meetings, residential treatment, detoxification, methadone maintenance program).

Duration and Treatment Goals

The treatment of individuals with PDs can be a long-term process. The added problems of reduced treatment retention and compliance associated with substance abuse raise questions of what the appropriate treatment goals are for this group. The goal should not be to accomplish deep and permanent change in personality structure within a relatively short term. If facilities or resources are limited, a more practical aim might be to improve substance abuse treatment outcomes by teaching patients how to cope with or modulate maladaptive personality processes.

Required Therapist Training

Patients with comorbid SUD and PD can put a strain on the resources of many treatment programs. Therapists treating these patients should have thorough education and training in PDs, addiction, and therapy in general. More experienced therapists may be more appropriate given the complex array of presenting problems, although even seasoned therapists would likely benefit from consultation on difficult cases.

Essential Ingredients

The dual focus of treatment should be clear from the beginning of treatment, even if different problems are targeted at different points in treatment. The trait-based approach to personality pathology introduced in the Alternative DSM-5 Model for Personality Disorders (American Psychiatric Association 2013) may aid the therapist in treatment planning. Use of motivational interviewing (Martino et al. 2002) during the admission phase and throughout the treatment process may be beneficial with dual-diagnosis patients. Regular individual therapy is helpful in establishing a therapeutic alliance and fostering commitment to treatment. Direct therapeutic attention to maladaptive personality traits may increase cognitive and coping skills, which in turn may improve symptomatology and reduce the risk for relapse. Participation in some modality of aftercare (ongoing outpatient therapy, Alcoholics Anonymous or Narcotics Anonymous meetings) could be beneficial to patients who have completed more intensive treatment.

Pharmacotherapy

To date, no medications have been approved by the U.S. Food and Drug Administration (FDA) or the European Medicines Agency for the treatment of PDs (Bozzatello et al. 2017). As a result, the use of medications for treating PDs remains off-label, and patients' informed consent should be documented. It is also important to note that pharmacotherapy focused on particular symptom domains, such as cognitive-perceptual symptoms (e.g., hallucinations), impulsive-behavioral dyscontrol (e.g., self-injury), and affective dysregulation (e.g., depressed mood), has been shown to be more effective than strategies focused on PD diagnoses alone (Nelson 2018; Soloff 1998). Still, many placebo-controlled trials of pharmacotherapy for PDs to date have focused on specific disorders. In the following review, we focus on placebo-controlled trials of pharmacotherapeutic treatments for PDs and SUDs by diagnostic category, and then provide a review of studies assessing pharmacotherapy for comorbid PDs and SUDs. More details regarding the pharmacotherapy of PDs can be found in Chapter 17, "Pharmacological Management."

Personality Disorders

Overall, evidence for pharmacotherapy for PDs is scarce, and limited by small sample sizes, comorbid psychopathology, short follow-up periods, inconsistent outcome measures, and a bias toward BPD (Bozzatello et al. 2017). For example, placebo-controlled trials have been conducted for only three PDs—schizotypal, borderline, and antisocial—with more than twice as many studies on BPD than on all other PDs (Bozzatello et al. 2017). A detailed overview of randomized controlled trials (RCTs) of pharmacotherapy for PDs is presented in Table 21–2 (see also Chapter 17, "Pharmacological Management," in this volume).

TABLE 21–2. Placebo-controlled trials of pharmacotherapy for personality disorders

Diagnostic group	Medication	Trials	Benefit	Study/drug limitations
Schizotypal PD	Risperidone	Koenigsberg et al. 2003; McClure et al. 2009	Improved Positive and Negative Syndrome Scale score No improvement in Hamilton Depression Rating Scale, Clinical Global Impression, Schizotypal Personality Disorder Questionnaire, spatial and verbal working memory, spatial memory, vigilance, or work list learning	Small *N* High dropout rate due to side effects
	Guanfacine	McClure et al. 2007	Improved content processing	Small *N*
	Pergolide	McClure et al. 2010	Improved visual spatial working memory, executive functioning, and verbal learning and memory	Small *N* Trial halted due to evidence of heart problems related to use
Borderline PD	Fluoxetine	Markovitz 1995; Salzman et al. 1995; Coccaro and Kavoussi 1997	Improved anger, aggression, anxious-depressive symptoms, and global symptoms Improved impulsive-aggressive behaviors and irritability among patients with PDs and comorbid dysthymic, anxiety, and substance use disorders	Insufficient control for comorbidity of affective and anxiety disorders Salzmann et al. included a mixed sample of PD patients (one-third with BPD)
	Fluvoxamine	Rinne et al. 2002	Improved rapid mood shifts No improvement in impulsivity and aggression	Sample included only females
	Lithium	Links et al. 1990	Improved anger and suicidality No improvement in mood symptoms	Small *N* All patients also receiving concomitant therapy High risk of toxicity No regular blood level controls Not recommended

TABLE 21–2. Placebo-controlled trials of pharmacotherapy for personality disorders *(continued)*

Diagnostic group	Medication	Trials	Benefit	Study/drug limitations
Borderline PD *(continued)*	Carbamazepine	De la Fuente and Lotstra 1994	No significant differences in clinical benefits compared to placebo	Trial of limited duration (5 weeks) High risk of adverse events (e.g., agranulocytosis) Not recommended
	Valproate sodium	Hollander et al. 2001; Frankenburg and Zanarini 2002; Hollander et al. 2003	Improved interpersonal sensitivity, anger, hostility, and aggressiveness No significant improvement in global symptomatology, affective dysregulation, or behavioral disinhibition	Small N and high dropout rate Frankenburg and Zanarini sample included only females
	Divalproex ER	Moen et al. 2012	No significant differences in clinical benefits compared to placebo	Small N Trial began after 4 weeks of DBT
	Topiramate	Loew et al. 2006; Nickel 2007a, 2007b; Nickel and Loew 2008; Nickel et al. 2004, 2005	Improved anger, irritability, aggression, somatization symptoms, interpersonal sensitivity, hostility, and global functioning after 8 weeks and at 18-month follow-up No improvement on obsessive-compulsive, depression, paranoid ideation, and psychoticism scales Weight loss is to be expected	Short trial duration (8–10 weeks) in Nickel et al. (2007a, 2007b) and Lowe et al.
	Lamotrigine	Tritt et al. 2005; Reich et al. 2009	Improved anger No improvement in overall score on Zanarini Rating Scale for Borderline Personality Disorder	Small N Tritt et al. sample included only females Reich et al. did not control for comorbidity of affective and anxiety disorders or antidepressant use

TABLE 21–2. Placebo-controlled trials of pharmacotherapy for personality disorders *(continued)*

Diagnostic group	Medication	Trials	Benefit	Study/drug limitations
Borderline PD *(continued)*	Haloperidol	Soloff et al. 1993; Cornelius et al. 1993	Mixed results regarding effect on hostility and impulsive-aggressive behaviors No improvement of global severity, anger, or psychoticism May worsen depressive symptoms	Short trial duration (5 weeks) High dropout rate
	Risperidone	Schulz et al. 1998	Improved psychoticism, paranoid ideas, phobic anxiety, and interpersonal sensitivity No improvement in global functioning	Small *N* Short trial duration (5 weeks)
	Olanzapine	Zanarini and Frankenburg 2001; Bogenschutz and Nurnberg 2004; Soler et al. 2005; Schulz et al. 2008; Linehan et al. 2008; Zanarini et al. 2011b	Improved interpersonal sensitivity, anxiety, anger, hostility, paranoia, psychoticism, and global functioning Somewhat mixed results regarding effect on BPD symptomatology, although some results suggest that olanzapine is associated with a higher response rate and shorter time to response compared to other treatments Consistent improvements among patients receiving simultaneous DBT Risk of adverse events (particularly weight gain) exhibits a dose-response trend	
	Aripiprazole	Nickel et al. 2006, 2007	Improved psychotic symptoms, depression, anxiety, and hostility Improvements confirmed at 18-month follow-up	Small *N* Short trial duration (8 weeks)
	Ziprasidone	Pascual et al. 2006, 2008	No improvement in psychoticism, depression, anxiety, impulsivity, or hostility	Small *N*

TABLE 21–2. Placebo-controlled trials of pharmacotherapy for personality disorders *(continued)*

Diagnostic group	Medication	Trials	Benefit	Study/drug limitations
Borderline PD *(continued)*	Quetiapine	Black et al. 2014; Lee et al. 2016	Low-dose (150 mg/day) quetiapine improved affective instability, cognitive-perceptual symptoms, aggressiveness, overall psychological distress, interpersonal sensitivity, depression, and hostility Improved time to response	Higher dose (300 mg/day) associated with more adverse effects and higher dropout rate
	Naloxone (for acute dissociative states)	Philipsen et al. 2004b	No difference in dissociative symptoms compared to placebo	Small *N*
	Naltrexone (for dissociative symptoms)	Schmahl et al. 2012	Intensity and duration of dissociative symptoms were improved but did not achieve statistical significance	Small *N* Short trial duration (3 weeks)
	Clonidine (for strong aversive inner tension, dissociative symptoms, and hyperarousal)	Philipsen et al. 2004a; Ziegenhorn et al. 2009	Improvement in dissociative symptoms, urge to commit self-injurious behaviors, hyperarousal (including sleep problems, irritability, concentration problems, hypervigilance, and exaggerated startle), and suicidal ideation, with the strongest effect between 30 and 60 minutes	Small *N* Philipsen et al. sample included only females Ziegenhorn et al. included participants with comorbid PTSD
Antisocial PD	Desipramine	Leal et al. 1994; Arndt et al. 1994	No improvement in percent of cocaine-free urines among patients with antisocial PD	Leal et al. included only patients with opioid and cocaine dependency Arndt et al. sample included only methadone-maintained outpatient males with cocaine dependency
	Nortriptyline	Powell et al. 1995	Reduced mean drinking days, alcohol dependence, and anxiety levels No improvement in severity of alcohol use	Small *N* Sample included only males

TABLE 21–2. Placebo-controlled trials of pharmacotherapy for personality disorders *(continued)*

Diagnostic group	Medication	Trials	Benefit	Study/drug limitations
Antisocial PD *(continued)*	Phenytoin	Barratt et al. 1997; Stanford et al. 2005	Improved frequency and intensity of aggressive behaviors	Sample included only male prisoners with impulsive aggression
	Valproate	Hollander et al. 2003; Stanford et al. 2005	Improved impulsive aggression, irritability, and global severity	Hollander et al. included all Cluster B disorders High dropout rate in Hollander et al. due to adverse effects Stanford et al. sample included only males
	Carbamazepine	Stanford et al. 2005	Improved impulsive aggression compared to placebo Effect was slightly delayed compared with phenytoin and valproate	Small *N* Sample included only males
	Amantadine	Leal et al. 1994	No improvement in percent of cocaine-free urines among patients with antisocial PD	Sample included only males with opioid and cocaine dependency
	Bromocriptine	Powell et al. 1995	Improved alcohol use disorder severity Anxiety and depressive symptoms improved somewhat but did not achieve statistical significance	Sample included only males with alcohol addiction
	Naltrexone	Ralevski et al. 2007	Improvement in alcohol dependence severity was equivalent to that in non–antisocial PD controls	Sample included a mix of BPD and antisocial PD patients with alcohol dependence

Note.   BPD=borderline personality disorder; DBT=dialectical behavior therapy; ER=extended release; PD=personality disorder; PTSD=posttraumatic stress disorder.
Source of studies.   Bozzatello et al. 2017.

Schizotypal PD.   Four small placebo-controlled trials have examined risperidone, guanfacine, and pergolide for schizotypal PD (for review, see Bozzatello et al. 2017). In two trials, risperidone was found to improve positive and negative symptoms, but not to improve depression, schizotypal symptoms, working memory, vigilance, or clinical global impression. There was also a high dropout rate due to adverse effects. Guanfacine was found to improve content processing. Pergolide was found to improve working memory, executive functioning, and verbal learning; however, this trial was halted due to evidence of heart problems related to pergolide use.

Borderline PD.   A number of trials have examined pharmacotherapeutic treatments for BPD, including antidepressants, mood stabilizers, and antipsychotics, with ranging efficacy and study quality. Overall, antidepressants, including fluoxetine and fluvoxamine, have shown efficacy in reducing internalizing symptoms (for review, see Bozzatello et al. 2017). Specifically, fluoxetine was associated with reduced anger, aggression, anxious-depressive symptoms, and global symptoms, whereas fluvoxamine was associated with reduced rapid mood shifts. However, trials with fluoxetine did not control for comorbid affective and anxiety disorders.

Mood stabilizers have shown mixed efficacy in reducing BPD symptoms (for review, see Bozzatello et al. 2017). In one trial each, carbamazepine and extended-release divalproex showed no significant clinical benefits compared to placebo. However, valproate sodium, topiramate, and lamotrigine were all shown to reduce anger and aggression.

Antipsychotics have shown similarly mixed efficacy (for review, see Bozzatello et al. 2017). In two trials, haloperidol had an inconsistent effect on hostility and impulsive aggression; in one case, the authors concluded that haloperidol may worsen depressive symptoms. Ziprasidone was similarly associated with no improvement in psychoticism, depression, anxiety, impulsivity, or hostility. However, risperidone, olanzapine, aripiprazole, and low-dose quetiapine all showed efficacy in reducing a range of psychiatric symptoms. Olanzapine, in particular, has been associated with improved interpersonal sensitivity, anger, anxiety, hostility, paranoia, psychoticism, and global functioning in a number of trials.

Finally, two trials examined clonidine and one trial examined naltrexone for treating acute dissociative symptoms (for review, see Bozzatello et al. 2017). Clonidine was associated with reductions in dissociative symptoms, urge to commit self-injurious behaviors, hyperarousal, and suicidal ideation, with the strongest effect between 30 and 60 minutes. Naltrexone was similarly associated with reduced intensity and duration of dissociative symptoms, although it did not reach statistical significance, potentially as a result of small sample size.

Antisocial PD.   Evidence around pharmacotherapy for antisocial PD is extremely limited (for review, see Bozzatello et al. 2017). One placebo-controlled trial of male prisoners with impulsive aggression found phenytoin to decrease the frequency and intensity of aggressive behaviors. Two trials found valproate to similarly reduce impulsive aggression, irritability, and global severity; however, one of these trials included all Cluster B disorders and reported a high dropout rate due to adverse effects. Carbamazepine was also associated with reduced impulsive aggression, but this effect was slightly delayed compared with phenytoin and valproate. In general, it is suggested that medication not be used to treat antisocial PD (Nelson 2018).

Substance Use Disorders

Strong evidence exists supporting pharmacotherapy for certain SUDs. Below, we review the evidence for medications for alcohol use, opioid use, and other SUDs.

Alcohol use disorder. As of 2019, three medications have FDA approval for the treatment of AUD: disulfiram, naltrexone, and acamprosate. Disulfiram, a competitive inhibitor of acetaldehyde dehydrogenase, causes severe nausea, vomiting, sweating, and headache when combined with alcohol. Success of this medication has been primarily observed in open-label studies, with no evidence of sustained abstinence compared to placebo in blinded trials (Knox et al. 2019). Naltrexone, a μ-opioid receptor antagonist, works to block the rewarding effects of alcohol. Placebo-controlled trials of oral naltrexone have demonstrated a significantly reduced risk of relapse for any drinking and heavy drinking with treatment (Knox et al. 2019). Long-acting injectable naltrexone has similarly been found to decrease the percentage of heavy drinking days. Finally, acamprosate has been associated with decreased risk of relapse to any drinking but has no effect on relapse to heavy drinking (Knox et al. 2019).

Two additional medications, nalmefene and baclofen, have been approved by the European Medicines Agency for the treatment of AUD and may be used off-label in the United States. Both have been shown to be effective in decreasing binge drinking and reducing relapse rates (Knox et al. 2019). Other non-approved but effective medications, including gabapentin and topiramate, may be used off-label when other medications fail (Knox et al. 2019). Despite its demonstrated efficacy, pharmacotherapy for AUD is heavily underutilized in clinical practice, and patients would benefit from wider consideration and use of such medications (Knox et al. 2019).

Opioid use disorder. Methadone, buprenorphine, and naltrexone are currently the three approved medications for opioid use disorder (MOUD). MOUD are prescribed on a long-term basis (6 or more months) and have been shown to reduce the risk of death and disease from opioid use disorder (Bell and Strang 2020). Methadone is a full opioid agonist with a variable half-life of 13–50 hours. Methadone is viewed as the gold standard for MOUD, and has been demonstrated to reduce cravings, withdrawal symptoms, and relapse (Bell and Strang 2020). A dose of 30 mg/day is sufficient to block opioid withdrawal for at least 24 hours; however, a dose of 60–100 mg/day is most effective in promoting abstinence (Bell and Strang 2020). In a dose-response fashion, a longer duration of methadone treatment has been linked to better outcomes. However, methadone may be dispensed only by licensed clinics and requires daily clinic visits, which can be a barrier to compliance (Bell and Strang 2020). Buprenorphine, a partial opioid agonist, binds tightly to the μ-opioid receptor, thereby blocking the effects of other, nonsynthetic opioids. Similar to methadone, buprenorphine is demonstrated to reduce cravings, withdrawal, and relapse (Bell and Strang 2020). Frequently, this medication is combined with naloxone (known commercially as Suboxone) to deter potential abuse. Doses of more than 16 mg/day are demonstrated to have the highest efficacy in retaining patients in treatment (Bell and Strang 2020). Physicians who wish to prescribe buprenorphine must obtain a waiver, most often through completion of an 8-hour course. Naltrexone, an opioid antagonist, also blocks the effects of opioids, but lacks the reinforcing properties of methadone and buprenorphine. It also requires a 7- to 10-day period of abstinence prior to initiation; as a result, naltrexone compliance is low, and dropout rates during induction are often above 50% (Bell and

Strang 2020). Still, naltrexone may be beneficial for particularly motivated patients, and can be prescribed by any health care provider who is licensed to prescribe.

Overall, MOUD are associated with reduced risk of overdose, with longer MOUD duration corresponding to lower risk. However, in the month after leaving treatment, risk of fatal overdose is elevated, as is risk among patients who concurrently use benzodiazepines and methadone. Therefore, when initiating and continuing patients on MOUD, clinicians should consistently emphasize the importance of medication adherence and limiting concurrent substance use (Bell and Strang 2020). Like medications for AUD, MOUD are heavily underutilized; wider adoption of these medications in practice would undoubtedly work to retain a greater number of patients in care and reduce overdose deaths.

Other substance use disorders.   As of 2019, no effective pharmacological treatments have been found for stimulant, cocaine, or cannabis use disorders. However, laboratory and clinical trials are under way to develop effective medications for these SUDs.

Comorbid PDs and SUDs

Few placebo-controlled trials to date have examined pharmacotherapy for patients with comorbid PDs and substance use. Moreover, to our knowledge, all of these studies have focused specifically on antisocial PD. In a sample of patients with comorbid antisocial PD and cocaine or opioid dependency, desipramine and amantadine were found to have no effect on the percentage of cocaine-free urine samples (Arndt et al. 1994; Leal et al. 1994). In a small sample of males with comorbid alcohol dependence and antisocial PD, nortriptyline was associated with reduced mean drinking days, alcohol dependence severity, and anxiety levels (Powell et al. 1995). Bromocriptine was similarly associated with reduced AUD severity, as well as some improvement in anxiety and depression (Powell et al. 1995). Finally, an RCT of naltrexone among patients with comorbid antisocial PD and alcohol dependence demonstrated reductions in AUD severity that was equivalent to that in non-PD controls (Ralevski et al. 2007).

Summary

In the subsections above, we reviewed the evidence for pharmacotherapy for treating PDs and SUDs individually and as co-occurring disorders. In accordance with the majority of placebo-controlled trials, we have focused on diagnosis-specific medication strategies; however, another approach is to focus on specific symptom domains (Nelson 2018; Soloff 1998). Overall, affective dysregulation and cognitive or perceptual disturbances are best managed with low-dose antipsychotics, whereas impulsivity and behavioral dyscontrol are best managed with mood stabilizers (Nelson 2018). Because there is increased risk of suicidality among patients with severe PDs, and particularly BPD, prescribing disinhibiting or potentially toxic medications such as benzodiazepines should be avoided (Nelson 2018).

Using DSM-5

In this section, we review the DSM-IV and DSM-5 approaches to diagnosing SUDs and PDs. DSM-IV defined two SUD types: abuse and dependence. Although dependence was consistently shown to be reliable and valid, abuse had inconsistent reliability and validity (Hasin et al. 2006). Thus, in DSM-5, abuse and dependence were replaced by a single diagnosis of substance use disorder (Hasin et al. 2013), defined by 11 criteria: all seven of the DSM-IV dependence criteria, three of the four DSM-IV abuse criteria (legal problems was dropped), and craving. (Several substances, such as phencyclidine, other hallucinogens, and inhalants, do not have established withdrawal signs and symptoms, so the criterion for withdrawal does not apply to these SUDs.) A threshold of two or more criteria for the diagnosis of SUD was selected, with mild, moderate, and severe SUD indicated by 2–3, 4–5, and ≥6 criteria, respectively. The newly defined SUD was based on extensive research showing that each of the 11 criteria is an indicator of the same underlying latent trait (Hasin et al. 2013).

Overall, measurement properties of the DSM-5 SUD diagnosis have been fair to excellent. Using DSM-IV as a gold standard, Compton et al. (2013) found that the sensitivity, specificity, positive and negative predictive values, and concordance of the new DSM-5 SUD diagnoses were excellent. Goldstein et al. (2015) found that prevalence rates of various SUDs were similar using the two diagnoses, and Grant et al. (2015b, 2016) found that DSM-5 had fair to good reliability for alcohol and most drug-specific use disorders (κ=0.41–0.62). Studies of clinical, rather than general population, samples have yielded similar reliability and validity estimates for DSM-5 SUDs (Denis et al. 2015; Kelly et al. 2014; Peer et al. 2013); however, further evidence using larger samples is needed. Because DSM-5 diagnostic criteria are often used in clinical settings, this is an important area for future research.

In DSM-5 Section II, the definitions of PDs remained the same as they were in DSM-IV. However, an alternative model for conceptualizing and diagnosing PDs based on impairments in personality functioning and pathological personality traits was developed for DSM-5 Section III (See Chapter 5, "Manifestations, Assessment, Diagnosis, and Differential Diagnosis," and Chapter 4, "The Alternative DSM-5 Model for Personality Disorders," in this volume.) Interestingly, Grant et al. (2015b) found that the reliabilities of antisocial, borderline, and schizotypal PD diagnoses in DSM-5 Section II were greater when the social/occupational dysfunction or distress criterion was excluded. Future research into the validity and reliability of DSM-5 PD diagnoses in clinical and community samples is warranted.

Conclusion

SUDs are highly prevalent among individuals with PDs, and vice versa. Although PDs can be measured reliably and validly in patients with SUDs, it can be difficult to distinguish the symptoms and pathologies of each.

With respect to causal pathways, evidence supports multiple pathways from personality (and potentially PDs) to SUD, including behavioral disinhibition, stress reduction, and reward sensitivity. However, the latest findings from genetic epidemiology and molecular genetics supports a common factor model.

Although evidence is somewhat equivocal, several studies suggest that individuals with comorbid SUDs and PDs benefit from SUD treatment as much as do those with only SUDs, emphasizing the importance of providing treatment to individuals with comorbidities. However, these individuals may improve only to a level of problem severity that still leaves them at considerable risk for relapse. More research is needed to determine whether patients with PDs and comorbid SUDs benefit from treatments focusing on PDs as much as do patients with PDs but not SUDs. Dual-focus treatments consisting of an integrated package of elements targeting both the SUD and maladaptive personality traits could provide more benefit to patients than therapies with a single focus. Some preliminary data support certain dual-focus treatments, but more research is needed.

Psychotherapy with pharmacotherapy targeted to specific symptoms is recommended for the treatment of PDs, and we see no reason to substantially deviate from this recommendation for patients with co-occurring SUDs. That said, effective treatment of these patients often requires modifications to traditional programs and methods.

References

Aliev F, Wetherill L, Bierut L, et al: Genes associated with alcohol outcomes show enrichment of effects with broad externalizing and impulsivity phenotypes in an independent sample. J Stud Alcohol Drugs 76:38–46, 2015

American Psychiatric Association: Diagnostic and Statistical Manual: Mental Disorders. Washington, DC, American Psychiatric Association, 1952

American Psychiatric Association: Diagnostic and Statistical Manual of Mental Disorders, 2nd Edition. Washington, DC, American Psychiatric Association, 1968

American Psychiatric Association: Diagnostic and Statistical Manual of Mental Disorders, 3rd Edition. Washington, DC, American Psychiatric Association, 1980

American Psychiatric Association: Diagnostic and Statistical Manual of Mental Disorders, 4th Edition. Washington, DC, American Psychiatric Association, 1994

American Psychiatric Association: Diagnostic and Statistical Manual of Mental Disorders, 5th Edition. Washington, DC, American Psychiatric Association, 2013

Arndt IO, McClellan AT, Dorozynsky L, et al: Desipramine treatment for cocaine dependence: role of antisocial personality disorder. J Nerv Ment Dis 182:151–156, 1994

Axelrod SR, Perepletchikova F, Holtzman K, et al: Emotion regulation and substance use frequency in women with substance dependence and borderline personality disorder receiving dialectical behavior therapy. Am J Drug Alcohol Abuse 37:37–42, 2011

Bahlmann M, Preuss UW, Soyka M: Chronological relationship between antisocial personality disorder and alcohol dependence. Eur Addict Res 8:195–200, 2002

Ball SA: Manualized treatment for substance abusers with personality disorders: dual focus schema therapy. Addict Behav 23:883–891, 1998

Ball SA: Comparing individual therapies for personality disordered opioid dependent patients. J Pers Disord 21:305–321, 2007

Ball SA, Young JE: Dual focus schema therapy for personality disorders and substance dependence: case study results. Cogn Behav Pract 7:270–281, 2000

Ball SA, Rounsaville BJ, Tennen H, et al: Reliability of personality disorder symptoms and personality traits in substance-dependent inpatients. J Abnorm Psychol 110:341–352, 2001

Ball SA, Cobb-Richardson P, Connolly AJ, et al: Substance abuse and personality disorders in homeless drop-in center clients: symptom severity and psychotherapy retention in a randomized clinical trial. Compr Psychiatry 46:371–379, 2005

Ball SA, Maccarelli LM, LaPaglia DM, et al: Randomized trial of dual-focused vs. single-focused individual therapy for personality disorders and substance dependence. J Nerv Ment Dis 199:319–328, 2011

Barker V, Romaniuk L, Cardinal RN, et al: Impulsivity in borderline personality disorder. Psychol Med 45:1955–1964, 2015

Barratt ES, Stanford MS, Felthous AR, et al: The effects of phenytoin on impulsive and premeditated aggression: a controlled study. J Clin Psychopharmacol 17:341–349, 1997

Bateman AW, Gunderson J, Mulder R: Treatment of personality disorder. Lancet 385:735–743, 2015

Bazanis E, Rogers RD, Dowson JH, et al: Neurocognitive deficits in decision-making and planning of patients with DSM-III-R borderline personality disorder. Psychol Med 32:1395–1405, 2002

Beckstead DJ, Lambert MJ, DuBose AP, et al: Dialectical behavior therapy with American Indian/Alaska Native adolescents diagnosed with substance use disorders: combining an evidence-based treatment with cultural, traditional, and spiritual beliefs. Addict Behav 51:84–87, 2015

Begleiter H, Porjesz B, Bihari B, et al: Event-related brain potentials in boys at risk for alcoholism. Science 225:1493–1496, 1984

Bell J, Strang J: Medication treatment of opioid use disorder. Biol Psychiatry 87:82–88, 2020

Bernstein DP, Handelsman L: The neurobiology of substance abuse and personality disorders, in Neuropsychiatry of Personality Disorders. Edited by Ratey J. Cambridge, UK, Blackwell Science, 1995, pp 120–148

Black DW, Zanarini MC, Romine A, et al: Comparison of low and moderate dosages of extended-release quetiapine in borderline personality disorder: a randomized, double-blind, placebo-controlled trial. Am J Psychiatry 171:1174–1182, 2014

Blanco C, Flórez-Salamanca L, Secades-Villa R, et al: Predictors of initiation of nicotine, alcohol, cannabis, and cocaine use: results of the National Epidemiologic Survey on Alcohol and Related Conditions (NESARC). Am J Addict 27:477–484, 2018

Bogenschutz MP, Nurnberg GH: Olanzapine versus placebo in the treatment of borderline personality disorder. J Clin Psychiatry 65(1):104–109, 2004

Borman PD, Zilberman ML, Tavares H, et al: Personality changes in women recovering from substance-related dependence. J Addict Dis 25:59–66, 2006

Bornovalova MA, Hicks BM, Iacono WG, et al: Longitudinal twin study of borderline personality disorder traits and substance use in adolescence: developmental change, reciprocal effects, and genetic and environmental influences. Personal Disord 4:23–32, 2013

Bozzatello P, Ghirardini C, Uscinska M, et al: Pharmacotherapy of personality disorders: what we know and what we have to search for. Future Neurology 12:199–222, 2017

Cacciola JS, Alterman AI, Rutherford MJ, et al: Treatment response of antisocial substance abusers. J Nerv Ment Dis 183:166–171, 1995

Cackowski S, Reitz AC, Ende G, et al: Impact of stress on different components of impulsivity in borderline personality disorder. Psychol Med 44:3329–3340, 2014

Carr CP, Martins CMS, Stingel AM et al: The role of early life stress in adult psychiatric disorders: a systematic review according to childhood trauma subtypes. J Nervous Mental Dis 201:1007–1020, 2013

Casadio P, Olivoni D, Ferrari B, et al: Personality disorders in addiction outpatients: prevalence and effects on psychosocial functioning. Subst Abuse 8:17–24, 2014

Caspi A, Begg D, Dickson N, et al: Personality differences predict health-risk behaviors in young adulthood: evidence from a longitudinal study. J Pers Soc Psychol 73:1052–1063, 1997

Cavicchioli M, Movalli M, Vassena G, et al: The therapeutic role of emotion regulation and coping strategies during a stand-alone DBT Skills training program for alcohol use disorder and concurrent substance use disorders. Addict Behav 98:106035, 2019

Clarke TK, Adams MJ, Davies G, et al: Genome-wide association study of alcohol consumption and genetic overlap with other health-related traits in UK Biobank (N=112,117). Mol Psychiatry 22:1376–1384, 2017

Cloninger CR, Sigvardsson S, Bohman M: Childhood personality predicts alcohol abuse in young adults. Alcohol Clin Exp Res 12:494–505, 1988

Coccaro EF, Kavoussi RJ: Fluoxetine and impulsive aggressive behavior in personality-disordered subjects. Arch Gen Psychiatry 54:1081–1088, 1997

Cohen P, Chen H, Crawford TN, et al: Personality disorders in early adolescence and the development of later substance use disorders in the general population. Drug Alcohol Depend 88 (suppl 1):S71–S84, 2007

Compton WM, Dawson DA, Goldstein RB, et al: Crosswalk between DSM-IV dependence and DSM-5 substance use disorders for opioids, cannabis, cocaine and alcohol. Drug Alcohol Depend 132:387–390, 2013

Conrod PJ, Pihl RO, Vassileva J: Differential sensitivity to alcohol reinforcement in groups of men at risk for distinct alcoholism subtypes. Alcohol Clin Exp Res 22:585–597, 1998

Cornelius JR, Soloff PH, Perel JM, et al: Continuation pharmacotherapy of borderline personality disorder with haloperidol and phenelzine. Am J Psychiatry 150:1843–1848, 1993

Daughters SB, Stipelman BA, Sargeant MN, et al: The interactive effects of antisocial personality disorder and court-mandated status on substance abuse treatment dropout. J Subst Abuse Treat 34:157–164, 2008

De la Fuente J, Lotstra F: A trial of carbamazepine in borderline personality disorder. Eur Neuropsychopharmacol 4:479–486, 1994

DeMarce JM, Lash SJ, Parker JD, et al: Validity of the structured clinical interview for DSM-IV among veterans seeking treatment for substance use disorders. Int J Ment Health Addict 11:546–556, 2013

Denis CM, Gelernter J, Hart AB, et al: Inter-observer reliability of DSM-5 substance use disorders. Drug Alcohol Depend 153:229–235, 2015

Dimeff L, Rizvi SL, Brown M, et al: Dialectical behavior therapy for substance abuse: a pilot application to methamphetamine-dependent women with borderline personality disorder. Cogn Behav Pract 7:457–468, 2000

Dom G, De Wilde B, Hulstijn W, et al: Decision-making deficits in alcohol-dependent patients with and without comorbid personality disorder. Alcohol Clin Exp Res 30:1670–1677, 2006

Easton CJ, Oberleitner LM, Scott MC, et al: Differences in treatment outcome among marijuana-dependent young adults with and without antisocial personality disorder. Am J Drug Alcohol Abuse 38:305–313, 2012

Eaton NR, Krueger RF, Keyes KM, et al: Borderline personality disorder comorbidity: relationship to the internalizing–externalizing structure of common mental disorders. Psychol Med 41:1041–1050, 2011

Elam KK, Wang FL, Bountress K, et al: Predicting substance use in emerging adulthood: a genetically informed study of developmental transactions between impulsivity and family conflict. Dev Psychopathol 28:673–688, 2016

Fenton MC, Keyes K, Geier T, et al: Psychiatric comorbidity and the persistence of drug use disorders in the United States. Addiction 107:599–609, 2012

Fernandez-Montalvo J, Lopez-Goni JJ: Comparison of completers and dropouts in psychological treatment for cocaine addiction. Addict Res Theory 18:433–441, 2010

Few LR, Grant JD, Trull TJ, et al: Genetic variation in personality traits explains genetic overlap between borderline personality features and substance use disorders. Addiction 109:2118–2127, 2014

Foulds JA, Boden JM, Newton-Howes GM, et al: The role of novelty seeking as a predictor of substance use disorder outcomes in early adulthood. Addiction 112:1629–1637, 2017

Frankenburg FR, Zanarini MC: Divalproex sodium treatment of women with borderline personality disorder and bipolar II disorder: a double-blind placebo-controlled pilot study. J Clin Psychiatry 63:442–426, 2002

Galen LW, Brower KJ, Gillespie BW, et al: Sociopathy, gender, and treatment outcome among outpatient substance abusers. Drug Alcohol Depend 61:23–33, 2000

Gill K, Nolimal D, Crowley TJ: Antisocial personality disorder, HIV risk behavior and retention in methadone maintenance therapy. Drug Alcohol Depend 30:247–252, 1992

Gillespie NA, Aggen SH, Neale MC, et al: Associations between personality disorders and cannabis use and cannabis use disorder: a population-based twin study. Addiction 113:1488–1498, 2018

Gilmore CS, Malone SM, Iacono WG: Brain electrophysiological endophenotypes for externalizing psychopathology: a multivariate approach. Behav Genet 40:186–200, 2010

Goldman D, Oroszi G, Ducci F: The genetics of addictions: uncovering the genes. Nat Rev Genet 6:521–532, 2005

Goldman GA, Gregory RJ: Relationships between techniques and outcomes for borderline personality disorder. Am J Psychother 64:359–371, 2010

Goldstein RB, Compton WM, Pulay AJ, et al: Antisocial behavioral syndromes and DSM-IV drug use disorders in the United States: results from the National Epidemiologic Survey on Alcohol and Related Conditions. Drug Alcohol Depend 90:145–158, 2007a

Goldstein RB, Dawson DA, Saha TD, et al: Antisocial behavioral syndromes and DSM-IV alcohol use disorders: results from the National Epidemiologic Survey on Alcohol and Related Conditions. Alcohol Clin Exp Res 31:814–828, 2007b

Goldstein RB, Chou SP, Smith SM, et al: Nosologic comparisons of DSM-IV and DSM-5 alcohol and drug use disorders: results from the National Epidemiologic Survey on Alcohol and Related Conditions–III. J Stud Alcohol Drugs 76:378–388, 2015

Goldstein RB, Chou SP, Saha TD, et al: The epidemiology of antisocial behavioral syndromes in adulthood: results from the National Epidemiologic Survey on Alcohol and Related Conditions–III. J Clin Psychiatry 78:90–98, 2017

Grant BF, Dawson DA, Stinson FS, et al: The Alcohol Use Disorder and Associated Disabilities Interview Schedule–IV (AUDADIS-IV): reliability of alcohol consumption, tobacco use, family history of depression and psychiatric diagnostic modules in a general population sample. Drug Alcohol Depend 71:7–16, 2003

Grant BF, Stinson FS, Dawson DA, et al: Co-occurrence of 12-month alcohol and drug use disorders and personality disorders in the United States: results from the National Epidemiologic Survey on Alcohol and Related Conditions. Arch Gen Psychiatry 61:361–368, 2004

Grant BF, Chou SP, Goldstein RB, et al: Prevalence, correlates, disability, and comorbidity of DSM-IV borderline personality disorder: results from the Wave 2 National Epidemiologic Survey on Alcohol and Related Conditions. J Clin Psychiatry 69:533–545, 2008

Grant BF, Goldstein RB, Saha TD, et al: Epidemiology of DSM-5 alcohol use disorder: results from the National Epidemiologic Survey on Alcohol and Related Conditions III. JAMA Psychiatry 72:757–766, 2015a

Grant BF, Goldstein RB, Smith SM, et al: The Alcohol Use Disorder and Associated Disabilities Interview Schedule-5 (AUDADIS-5): reliability of substance use and psychiatric disorder modules in a general population sample. Drug Alcohol Depend 148:27–33, 2015b

Grant BF, Saha TD, Ruan WJ, et al: Epidemiology of DSM-5 drug use disorder: results from the National Epidemiologic Survey on Alcohol and Related Conditions–III. JAMA Psychiatry 73:39–47, 2016

Grant JE, Chamberlain SR: Impulsive action and impulsive choice across substance and behavioral addictions: cause or consequence? Addict Behav 39:1632–1639, 2014

Gregory RJ, Chlebowski S, Kang D, et al: A controlled trial of psychodynamic psychotherapy for co-occurring borderline personality disorder and alcohol use disorder. Psychotherapy (Chic) 45:28–41, 2008

Grella CE, Joshi V, Hser YI: Followup of cocaine-dependent men and women with antisocial personality disorder. J Subst Abuse Treat 25:155–164, 2003

Harford TC, Chen CM, Kerridge BT, et al: Self- and other-directed forms of violence and their relationship with lifetime DSM-5 psychiatric disorders: results from the National Epidemiologic Survey on Alcohol Related Conditions–III (NESARC-III). Psychiatry Res 262:384–392, 2018

Harned MS, Chapman AL, Dexter-Mazza ET, et al: Treating co-occurring Axis I disorders in recurrently suicidal women with borderline personality disorder: a 2-year randomized trial of dialectical behavior therapy versus community treatment by experts. J Consult Clin Psychol 76:1068–1075, 2008

Haro G, Mateu C, Martinez-Raga J, et al: The role of personality disorders on drug dependence treatment outcomes following inpatient detoxification. Eur Psychiatry 19:187–192, 2004

Hasin D, Hatzenbuehler ML, Keyes K, et al: Substance use disorders: Diagnostic and Statistical Manual of Mental Disorders, fourth edition (DSM-IV) and International Classification of Diseases, tenth edition (ICD-10). Addiction 101 (suppl 1):59–75, 2006

Hasin DS, Stinson FS, Ogburn E, et al: Prevalence, correlates, disability, and comorbidity of DSM-IV alcohol abuse and dependence in the United States: results from the National Epidemiologic Survey on Alcohol and Related Conditions. Arch Gen Psychiatry 64:830–842, 2007

Hasin D, Fenton MC, Skodol A, et al: Personality disorders and the 3-year course of alcohol, drug, and nicotine use disorders. Arch Gen Psychiatry 68:1158–1167, 2011

Hasin D, O'Brien CP, Auriacombe M, et al: DSM-5 criteria for substance use disorders: recommendations and rationale. Am J Psychiatry 170:834–851, 2013

Hasin DS, Kerridge BT, Saha TD, et al: Prevalence and correlates of DSM-5 cannabis use disorder, 2012–2013: findings from the National Epidemiologic Survey on Alcohol and Related Conditions–III. Am J Psychiatry 173:588–599, 2016

Hollander E, Allen A, Lopez RP, et al: A preliminary double-blind, placebo-controlled trial of divalproex sodium in borderline personality disorder. J Clin Psychiatry 62:199–203, 2001

Hollander E, Tracy KA, Swann AC, et al: Divalproex in the treatment of impulsive aggression: efficacy in Cluster B personality disorders. Neuropsychopharmacology 28:1186–1197, 2003

Iacono WG, Carlson SR, Taylor J, et al: Behavioral disinhibition and the development of substance-use disorders: findings from the Minnesota Twin Family Study. Dev Psychopathol 11:869–900, 1999

Iacono WG, Carlson SR, Malone SM, et al: P3 event-related potential amplitude and the risk for disinhibitory disorders in adolescent boys. Arch Gen Psychiatry 59:750–757, 2002

Jensen M, Chassin L, Gonzales NA: Neighborhood moderation of sensation seeking effects on adolescent substance use initiation. J Youth Adolesc 46:1953–1967, 2017

Kaiser A, Bonsu JA, Charnigo RJ, et al: Impulsive personality and alcohol use: bidirectional relations over one year. J Stud Alcohol Drugs 77:473–482, 2016

Karterud S, Arefjord N, Andresen NE, et al: Substance use disorders among personality disordered patients admitted for day hospital treatment: implications for service developments. Nord J Psychiatry 63:57–63, 2009

Kelly SM, Gryczynski J, Mitchell SG, et al: Concordance between DSM-5 and DSM-IV nicotine, alcohol, and cannabis use disorder diagnoses among pediatric patients. Drug Alcohol Dependence 140:213–216, 2014

Kendler KS, Aggen SH, Knudsen GP, et al: The structure of genetic and environmental risk factors for syndromal and subsyndromal common DSM-IV Axis I and all Axis II disorders. Am J Psychiatry 168:29–39, 2011

Keyes KM, Eaton NR, Krueger RF, et al: Thought disorder in the meta-structure of psychopathology. Psychol Med 43:1673–1683, 2013

Knox J, Hasin DS, Larson F, et al: Prevention, screening, and treatment for heavy drinking and alcohol use disorder. Lancet Psychiatry 6:1054–1067, 2019

Koenigsberg HW, Reynolds D, Goodman M, et al: Risperidone in the treatment of schizotypal personality disorder. J Clin Psychiatry 64:628–634, 2003

Krampe H, Wagner T, Stawicki S, et al: Personality disorder and chronicity of addiction as independent outcome predictors in alcoholism treatment. Psychiatr Serv 57:708–712, 2006

Kranzler HR, Zhou H, Kember RL, et al: Genome-wide association study of alcohol consumption and use disorder in 274,424 individuals from multiple populations. Nat Commun 10:1499, 2019

Krueger RF: The structure of common mental disorders. Arch Gen Psychiatry 56:921–926, 1999

Krueger RF, Caspi A, Moffitt TE, et al: Personality traits are differentially linked to mental disorders: a multitrait-multidiagnosis study of an adolescent birth cohort. J Abnorm Psychol 105:299–312, 1996

Lawrence KA, Allen JS, Chanen AM: Impulsivity in borderline personality disorder: reward-based decision-making and its relationship to emotional distress. J Pers Disord 24:785–799, 2010

Leal J, Ziedonis D, Kosten T: Antisocial personality disorder as a prognostic factor for pharmacotherapy of cocaine dependence. Drug Alcohol Depend 35:31–35, 1994

Lee SS, Allen J, Black DW, et al: Quetiapine's effect on the SCL-90-R domains in patients with borderline personality disorder. Ann Clin Psychiatry 28:4–10, 2016

Linehan MM, Dimeff LA: Dialectical Behavior Therapy Manual of Treatment Interventions for Drug Abusers With Borderline Personality Disorder. Seattle, University of Washington, 1997

Linehan MM, Korslund KE: Dialectical behavior therapy: from soup to nuts. Workshop presentation at the annual meeting of the Association for Behavioral and Cognitive Therapies. Chicago, IL, November 15–16, 2006

Linehan MM, Schmidt H III, Dimeff LA, et al: Dialectical behavior therapy for patients with borderline personality disorder and drug-dependence. Am J Addict 8:279–292, 1999

Linehan MM, Dimeff LA, Reynolds SK, et al: Dialectical behavior therapy versus comprehensive validation therapy plus 12-step for the treatment of opioid dependent women meeting criteria for borderline personality disorder. Drug Alcohol Depend 67:13–26, 2002

Linehan MM, McDavid JD, Brown MZ, et al: Olanzapine plus dialectical behavior therapy for women with high irritability who meet criteria for borderline personality disorder: a double blind, placebo-controlled pilot study. J Clin Psychiatry 69:999–1005, 2008

Links PS, Steiner M, Boiago I, Irwin D: Lithium therapy for borderline patients: preliminary findings. Journal of Personality Disorders, 4:173-181, 1990

Liu M, Jiang Y, Wedow R, et al: Association studies of up to 1.2 million individuals yield new insights into the genetic etiology of tobacco and alcohol use. Nat Genet 51:237–244, 2019

Loew TH, Nickel MK, Muehlbacher M, et al: Topiramate treatment for women with borderline personality disorder: a double-blind, placebo-controlled study. J Clin Psychopharmacol 26:61–66, 2006

Long EC, Aggen SH, Neale MC, et al: The association between personality disorders with alcohol use and misuse: a population-based twin study. Drug Alcohol Depend 174:171–180, 2017

Longabaugh R, Rubin A, Malloy P, et al: Drinking outcomes of alcohol abusers diagnosed as antisocial personality disorder. Alcohol Clin Exp Res 18:778–785, 1994

Lu RB, Lee JF, Huang SY, et al: Interaction between ALDH2*1*1 and DRD2/ANKK1 TaqI A1A1 genes may be associated with antisocial personality disorder not co-morbid with alcoholism. Addict Biol 17:865–874, 2012

MacKillop J, Amlung MT, Few LR, et al: Delayed reward discounting and addictive behavior: a meta-analysis. Psychopharmacology (Berl) 216:305–321, 2011

Maffei C, Cavicchioli M, Movalli M, et al: Dialectical behavior therapy skills training in alcohol dependence treatment: findings based on an open trial. Subst Use Misuse 53:2368–2385, 2018

Marlowe DB, Kirby KC, Festinger DS, et al: Impact of comorbid personality disorders and personality disorder symptoms on outcomes of behavioral treatment for cocaine dependence. J Nerv Ment Dis 185:483–490, 1997

Markovitz PA: Pharmacotherapy of impulsivity, aggression, and related disorders, in Impulsivity and Aggression. Edited by Oldham JM, Hollander E, Skodol AE. Washington, DC, American Psychiatric Press, 1995, pp 263–287

Martino S, Carroll K, Kostas D, et al: Dual diagnosis motivational interviewing: a modification of motivational interviewing for substance-abusing patients with psychotic disorders. J Subst Abuse Treat 23:297–308, 2002

Masse LC, Tremblay RE: Behavior of boys in kindergarten and the onset of substance use during adolescence. Arch Gen Psychiatry 54:62–68, 1997

Mather DB: The role of antisocial personality in alcohol rehabilitation treatment effectiveness. Mil Med 152:516–518, 1987

McClure MM, Barch DM, Romero MJ, et al: The effects of guanfacine on context processing abnormalities in schizotypal personality disorder. Biol Psychiatry 61:1157–1160, 2007

McClure MM, Koenigsberg HW, Reynolds D, et al: The effects of risperidone on the cognitive performance of individuals with schizotypal personality disorder. J Clin Psychopharmacol 29:396–398, 2009

McClure MM, Harvey PD, Goodman M, et al: Pergolide treatment of cognitive deficits associated with schizotypal personality disorder: continued evidence of the importance of the dopamine system in the schizophrenia spectrum. Neuropsychopharmacology 35:1356–1362, 2010

McGlashan TH, Grilo CM, Skodol AE, et al: The Collaborative Longitudinal Personality Disorders Study: baseline Axis I/II and II/II diagnostic co-occurrence. Acta Psychiatr Scand 102:256–264, 2000

Messina NP, Wish ED, Hoffman JA, et al: Antisocial personality disorder and TC treatment outcomes. Am J Drug Alcohol Abuse 28:197–212, 2002

Moen R, Freitag M, Miller M, et al: Efficacy of extended-release divalproex combined with "condensed" dialectical behavior therapy for individuals with borderline personality disorder. Ann Clin Psychiatry 24:255–260, 2012

Myers MG, Stewart DG, Brown SA: Progression from conduct disorder to antisocial personality disorder following treatment for adolescent substance abuse. Am J Psychiatry 155:479–485, 1998

Nelson KJ: Pharmacotherapy for personality disorders. UpToDate Last updated June 26, 2018. Available at: https://www.uptodate.com/contents/pharmacotherapy-for-personality-disorders. Accessed June 2019.

Nickel MK: Topiramate reduced aggression in female patients with borderline personality disorder. Eur Arch Psychiatry Clin Neurosci 257:432–433, 2007a

Nickel MK: Topiramate treatment of aggression in male borderline patients. Aust NZ J Psychiatry 41:461–462, 2007b

Nickel MK, Loew TH: Treatment of aggression with topiramate in male borderline patients, part II: 18-month follow-up. Eur Psychiatry 23:115–117, 2008

Nickel MK, Nickel C, Mitterlehner FO, et al: Topiramate treatment of aggression in female borderline personality disorder patients: a double-blind, placebo-controlled study. J Clin Psychiatry 65:1515–1519, 2004

Nickel MK, Nickel C, Kaplan P, et al: Treatment of aggression with topiramate in male borderline patients: a double-blind, placebo-controlled study. Biol Psychiatry 57:495–499, 2005

Nickel MK, Muehlbacher M, Nickel C, et al: Aripiprazole in the treatment of patients with borderline personality disorder: a double-blind, placebo-controlled study. Am J Psychiatry 163:833–838, 2006

Nickel MK, Loew TH, Pedrosa Gil F: Aripiprazole in treatment of borderline patients, part II: an 18-month follow-up. Psychopharmacology (Berl) 19:1023–1026, 2007

Nielsen P, Rojskjaer S, Hesse M: Personality-guided treatment for alcohol dependence: a quasi-randomized experiment. Am J Addict 16:357–364, 2007

Ogloff JR, Talevski D, Lemphers A, et al: Co-occurring mental illness, substance use disorders, and antisocial personality disorder among clients of forensic mental health services. Psychiatr Rehabil J 38:16–23, 2015

Ouimette PC, Gima K, Moos RH, et al: A comparative evaluation of substance abuse treatment, IV: the effect of comorbid psychiatric diagnoses on amount of treatment, continuing care, and 1-year outcomes. Alcohol Clin Exp Res 23:552–557, 1999

Pascual JC, Madre M, Soler J, et al: Injectable atypical antipsychotics for agitation in borderline personality disorder. Pharmacopsychiatry 39:117–118, 2006

Pascual JC, Soler J, Puigdemont D, et al: Ziprasidone in the treatment of borderline personality disorder: a double blind, placebo controlled, randomized study. J Clin Psychiatry 69:603–608, 2008

Peer K, Rennert L, Lynch KG, et al: Prevalence of DSM-IV and DSM-5 alcohol, cocaine, opioid, and cannabis use disorders in a largely substance dependent sample. Drug Alcohol Depend 127:215–219, 2013

Petry NM: Discounting of delayed rewards in substance abusers: relationship to antisocial personality disorder. Psychopharmacology (Berl) 162:425–432, 2002

Philipsen A, Richter H, Schmahl C, et al: Clonidine in acute aversive inner tension and self-injurious behavior in female patients with borderline personality disorder. J Clin Psychiatry 65:1414–1419, 2004a

Philipsen A, Schmahl C, Lieb K: Naloxone in the treatment of acute dissociative states in female patients with borderline personality disorder. Pharmacopsychiatry 37:196–199, 2004b

Polich J, Pollock VE, Bloom FE: Meta-analysis of P300 amplitude from males at risk for alcoholism. Psychol Bull 115:55–73, 1994

Porjesz B, Begleiter H: Human brain electrophysiology and alcoholism, in Alcohol and the Brain. Edited by Tarter DV, Thiel DV. New York, Plenum, 1985, pp 139–182

Porjesz B, Rangaswamy M, Kamarajan C, et al: The utility of neurophysiological markers in the study of alcoholism. Clin Neurophysiol 116:993–1018, 2005

Powell BJ, Campbell JL, Landon JF, et al: A double-blind, placebo-controlled study of nortriptyline and bromocriptine in male alcoholics subtyped by comorbid psychiatric disorders. Alcohol Clin Exp Res 19:462–468, 1995

Pulay AJ, Dawson DA, Ruan WJ, et al: The relationship of impairment to personality disorder severity among individuals with specific Axis I disorders: results from the National Epidemiologic Survey on Alcohol and Related Conditions. J Pers Disord 22:405–417, 2008

Pulay AJ, Stinson FS, Dawson DA, et al: Prevalence, correlates, disability, and comorbidity of DSM-IV schizotypal personality disorder: results from the Wave 2 National Epidemiologic Survey on Alcohol and Related Conditions. Prim Care Companion J Clin Psychiatry 11:53–67, 2009

Pulay AJ, Stinson FS, Ruan WJ, et al: The relationship of DSM-IV personality disorders to nicotine dependence—results from a national survey. Drug Alcohol Depend 108:141–145, 2010

Ralevski E, Ball S, Nich C, et al: The impact of personality disorders on alcohol-use outcomes in a pharmacotherapy trial for alcohol dependence and comorbid Axis I disorders. Am J Addict 16:443–449, 2007

Reich DB, Zanarini MC, Bieri KA: A preliminary study of lamotrigine in the treatment of affective instability in borderline personality disorder. Int Clin Psychopharmacol 24:270–275, 2009

Ridgely MS, Goldman HH, Willenbring M: Barriers to the care of persons with dual diagnoses: organizational and financing issues. Schizophr Bull 16:123–132, 1990

Rinne T, van den Brink W, Wouters L, et al: SSRI treatment of borderline personality disorder: a randomized, placebo-controlled clinical trial for female patients with borderline personality disorder. Am J Psychiatry 159:2048–2054, 2002

Rizvi SL, Dimeff LA, Skutch J, et al: A pilot study of the DBT coach: an interactive mobile phone application for individuals with borderline personality disorder and substance use disorder. Behav Ther 42:589–600, 2011

Rounsaville BJ, Kranzler HR, Ball S, et al: Personality disorders in substance abusers: relation to substance use. J Nerv Ment Dis 186:87–95, 1998

Roysamb E, Kendler KS, Tambs K, et al: The joint structure of DSM-IV Axis I and Axis II disorders. J Abnorm Psychol 120:198–209, 2011

Ruan WJ, Goldstein RB, Chou SP, et al: The Alcohol Use Disorder and Associated Disabilities Interview Schedule–IV (AUDADIS-IV): reliability of new psychiatric diagnostic modules and risk factors in a general population sample. Drug Alcohol Depend 92:27–36, 2008

Rubio G, Jiménez M, Rodríguez-Jiménez R, et al: Varieties of impulsivity in males with alcohol dependence: the role of cluster-B personality disorder. Alcohol Clin Exp Res 31:1826–1832, 2007

Salzman C, Wolfson AN, Schatzberg A, et al: Effect of fluoxetine on anger in symptomatic volunteers with borderline personality disorder. J Clin Psychopharmacol 15:23–29, 1995

Samuel DB, LaPaglia DM, Maccarelli LM, et al: Personality disorders and retention in a therapeutic community for substance dependence. Am J Addict 20:555–562, 2011

Sanchez-Roige S, Palmer AA, Fontanillas P, et al: Genome-wide association study meta-analysis of the Alcohol Use Disorders Identification Test (AUDIT) in two population-based cohorts. Am J Psychiatry 176:107–118, 2019

Schmahl C, Kleindienst N, Limberger M, et al: Evaluation of naltrexone for dissociative symptoms in borderline personality disorder. Int Clin Psychopharmacol 27:61–68, 2012

Schuckit MA, Klein J, Twitchell G, et al: Personality test scores as predictors of alcoholism almost a decade later. Am J Psychiatry 151:1038–1042, 1994

Schulz SC, Camlin KL, Barry S, et al: Risperidone for borderline personality disorder: a double-blind study. Presentation at the 37th Annual Meeting of the American College of Neuropsychopharmacology, December 14–18, 1998

Schulz SC, Zanarini MC, Bateman A, et al: Olanzapine for the treatment of borderline personality disorder: variable-dose, 12-week, randomised double-blind placebo-controlled study. Br J Psychiatry 193:485–492, 2008

Sher KJ, Trull TJ: Personality and disinhibitory psychopathology: alcoholism and antisocial personality disorder. J Abnorm Psychol 103:92–102, 1994

Sher KJ, Bartholow BD, Wood MD: Personality and substance use disorders: a prospective study. J Consult Clin Psychol 68:818–829, 2000

Siever LJ, Davis KL: A psychobiological perspective on the personality disorders. Am J Psychiatry 148:1647–1658, 1991

Skeem JL, Cooke DJ: Is criminal behavior a central component of psychopathy? Conceptual directions for resolving the debate. Psychol Assess 22:433–445, 2010

Skeem JL, Manchak S, Peterson JK: Correctional policy for offenders with mental illness: creating a new paradigm for recidivism reduction. Law Hum Behav 35:110–126, 2011

Skodol AE, Oldham JM, Gallaher PE: Axis II comorbidity of substance use disorders among patients referred for treatment of personality disorders. Am J Psychiatry 156:733–738, 1999

Soler J, Pascual JC, Barrachina J, et al: Double-blind, placebo-controlled study of dialectical behavior therapy plus olanzapine for borderline personality disorder. Am J Psychiatry 162:1221–1224, 2005

Soloff PH: Algorithms for pharmacological treatment of personality dimensions: symptom-specific treatments for cognitive-perceptual, affective, and impulsive-behavioral dysregulation. Bull Menninger Clin 62:195–214, 1998

Soloff PH, Cornelius J, George A, et al: Efficacy of phenelzine and haloperidol in borderline personality disorder. Arch Gen Psychiatry 50:377–385, 1993

Stanford MS, Helfritz LE, Conklin SM, et al: A comparison of anticonvulsants in the treatment of impulsive aggression. Exp Clin Psychopharmacol 13:72–77, 2005

Stinson FS, Dawson DA, Goldstein RB, et al: Prevalence, correlates, disability, and comorbidity of DSM-IV narcissistic personality disorder: results from the Wave 2 National Epidemiologic Survey on Alcohol and Related Conditions. J Clin Psychiatry 69:1033–1045, 2008

Swendsen J, Burstein M, Case B, et al: Use and abuse of alcohol and illicit drugs in U.S. adolescents: results of the National Comorbidity Survey—Adolescent Supplement. Arch Gen Psychiatry 69:390–398, 2012

Tarter RE, Vanyukov M: Alcoholism: a developmental disorder. J Consult Clin Psychol 62:1096–1107, 1994

Thomas VH, Melchert TP, Banken JA: Substance dependence and personality disorders: comorbidity and treatment outcome in an inpatient treatment population. J Stud Alcohol 60:271–277, 1999

Tritt K, Nickel C, Lahmann C, et al: Lamotrigine treatment of aggression in female borderline patients: a randomized, double-blind, placebo-controlled study. J Psychopharmacol 19:287–291, 2005

Trucco EM, Hicks BM, Villafuerte S, et al: Temperament and externalizing behavior as mediators of genetic risk on adolescent substance use. J Abnormal Psychol 125:565–575, 2016

Trull TJ, Jahng S, Tomko RL, et al: Revised NESARC personality disorder diagnoses: gender, prevalence, and comorbidity with substance dependence disorders. J Pers Disord 24:412–26, 2010

Tull MT, Gratz KL: The impact of borderline personality disorder on residential substance abuse treatment dropout among men. Drug Alcohol Depend 121:97–102, 2012

van den Bosch LM, Verheul R: Personality disorders, in Drug Abuse and Addiction in Medical Illness: Causes, Consequences, and Treatment. New York, Springer, 2012, pp 311–321

van den Bosch LM, Verheul R, Schippers GM, et al: Dialectical behavior therapy of borderline patients with and without substance use problems: implementation and long-term effects. Addict Behav 27:911–923, 2002

van Dijk FE, Lappenschaar M, Kan CC, et al: Symptomatic overlap between attention-deficit/hyperactivity disorder and borderline personality disorder in women: the role of temperament and character traits. Compr Psychiatry 53:39–47, 2012

van Wamel A, Jansen H, Kuijpers E: Addiction and personality disorders: towards integrated treatment. Implementation in an Axis II treatment team. Ment Health Subst Use 3:219–226, 2010

Verheul R: Co-morbidity of personality disorders in individuals with substance use disorders. Eur Psychiatry 16:274–282, 2001

Verheul R, van den Brink W, Hartgers C: Personality disorders predict relapse in alcoholic patients. Addict Behav 23:869–882, 1998

Verheul R, van den Brink W, Koeter MW, et al: Antisocial alcoholic patients show as much improvement at 14-month follow-up as non-antisocial alcoholic patients. Am J Addict 8:24–33, 1999

Verheul R, Kranzler HR, Poling J, et al: Axis I and Axis II disorders in alcoholics and drug addicts: fact or artifact? J Stud Alcohol 61:101–110, 2000

Vincent AS, Sorocco KH, Carnes B, et al: Antisocial characteristics and early life adversity predict substance use disorders in young adults: the Oklahoma Family Health Patterns Project. J Subst Abus Alcohol 5:1059, 2017

Walters RK, Polimanti R, Johnson EC, et al: Transancestral GWAS of alcohol dependence reveals common genetic underpinnings with psychiatric disorders. Nat Neurosci 21:1656–1669, 2018

Wetterborg D, Långström N, Andersson G, et al: Borderline personality disorder: prevalence and psychiatric comorbidity among male offenders on probation in Sweden. Compr Psychiatry 62:63–70, 2015

Wills TA, Windle M, Cleary SD: Temperament and novelty seeking in adolescent substance use: convergence of dimensions of temperament with constructs from Cloninger's theory. J Pers Soc Psychol 74:387–406, 1998

Zanarini MC: Borderline personality disorder as an impulse spectrum disorder, in Borderline Personality Disorder: Etiology and Treatment. Edited by Paris J. Washington, DC, American Psychiatric Press, 1993, pp 67–86

Zanarini MC, Frankenburg FR: Olanzapine treatment of female borderline personality disorder patients: a double-blind, placebo-controlled pilot study. J Clin Psychiatry 62:849–854, 2001

Zanarini MC, Frankenburg FR, Weingeroff JL, et al: The course of substance use disorders in patients with borderline personality disorder and Axis II comparison subjects: a 10-year follow-up study. Addiction 106:342–348, 2011a

Zanarini MC, Schulz SC, Detke HC, et al: A dose comparison of olanzapine for the treatment of borderline personality disorder: a 12-week randomized, double-blind, placebo-controlled study. J Clin Psychiatry 72:1353–1362, 2011b

Ziegenhorn AA, Roepke S, Schommer NC, et al: Clonidine improves hyperarousal in borderline personality disorder with or without comorbid posttraumatic stress disorder: a randomized, double-blind, placebo-controlled trial. J Clin Psychopharmacol 29:170–173, 2009

Zimmerman M: Diagnosing personality disorders: a review of issues and research methods. Arch Gen Psychiatry 51:225–245, 1994

Zimmerman M, Coryell WH: Diagnosing personality disorders in the community: a comparison of self-report and interview measures. Arch Gen Psychiatry 47:527–531, 1990

Zuckerman M: Vulnerability to Psychopathology: A Biosocial Model. Washington, DC, American Psychological Association, 1999

CHAPTER 22

Antisocial Personality Disorder and Other Antisocial Behavior

Donald W. Black, M.D.

Nancee S. Blum, M.S.W.

In this chapter, we summarize much of what has been learned about antisocial personality disorder (ASPD) and other forms of antisocial behavior, including childhood conduct disorder, adult antisocial behavior, and psychopathy. ASPD is perhaps the most troublesome form of antisocial behavior and wreaks more havoc on society than most other mental disorders because it primarily involves actions directed against the social environment. Antisocial criminals are responsible for untold financial losses and require additional billions to police and punish them. The despair and anxiety wrought by antisocial persons tragically affect families and communities. Many people with ASPD live in poverty or draw on the social welfare system, hampered by poor school and work performance and an inability to establish a life plan. Despite high public health significance, ASPD is largely ignored or misunderstood by many clinicians and researchers.

ASPD is associated with a pattern of socially irresponsible, exploitative, and guiltless behavior resulting in disturbances in many areas of life, including family relations, schooling, work, military service, and marriage (North and Yutzy 2010). Behaviors include criminal acts and failure to conform to the law, failure to sustain consistent employment, manipulation and deception of others for personal gain, and failure to develop or sustain stable interpersonal relationships. Other attributes of ASPD include a lack of empathy for others, rare experiences of remorse, and failure to learn from the negative results of one's behavior. The spectrum of behaviors seen in people with ASPD ranges from relatively minor acts at one end (e.g., lying, cheating) to heinous acts at the other (e.g., rape, murder). Common and widespread, the presence of ASPD is rarely acknowledged, and determining its causes is as elusive as understanding its treatment.

Diagnostic Issues

Historical Overview

Clinical descriptions of antisocial behavior date to the early nineteenth century when Philippe Pinel, a leader in the French Revolution and founding father of modern psychiatry, used the term *manie sans délire* to describe people with irrational outbursts of rage and violence (North and Yutzy 2010). English physician James Pritchard wrote about *moral insanity*, a condition in which a person's intellectual faculties were unimpaired but moral principles were "depraved or perverted." His term foreshadowed the later focus on the moral dimensions of ASPD. German psychiatrist Julius Koch introduced the term *psychopathic inferiority* in the late nineteenth century to replace moral insanity as a diagnosis. The term described a broad range of deviant behaviors and eccentricities and implied that the disorder resulted from constitutional factors (Black 2013).

Scottish psychiatrist David Henderson (1939) and American psychiatrist Hervey Cleckley (1941/1976), working independently at about the same time, each used the term *psychopathy*. In *Mask of Sanity: An Attempt to Clarify Some Issues About the So-Called Psychopathic Personality*, Cleckley (1941/1976) provided a detailed description of psychopathic behavior, which he set apart from other psychiatric conditions and behavioral abnormalities. Through a series of case vignettes, Cleckley showed how the disorder transcends social class. Both Cleckley and Henderson considered psychopathy a true illness, and our present understanding reflects much of their early work.

DSM Classifications

Cleckley (1941/1976) inspired the creation of a new diagnostic category, *sociopathic personality disturbance*, in DSM-I (American Psychiatric Association 1952). Generally abbreviated as *sociopathy*, the term was used to describe persons whose abnormal behavior was directed toward the social environment: "Individuals to be placed in this category are ill primarily in terms of society and of conformity with the prevailing cultural milieu, and not only in terms of personal discomfort and relations with other individuals" (American Psychiatric Association 1952, p. 38). Subtypes included *antisocial reaction, dyssocial reaction, sexual deviation*, and *addiction*, which included alcoholism and drug addiction. *Antisocial reaction* referred to the behavior of chronically antisocial individuals who were always in trouble and without loyalties to other persons, groups, or codes. *Dyssocial reaction* referred to those with disregard for the usual social codes, having lived in an "abnormal moral environment, but who [were] capable of strong loyalties" (American Psychiatric Association 1952, p. 38). The term *antisocial personality disorder* was introduced in DSM-II (American Psychiatric Association 1968), and the new definition combined elements of the antisocial and dyssocial reactions of DSM-I. Listed among other personality disturbances, the disorder was no longer linked with addictions or deviant sexuality. As defined in DSM-II, the term was "reserved for individuals who are basically unsocialized and whose behavior pattern brings them repeatedly into conflict with society" (American Psychiatric Association 1968, p. 43).

Diagnostic criteria introduced in DSM-III (American Psychiatric Association 1980) were inspired by the work of Robins (1966), as well as both the Washington University ("Feighner") criteria (Feighner et al. 1972) and the Research Diagnostic Criteria (Spitzer et al. 1978), and emphasized the continuity between adult and childhood behavioral problems. The criteria were simplified in subsequent editions, including DSM-III-R (American Psychiatric Association 1987) and DSM-IV (American Psychiatric Association 1994), and no changes were made in the DSM-5 Section II criteria (American Psychiatric Association 2013).

The DSM-5 Section II criteria require that a person have at least three of these seven pathological personality traits: failure to conform to social norms with respect to lawful behaviors, deceitfulness, impulsivity, irritability or aggressiveness, reckless disregard for safety of self or others, irresponsibility, and lack of remorse. The person must be age 18 years or older, and there should be evidence of conduct disorder with onset before age 15. Schizophrenia and bipolar disorder must be ruled out as causes of the disturbance.

The Alternative DSM-5 Model for Personality Disorders (AMPD), created during the development of DSM-5, appears in DSM-5 Section III, "Emerging Measures and Models." All the personality disorders (PDs)—including ASPD—are defined in terms of impairments in self functioning (identity and self-direction) and interpersonal functioning (empathy and intimacy), as well as pathological personality traits shown to be empirically related to the disorder. The personality functioning criterion (Criterion A) focuses on the egocentrism, absence of prosocial internal standards, lack of empathy, and exploitative interpersonal relationships characteristics of ASPD, and the personality traits criterion (Criterion B) requires six or more of the following pathological traits from the domains of Antagonism and Disinhibition: manipulativeness, callousness, deceitfulness, hostility, risk taking, impulsivity, and irresponsibility. The presence of conduct disorder before age 15, which is required in the criteria set in DSM-5 Section II, is not required in the AMPD. Newer research has not supported the requirement of a history of conduct disorder (McGonigal et al. 2019).

Table 22–1 presents a comparison of the DSM-5 Section II ("Diagnostic Criteria and Codes") criteria (left column) with the AMPD (right column). (For additional details on the AMPD, see Chapter 3, "Articulating a Core Dimension of Personality Pathology," Chapter 4, "The Alternative DSM-5 Model for Personality Disorders," and Chapter 5, "Manifestations, Assessment, Diagnosis, and Differential Diagnosis," in this volume.)

Relationship of ASPD to Psychopathy

Although the word *psychopathy* predates the word *antisocial*, the terms initially were used interchangeably. The term *psychopathy* gradually came to be used in a restricted fashion defined by a constellation of psychological manifestations and traits to describe a clinical entity distinct from ASPD. Many clinicians and researchers were dissatisfied with the DSM-III criteria for ASPD and its focus on behaviors (e.g., criminality, aggression) rather than underlying psychological traits. Although DSM-III proved to be reliable, critics felt that validity had been sacrificed in favor of reliability because of the failure to include all the traits of psychopathy identified by Cleckley (1941/1976) (Widiger 2006). In response, the authors of DSM-III-R added lack of remorse as a criterion for ASPD; then in DSM-IV, the criteria were simplified and became more

TABLE 22–1. Comparison of DSM-5 Section II and Section III criteria for antisocial personality disorder (ASPD)

DSM-5 Section II ASPD	DSM-5 Section III ASPD
A. A pervasive pattern of disregard for and violation of the rights of others, occurring since age 15 years, as indicated by three (or more) of the following: 1. Failure to conform to social norms with respect to lawful behaviors, as indicated by repeatedly performing acts that are grounds for arrest. 2. Deceitfulness, as indicated by repeated lying, use of aliases, or conning others for personal profit or pleasure. 3. Impulsivity or failure to plan ahead. 4. Irritability and aggressiveness, as indicated by repeated physical fights or assaults. 5. Reckless disregard for safety of self or others. 6. Consistent irresponsibility, as indicated by repeated failure to sustain consistent work behavior or honor financial obligations. 7. Lack of remorse, as indicated by being indifferent to or rationalizing having hurt, mistreated, or stolen from another. B. The individual is at least age 18 years.	Typical features of antisocial personality disorder are a failure to conform to lawful and ethical behavior and an egocentric, callous lack of concern for others, accompanied by deceitfulness, irresponsibility, manipulativeness, and/or risk taking. Characteristic difficulties are apparent in identity, self-direction, empathy, and/or intimacy, as described below, along with specific maladaptive traits in the domains of Antagonism and Disinhibition. A. Moderate or greater impairment in personality functioning, manifested by characteristic difficulties in two or more of the following four areas: 1. *Identity:* Egocentrism; self-esteem derived from personal gain, power, or pleasure. 2. *Self-direction:* Goal setting based on personal gratification; absence of prosocial internal standards, associated with failure to conform to lawful or culturally normative ethical behavior. 3. *Empathy:* Lack of concern for feelings, needs, or suffering of others; lack of remorse after hurting or mistreating another. 4. *Intimacy:* Incapacity for mutually intimate relationships, as exploitation is a primary means of relating to others, including by deceit and coercion; use of dominance or intimidation to control others. B. Six or more of the following seven pathological personality traits: 1. *Manipulativeness* (an aspect of Antagonism): Frequent use of subterfuge to influence or control others; use of seduction, charm, glibness, or ingratiation to achieve one's ends. 2. *Callousness* (an aspect of Antagonism): Lack of concern for feelings or problems of others; lack of guilt or remorse about the negative or harmful effects of one's actions on others; aggression; sadism. 3. *Deceitfulness* (an aspect of Antagonism): Dishonesty and fraudulence; misrepresentation of self; embellishment or fabrication when relating events. 4. *Hostility* (an aspect of Antagonism): Persistent or frequent angry feelings; anger or irritability in response to minor slights and insults; mean, nasty, or vengeful behavior.

TABLE 22–1.   **Comparison of DSM-5 Section II and Section III criteria for antisocial personality disorder (ASPD)** *(continued)*

DSM-5 Section II ASPD	DSM-5 Section III ASPD
	5. *Risk taking* (an aspect of Disinhibition): Engagement in dangerous, risky, and potentially self-damaging activities, unnecessarily and without regard for consequences; boredom proneness and thoughtless initiation of activities to counter boredom; lack of concern for one's limitations and denial of the reality of personal danger.
	6. *Impulsivity* (an aspect of Disinhibition): Acting on the spur of the moment in response to immediate stimuli; acting on a momentary basis without a plan or consideration of outcomes; difficulty establishing and following plans.
	7. *Irresponsibility* (an aspect of Disinhibition): Disregard for—and failure to honor—financial and other obligations or commitments; lack of respect for—and lack of follow-through on—agreements and promises.
C. There is evidence of conduct disorder [see DSM-5 diagnostic criteria for conduct disorder] with onset before age 15 years.	C. The impairments in personality functioning and the individual's personality trait expression are relatively inflexible and pervasive across a broad range of personal and social situations.
D. The occurrence of antisocial behavior is not exclusively during the course of schizophrenia or bipolar disorder.	D. The impairments in personality functioning and the individual's personality trait expression are relatively stable across time, with onsets that can be traced back to at least adolescence or early adulthood.
	E. The impairments in personality functioning and the individual's personality trait expression are not better explained by another mental disorder.
	F. The impairments in personality functioning and the individual's personality trait expression are not solely attributable to the physiological effects of a substance or another medical condition (e.g., severe head trauma).
	G. The impairments in personality functioning and the individual's personality trait expression are not better understood as normal for the individual's developmental stage or sociocultural environment.

Note. The individual is at least 18 years of age.

Source. Criteria reprinted from American Psychiatric Association: *Diagnostic and Statistical Manual of Mental Disorders*, 5th Edition. Arlington, VA, American Psychiatric Association, 2013. Copyright © 2013. American Psychiatric Association. Used with permission.

trait-based. Of note, in the AMPD, all of the B criteria for ASPD (and other PDs) are described in trait terms.

Motivated by concerns that the DSM approach emphasized delinquent and antisocial symptoms to the exclusion of psychological traits, Hare created the Psychopathy Checklist (PCL) to assess traits he and others have associated with psychopathy as a distinct clinical syndrome (e.g., glibness, callousness, lack of emotional connection to others, incapacity for guilt or remorse) (Hare 1983; Hare and Neumann 2006). Much of his work in validating the questionnaire, or its revision, the PCL-R (Hare 1991), has taken place in correctional settings, where the instrument has proven reliable in identifying people with these traits, as well as predicting recidivism, parole violations, and violence in offenders and psychiatric patients (Hare and Neumann 2006). The following traits are included in the AMPD: manipulativeness, callousness, impulsivity, irresponsibility, deceitfulness, risk taking.

Psychopathy has gained support as a topic of investigation, perhaps because it is measurable and identifies a homogeneous group of people. However, it also has contributed to confusion among clinicians and researchers, who have difficulty distinguishing ASPD and psychopathy. The two syndromes overlap, and although Hare (1983) noted that most antisocial persons are not "psychopaths" as defined by his checklist, *nearly all* psychopathic individuals exhibit antisocial traits and behavior that meet the criteria for ASPD. This overlap has been assessed in prisoners, in whom the prevalence of both conditions is high. Nearly one-third of incarcerated men with ASPD are psychopathic individuals. Coid and Ulrich (2010) have suggested that psychopathy lies along a continuum of severity with ASPD and likely constitutes its most severe variant.

The AMPD includes the specifier "with psychopathic features" to denote individuals who are also characterized by low anxiety and a particularly dominant interpersonal style.

Conduct Disorder

Conduct disorder was introduced in DSM-III and included four subtypes based on a 2×2 matrix on the axes of socialization and aggressivity. This scheme was dropped from DSM-III-R and subsequent editions because the subtyping was judged to lack clinical utility and to be at variance with research findings. *Conduct disorder* is defined as "a repetitive and persistent pattern of behavior in which the basic rights of others or major age-appropriate societal norms or rules are violated" (American Psychiatric Association 2013, p. 469). In DSM-5, conduct disorder has been moved from the DSM-IV chapter "Disorders Usually First Diagnosed in Infancy, Childhood, or Adolescence" to "Disruptive, Impulse-Control, and Conduct Disorders."

Conduct disorder is a predominantly male disorder and affects approximately 5%–15% of children (Black 2013). The disorder has an early onset and is, in general, present by the preschool years, usually by age 8. In 80% of future cases, a first symptom has appeared by age 11 years (Robins and Price 1991). Most children with conduct disorder do not develop adult ASPD, although they remain at high risk, with an estimated 25% of girls and 40% of boys with conduct disorder eventually developing ASPD (Robins 1987). Rates for the progression from conduct disorder to ASPD are much higher in adolescents with conduct disorder who also abuse substances (Myers et al. 1998). Follow-up studies show that the likelihood of a child's developing ASPD is associated with early onset of behavioral problems, a history of physical violence, and both variety and severity of childhood misbehaviors (Loeber et al. 2002a, 2002b; Robins 1966). Childhood attention-deficit/hyperactivity disorder (ADHD) also increases risk for ASPD (Storebø and Simonsen 2016).

The diagnosis of conduct disorder requires that at least 3 of 15 problematic behaviors were present in the previous 12 months, with at least one criterion present in the past 6 months. Although the diagnosis can be made in adults, the symptoms usually emerge in childhood or adolescence, and onset is rare after age 16 years. The criteria specify a childhood-onset type (prior to age 10 years) and an adolescent-onset type (after age 10 years), in recognition of the fact that early onset is one of the strongest predictors of poor outcome. Using data from the National Epidemiologic Survey of Alcohol and Related Conditions (NESARC), Goldstein et al. (2006) reported that childhood-onset conduct disorder was more likely than adolescent-onset conduct disorder to be associated with violent behaviors including those against persons, animals, and property.

When considering the diagnosis, clinicians should note misbehaviors in four main areas: aggression toward people or animals, destruction of property, deceitfulness or theft, and serious violations of rules. Childhood symptoms include fights with peers, conflicts with parents and other authority figures, stealing, vandalism, fire setting, and cruelty to animals or other children. School-related behavior problems are common, as is poor academic performance. In addition, many of these children have a history of running away from home. These behavior problems must significantly impair the child's social, academic, or occupational functioning. Boys with conduct disorder are more likely to exhibit physical aggression, whereas girls are more likely to show relational aggression—that is, behavior that harms social relationships (American Psychiatric Association 2013).

Moffitt (1993a, 2015) differentiated adolescence-limited and life-course-persistent antisocial behaviors. Youths with adolescence-limited antisocial behaviors have little or no history of earlier antisocial behavior, and they tend to spontaneously improve, which explains why most children and adolescents with conduct disorder never develop adult ASPD. A small proportion of men with extreme behavioral problems have life-course-persistent antisocial behaviors; these men have an early onset of antisocial behavior, develop more severe behavioral problems, and have a greater variety of problems. In contrast, most antisocial youths develop adolescence-limited antisocial behavior, which is less severe and typically arises in the context of teenage peer group pressure.

Adult Antisocial Behavior

DSM-5 includes adult antisocial behavior in the section "Other Conditions That May Be a Focus of Clinical Attention." This designation is used when adult antisocial behavior is the focus of clinical attention and is not considered due to a mental disorder even though the condition may be troublesome to the individual and community (American Psychiatric Association 2013, p. 726). The category is used to describe persons who manifest antisocial behavior but do not otherwise meet criteria for ASPD or other disorders that could explain the behavior (e.g., professional thieves, racketeers, dealers of illegal substances). Individuals with adult antisocial behavior are presumed to be fundamentally normal people whose choices and decisions have led them astray.

Typically, individuals with adult antisocial behavior have no history of childhood conduct disorder. They tend to have milder syndromes compared with individuals who meet criteria for ASPD (Black and Braun 1998; Goldstein et al. 2007, 2008; McGonigal et al. 2019).

Epidemiology

Surveys in the United States and United Kingdom indicate that between 2% and 5% of the general adult population have antisocial features that meet the criteria for lifetime ASPD. The National Institute of Mental Health's Epidemiologic Catchment Area (ECA) survey was the first large study conducted in the United States (Robins et al. 1984). Data from nearly 15,000 subjects at five sites showed that 2%–4% of men and 0.5%–1% of women have antisocial features that meet the criteria for ASPD. The National Comorbidity Survey, a probability survey of more than 8,000 American adults, found an overall rate of 3.5% (Kessler et al. 1994). More recently, the NESARC, involving over 43,000 Americans, reported an overall rate of 3.6% (5.5% for men, 1.9% for women) (Compton et al. 2005). The British National Survey of Psychiatric Morbidity reported a prevalence rate of 2.9% for ASPD in the United Kingdom (Ullrich and Coid 2009). These surveys possibly *underestimate* the prevalence of ASPD, however, because they do not include data on institutionalized and incarcerated persons, who are likely to have higher rates of ASPD.

NESARC researchers also reported rates for other antisocial syndromes. The prevalence in adults for lifetime conduct disorder (in the absence of adult antisocial behavior) was 1.1% (1.5% for men, 0.7% for women). Lifetime adult antisocial behavior without a history of conduct disorder was found in 12.3% (16.5% for men, 8.5% for women). These data suggest that antisocial behavioral syndromes occur along a continuum of severity (Compton et al. 2005; Goldstein et al. 2007, 2008).

ASPD is overrepresented among men and women in jails and prisons (Black et al. 2010). An early study showed that up to 80% of incarcerated men and 65% of incarcerated women were judged to have ASPD based on the Feighner criteria (Guze 1976). More recent work has suggested that prevalence may have declined as the prison population has grown. A prison-based study that used a structured interview to identify ASPD found that 35% of offenders had antisocial features that met the criteria for ASPD (Black et al. 2010). The ASPD rate is also high in particular patient groups. For example, the prevalence of ASPD in persons undergoing residential drug treatment may reach 55% (Goldstein et al. 1996). The rate of ASPD among homeless persons is also high (North et al. 1993).

ASPD is associated with low socioeconomic status, which can be attributed in part to poor educational achievement, poor job performance, and frequent unemployment. In the NESARC, respondents with lower educational levels and lower income levels were more likely to have ASPD (Compton et al. 2005). According to Robins (1987), persons with ASPD begin life at a disadvantaged level and their adult social class continues to decline, even falling below that of their parents. However, low social class itself is not responsible for ASPD, as demonstrated in a study of African American youths by Robins et al. (1971). The authors showed that children without conduct disorder symptoms were not at risk for ASPD when raised in impoverished families, but that children with high rates of conduct symptoms were at risk for ASPD even when reared in "white-collar" families.

The question of whether ASPD is more common in certain racial or ethnic groups is unsettled. The ECA survey showed that African American respondents were more likely than Caucasians to exhibit antisocial symptoms that could lead to arrest and incarceration, although there were no racial differences in ASPD prevalence (Robins 1987). In the NESARC, Native Americans were at increased risk for ASPD, whereas Asian American and Hispanic/Latino respondents were at lower risk for ASPD than Caucasians (Compton et al. 2005).

ASPD is primarily a disorder of younger persons. According to both the ECA and NESARC surveys, rates of ASPD diminish with advancing age (Compton et al. 2005; Robins et al. 1984). Lower prevalence in older adults could be attributable to improvement in or remission of the syndrome; to forgetfulness (i.e., not recalling past misbehaviors) or denial of symptoms; or to high mortality rates (i.e., many with ASPD die prematurely and are therefore not available for late-life surveys). Some have argued that ASPD could be less common because the crime-based criteria fail to capture the behavioral problems of older adults (Holzer and Vaughn 2017).

Clinical Manifestations

The clinical manifestations of ASPD begin early, often leading to the diagnosis of conduct disorder (Black 2013; North and Yutzy 2010). As antisocial youth attain adult status, problems develop in other areas of life reflecting age-appropriate responsibilities. These problems include uneven job performance, unreliability, frequent job changes, and losing jobs through quitting or being fired. Pathological lying and the use of aliases are common. Many persons with ASPD are sexually promiscuous and become sexually active at a younger age than their peers. Marriages are often unstable, leading to high rates of divorce, and may be accompanied by domestic violence.

People with ASPD who join the armed forces often have unsatisfactory experiences because of their inability to accept military discipline (Black et al. 1995b; Robins 1966). They are more likely than others to be absent without leave, court-martialed, or dishonorably discharged. Criminality is common among people with ASPD. Offenses vary but range from nonviolent property offenses to acts of extreme violence, which may include sodomy, rape, or murder. Clinical symptoms of ASPD, as found in the NESARC (Goldstein et al. 2007), are shown in Table 22–2.

Gender Differences

There are differences between men and women in ASPD prevalence, onset, and symptoms. Rates are much higher in men than women, leading some to suggest that the ASPD criteria are biased because of their focus on criminal and aggressive behaviors

TABLE 22–2. Antisocial personality disorder (ASPD) symptoms in 305 women and 750 men in the NESARC study

Symptoms	Women	Men	Total
Repeated unlawful behaviors, %	81	85	84
Deceitfulness, %	56	46	49
Impulsivity/failure to plan ahead, %	62	54	56
Irritability/aggressiveness, %	74	75	75
Recklessness, %	62	85	79
Consistent irresponsibility, %	89	86	87
Lack of remorse, %	53	52	52
Total ASPD criteria met since age 15, mean	4.8	4.8	4.8
Lifetime violent symptoms, mean	3.0	3.3	3.2

Note. NESARC=National Epidemiologic Survey on Alcohol and Related Conditions.
Source. Adapted from Goldstein et al. 2007.

that are less common in women (Dolan and Völlm 2009; Goldstein et al. 1996). Another possibility is that the syndromes in men and women are etiologically distinct.

Robins (1966) observed that troubled girls later diagnosed as antisocial were more likely than boys to have engaged in sexual misbehavior and had a later onset of behavioral problems. As women, they married at a younger age than their nonantisocial peers, and they chose husbands "who drank, were arrested, were unfaithful, deserted, or failed to support them" (p. 49). Those with children had more children than did nonantisocial women, and their children tended to be difficult, perhaps sadly destined to follow their parents' path in life. Like her male counterpart, a woman with ASPD has low earning potential, is often financially dependent on others (or the government), and sometimes exhibits aggressive behavior. Women with ASPD are disconnected from the community and have high rates of depression, anxiety disorders, and substance use disorders.

Other data on gender differences suggest that antisocial boys are more likely than antisocial girls to engage in fighting, use weapons, engage in cruelty to animals, and set fires. Girls are more often involved in "victimless" antisocial behaviors, such as running away. As adults, women with ASPD are more likely to have problems that center on the home and family, such as irresponsibility as a parent, neglectful or abusive treatment of their children, and physical violence toward husbands and partners (Goldstein et al. 1996).

Etiology

Genetics of Antisocial Behavior

Research supports a genetic diathesis for antisocial behavior, with a relatively recent large-scale study estimating heritability at 51% (Rosenstrom et al. 2017). Additionally, results from more than 100 family, twin, and adoption studies strongly indicate that antisocial behavior runs in families, in part due to the transmission of genes (Slutske 2001). In fact, nearly 20% of first-degree relatives of persons with ASPD will have the disorder themselves (Guze et al. 1967). A review of twin study data reported monozygotic concordance for antisocial behavior of nearly 67%, compared with 31% concordance for dizygotic twins (Brennan and Mednick 1993). Adoption studies have shown that ASPD is more frequent in adoptees with antisocial biological relatives than adoptees without antisocial relatives (Cadoret et al. 1985).

These same studies also suggest that much of the risk for becoming antisocial could be due to family experiences or to experiences specific to an individual (Slutske 2001). An important study in the new era of molecular genetics points to the influence of the monoamine oxidase A gene *MAOA*. (Monoamine oxidase is an enzyme that breaks down the neurotransmitter serotonin.) The low-activity variant of the gene has been found in antisocial persons who had been severely abused as children (Caspi et al. 2002). In contrast, children who had a high-activity variant of the gene rarely became antisocial, despite the presence of abuse.

Tielbeek et al. (2012) conducted a genome-wide association study of adult antisocial behavior in nearly 5,000 persons, but the researchers were unable to link any genes with antisocial behavior. This report was followed by a similar study of 370 offenders with ASPD; Rautiainen et al. (2016) identified two polymorphisms at the 6p21.2 *LINC00951–LRFN2* gene region, although the functional significance of the region is unknown.

Psychophysiology and Neurodevelopment

Autonomic underarousal has been posited as underlying psychopathy; this condition likely constitutes a poor-prognosis subset of individuals with ASPD (Hare 1986). Briefly, compared with subjects without psychopathology, psychopathic persons require greater sensory input to produce normal brain functioning, possibly leading these individuals to seek potentially dangerous or risky situations to raise their level of arousal to desired levels. Evidence supporting this theory includes the finding that antisocial adults (and youth with conduct disorder) have low resting pulse rates, low skin conductance, and increased amplitude on event-related potentials (Scarpa and Raine 1997). A study of 15-year-old English schoolchildren found that those who committed crimes during the subsequent 9 years were more likely to have a low resting pulse at baseline, reduced skin conductance, and more slow-wave electroencephalographic (EEG) activity than the others (Raine et al. 1990).

The presence of EEG abnormalities in nearly half of antisocial persons, along with high rates of minor facial anomalies, learning disorders, enuresis, and behavioral hyperactivity, further suggests that ASPD is a neurodevelopmental syndrome (Moffitt 1993b). Maternal smoking and starvation have also been linked with antisocial behavior (Neugebauer et al. 1999; Wakschlag et al. 1997). The mechanism behind these relationships is unclear, but it could be that subtle brain injury contributing to antisocial behavior results from lower levels of oxygen available to the fetus, from fetal exposure to chemicals generated from tobacco smoke, or from the deleterious effect of malnutrition on the developing brain (Raine 2018).

Neurotransmission

Central nervous system (CNS) neurotransmitters are thought to have a role in mediating antisocial behavior. Serotonin in particular has been linked with impulsive and aggressive behavior. Low levels of its metabolite 5-hydroxyindoleacetic acid have repeatedly been found in cerebrospinal fluid of persons with violent or impulsive behavior (Åsberg et al. 1976; Virkkunen et al. 1987). It is thought that the presence of serotonin may curb impulsive and aggressive behaviors. Genetic disturbances in serotonin function may predispose a person to have impulsive and aggressive behavior (Nielsen et al. 1994).

Neuroimaging

Abnormal CNS functioning in antisocial individuals has been suggested from brain imaging studies (Dolan 2010; Yang et al. 2008). Several crucial brain regions have been implicated, including the prefrontal cortex, the superior temporal cortex, the amygdala–hippocampal complex, and the anterior cingulate cortex.

Using positron emission tomography to measure glucose uptake in murderers, many of whom were likely antisocial, Raine et al. (1997) found impairments in the prefrontal cortex and other underlying structures. Raine et al. (2000) also reported that according to results from magnetic resonance imaging, antisocial men had reduced gray matter volume in the prefrontal lobes; this was the first indication that anomalies in these structures may underlie some antisocial behavior. Subsequent studies have suggested that the finding of reduced gray matter volumes could be influenced by comorbid conditions such as psychopathy or substance abuse, both of which are difficult to disentangle from ASPD (Raine 2018).

In an attempt to localize symptoms, Yang et al. (2007) looked at a group of individuals who pathologically lie—a common characteristic of individuals with ASPD. The liars had an *increase* in prefrontal white matter volume; repeated lying activates the prefrontal circuitry, leading to permanent changes in brain structure, prompting the authors to compare this finding with "Pinocchio's nose." Yang et al. (2009) also found smaller amygdalae in psychopathic individuals compared with controls, possibly explaining the shallow emotions observed in psychopathic persons.

Kiehl et al. (2001) used functional magnetic resonance imaging to investigate brain activity in psychopathic individuals during various emotional and cognitive experiments. They reported reduced activity in the amygdala in psychopathic individuals in response to hearing emotionally charged words; this finding might help explain why these individuals have difficulty learning to avoid behaviors with unwanted or negative outcomes. A subsequent study, conducted under similar conditions but using a different experimental task, showed that psychopathic individuals had *increased* activation in the right temporal lobe, suggesting that a malfunction in this brain region could contribute to the fearlessness that characterizes psychopathy (Kiehl et al. 2004).

Although research points to evidence of subtle structural and functional deficits in the neural circuits that may help mediate antisocial behavior, their clinical significance remains unclear, and data interpretation is hampered by variation among the studies in terms of imaging method and study population. Nonetheless, it is possible that frontal deficits (prefrontal cortex and anterior cingulate cortex) contribute to impulsivity, poor judgment, and irresponsible behavior, whereas dysfunction in temporal regions (amygdala–hippocampal and superior temporal cortex) predisposes to antisocial features such as inability to follow rules and deficient moral judgment (Yang et al. 2009). Taken together, these findings suggest a link between cortical dysfunction and antisocial behavior.

Family and Social Factors

Child abuse is reported to contribute to the development of ASPD. Parents of persons who develop ASPD are often incompetent, absent, or abusive (Robins 1966, 1987). They are often significantly troubled themselves, showing high levels of antisocial behavior; furthermore, some have alcohol use disorder, are divorced or separated, or exhibit antisocial behavior. Erratic or inappropriate parental discipline and inadequate supervision have been linked with antisocial behavior (Reti et al. 2002). Antisocial parents are unlikely to effectively monitor their child's behavior, set rules and ensure that they are obeyed, check on the child's whereabouts, or steer the child away from troubled playmates. However, having an antisocial child also may induce negative, neglectful responses in parents (Bell and Chapman 1986).

Individuals with ASPD are more likely than others to report histories of childhood maltreatment, including abuse (emotional, physical, sexual) and neglect (Krastins et al. 2014; Luntz and Widom 1994). In some instances, abuse may become a learned behavior that formerly abused adults perpetuate with their own children, leading to an intergenerational cycle of abuse.

Peer Relationships

Disturbed peer relationships were first identified as contributing to the development of antisocial behavior in the pioneering studies of Glueck and Glueck (1950). They reported that 98% of 500 delinquent boys had delinquent friends, compared with 7% of 500 nondelinquent peers. The delinquent boys were also more likely than nondelinquent peers to report that they had been gang members (56% vs. 1%). This pattern of association (i.e., the "birds of a feather" phenomenon) usually begins during the elementary school years. More recently, Juvonen and Ho (2008) found that youths who are attracted to antisocial peers often engage in antisocial behavior themselves to gain acceptance. These relationships can reward aggressive behavior and encourage gang membership. Gangs may be attractive to those individuals who feel rejected by their families and peer group.

Media Influence

Since the advent of television, media depictions of violence have long been thought to foster the development of antisocial behavior. Huesmann and Taylor (2006) concluded that through repeated exposure, children become desensitized to violence and learn to accept a more hostile view of the world. Those most vulnerable to the media onslaught appear to be those who already live in a "culture of violence," in which there are few barriers to aggressive behavior. That said, it is not known whether violent media depictions are a risk factor for ASPD or other antisocial syndromes.

A related issue is the effect of violent video games. In a study of juvenile offenders, violent video games were associated with delinquency and violent behavior, yet the researchers concluded that the association could be another indicator of antisociality, and not represent a causal link (DeLisi et al. 2012).

Course and Outcome

ASPD is a lifelong disorder that usually has an onset in childhood and is fully expressed by the late teens or early 20s. In a 30-year follow-up of 82 antisocial persons originally seen in a child guidance clinic, Robins (1966) found that the disorder was more severe early in its course and that antisocial persons tended to improve with advancing age. She observed that at a mean age of 45 years at follow-up, 12% of the subjects had remitted (defined as no symptoms of ASPD) and another 20% had improved; the rest were as disturbed as (or more disturbed than) at study intake. The median age for improvement was 35 years, although Robins pointed out that improvement can occur at any age.

Black et al. (1995b) followed 71 antisocial men (mean age 54 years) who had been admitted to an academic hospital a mean of 29 years earlier. Of these individuals, 27% were rated as having experienced remission of their antisocial symptoms, 31% as improved, and 42% as unimproved. Those most likely to have improved were the least deviant at baseline and were older at follow-up. The course for the men was compared with previously published data from the "Iowa 500" study of individuals with schizophrenia and depression, as well as normal control subjects, all hospitalized at the same facility during an overlapping period (Black et al. 1995a). Antisocial men fared less well than depressed subjects and control subjects in their marital, occupational, and psychiatric adjustment. They functioned better than people with schizophrenia in their marital status and housing, but not in their occupational status or aggregate psychiatric symptoms. In other words, antisocial persons were more likely than those with schizophrenia to be married and to have their own housing, but they were just as likely to perform poorly in the workplace and to have disabling psychiatric symptoms (but not psychotic symptoms).

The studies of Robins (1966) and Black et al. (1995a, 1995b) show that while the most dangerous and destructive behaviors associated with ASPD may improve or remit, other troublesome problems remain. Although older people with ASPD are less likely to commit crimes or become violent than when they were younger, many remain troublesome to their families and the community. Some fail to improve at all. When improvement occurs, it typically follows many years of antisocial behavior that has stunted the individuals' educational and work achievement, thus limiting their potential achievement.

Marriage is another moderating variable. In Robins's (1966) study, more than half of married antisocial persons improved, but few unmarried persons did so. More recently, Burt et al. (2010) used twin data to show that men with lower levels of antisocial behavior were more likely to marry and that those who married engaged in less antisocial behavior than their unmarried co-twin. These data appear to confirm Robins's (1966) observation that marriage has a buffering effect on antisocial behavior and are largely consistent with findings reported by Glueck and Glueck (1950), later reanalyzed by Sampson and Laub (1993). Sampson and Laub's study found that job stability and marital attachment were linked with improvement.

Antisocial persons often die prematurely from accidental deaths, suicides, or homicides (Black et al. 1996; Robins 1966). A recent study using follow-up data from the ECA survey found that antisocial persons were specifically at risk for early death from all causes, but particularly from suicide, malignancies, lung disease, and HIV infections (Krasnova et al. 2019). The following vignette demonstrates the continuity of antisocial behavior over time, the high frequency of co-occurring substance use disorders, and the toll ASPD takes on individuals, society, and family members (Black and Andreasen 2021, p. 413).

Case Example

Russell, age 18, was admitted for evaluation of antisocial behavior. His early childhood was chaotic and abusive. His alcoholic father had married five times and abandoned his family when Russell was age 6. Because his mother had a history of incarceration and was unable to care for him, Russell was placed in foster care until he was adopted at age 8. His adoptive father was a university professor; his adoptive mother was described as compulsive and strict.

Russell had a criminal streak from early childhood. He lied, cheated at games, shoplifted, and stole money from his mother's purse. He once burglarized a church and, when older, stole an automobile. Despite an above-average IQ of 112, Russell's school performance was poor, and he was frequently in detention for breaking rules. Because of continued law breaking, he was sent to a juvenile reformatory at age 16 for 2 years. While in the reformatory, he slashed another boy with a razor blade in a fight. Russell had his first sexual experience before his peers, and after leaving the reformatory, he had several different sexual partners. He chain-smoked and admitted to abusing alcohol. An electroencephalogram was normal. He was discharged from the hospital after a 16-day stay and was considered unimproved. He had been poorly cooperative with attempts at both individual and group therapy during the hospital stay.

Russell was interviewed 30 years later. He used an alias and lived in an impoverished community. Now age 48, Russell appeared ill and haggard. He admitted to more than 20 arrests and more than five felony convictions on charges ranging from attempted murder and armed robbery to driving while intoxicated. He had spent more than 17 years in prison. His most recent arrest occurred within the past year and was for public intoxication and simple assault.

Russell reported over nine hospitalizations for alcohol detoxification, the latest occurring earlier that year. He admitted to past use of marijuana, amphetamines, tranquilizers, cocaine, and heroin.

Russell had never held a full-time job in his life. The longest job he had held lasted only 60 days. He was currently doing bodywork on cars in his own garage to earn a living but had not done any work for several months. He had lived in six different states and had moved more than 20 times in 10 years.

Russell reported that nine persons lived in his home, including his four children. He had met his common-law wife in a psychiatric hospital. She used tranquilizers for emotional problems, and the marriage was unsatisfactory. He reported occasionally attending Alcoholics Anonymous at a local church but otherwise did not socialize outside his family.

Russell admitted that he had not yet settled down and told us that he still spent money foolishly, was frequently reckless, and got into frequent fights and arguments. He said that he got a "charge out of doing dangerous things."

Assessment

The diagnosis of a patient rests on a history of chronic and repetitive behavioral problems beginning in childhood or early adolescence that continue into adulthood (Black 2013). Because antisocial individuals may not be forthcoming regarding their past symptoms, family members and friends can be helpful informants if available (and the patient has consented to their participation). Family members may be more accurate in describing their relatives' antisocial behavior than the patients themselves (Andreasen et al. 1986). Records of previous clinic or hospital visits can provide important diagnostic clues.

Psychological tests can be helpful, particularly when a patient refuses to allow interviews with relatives or when informants are unavailable. The Minnesota Multiphasic Personality Inventory, and subsequent revisions, yields a broad profile of personality functioning, and a certain pattern of results is typical of ASPD (Butcher et al. 1989; Dahlstrom et al. 1972; Tellegen et al. 2003). The PCL-R can be used to measure the presence and severity of psychopathic traits and can be useful particularly if the antisocial person is being assessed in a forensic setting (Hare 1991). There are many structured interviews and paper-and-pencil questionnaires that assess PDs, including ASPD, but they are mainly used by researchers. Formal neuropsychological assessment of cognition, memory, and attention can help to pinpoint specific learning or other cognitive deficits that are common in ASPD. Antisocial persons generally score about 10 points lower than people without ASPD on traditional IQ tests and are also more likely to show evidence of learning disabilities (Moffitt 1993b; Raine 2018). Understanding a patient's specific learning disabilities may help identify goals for therapy or rehabilitation.

A medical history is helpful because of the antisocial person's tendency to engage in impulsive or risky behavior. This behavior places the individual at risk for accidental injuries, closed-head injuries, and sexually transmitted diseases, including HIV and hepatitis C (Brooner et al. 1993). The presence of tattoos has traditionally been associated with ASPD. Even as their frequency in the general population has increased, tattoos continue to be associated with risk-taking behaviors, such as greater use of alcohol or other drugs and criminality (Laumann and Derick 2006). Tattoos are especially prevalent in prison populations, where they may have special significance by indicating individual or group identity (Cardasis et al. 2008).

Differential Diagnosis

The differential diagnosis of ASPD includes other PDs (e.g., borderline PD, narcissistic PD), substance use disorders, psychotic and mood disorders, intermittent explosive disorder, and medical conditions such as temporal lobe epilepsy (Black 2013). Chronic or intermittent alcohol or drug use can contribute to the development of antisocial behavior, either as a by-product of the intoxication itself or as a result of a drug habit that needs financial support. Psychoses or bipolar disorder can also lead to violent or assaultive behavior and should be considered as a cause of antisocial behavior. Psychotic patients occasionally commit criminal offenses, but such behavior typically results from psychotic thought processes. Intermittent explosive disorder involves isolated episodes of assaultive or destructive behavior, but there is usually no history of childhood conduct disorder or other features of ASPD, such as a pattern of chronic irresponsibility or failure to honor obligations. Medical explanations for antisocial behavior that need to be ruled out include temporal lobe epilepsy, which can cause random outbursts of violence, and tumors or strokes, which could lead to personality changes.

ASPD needs to be distinguished from borderline PD, a syndrome characterized by the presence of unstable moods, relationships, and behaviors (e.g., self-harm) diagnosed predominantly in women. Although ASPD and borderline PD are often comorbid, they are fundamentally distinct (Paris et al. 2013).

The differential diagnosis in children with conduct disorder includes oppositional defiant disorder, ADHD, autism spectrum disorder, and psychotic and mood disorders, all of which can be associated with sporadic verbal outbursts or physical assaults. Arguably the most difficult differentiation is that between conduct disorder and oppositional defiant disorder. The child with oppositional defiant disorder is difficult and uncooperative, but his or her behavior generally does not involve outright aggression, destruction of property, theft, or deceit, as with conduct disorder. A child with ADHD may be inattentive, hyperactive, or disruptive but usually does not violate the rights of others or societal norms.

Both ASPD and conduct disorder are distinguishable from normal behavior. Most children experience episodes of rambunctious behavior that can be accompanied by inappropriate language or destructive acts. Similarly, many children or adolescents engage in reckless behavior, vandalism, or even minor criminal activity such as shoplifting, often involving peers. Isolated acts of misbehavior are inconsistent with the diagnosis of either conduct disorder or ASPD, which involve repetitive acts of misbehavior over time. Adults with criminal or antisocial behavior who do not meet criteria for ASPD should be designated as having adult antisocial behavior (see "Other Conditions That May Be a Focus of Clinical Attention" in DSM-5, p. 726).

Clinical Management

The ECA study showed that nearly 20% of participants with ASPD had sought mental health care in the past year (Shapiro et al. 1984), whereas a survey from the United Kingdom showed that nearly 25% of persons with ASPD had sought care in the past year (Ullrich and Coid 2009). Antisocial persons who seek care usually do so for accompanying depression or substance misuse, marital or family issues, anger dyscontrol, or suicidal behavior (Black and Braun 1998), and not ASPD per se.

The mental health care needs of a person with ASPD can generally be addressed in outpatient settings via an array of services (e.g., medication management, individual and family therapy). There is generally little reason to psychiatrically hospitalize antisocial persons, who can be disruptive to the ward milieu (Black 2013). The exception is when a person needs a safe environment because of recent (or imminent) suicidal behavior or recent violent or assaultive acts, or for the treatment of alcohol or drug withdrawal.

Pharmacotherapy

No medications have been approved by the U.S. Food and Drug Administration to treat ASPD. Medications are sometimes used "off-label" to treat antisocial persons, generally for their aggressive behaviors and irritability, or, more often, for their co-occurring disorders, such as major depression or an anxiety disorder (Black 2017).

The use of psychotropic medications to treat ASPD was reviewed by the National Institute for Health and Care Excellence (NICE) in the United Kingdom (National Collaborating Centre for Mental Health 2009). The review was unable to identify any randomized controlled trials conducted in persons with ASPD. The report concluded that the sparse evidence did not support the routine use of medication for antisocial persons, but that medication for co-occurring disorders should be used according to guidelines for the disorder in question (e.g., major depression). NICE cautioned clinicians to be aware of the poor adherence, high attrition, and potential for misuse of prescription medication common to these patients. Similarly, a Cochrane Database review found that the body of evidence was insufficient to allow conclusions about the use of drug treatments for ASPD (Khalifa et al. 2010).

Nonetheless, several drugs have been shown to reduce aggression, a target symptom of many antisocial persons, and these drugs may be helpful in carefully selected patients. Lithium carbonate has been found to reduce anger, threatening behavior, and assaults in prison inmates (Sheard et al. 1976), as well as bullying, fighting, and temper outbursts in aggressive children (Campbell et al. 1995). The anticonvulsant phenytoin has been shown to reduce impulsive aggression in prison settings (Barratt et al. 1991), whereas divalproex has been found to reduce temper outbursts and mood lability in disruptive youths (Donovan et al. 2000).

Antipsychotic medications have also been shown to deter aggression in adults as well as youths with conduct disorder (Reyes et al. 2006; Walker et al. 2003). Although there are no trials of second-generation antipsychotics in individuals with ASPD, case reports suggest that these medications may be helpful. In one report, four antisocial men with aggressive behavior received quetiapine (Walker et al. 2003). Following treatment, the men were less irritable, impulsive, and aggressive. In a single case report, a man with ASPD improved after being given risperidone for violent behavior (Hirose 2001).

Other drugs, including carbamazepine, valproate, propranolol, buspirone, and trazodone, have been used to treat aggression in persons with brain injury, intellectual disability, or impulsive-aggressive PDs (Black 2013). Response to medication is variable, and although some patients improve, others fail to improve at all. When improvement occurs, it tends to be partial; improvement may mean only that the individual has fewer outbursts than before or has a "longer fuse," giving him or her more time to reflect before lashing out. Because these drugs target symptoms found in ASPD, it is possible that they may be effective in antisocial persons.

As recommended by NICE (National Collaborating Centre for Mental Health 2009), psychotropic medication can be targeted to treat co-occurring disorders. Mood and anxiety disorders are common in persons with ASPD. These disorders may respond to treatment with antidepressant or tranquilizing medications. Similarly, bipolar patients with antisocial behavior can be treated with mood stabilizers, such as lithium carbonate, carbamazepine, or valproate. Benzodiazepines should be avoided because they have the potential to increase "acting-out" behaviors (e.g., aggressive outbursts), as has been shown in patients with borderline PD (Cowdry and Gardner 1988). Furthermore, the drugs can be habit forming and should be avoided in patients prone to addiction, such as people with ASPD. Stimulant medications can be used to reduce symptoms of co-occurring ADHD. Caution should be used before prescribing potentially addictive stimulants such as methylphenidate or dextroamphetamine. Use of these agents should be preceded by trials with nonaddicting alternatives, such as bupropion, clonidine, or atomoxetine (Black 2017).

Psychological Treatments

According to NICE and the Cochrane Database reviews, insufficient data are available to assess the value of psychotherapy in persons with ASPD (Gibbon et al. 2010). Complicating these reviews is the fact that most studies reviewed involved participants other than those with ASPD. NICE identified one randomized controlled trial involving subjects with ASPD: Davidson et al. (2009) compared cognitive-behavioral therapy (CBT) with "usual care" in 52 antisocial men but found no effect of CBT on anger or verbal aggression. Nonetheless, Davidson et al. (2010) reported, "The view from the ground…was that doing [CBT] was helpful in reducing antisocial behaviours and changing thinking" (p. 94). They recommended that therapists be aware of personal risks while carrying out therapy and be skilled at modifying session content and their behavior to control levels of "high affect." Although this research and other early data suggest that CBT can be helpful, only larger and longer-term studies will reveal its true effectiveness.

Individual psychotherapy has long been used with antisocial patients, and CBT models, such as that employed by Davidson et al. (2009), have been developed for individuals with PDs and patterned after those models created for the treatment of major depression or the anxiety disorders. According to Beck et al. (2004), the goal of CBT is to "improve moral and social behavior through enhancement of cognitive functioning" (p. 168). To achieve these aims, the therapist focuses on evaluating situations in which a patient's distorted beliefs and attitudes may have interfered with interpersonal functioning or in achieving goals. Once the patient has gained an understanding of how he or she has contributed to his or her own problems, the therapist can help the patient to gradually make sensible changes in his or her thinking and behavior. Guidelines are set for the patient's involvement, including regular attendance, active participation, and completion of homework outside of office visits. CBT may be helpful to persons with mild antisocial disorders who possess some insight and have reason to improve—for example, those who risk losing a spouse or job if their behavior is not controlled.

The CBT model described by Beck et al. (2004) for antisocial persons focuses on evaluating situations in which a patient's distorted beliefs and attitudes interfere with functioning or achieving success. For example, unable to assess his actions critically, an antisocial man may attribute a history of work conflicts to unjust persecution or other factors beyond his control, never pausing to examine the consequences of his actions. Working together, patient and therapist develop a problem list to help clarify problems and expose tensions, and to show how—and when—they interfere with daily life. Once identified, cognitive distortions that underlie each problem are systematically exposed and challenged. Some of the distortions most common to ASPD, as outlined by Beck et al. (2004), include the following:

- *Justification*—the patient's belief that his desires are adequate grounds for his actions
- *Thinking is believing*—a tendency to assume that his thoughts and feelings are correct simply because they occur to him
- *Personal infallibility*—the idea that he can do no wrong
- *Feelings make facts*—the conviction that his decisions are always right when they feel good
- *The impotence of others*—a belief that everyone else's views are irrelevant unless they directly affect the patient's immediate circumstances
- *Low-impact consequences*—the notion that the results of his behaviors will not affect him

More recently, Mitchell et al. (2015) have emphasized the need to reduce the individual's criminal and manipulative behaviors because of the harm they cause to others and society, even though such behaviors can be perceived as rewarding, legitimate, and justifiable by the patient. They recommend a collaborative strategy employing motivational interviewing techniques to encourage the patient to make needed changes.

Another therapy model for antisocial persons that has shown promise is mentalization-based therapy (MBT; Bateman and Fonagy 2019), which has a theoretical basis in attachment theory. Mentalizing is considered a key component of self-identity and a central aspect of interpersonal relationships and social function. Developed for people with borderline PD, MBT has been adapted to focus on the unique mentalizing problems of ASPD, such as showing overcontrol of their "emotional states within well-structured, schematic attachment relationships" (pp. 182–183). A subanalysis of data from a trial of MBT in persons with borderline PD, some of whom had comorbid ASPD, showed that MBT was more effective than a control condition (Bateman 2013; Bateman and Fonagy 2019).

Antisocial persons often possess traits that interfere with the process of psychotherapy and make working with them difficult; these traits include their tendency to be impulsive, blame others, and have difficulty in developing trust (Strasburger 1986). Therapists must be aware of their own feelings and remain vigilant to prevent countertransference from disrupting therapy. No matter how determined the therapist may be to help an antisocial patient, it is possible that the patient's criminal past, irresponsibility, and unpredictable tendency toward violence may render him or her thoroughly unlikable (Black 2013). Mental health professionals should anticipate their emotions and display an attitude of acceptance without moralizing.

Persons at the extreme end of the antisocial spectrum may be even more difficult to engage in therapy. According to Hare (1993), the rigid personality structure of psychopathic persons generally resists outside influence. He has observed that in therapy, many such persons simply go through the motions and may even learn skills that help them better manipulate others. Hare is particularly skeptical of group therapy for these individuals. There is no evidence, however, that therapy makes psychopathic persons worse (D'Silva et al. 2004).

Although therapy may not help those at the extreme end of the antisocial spectrum, Beck et al. (2004) point out that antisocial people are unfairly labeled as unable to profit from therapy, which they call the "untreatability myth." Treatment may be challenging, but CBT is one approach that may help some antisocial persons develop the capacity to make appropriate decisions and get their lives on track.

Abuse of alcohol and drugs is common among antisocial persons and may aggravate antisocial symptoms. Once withdrawal has been medically managed, the patient can be referred to a specialized treatment program, the goal of which should be abstinence. Antisocial individuals who abuse substances and who achieve abstinence are less likely to engage in antisocial or criminal behaviors, and also have fewer family conflicts and emotional problems (Cacciola et al. 1996). Patients should be encouraged to attend meetings of Alcoholics Anonymous or similar organizations (e.g., Narcotics Anonymous). Gambling disorder is also common in those with ASPD; these patients should be encouraged to attend Gamblers Anonymous (Black 2013).

Antisocial people with spouses and families may benefit from marriage and family counseling. Allowing family members into the process may help antisocial persons realize the impact of their disorder on others. Therapists who specialize in family counseling may address the antisocial person's difficulties in maintaining enduring attachments, inability to be an effective parent, problems with dishonesty and irresponsibility, and anger and hostility that can contribute to domestic violence (Dutton and Golant 1995).

For juvenile offenders, treatment programs that emphasize behavior modification or skills training may produce modest benefits and reduce recidivism (Lipsey 1992). Traditional counseling and deterrent strategies such as "shock" incarceration have generally been unhelpful. With shock incarceration, offenders receive stiff sentences to "shock" them into improving; once they are incarcerated, the sentence is reduced. "Scared straight"–type programs, in which troubled youth visit prisons to frighten them out of crime, are also unsuccessful (Gibbons 1981). More recently, "boot camps" or "wilderness" programs have garnered attention; in an attempt to foster prosocial behavior, troubled youth are placed in isolated "camps" away from negative influences for experiences that foster bonding and trust with similarly disturbed kids. Whether these programs offer more than transitory benefit has not been demonstrated (Bottcher and Ezell 2005).

Family therapy may offer the best help for dealing with children with a conduct disorder (Sholevar 2001). Treatment should focus on enhancing parental management skills to improve communication and to provide more effective and consistent discipline. Parents can learn to supervise the child more effectively, and to steer impressionable children away from troubled peers. Parents also can learn skills to help stop misbehavior before it escalates to violence, which may eventually help reduce their child's risk for ASPD.

Perhaps the best-known family intervention for targeting violence in antisocial youth is multisystemic therapy (MST), developed by Henggeler et al. (1996). Treatment goals are developed in collaboration with the youth and parents. A meta-analysis by van der Stouwe et al. (2014) showed that MST had significant treatment effects on delinquency and psychopathology, substance use, and family and peer factors.

Conclusion

Antisocial behavior has been clinically recognized for over two centuries, is common, and is disruptive to individuals, families, and society. There is a full spectrum of severity, ranging from psychopathic behavior at the severe end to milder adult antisocial behavior at the other. The disorder is common in the general population, with a male preponderance. Although antisocial behaviors improve or even remit in some persons, the majority of individuals with these behaviors have lifelong, recurrent behavioral problems, including criminality. The cause of antisocial behavior is unknown, but it is likely that both genetic and environmental factors are involved in its development. There are no standard or proven treatments. Anticonvulsants, lithium, and antipsychotics have been shown to reduce aggression and may benefit some antisocial persons. Pharmacological treatment should focus on targeting co-occurring disorders such as major depression or bipolar disorder. Substance use disorders should be treated with the aim of achieving abstinence; this may reduce antisocial symptoms. CBT and mentalizing models have been developed for antisocial persons and may help those with milder syndromes. Prevention strategies targeting troubled children may offer hope to parents and their troubled offspring.

References

American Psychiatric Association: Diagnostic and Statistical Manual: Mental Disorders. Washington, DC, American Psychiatric Association, 1952

American Psychiatric Association: Diagnostic and Statistical Manual of Mental Disorders, 2nd Edition. Washington, DC, American Psychiatric Association, 1968

American Psychiatric Association: Diagnostic and Statistical Manual of Mental Disorders, 3rd Edition. Washington, DC, American Psychiatric Association, 1980

American Psychiatric Association: Diagnostic and Statistical Manual of Mental Disorders, 3rd Edition, Revised. Washington, DC, American Psychiatric Association, 1987

American Psychiatric Association: Diagnostic and Statistical Manual of Mental Disorders, 4th Edition. Washington, DC, American Psychiatric Association, 1994

American Psychiatric Association: Diagnostic and Statistical Manual of Mental Disorders, 5th Edition. Arlington, VA, American Psychiatric Association, 2013

Andreasen NC, Rice J, Endicott J, et al: The family history approach to diagnosis: how useful is it? Arch Gen Psychiatry 43:421–429, 1986

Åsberg M, Träskman L, Thoren P: 5-HIAA in the cerebrospinal fluid: a biochemical suicide predictor? Arch Gen Psychiatry 33:1193–1197, 1976

Barratt ES, Kent TA, Bryant SG, et al: A controlled trial of phenytoin in impulsive aggression. J Clin Psychopharmacology 11:388–389, 1991

Bateman A: Antisocial personality disorder: a mentalizing framework. Focus 11:178–186, 2013

Bateman A, Fonagy P: Mentalization-based treatment of borderline and antisocial personality disorder, in Contemporary Psychodynamic Psychotherapy. Edited by Kealy D, Ogrodniczuk JS. Cambridge, MA, Academic Press, 2019, pp 133–148

Beck A, Freeman A, Davis D: Antisocial personality disorder, in Cognitive Therapy of Personality Disorders, 2nd Edition. Edited by Beck AT, Freeman A, Davis DD. New York, Guilford, 2004, pp 162–176

Bell RQ, Chapman M: Child effect in studies using experimental or brief longitudinal approaches to socialization. Dev Psychol 22:595–603, 1986

Black DW: Bad Boys, Bad Men: Confronting Antisocial Personality Disorder (Sociopathy), Revised and Updated. New York, Oxford University Press, 2013

Black DW: Treatment of antisocial personality disorder. Curr Treat Options Psychiatry, 4:295–302, 2017

Black DW, Andreasen NC: Introductory Textbook of Psychiatry, 7th Edition. Washington, DC, American Psychiatric Association Publishing, 2021

Black DW, Braun D: Antisocial patients: a comparison of persons with and persons without childhood conduct disorder. Ann Clin Psychiatry 10:53–57, 1998

Black DW, Baumgard CH, Bell SE: The long-term outcome of antisocial personality disorder compared with depression, schizophrenia, and surgical conditions. Bull Am Acad Psychiatry Law 23:43–52, 1995a

Black DW, Baumgard CH, Bell SE: A 16- to 45-year follow-up of 71 men with antisocial personality disorder. Compr Psychiatry 36:130–140, 1995b

Black DW, Baumgard CH, Bell SE, et al: Death rates in 71 men with antisocial personality disorder: a comparison with general population mortality. Psychosomatics 37:131–136, 1996

Black DW, Gunter T, Loveless P, et al: Antisocial personality disorder in incarcerated offenders: clinical characteristics, comorbidity, and quality of life. Ann Clin Psychiatry 22:113–120, 2010

Bottcher J, Ezell ME: Examining the effectiveness of boot camps: a randomized experiment with a long-term follow-up. Journal of Research in Crime and Delinquency 42: 309-332, 2005

Brennan PA, Mednick SA: Genetic perspectives on crime. Acta Psychiatr Scand Suppl 370:19–26, 1993

Brooner RK, Greenfield L, Schmidt CW, et al: Antisocial personality disorder and HIV infection among intravenous drug abusers. Am J Psychiatry 150:53–58, 1993

Burt SA, Donnellan MB, Humbad MN, et al: Does marriage inhibit antisocial behavior? An examination of selection vs causation via a longitudinal twin design. Arch Gen Psychiatry 67:1309–1315, 2010

Butcher JN, Dahlstrom WG, Graham JR, et al: The Minnesota Multiphasic Personality Inventory–2 (MMPI-2): Manual for Administration and Scoring. Minneapolis, University of Minnesota, 1989

Cacciola JS, Alterman AI, Rutherford MJ, et al: Treatment response of antisocial substance abusers. J Nerv Ment Dis 183:166–171, 1996

Cadoret RJ, O'Gorman TW, Troughton E, et al: Alcoholism and antisocial personality: interrelationships, genetic and environmental factors. Arch Gen Psychiatry 42:161–167, 1985

Campbell M, Adams PB, Small AM, et al: Lithium in hospitalized aggressive children with conduct disorder: a double-blind and placebo-controlled study. J Am Acad Child Adolesc Psychiatry 34:445–453, 1995

Cardasis W, Huth-Bocks A, Silk KR: Tattoos and antisocial personality disorder. Personal Ment Health 2:171–182, 2008

Caspi A, McClay J, Moffitt TE, et al: Role of genotype in the cycle of violence in maltreated children. Science 297:851–854, 2002

Cleckley H: Mask of Sanity: An Attempt to Clarify Some Issues About the So-Called Psychopathic Personality, 5th Edition (1941). St Louis, MO, Mosby, 1976

Coid J, Ullrich S: Antisocial personality disorder is on a continuum with psychopathy. Compr Psychiatry 51:426–433, 2010

Compton WM, Conway KP, Stinson FS, et al: Prevalence, correlates, and comorbidity of DSM-IV antisocial personality syndromes and alcohol and specific drug use disorders in the United States: results from the National Epidemiologic Survey on Alcohol and Related Conditions. J Clin Psychiatry 66:677–685, 2005

Cowdry RW, Gardner DL: Pharmacotherapy of borderline personality disorder: alprazolam, carbamazepine, trifluoperazine, and tranylcypromine. Arch Gen Psychiatry 45:111–119, 1988

Dahlstrom WG, Welsh GS, Dahlstrom LE: An MMPI Handbook. Minneapolis, University of Minnesota Press, 1972

Davidson KM, Tyrer P, Tata P, et al: Cognitive behaviour therapy for violent men with antisocial personality disorder in the community: an exploratory randomized controlled trial. Psychol Med 39:569–577, 2009

Davidson KM, Halford J, Kirkwood L, et al: CBT for violent men with antisocial personality disorder: reflections on the experience of carrying out therapy in MASCOT, a pilot randomized controlled trial. Personal Ment Health 4:86–95, 2010

DeLisi M, Vaughn MG, Gentile DA, et al: Violent video games, delinquency, and youth violence: new evidence. Youth Violence and Juvenile Justice 11:132–142, 2012

Dolan MC: What imaging tells us about violence in antisocial men. Crim Behav Ment Health 20:199–214, 2010

Dolan M, Völlm B: Antisocial personality disorder and psychopathy in women: a literature review on the reliability and validity of assessment instruments. Int J Law Psychiatry 32:2–9, 2009

Donovan SJ, Stewart JW, Nunes EV, et al: Divalproex treatment for youth with explosive temper and mood lability: a double-blind, placebo-controlled crossover design. Am J Psychiatry 157:818–820, 2000

D'Silva K, Duggan C, McCarthy L: Does treatment really make psychopaths worse? A review of the evidence. J Pers Disord 18:163–177, 2004

Dutton DG, Golant SK: The Batterer: A Psychological Profile. New York, Basic Books, 1995

Feighner JP, Robins E, Guze SB, et al: Diagnostic criteria for use in psychiatric research. Arch Gen Psychiatry 26:57–63, 1972

Gibbon S, Duggan C, Stoffers J, et al: Psychological interventions for antisocial personality disorder. Cochrane Database Syst Rev (6):CD007668, 2010

Gibbons DC: Delinquent Behavior, 3rd Edition. Englewood Cliffs, NJ, Prentice Hall, 1981

Glueck S, Glueck E: Unraveling Juvenile Delinquency. Cambridge, MA, Harvard University Press, 1950

Goldstein RB, Powers SI, McCusker J, et al: Gender differences in manifestations of antisocial personality disorder among residential drug abuse treatment clients. Drug Alcohol Depend 41:35–45, 1996

Goldstein RB, Grand BF, Ruan J, et al: Antisocial personality disorder with childhood- vs adolescence-onset conduct disorder: results from the National Epidemiologic Survey on Alcohol and Related Conditions. J Nerv Ment Dis 194:667–675, 2006

Goldstein RB, Dawson DA, Saha TD, et al: Antisocial behavioral syndromes and DSM-IV alcohol use disorders: results from the National Epidemiologic Survey on Alcohol and Related Conditions. Alcohol Clin Exp Res 31:814–828, 2007

Goldstein RB, Dawson DA, Chou P, et al: Antisocial behavioral syndromes and past-year physical health among adults in the United States: results from the National Epidemiologic Survey on Alcohol and Related Conditions. J Clin Psychiatry 69:368–380, 2008

Guze S: Criminality and Psychiatric Disorders. New York, Oxford University Press, 1976

Guze SB, Wolfgram ED, McKinney JK, et al: Psychiatric illness in the families of convicted criminals: a study of 519 first degree relatives. Dis Nerv Syst 28:651–659, 1967

Hare RD: Diagnosis of antisocial personality disorder in two prison populations. Am J Psychiatry 140:887–890, 1983

Hare RD: Twenty years of experience with the Cleckley psychopath, in Unmasking the Psychopath: Antisocial Personality and Related Syndromes. Edited by Reid WJ, Dorr D, Walker JI, et al. New York, WW Norton, 1986, pp 3–27

Hare RD: The Hare Psychopathy Checklist—Revised. North Tonawanda, NY, Multi-Health Systems, 1991

Hare RD: Without Conscience: The Disturbing World of Psychopaths Among Us. New York, Pocket Books, 1993

Hare RD, Neumann CS: The PCL-R assessment of psychopathy: development, structural properties, and new developments, in Handbook of Psychopathy. Edited by Patrick CJ. New York, Guilford, 2006, pp 58–90

Henderson D: Psychopathic States. New York, WW Norton, 1939

Henggeler SW, Cunningham, PB, Pickrel SG, et al: Multisystemic therapy: an effective violence prevention approach for serious juvenile offenders. J Adolesc 19:47–61, 1996

Hirose S: Effective treatment of aggression and impulsivity in antisocial personality disorder with risperidone. Psychiatry Clin Neurosci 55:161–162, 2001

Holzer KJ, Vaughn MG: Antisocial personality disorder in older adults: a critical appraisal. J Geriatr Psychiatry Neurol 30:291–301, 2017

Huesmann LR, Taylor LD: The role of media violence in violent behavior. Annu Rev Public Health 27:393–415, 2006

Juvonen J, Ho AY: Social motives underlying antisocial behavior across middle school grades. J Youth Adolesc 37:747–756, 2008

Kessler RC, McGonagle KA, Zhao S: Lifetime and 12-month prevalence of DSM-III-R psychiatric disorders in the United States: results from the National Comorbidity Survey. Arch Gen Psychiatry 51:8–19, 1994

Khalifa N, Duggan C, Stoffers J, et al: Pharmacological interventions for antisocial personality disorder. Cochrane Database Syst Rev (8):CD007667, 2010

Kiehl KA, Smith AM, Hare RD, et al: Limbic abnormalities in affective processing by criminal psychopaths as revealed by functional magnetic resonance imaging. Biol Psychiatry 50:677–684, 2001

Kiehl KA, Smith AM, Mendrek A, et al: Temporal lobe abnormalities in semantic processing by criminal psychopaths as revealed by functional magnetic resonance imaging. Psychiatry Res 130:27–42, 2004

Krasnova A, Eaton WW, Samuels JF: Antisocial personality and risks of cause-specific mortality: results from the Epidemiologic Catchment Area study with 27 years of follow up. Soc Psychiatry Psychiatr Epidemiol 54:617–625, 2019

Krastins A, Francis AJP, Field AM, et al: Childhood predictors of adulthood antisocial personality disorder symptomatology. Austral Psychol 49:142–150, 2014

Laumann AE, Derick AJ: Tattoos and body piercings in the United States: a national data set. J Am Acad Dermatol 55:413–421, 2006

Lipsey MW: The effect of treatment on juvenile delinquents: results from meta-analysis, in Psychiatry and the Law. Edited by Lösel F, Bender D, Bliesener T. Berlin, De Gruyter, 1992, pp 131–143

Loeber R, Burke JD, Lahey BB: What are adolescent antecedents to antisocial personality disorder? Crim Behav Ment Health 12:24–36, 2002a

Loeber R, Stouthamer-Loeber M, Farrington DP, et al: Editorial introduction: three longitudinal studies of children's development in Pittsburgh: the Developmental Trends Study, the Pittsburgh Youth Study, and the Pittsburgh Girls Study. Crim Behav Ment Health 12:1–23, 2002b

Luntz BK, Widom CS: Antisocial personality disorder in abused and neglected children grown up. Am J Psychiatry 101:670–674, 1994

McGonigal PK, Kerr S, Morgan T, et al: Should childhood conduct disorder be necessary to diagnose antisocial personality disorder in adults? Ann Clin Psychiatry 31:36–43, 2019

Mitchell D, Tafrate RC, Freeman A: Antisocial personality disorder, in Cognitive Therapy of Personality Disorders, 3rd Edition. Edited by Beck AT, Davis DD, Freeman A. New York, Guilford, 2015, pp 346–365

Moffitt T: Adolescence limited and life-course persistent antisocial behavior: a developmental taxonomy. Psychol Rev 100:674–701, 1993a

Moffitt T: The neuropsychology of conduct disorder. Dev Psychopathol 5:135–151, 1993b

Moffitt TE: Life-course persistent versus adolescence limited antisocial behavior, in Developmental Psychopathology, Vol 3: Risk, Disorder, and Adaptation, Second Edition. Edited by Cicchetti D, Cohen DJ. New York, Wiley, 2015, pp 570–598

Myers MG, Stewart DG, Brown SA: Progression from conduct disorder to antisocial personality disorder following treatment for adolescent substance abuse. Am J Psychiatry 155:479–485, 1998

National Collaborating Centre for Mental Health: Antisocial Personality Disorder: Treatment, Management, and Prevention. The National Institute for Health and Clinical Excellence (NICE) Guidelines. National Clinical Practice Guideline No 77. London, RCPsych Publications, 2009

Neugebauer R, Hoek HW, Susser E: Prenatal exposure to wartime famine and development of antisocial personality disorder in early adulthood. JAMA 282:455–462, 1999

Nielsen DA, Goldman D, Virkkunen M, et al: Suicidality and 5-hydroxyindoleacetic acid concentration associated with tryptophan hydroxylase polymorphism. Arch Gen Psychiatry 51:34–38, 1994

North CS, Yutzy SH: Goodwin and Guze's Psychiatric Diagnosis, 6th Edition. New York, Oxford University Press, 2010

North CS, Smith EM, Spitsnagel EL: Is antisocial personality a valid diagnosis in the homeless? Am J Psychiatry 150:578–583, 1993

Paris J, Chenard-Poirier MP, Biskin R: Antisocial and borderline disorders revisited. Compr Psychiatry 54:321–325, 2013

Raine A: Antisocial personality disorder as a neurodevelopmental disorder. Ann Rev Clin Psychol 14:259–289, 2018

Raine A, Venables PH, Williams M: Relationship between central and autonomic measures of arousal at age 15 years and criminality at age 24 years. Arch Gen Psychiatry 47:1003–1007, 1990

Raine A, Lencz T, Bihrle S, et al: Reduced prefrontal grey matter volume and reduced autonomic activity and antisocial personality disorder. Arch Gen Psychiatry 57:119–127, 2000

Raine R, Buchsbaum MS, LaCasse L: Brain abnormalities in murderers indicated by positron emission tomography. Biol Psychiatry 42:495–508, 1997

Rautiainen M-R, Paunio T, Repo-Tiihonen E, et al: Genome-wide association study of antisocial personality disorder. Transl Psychiatry 6:e883, Sep 2016

Reti IM, Samuels JF, Eaton WW, et al: Adult antisocial personality traits are associated with experiences of low paternal care and maternal over-protection. Acta Psychiatr Scand 106:126–133, 2002

Reyes M, Buitelaar J, Toren P, et al: A randomized, double-blind, placebo-controlled study of risperidone maintenance treatment in children and adolescents with disruptive behavior disorders. Am J Psychiatry 163:402–410, 2006

Robins LN: Deviant Children Grown Up: A Sociological and Psychiatric Study of Sociopathic Personality. Baltimore, MD, Williams & Wilkins, 1966

Robins LN: The epidemiology of antisocial personality disorder, in Psychiatry, Vol 3. Edited by Michels RO, Cavenar JO. Philadelphia, PA, Lippincott, 1987, pp 1–14

Robins LN, Price RK: Adult disorders predicted by childhood conduct problems: results from the NIMH Epidemiologic Catchment Area project. Psychiatry 54:116–132, 1991

Robins LN, Murphy GE, Woodruff RA, et al: Adult psychiatric status of black school boys. Arch Gen Psychiatry 24:338–345, 1971

Robins L, Helzer JE, Weissman MM, et al: Lifetime prevalence of specific psychiatric disorders in three sites. Arch Gen Psychiatry 41:949–958, 1984

Rosenstrom T, Ystrom E, Torvik AK, et al: Genetic and environmental structure of DSM-IV criteria for antisocial personality disorder: a twin study. Behav Genet 47:265–277, 2017

Sampson R, Laub J: Crime in the Making: Pathways and Turning Points Through Life. Cambridge, MA, Harvard University Press, 1993

Scarpa A, Raine A: Psychophysiology of anger and violent behavior. Psychiatr Clin North Am 20:375–403, 1997

Shapiro S, Skinner EA, Kesler LG, et al: Utilization of health and mental health services. Arch Gen Psychiatry 14:971–978, 1984

Sheard MH, Marini JL, Bridges CI, et al: The effect of lithium on impulsive aggressive behavior in man. Am J Psychiatry 133:1409–1413, 1976

Sholevar GP: Family therapy for conduct disorders. Child Adolesc Psychiatry Clin N Am 10:501–517, 2001

Slutske WS: The genetics of antisocial behavior. Curr Psychiatry Rep 3:158–162, 2001

Spitzer RL, Endicott J, Robins E: Research diagnostic criteria: rationale and reliability. Arch Gen Psychiatry 35:773–782, 1978

Storebø OJ, Simonsen E: The association between ADHD and antisocial personality disorder. (ASPD): a review. J Atten Disord 20:815–824, 2016

Strasburger LH: The treatment of antisocial syndromes: the therapist's feelings, in Unmasking the Psychopath: Antisocial Personality and Related Syndromes. Edited by Reid WH, Dorr D, Walker JI, et al. New York, WW Norton, 1986, pp 191–207

Tellegen A, Ben-Porath YS, McNulty JL, et al: The MMPI-2 Restructured Clinical Scales: Development, Validation, and Interpretation. Minneapolis, University of Minnesota Press, 2003

Tielbeek JJ, Medland SE, Benyamin B, et al: Unraveling the genetic etiology of adult antisocial behavior: a genome-wide association study. PloS One 7:e45086, 2012

Ullrich S, Coid J: Antisocial personality disorder: comorbid Axis I mental disorders and health service use among a national household population. Personal Ment Health 3:151–164, 2009

Van der Stouwe T, Asscher JJ, Stams GJJM, et al: The effectiveness of Multisystemic Therapy (MST): a meta-analysis. Clin Psychol Rev 34:468–481, 2014

Virkkunen M, Nuutila A, Goodwin FK, et al: Cerebrospinal fluid monoamine metabolite levels in male arsonists. Arch Gen Psychiatry 44:241–247, 1987

Wakschlag LS, Lahey BB, Loeber R, et al: Maternal smoking during pregnancy and risk of conduct disorder in boys. Arch Gen Psychiatry 54:670–676, 1997

Walker C, Thomas J, Allen TS: Treating impulsivity, irritability, and aggression of antisocial personality disorder with quetiapine. Int J Offender Ther Comp Criminol 47(5):556–567, 2003

Widiger TA: Psychopathy and DSM-IV psychopathology, in Handbook of Psychopathy. Edited by Patrick CJ. New York, Guilford, 2006, pp 156–171

Yang Y, Raine A, Narr KL, et al: Localisation of prefrontal white matter in pathological liars. Br J Psychiatry 190:174–175, 2007

Yang Y, Glenn AL, Raine A: Brain abnormalities in antisocial individuals: implications for the law. Behav Sci Law 26:65–83, 2008

Yang Y, Raine A, Narr KL, et al: Localization of deformations within the amygdala of individuals with psychopathy. Arch Gen Psychiatry 66:986–994, 2009

CHAPTER 23

Personality Disorders in the Medical Setting

Sara Siris Nash, M.D., FACLP, FAPA

Jennifer Sotsky, M.D.

Christian Hicks, M.D.

Philip R. Muskin, M.D., M.A., DLFAPA, LFACLP

The challenges of managing patients with maladaptive personality traits or disorders in the medical setting are numerous and long-standing. In the ancient world, Hippocrates and Galen identified disease as a misalignment of the four humors. Importantly, they connected a temperament to each humor: choleric (yellow bile), melancholic (black bile), sanguine (blood), and phlegmatic (phlegm) (Friedman 1990). In the late nineteenth and early twentieth centuries, Jean-Martin Charcot, Pierre Janet, and Sigmund Freud recognized the psychological underpinnings of what was seen as neurological illness. By the 1940s, Helen Flanders Dunbar established the field of psychosomatic medicine, connecting personality types with medical symptoms (Dunbar 1948; Gorfinkle and Tager 2003). In the following decades, Franz Alexander, Grete Bibring, and Ralph Kahana related illness and illness behavior to psychodynamics and personality styles (Kahana and Bibring 1964). From these insights into how patients respond to illness grew a field that explored the meaning of illness to patients. The subjective experience of and response to illness can be exhibited in objective maladaptive behaviors that are fundamentally connected to patients' underlying attachment styles, coping mechanisms, and defense utilization strategies.

Personality disorders (PDs) are common, occurring in approximately 10% of the general population (Lenzenweger 2008). Some studies have reported rates ranging from 19.7% to 64% when clinical populations are sampled (Diefenbacher et al. 2009; Torgersen 2012). In the general hospital setting, an estimated 20% of patients presenting to consultation-liaison psychiatry services have a PD diagnosis (Laugharne and Flynn 2013). Maladaptive personality patterns may be a symptom of an underlying medical condition, part of a categorical diagnosis of PD, or features of a broader dimensional consideration of a patient's personality. Generally, according to DSM-5 (American Psychiatric Association 2013), all maladaptive personality traits lead to "clinically significant distress or impairment in social, occupational, or other important areas of functioning."

The most prevalent PDs encountered in the medical setting, as aggregated by Torgersen (2012), included borderline (28.5% of patients), avoidant (24.6%), dependent (15%), and obsessive-compulsive (10.5%) PDs. The data emphasize the prevalence of PDs in populations of patients seeking medical care. Important possible sequelae of maladaptive personality were reviewed by Skodol (2018) and remind the clinician of the potential downstream effects of PDs; these include physical injuries due to impulsive and reckless behavior, self-harm, high-risk sexual behavior, comorbid psychiatric disorders, and functional impairment in self-care, work, and interpersonal relationships. In addition, people with PDs are at risk for shortened life spans (Fok et al. 2012). They have increased risks of obesity, pain disorders, and complaints of insomnia (Dixon-Gordon et al. 2018). Cardiovascular disease and arthritis are associated with DSM-IV Cluster A and B PDs (Quirk et al. 2016). Therefore, people with PDs are potentially high utilizers of primary care.

Recognizing and correctly identifying features of maladaptive personality are important for several reasons. Doing so helps to establish all presenting medical and psychiatric diagnoses, to predict possible sequelae, and to formulate effective short- and long-term treatment strategies.

Psychiatric consultation in the medical setting for patients with complex character pathology is often targeted to the management of the "difficult patient." To understand what makes a patient "difficult," a consultant needs to consider not only the vagaries of a particular patient but also the subjective experience of the medical environment. This deliberation allows the consultant to comprehend the effect of the medical setting on the patient, and to appreciate the relationship between the patient's "difficult" behavior and his or her personal history (Lipowski 1970; Lloyd 1977). As detailed by Groves and Muskin (2019), "The importance of individual subjectivity is emphasized through the placement of coping styles, defense mechanisms, personality types, and the appraised meaning of illness as central mediators of the behavioral and emotional responses to the stresses of medical illness" (p. 54).

In this chapter, we explore the role of PDs in the inpatient medical setting. Although inpatient and outpatient environments vary significantly, the ways in which patients behave and the complexities caused by these behavioral manifestations are actually quite similar. First, we examine how the medical hospital provides a uniquely stressful and regressive environment for patients, and how their history of attachment, trauma, and problem solving results in more or less adaptive responses. Second, we use case vignettes to review the commonly experienced behaviors associated with different personality styles in the medical setting. Finally, we consider possible diagnostic patterns associated with personality pathology frequently seen in medical environments.

The Medical Setting

Unique Challenges of the Medical Setting

The hospital is an intrinsically stressful environment. Into this setting arrive individuals already vulnerable due to their underlying illnesses. The hospital can be isolating, frightening, and depersonalizing. Patients are separated from their usual support systems, deprived of privacy, and forced to relinquish control over many highly personal aspects of their lives: what they wear; what, when, and sometimes how they eat; even how they go to the bathroom (Gazzola and Muskin 2003). The seven broad areas of psychological stress for hospitalized patients outlined by Strain and Grossman (1975) remain valid decades after their original paper: the basic threat to narcissistic integrity; fear of strangers; separation anxiety; fear of the loss of love and approval; fear of the loss of control of developmentally achieved functions; fear of loss of or injury to body parts; and reactivation of feelings of guilt and shame and accompanying fears of retaliation for previous transgressions. Pain, sleep disruption, physical disability, and the threat of bodily invasion or even death evoke anxiety and fear (Groves and Muskin 2019). In the frightening environment of the medical hospital, regression is the norm. All patients, regardless of their psychological strengths or weaknesses, experience regression; for those with underlying personality pathology, regression can become problematic, especially around issues such as trust, self-control, and dependency (Geringer and Stern 1986).

Perry and Viederman (1981) described three critical tasks that patients must navigate to successfully cope with a medical illness: 1) patients must admit to themselves and to others that they are ill; 2) they must allow themselves to regress, consciously or unconsciously, and depend on others for care; and 3) they must embrace recovery and resume normal functioning. Each of these undertakings is associated with its own inherent stresses that must be managed. It is important to recognize that the acceptance of illness, psychological regression, and dependency need not be negative states. Health care providers need to understand the meaning of the illness experience for the patient in question so they can deliver care in a way most consistent with and beneficial to the patient's needs.

Patient Responses to Illness and the Medical Setting: The Role of Attachment

How patients manage, both adaptively and maladaptively, in the medical setting derives from their underlying attachment style, coping strategies, and defense mechanisms (Groves and Muskin 2019). Personality styles, personality organization, and PDs are influenced by early life experiences, including trauma and other encounters that heighten or protect against a sense of problematic vulnerability. John Bowlby (1969) recognized patterns of behavior in children separated from their parents during a hospitalization. Attachment theory, the ultimate development of these observations, suggests that the experience of an individual's earliest parent-child relationships directly influences subsequent behavior and the individual's ability to create and maintain other meaningful relationships over time. Dimensions of attachment include interconnected concepts of self-esteem, affect modulation and expression, mentalization, and the ability to develop intimate, cohesive relationships. (See Chapter 7, "Development, Attachment, and Childhood Experiences: A Mentalizing Perspective," in this volume for more on this topic.)

Individuals may have secure or insecure attachment types. Securely attached individuals possess a fundamental sense of self-assurance and the ability to trust others. Their behavior, as seen in both the expression and modulation of affect, reflects an intrinsic sense that attachment figures are reliable and will be helpful in times of stress (Hunter and Maunder 2001). For these people, then, the regression and challenges faced during a medical hospitalization do not necessarily need to be threatening, even if they are difficult. Hospital staff readily empathize with securely attached patients given their ease in flexibly transitioning between their regressed and independent, confident selves (Maunder and Hunter 2009). About 55% of the general population is securely attached (Mickelson et al. 1997). The remainder of the population experiences insecure attachment, which is further subdivided into three categories: avoidant/dismissive, anxious/preoccupied, and disorganized/fearful styles. Each of these subdivisions can be understood by considering a particular self-object dyad, and how that relationship in turn results in affect expression and modulation. Not surprisingly, the types of insecure attachment have a profound effect on the experience of patients and caregivers in the medical setting. Hunter and Maunder have explored attachment theory in the medical setting and considered how insecure attachment styles can be used to understand illness behavior (Hunter and Maunder 2001) as well as health risk and disease (Maunder and Hunter 2001). Their work suggested that "[t]he data can be organized into a model that describe[s] attachment insecurity leading to disease risk through three mechanisms. These are increased susceptibility to stress, increased use of external regulators of affect, and altered help-seeking behavior" (Maunder and Hunter 2001, p. 556).

Individuals with an avoidant/dismissive attachment style see themselves as fundamentally self-confident and self-reliant; it is the other who is untrustworthy, not dependable, or incompetent. This response grows out of the experience of a distant or unreliable caregiver in early life. Avoidant/dismissive individuals tend to eschew distressing situations, and may overregulate and underexpress affect. Because of their fundamental mistrust, patients with this style may underreport symptoms or underutilize care. To successfully help patients with avoidant/dismissive attachment to navigate serious medical illness, medical providers must take great care to ensure the patients' sense of control and independence. Providers must demonstrate flexibility to counteract the often rigid, fixed views of these patients. Because these patients may resent being proscribed treatments, careful attention to relationship building in the hospital may pay dividends later, especially if chronic illness requiring ongoing care is at play (Hunter and Maunder 2001).

Persons with an anxious/preoccupied attachment style do not feel internally secure but do identify the other as being reliable and dependable. The anxiously attached individual is highly needy and dependent, furiously clings to others in an attempt to manage distress, and is difficult to reassure. Affect is underregulated and overexpressed. These patients may experience increased somatization, hypervigilance, and medically unexplained symptoms. They tend to overutilize medical resources, fragment their care, and exhaust their physicians (Maunder and Hunter 2009). Successful management of these patients requires that caregivers are consistent and reliable, meet regularly with the patients (and avoid the inevitable countertransference desire to abandon the patient), and set firm limits and boundaries (Hunter and Maunder 2001).

Patients with disorganized/fearful attachment view neither the self nor the object as safe or tolerable. This style tends to follow early interactions with an unpredictable and hurtful or abusive caretaker. These individuals have difficulty in terms of both self-reflection and the ability to understand the thoughts and behaviors of others. In disorganized attachment, regulation and expression of affect are characteristically inconsistent (Hunter and Maunder 2001). Patients may experience a high level of medically unexplained symptoms while simultaneously underutilizing care (Maunder and Hunter 2009). They may look for increasing amounts of care while at the same time rejecting it. They feel hopelessly unable to fend for themselves and greatly resent their dependency (Hunter and Maunder 2001). Treatment in the medical hospital is thus extremely complicated. In terms of obtaining a therapeutic outcome, Hunter and Maunder (2001) suggest that a

> more realistic goal is to limit the degree to which the patient disorganizes the treatment team, so the team can potentially maintain its function as an effective external regulator and care provider. By conveying, in a sense, that "at least this place operates by these rules" one can reduce the experience of unreliability that will exacerbate their expectation of threat. There is little advantage in interpreting their internal conflict, given their low ability to reflect upon their own or other's mental states. It is better to acknowledge the hostility, but put clear limits around the acceptable expressions of anger. Clarify that there will be no inappropriate closeness, but also clarify what they may realistically expect from staff. (p. 181)

Coping, Defense Mechanisms, and Personality Styles: How to Manage in the Medical Hospital

Coping, which tends to be more active and conscious, and defense mechanisms, which tend to be intrapsychic and unconscious, both play a critical role in how patients respond to conflict and threat. Both responses are regularly utilized in the medical setting, and each can be employed in more or less adaptive ways. Geringer and Stern (1986) reflect on how each distinctive personality style has particular associated coping and defensive mechanisms based in an individual's ability to utilize cognitive, affective, and behavioral defenses. As they explain, "The ways in which patients successfully cope with the psychological tasks associated with medical illness are based on their habitual defensive styles. These defensive patterns are the hallmarks of a patient's character type. Assessment of a patient's character style when supplemented by an understanding of the unique meaning of an illness to each individual can lead to a specific therapeutic intervention designed to help a person deal more successfully with the psychological ramifications of the illness" (Geringer and Stern 1986, p. 252). Groves and Muskin (2019) further explain that by understanding the combination of a patient's subjective experience, personality style, coping strategies, and defensive operations, health care teams can more optimally create a therapeutic alliance and provide interventions in a way that will be acceptable to and accepted by the patient. (See Chapter 11, "Therapeutic Alliance," for a full discussion of alliance building and maintaining with patients with personality pathology.)

Personality styles are universal, dimensional, and not necessarily pathological. They exist on a spectrum, with PDs at the far end (Oldham and Skodol 2000). When individuals are under stress in the medical setting, the more problematic qualities associated with each personality style often become increasingly apparent. This is not a new concept; more than 50 years ago, Kahana and Bibring (1964) wrote a paper, "Personality Styles in Medical Management," in which they highlighted seven archetypal personality styles—dependent, obsessional, histrionic, masochistic, paranoid, schizoid, and narcissistic—and described the associated characteristics, subjective meaning of the illness, and countertransference responses.

A decade and a half after Kahana and Bibring's (1964) paper, James Groves (1978) expanded on these styles as he explored the challenges of ministering to patients who summon dread in their physicians. Although there is some overlap with Kahana and Bibring's seven types, in "Taking Care of the Hateful Patient," Groves identified four pathological character styles of patients: "dependent clingers," "entitled demanders," "manipulative help-rejecters," and "self-destructive deniers." Over time, dependent clingers take initial expressions of genuine gratitude to an unhealthy degree that exhausts and even repulses the doctor who once felt special and powerful in their midst. Physicians must set limits and remind patients that care will continue, but only within the confines of these limits. "This approach is not cruelty or rejection," cautions Groves (1978). "It is in the best interest of patient care to protect the patient from promises that cannot be kept and from illusions that are bound to shatter" (p. 885).

Unlike dependent clingers, entitled demanders express their neediness using tactics such as "intimidation, devaluation and guilt-induction to place the doctor in the role of the inexhaustible supply depot" (Groves 1978, p. 885). Threats and hostility on the part of patients derive from their deep-seated fear of abandonment. By assuming an attitude of entitlement, these patients attempt to override their doctor's power. Physicians must recognize this pattern and not counterattack; after all, as Groves declares, "[e]ntitlement is such a patient's religion and should not be blasphemed" (p. 885). Instead, it is incumbent on physicians to help such patients recognize that what they deserve is excellent care, and that threats and intimidation interfere with that process.

The third style of hateful patient, manipulative help-rejecters, become progressively more pessimistic the more their doctors try to help them. "What is sought," explains Groves (1978), "is an undivorcible marriage with an inexhaustible caregiver" (p. 885). To help physicians avoid developing anxiety or depression (internalized from the patient), Groves suggests that doctors share, to some degree, in their patient's negative viewpoint while continuing to provide regular visits to assuage the patient's underlying fears of abandonment.

Self-destructive deniers are patients who engage in "unconsciously self-murderous behaviors" that lead to rage on the part of caregivers, who so intensely try to save their patients' lives. Physicians may come to embrace a secret desire for these patients to "die and get it over with." Groves (1978) recommends that with self-destructive deniers, physicians do their best to recognize the limitations of the situation and "work with diligence and compassion to preserve the denier as long as possible, just as one does with any other patient with a terminal illness" (p. 887).

Building on the work of Kahana, Bibring, and James Groves, Mark Groves and Philip Muskin (2019) break down the meaning of illness in patients with different personality traits and provide additional valuable management advice. To the dependent patient (at its extreme, the "dependent clinger"), illness is associated with the threat of abandonment. Although initially caregivers feel powerful and important, they quickly become averse to these patients, whom they experience as black holes of need. Recognizing this pattern allows the doctor to create limits, reassure (with the understanding that reassurance may not be easily accepted), schedule visits, and set expectations.

Obsessional patients fear a loss of control, because they enjoy order, organization, rationality, and morality. The unpredictable hospital schedule is disorienting and upsetting. Because the stress of medical illness and the hospital setting may lead to a fear-induced rigidity in patients with this personality type, offering detailed explanations and engaging patients in their care by providing choices and encouraging their input may help mitigate excessive frustration.

Histrionic patients are often entertaining but can be seductive and melodramatic. They are terrified that illness will result in a loss of attractiveness, attention, admiration, or love. Physicians may experience anxious or even erotic countertransference responses. A warm style coupled with firm boundaries from health care providers may reduce anxiety and help patients identify their fears rather than deny them.

Masochistic patients identify as long-suffering martyrs for whom illness represents an ego-syntonic punishment. Physicians typically feel helpless and hopeless, leading to frustration and self-doubt. For such "manipulative help-rejecters," there may be little to do except "share their pessimism" (Groves 1978). Medical interventions may be presented most effectively as yet another cross to bear (Gazzola and Muskin 2003) or as an opportunity to suffer to benefit others (Heiskell and Pasnau 1991), because these patients not only fail to respond to reassurance but may get worse if encouragement is offered.

Paranoid patients fear being attacked. Care teams themselves often feel attacked or accused, which can lead to the unconscious urge to counterattack. As detailed by Groves and Muskin (2011), "[a] calm, firm, direct stance is preferable to an angry, defensive stance or an intrusive, overly warm stance" (p. 53). Schizoid patients similarly may not regularly come to medical attention given their underlying aloof and avoidant style. They see illness as an intrusion, and are typically very difficult to engage in care. Respect for their privacy in the setting of a regular routine in which care is provided at a distance typically has the best results.

With their arrogant, demanding, and devaluing approach, narcissistic patients, such as the entitled demanders (Groves 1978), cause health care teams to bristle. Their seeming vanity and sense of exceptional importance cover an underlying vulnerability heightened by the threat that illness poses to their self-concept of perfection. Frustrated physicians, often made to feel inferior or unimportant, should not respond with anger. Instead, allying with such patients by agreeing that they deserve the best possible care is a more helpful approach.

All of these patient types, if managed adeptly, can be shepherded through the medical system such that they receive optimal care with the least disruption to themselves or others. When a patient's behaviors and the treatment team's approaches misalign, however, great difficulty—or even disaster—may ensue.

Commonly Experienced Behaviors: Case Examples

As described in the previous section, many more patients than those who meet full criteria for a disorder exhibit traits or behaviors associated with personality pathology in the setting of taking on the "sick role." When evaluating a patient for these behaviors, such as hostile outbursts and boundary issues, the clinician should keep in mind a broad differential diagnosis for such behaviors, including mood disorders, cognitive disorders, and medication side effects. Because the etiology of troubling behaviors is often multifactorial, an individual patient may exhibit features of multiple disorders, personality and otherwise. These behaviors represent critical opportunities to engage patients in psychiatric care, even if only briefly, while educating and supporting their other treatment providers. Understanding personality styles allows the psychiatric consultant to tailor a tolerable and therapeutic intervention to each unique patient (Nash et al. 2009). We present the following cases to illustrate commonly experienced behaviors seen by consultation-liaison psychiatrists and to propose management approaches to these situations.

Case Example 1

Ms. B is a 26-year-old intermittently homeless woman who supports herself with sex work. She has a history of type 1 diabetes, end-stage renal disease, depression, multiple past psychiatric hospitalizations, two prior suicide attempts by overdose, nonsuicidal self-injury, and arrest for assault. She has been admitted to the vascular surgery service for a partial foot amputation stemming from poorly controlled diabetes. Six months ago, she required a toe amputation, and ever since has been maintained on opiates for chronic pain. Despite appearing comfortable and being observed laughing and chatting on the phone with friends, she has been demanding intravenous opiate pain medications for severe pain and has threatened to harm herself if the team ignores her ultimatum. She was witnessed manually reopening a healing wound and pulling out an IV, which staff had required multiple attempts to insert. She surreptitiously took a vial of insulin from a nursing cart and later showed it to a staff member while threatening "to end it all because no one is helping me with my pain."

Demanding Pain Medications or Sedatives

In this case, Ms. B exhibits behaviors associated with borderline and antisocial PDs; these are among the most common and serious behaviors psychiatrists must address in hospitalized patients. There is a correlation between PDs and misuse of prescription medications in the hospital setting. Patients with borderline and antisocial PDs have a high degree of substance use and specifically pain medication overuse (Frankenburg and Zanarini 2006). In two studies of 419 internal medicine patients, Sansone and Sansone (2014) confirmed relationships between the self-reported misuse of prescription medications and borderline personality symptomatology.

Reasons for patient misuse of prescription medications are complex and may include sensation seeking, blocking of traumatic memories, experimenting with self-harming behavior, and avoidance of withdrawal in substance dependence (Frankenburg and Zanarini 2006; Sansone and Sansone 2014). Approaching a patient such as Ms. B in a firm and nonjudgmental way, with empathic listening, validation of the patient's frustration, and agreement that the patient is entitled to the best care, can be disarming and helpful. It is important not to neglect a thorough medical evaluation to identify sources of pain, and it is critical to probe for symptoms of an underlying substance use disorder. Motivational interviewing and offering medication-assisted treatment or psychotherapy for opioid use disorder, which is likely co-occurring with Ms. B's PD, would be appropriate. Working in a multidisciplinary fashion, in which the primary team, psychiatrist, and pain experts physically meet together with the patient to construct a detailed treatment plan, minimizes the risk for splitting and outbursts. Even in working with patients with borderline and antisocial traits, an emphasis on how collaboration with the treatment team can result in their needs being met is likely to increase cooperation (Leigh and Streltzer 2015).

Intentional Sabotage of Care, Including Self-Injurious Behavior

Ms. B deliberately interferes with her own care by manually reopening her wound and by pulling out her difficult-to-place IV. Intentional sabotage of medical care is a phenomenon that has long been recognized and discussed in the literature; links between medical sabotage and specific types of personality pathology, however, have not been clarified until more recently (Mergui et al. 2015; Sansone and Sansone 2014). Explanations for medical sabotage, as demonstrated by Ms. B, are complex and often multifactorial. Such self-injurious disruption may, for example, communicate the need to release feelings of tension, express the desire for care, or provide a rationale for increased analgesics. A high percentage of deliberately self-harming patients who presented in a general hospital were found to have Cluster B PDs, specifically borderline PD (BPD) (Mergui et al. 2015). In another study of 332 internal medicine outpatients, 16.7% of participants acknowledged intentionally making their medical situations worse (Sansone and Wiederman 2009b); this phenomenon showed a statistically significant relationship with the measure for BPD that was used in this study. The same research group also looked at a sample of 1,511 internal medicine outpatients and found that 2.9% of participants reported having exercised an injury "on purpose" (Sansone and Wiederman 2013). As expected, there were significant statistical correlations between the endorsement of self-injurious behavior and scores on two self-report measures for BPD, suggesting to the authors that exercising an injury on purpose may be an unusual and covert variant of self-harm behavior. In addition, they found a statistically significant relationship between intentionally preventing wounds from healing and BPD symptomatology (Sansone and Wiederman 2009a).

Management of self-sabotaging patients requires a multifaceted approach. Given the degree of Ms. B's behavioral disinhibition, she would require constant one-to-one observation and/or psychiatric admission. Mergui et al. (2015) note that in their study of hospitalized medical patients, 35% of patients under constant observation were diagnosed with a Cluster B PD. This result is similar to previous studies in which 22%–44% of patients under constant observation were found to be suffering from a PD. Psychotropic medication for impulsivity and mood symptoms may also be necessary. Ms. B is reminiscent of the entitled demander described by Groves (1978). She demonstrates a demanding hostility that can enrage and frighten others but likely masks a deep-seated fear of abandonment. Educating Ms. B's other providers on the meaning and functions of such behavior, and its connection to severe psychopathology, may create an opening for increased empathy. Although it would be difficult to conduct a full BPD-specific treatment, such as dialectical behavior therapy (Linehan 1993), in the acute medical setting, utilizing specific techniques from such treatments, such as safety planning, self-soothing skills, and validation, can be beneficial.

Case Example 2

Mr. A is a 59-year-old single man living alone and working for a nutraceuticals company. He has a long history of poorly controlled type 2 diabetes, hypertension, and heart failure, with chronic nonadherence to treatment. He was recently readmitted to the cardiology service for his third heart failure exacerbation episode in as many months. He has been intermittently refusing medications and expresses suspicion about his providers, including suggesting that they are "probably being paid off by big pharma." He is an avid conspiracy theorist and a self-proclaimed medical expert, spending large amounts of time online. Psychiatric consultations on past admissions have found the patient to have decision-making capacity. Mr. A has no other history of psychiatric treatments and considers himself staunchly "antipsychiatry." His sister, who lives in another state, says he has always been an odd and difficult person. He has been hostile with the primary care team, frequently yelling at them for perceived errors, threatening lawsuits, and making demeaning comments. Psychiatric consultation was requested for "paranoia" and because the patient refused a procedure.

Aggressive, Disruptive Behavior

Through his antagonism, grandiosity, isolation, and eccentricity, Mr. A exhibits features of several PDs. Aggressive or disruptive behavior by patients in the medical setting is closely linked to personality dysfunction. Although various aggressive and disruptive behaviors, such as refusal of treatment, outbursts disproportionate to the situation, or overt intimidation, have been noted in the clinical literature, little empirical research has been undertaken to examine the range of these behaviors (Sansone and Sansone 2014). In a survey of internal medicine patients, Sansone et al. (2011) described the prevalence of 17 disruptive behaviors as well as their relationship to borderline personality symptomatology. Patients with borderline personality behavior symptomatology were significantly more likely than participants without borderline personality behavior to report yelling, screaming, verbal threats, and/or refusing to talk to medical personnel (Sansone et al. 2011). Mr. A makes paranoid statements suggesting that others are trying to take advantage of him. His anger and grandiosity may well be defenses against the intense fear of the weakness and loss of control that accompany his illness. In the absence of substantial literature on recommendations for paranoid patients, practitioners should assume a neutral and calm attitude concerning suspicions, criticisms, and hostility. This patient would benefit from clear, detailed descriptions of interventions without ambiguous language (Nash et al. 2009). In the case of overt aggression or threats, patients such as Mr. A may require medication, such as benzodiazepines or antipsychotics, for agitation. Although borderline patients may experience disinhibition when prescribed benzodiazepines in the outpatient setting, the medication class is useful for rapid control of agitation in patients without delirium in the inpatient medical setting.

Treatment Nonadherence

Nonadherence to recommended treatments has been associated with personality dysfunction (Sansone and Sansone 2014). Although Mr. A likely has significant personality pathology, his background also warrants additional evaluation for other treatable psychiatric conditions that may contribute to nonadherence, such as substance use disorder, depression, or psychosis. Furthermore, an exploration of psychosocial factors leading to nonadherence, such as financial, housing, or relationship problems, may be helpful.

In approaching Mr. A, the clinician should attempt to understand what the illness means to the patient, and how his understanding translates into his perceived sense of threat. Nonadherence to medications and other treatments may function as a means to create medical instability and thus justify ongoing care and attention (Leigh and Streltzer 2015). It may also represent denial of an illness that is intolerably terrifying and overwhelming. Devaluing the treatment team's expertise by insulting them or by refusing their recommendations can be a form of projective identification in which physicians are made to feel powerless and helpless. Engaging in such maladaptive communication does not necessarily mean that the patient lacks capacity to refuse medical recommendations; instead, he may be sharing his anxieties, albeit in a nonproductive way. Mr. A is reminiscent of the self-destructive denier (Groves 1978). Mr. A induces feelings of anger, even murderous rage, and subsequent guilt in his caregivers. Management requires recognizing and discussing the intense countertransference reactions that this patient will inevitably generate. Allowing Mr. A to boast about his strengths, knowledge, and superiority may help him feel less weak and vulnerable, and therefore allow him to feel calmer and be more amenable to treatment. Taking a clear and firm approach to recommendations, and utilizing techniques of motivational interviewing when the patient seems to make decisions that are in conflict with his own interests, can also be useful.

Case Example 3

Ms. C is a 48-year-old divorced woman with two adult children. Her past medical history includes reported chronic Lyme disease, fibromyalgia, and multiple workups for medically unexplained symptoms. She was admitted to the inpatient neurology service for evaluation of headache, initially concerning for meningitis. Ms. C carries a binder with extensive previous records from other admissions. She does not have a primary care doctor, having summarily fired her previous several physicians because "they couldn't handle my complex problems." She is not currently in psychiatric care but was briefly in therapy 5 years ago after the death of her mother, for whom she was a caregiver. Ms. C pages the team throughout the day with numerous questions. She is flirtatious and overly familiar with her male doctors, telling them they are the best doctors with whom she has ever worked. She requested the male medical student's cell phone number, and she has repeatedly offered to set him up on a date with her daughter. The primary team believes that Ms. C is medically stable enough to be discharged, but she has refused; unsure of what else to do, they consulted psychiatry for "anxiety."

Overuse of Care

Ms. C paradoxically both overuses medical care by having multiple extensive workups and underuses it by not having a primary doctor. She exhibits features of dependent, masochistic, and histrionic personality styles, as well as hypochondriasis. Patients like Ms. C who have medically unexplained symptoms are common in the acute medical setting and have elevated rates of medical care utilization, including hospitalizations and total costs (Grover and Kate 2013). Such patients tend to "doctor shop," have higher rates of emergency visits, and are often noncompliant with scheduled appointments, engendering frustration in their physicians (Grover and Kate 2013). In a study of 62 patients with hypochondriasis, over 40% were determined to have PDs (Laugharne and Flynn 2013).

Although Ms. C likely has personality pathology, her case also warrants further evaluation for possible comorbidities such as anxiety and depression, which are found in 40% of patients with medically unexplained symptoms (Laugharne and Flynn 2013). Her masochism causes her to behave as if she were "born to suffer" and her life has been a long series of obligations and disappointments. Like many patients with these features, Ms. C has taken care of a sick family member, her mother, in the past. A helpful and therapeutic approach to working with Ms. C might entail addressing her symptom beliefs, and providing an explanation of physical symptoms that links to psychosocial issues when they are present (Grover and Kate 2013). In addition to reattribution, psychological treatments based on the principles of cognitive-behavioral therapy (CBT) have been evaluated for management of patients with medically unexplained symptoms. CBT has been shown to reduce the number of hospital visits and somatization severity in patients with medically unexplained symptoms (Grover and Kate 2013).

Boundary Issues

Patients with PDs or maladaptive behaviors often exhibit problems with boundaries in the medical setting. Ms. C's difficulty with boundaries appears to stem from her dependent, histrionic, and masochistic traits. Patients similar to Ms. C may initially appear polite and agreeable, but then, in their intense need for care, begin to engage in inappropriate behaviors, such as requesting the physician's personal cell phone number and calling repeatedly. Physicians may initially feel pulled to make special accommodations for such patients, but then become overwhelmed, angered, burned-out, and even desirous of escape.

Individuals with PDs often have intense needs to disrupt professional boundaries—perhaps to be uniquely known by the clinician, to be perceived as special, and to be loved (Sansone and Sansone 2014). These intense needs by the patient can manifest as overtly inappropriate behaviors, such as sexual innuendos or requests for social outings, but also may present more insidiously, such as by addressing the clinician by first name or gift giving. Clinicians need to be extremely wary of colluding with these types of boundary violations, even inadvertently, because doing so may lead to further deterioration of boundaries, culminating in negative clinical, personal, and even legal consequences. If the clinician is unsure about how to respond to a patient's provocative behavior, he or she should consider the "Headlines Test"—that is, how the clinician's behavior would appear to the public if it were publicized in the headlines of the local newspaper (Sansone and Sansone 2014). (See Chapter 19, "Boundary Issues," in this volume for further discussion.)

Akin to the dependent clinger described by Groves (1978), Ms. C appears to have a bottomless wish to be cared for and remain in the dependent sick role. Management of such patients involves creating a structure in which the patient feels cared for but also understands the limits of the doctor-patient relationship. It is useful to discuss in detail when and how it is most appropriate for the patient to reach the provider. The provider can empathically set limits by arranging predictable check-in times to alleviate the patient's distress. The patient will likely feel reassured by this attentiveness and caring without inappropriate closeness.

Masochistic patients suffer from an intense guilt that makes enjoyment of life difficult; the sick role can be addictive in how it functions as a means through which to forge close relationships with others. Such patients can react negatively to reassurances that might be perceived as minimizing their suffering and jeopardizing their relationships with others that are formed based on illness. Instead, physicians should give validation to these patients' suffering, and express appreciation for their courage and perseverance in the face of pain and hardship (Leigh and Streltzer 2015). Management may also involve discussing building a structure outside of the hospital in which the patient feels cared for and supported, which may prevent problems such as refusal of hospital discharge. This structure should ideally involve close follow-up with a primary doctor who is accustomed to regularly working with such patients and a psychotherapist. (See also Chapter 18, "Collaborative Treatment," in this volume.)

Diagnostic Considerations Related to Personality Pathology

Having outlined the challenges patients face in the medical setting and the types of personality pathology frequently seen, we now focus on important diagnostic considerations for clinicians to keep in mind when encountering abnormal personality or personality change in the general hospital. In this section, we address the strategies that will aid in identification of maladaptive personality traits, differential diagnosis of abnormal personality or personality change, and PDs related to certain medical and psychiatric pathologies seen in the general hospital.

Strategies That Will Aid in Identification of Maladaptive Personality Traits

Medical illness and personality are entangled in complex ways, and if left untreated, PDs can lead to adverse medical outcomes. Clinicians can detect personality pathology through a targeted history, observation of a patient's behavior in the hospital, and sensitivity to countertransference. PDs are common in certain clinical entities, and the role of personality in illness should be considered in these diagnoses. Once it is detected, medical causes of maladaptive personality symptoms should be ruled out. Accurate identification of PDs is important in formulating effective short- and long-term treatment strategies.

Identifying any of the behaviors described in the preceding sections will clue a clinician in to the possibility of personality pathology. As detailed in the earlier case examples, this includes medication or treatment nonadherence, abuse of prescription medications, aggressive and/or disruptive behaviors, intentional sabotage of medical care, boundary violations, and excessive health care utilization patterns (Sansone and Sansone 2014).

DSM-5 systematically outlines criteria for a general PD, which can be an important tool for identifying problematic personality traits. These are listed in Table 23–1.

Another important telltale clue to personality pathology in a patient is a strong countertransference reaction in the clinician (Colli and Ferri 2015; Grayer and Sax 1986; Kernberg 1976). Within the domain of countertransference, the clinician should be mindful of his or her own emotional responses, fantasies, and behaviors; if any of these become atypical, personality pathology within the patient should be strongly considered (Muskin and Haase 2001).

Kernberg (1965) first identified countertransference as a diagnostic tool in the *Journal of the American Psychoanalytic Association*:

> When dealing with borderline or severely regressed patients, as contrasted to those presenting symptomatic neuroses and many character disorders, the therapist tends to experience rather soon in the treatment intensive emotional reactions having more to do with the patient's premature, intense and chaotic transference, and with the therapist's capacity to withstand psychological stress and anxiety, than with any particular, specific problem of the therapist's past. In other words, given reasonably well-adjusted therapists, all hypothetically dealing with the same severely regressed and disorganized patient, their countertransference reactions will be somewhat similar, reflecting the patient's problems much more than any specific problem of the analyst's past....Thus, countertransference becomes an important diagnostic tool, giving information on the degree of regression in the patient and the predominant emotional position of the patient toward the therapist and the changes occurring in this position. (p. 43)

Differential Diagnosis of Abnormal Personality or Personality Change

Once maladaptive traits or personality changes have been identified, ruling out underlying medical pathology is paramount. If personality has changed acutely or subacutely, a comprehensive cognitive assessment should be performed in addition to a medical workup guided by a thorough history, review of systems, and physical examination. Table 23–2 highlights important potential medical causes of personality change and personality pathology, and Table 23–3 lists medications that have neuropsychiatric side effects. Each medical syndrome or medication will have its particular pattern of symptomatology, ranging from mood or anxiety symptoms to psychosis and delirium. Once medical causes of abnormal personality have been ruled out, a psychiatric formulation of abnormal personality traits can be made.

Personality Disorders Related to Medical and Psychiatric Pathologies

PDs have been shown to have epidemiological correlation with other medical and psychiatric diagnoses. Table 23–4 summarizes data on the comorbidity of PD with specific other diagnoses. This table is not intended to be a definitive or inclusive survey

---

TABLE 23–1.   **DSM-5 criteria for general personality disorder**

A. An enduring pattern of inner experience and behavior that deviates markedly from the expectations of the individual's culture. This pattern is manifested in two (or more) of the following areas:

   1. Cognition (i.e., ways of perceiving and interpreting self, other people, and events).

   2. Affectivity (i.e., the range, intensity, lability, and appropriateness of emotional response).

   3. Interpersonal functioning.

   4. Impulse control.

B. The enduring pattern is inflexible and pervasive across a broad range of personal and social situations.

C. The enduring pattern leads to clinically significant distress or impairment in social, occupational, or other important areas of functioning.

D. The pattern is stable and of long duration, and its onset can be traced back at least to adolescence or early adulthood.

E. The enduring pattern is not better explained as a manifestation or consequence of another mental disorder.

F. The enduring pattern is not attributable to the physiological effects of a substance (e.g., a drug of abuse, a medication) or another medical condition (e.g., head trauma).

Source. Criteria reprinted from American Psychiatric Association: *Diagnostic and Statistical Manual of Mental Disorders*, 5th Edition. Arlington, VA, American Psychiatric Association, 2013. Copyright © 2013. American Psychiatric Association. Used with permission.

of correlation or prevalence rates; rather, its utility will be for the diagnostician to consider a comorbid PD when the listed diagnoses are encountered.

Conclusion

Patients with PDs are commonly encountered in general medical settings. Frequently, psychiatric consultation is requested when the patients' behavior becomes difficult, uncomfortable, or frightening. In this chapter, we explored the reasons behind worsened regressive behavior in the hospital setting and identified the important ways that attachment theory, coping mechanisms, and personality style drive the meaning of the illness in sick patients. We reviewed commonly experienced behaviors and provided case examples to demonstrate how to parlay an academic understanding of personality pathology into useful strategies for managing problematic patient actions. Finally, we considered the complex interconnection between behavioral expression and medical illness, which is essential to the process of making accurate diagnoses and to the ultimate treatment of the patient.

TABLE 23–2.	Medical causes of personality change	

Infectious	Degenerative
Neurosyphilis	Alzheimer's dementia
HAND	Frontotemporal dementia
PANDAS	Dementia with Lewy bodies
Meningoencephalitis	Creutzfeldt-Jacob disease
Nutritional	Huntington's disease
B_{12} deficiency (pernicious anemia)	Vascular
Mercury, lead toxicity	Stroke
Endocrinological	Vascular dementia
Pituitary tumors	Traumatic
Hypo-/hyperthyroidism	Traumatic brain injury
Neoplastic	Seizure
Paraneoplastic syndromes	Temporal lobe epilepsy
CNS tumors	Other genetic
Autoimmune encephalitis	Wilson's disease
SLE, SREAT, anti-LGI1, anti-NMDA, CASPR2, GABA_B, AMPA, anti-Hu/Ma2	

Note. AMPA=α-amino-3-hydroxy-5-methyl-4-isoxazolepropionic acid; CASPR2=contactin associated protein 2; CNS=central nervous system; GABA_B=γ-aminobutyric acid type B; HAND=HIV-associated neurocognitive disorders; Hu/Ma2=example onconeural antibodies; LGI1=leucine-rich glioma-inactivated 1; NMDA=N-methyl-D-aspartate; PANDAS=pediatric autoimmune neuropsychiatric disorders associated with streptococcal infections; SLE=systemic lupus erythematosus; SREAT=steroid-responsive encephalopathy associated with auto-immune thyroiditis.
Source. Adapted from Muskin and Haase 2001; Wingfield et al. 2011.

TABLE 23–3.	Medications with neuropsychiatric side effects

Herbal medications

Steroids

Narcotics (especially meperidine and pentazocine)

Benzodiazepines

Stimulants (including theophylline)

Parkinson's treatments (dopa agonists)

Anticholinergics (including topical)

Antineoplastics

Barbiturates

Antiretrovirals

Cimetidine

Metoclopramide

Yohimbine

Metrizamide

Cardiac drugs (especially propranolol, captopril, clonidine, digitalis, lidocaine, methyldopa, mexiletine, reserpine, and disopyramide)

Source. Adapted from Muskin and Haase 2001.

TABLE 23–4.　**Prevalence of comorbid personality disorder (PD) in certain diagnoses**

Diagnosis	Prevalence of comorbid PD, %	Study
Substance use disorder	57.0	Rounsaville et al. 1998
Somatic symptom disorder	25	Bornstein and Gold 2008
Chronic pain	30 (with borderline personality disorder)	Sansone and Sansone 2012
Idiopathic chronic pelvic pain	13.3	Ehlert et al. 1999
Psychogenic nonepileptic seizures	50.6	Reuber et al. 2004
Factitious disorder	83	Ehlers and Plassmann 1994
Refractory chronic daily headache (inpatients)	26	Lake et al. 2009
Obesity	27	Sansone and Sansone 2013
Multiple allergies to medications	Anecdotal correlation	Sansone and Sansone 2014
HIV-positive status (men)	33	Perkins et al. 1993
Fibromyalgia	31.1	Uguz et al. 2010
Eating disorders	72	Wonderlich et al. 1990
Deliberate self-harm	46	Haw et al. 2001
Chronic fatigue syndrome	39	Henderson and Tannock 2004

References

American Psychiatric Association: Diagnostic and Statistical Manual of Mental Disorders, 5th Edition. Arlington, VA, American Psychiatric Association, 2013

Bornstein RF, Gold SH. Comorbidity of personality disorders and somatization disorder: a meta-analytic review. J Psychopathol Behav Assess 30:154–161, 2008

Bowlby J: Attachment and Loss, Vol. 1: Attachment. London, Hogarth Press/Institute of Psycho-Analysis, 1969

Colli A, Ferri M: Patient personality and therapist countertransference. Curr Opin Psychiatry 28:46–56, 2015

Diefenbacher A, Golombek U, Strain J: Personality disorders in consultation-liaison psychiatry: an empirical investigation. European Psychiatry 24:S1072, 2009

Dixon-Gordon KL, Conkey LC, Whalen DJ: Recent advances in understanding physical health problems in personality disorders. Curr Opin Psychol 21:1–5, 2018

Dunbar HF: Synopsis of Psychosomatic Diagnosis and Treatment. St Louis, MO, CV Mosby, 1948

Ehlers W, Plassmann R: Diagnosis of narcissistic self-esteem regulation in patients with factitious illness (Munchausen syndrome). Psychother Psychosom 62:69–77, 1994

Ehlert U, Heim C, Hellhammer DH: Chronic pelvic pain as a somatoform disorder. Psychother Psychosom 68:87–94, 1999

Fok ML, Hayes RD, Chang CK, et al: Life expectancy at birth and all-cause mortality among people with personality disorder. J Psychosom Res 73:104–107, 2012

Frankenburg FR, Zanarini MC: Personality disorders and medical comorbidity. Curr Opin Psychiatry 19:428–431, 2006

Friedman HS (ed): Personality and Disease. Oxford, UK, Wiley, 1990

Gazzola L, Muskin PR: The impact of stress and the objectives of psychosocial interventions, in Psychosocial Treatment for Medical Conditions: Principles and Techniques. Edited by Schein LA, Bernard HS, Spitz HI, et al. New York, Brunner-Routledge, 2003, pp 373–476

Geringer ES, Stern TA: Coping with medical illness: the impact of personality types. Psychosomatics 27:251–261, 1986

Gorfinkle KS, Tager F: Psychosocial factors affecting medical conditions, in Psychosocial Treatment for Medical Conditions: Principles and Techniques. Edited by Schein LA, Bernard HS, Spitz HI, et al. New York, Brunner-Routledge, 2003, pp 50–52

Grayer ED, Sax PR: A model for the diagnostic and therapeutic use of countertransference. Clin Soc Work J 14:295–309, 1986

Grover S, Kate N: Somatic symptoms in consultation-liaison psychiatry. Int Rev Psychiatry 25:52–64, 2013

Groves JE: Taking care of the hateful patient. N Engl J Med 298:883–887, 1978

Groves MA, Muskin PR: Psychological responses to illness, in The American Psychiatric Publishing Textbook of Psychosomatic Medicine: Psychiatric Care of the Medically Ill, 2nd Edition. Edited by Levenson JL. Washington, DC, American Psychiatric Publishing, 2011, pp 45–70

Groves MS, Muskin PR: Psychological responses to illness, in The American Psychiatric Association Publishing Textbook of Psychosomatic Medicine and Consultation-Liaison Psychiatry, 3rd Edition. Edited by Levenson JL. Washington, DC, American Psychiatric Association Publishing, 2019, pp 53–81

Haw C, Hawton K, Houston K, et al: Psychiatric and personality disorders in deliberate self-harm patients. Br J Psychiatry 178:48–54, 2001

Heiskell LE, Pasnau RO: Psychological reaction to hospitalization and illness in the emergency department. Emerg Med Clin North Am 9:207–218, 1991

Henderson M, Tannock C: Objective assessment of personality disorder in chronic fatigue syndrome. J Psychosom Res 56:251–254, 2004

Hunter JJ, Maunder RG: Using attachment theory to understand illness behavior. Gen Hosp Psychiatry 23:177–182, 2001

Kahana RJ, Bibring G: Personality types in medical management, in Psychiatry and Medical Practice in a General Hospital. Edited by Zinberg NE. New York, International Universities Press, 1964, pp 108–123

Kernberg OF: Notes on countertransference. J Am Psychoanal Assoc 13:38–56, 1965

Kernberg OF: Objects-Relations Theory and Clinical Psychoanalysis. New York, Jason Aronson, 1976

Lake A, Saper J, Hamel R: Comprehensive inpatient treatment of refractory chronic daily headache. Headache 49:555–562, 2009

Laugharne R, Flynn A: Personality disorders in consultation-liaison psychiatry. Curr Opin Psychiatry 26:84–89, 2013

Leigh H, Streltzer J: The patient's personality, personality types, traits, and disorders in the CL setting, in Handbook of Consultation-Liaison Psychiatry, 2nd Edition. Edited by Leigh H, Streltzer J. New York, Springer, 2015, pp 345–366

Lenzenweger MF: Epidemiology of personality disorders. Psychiatr Clin North Am 31:395–403, 2008

Linehan MM: Cognitive-Behavioral Treatment of Borderline Personality Disorder. New York, Guilford, 1993

Lipowski ZJ: Physical illness, the individual and the coping process. Psychiatry Med 1:91–102, 1970

Lloyd G: Psychological reactions to physical illness. Br J Hosp Med 18:352–358, 1977

Maunder RG, Hunter JJ: Attachment and psychosomatic medicine: developmental contributions to stress and disease. Psychosom Med 63:556–567, 2001

Maunder RG, Hunter JJ: Assessing patterns of adult attachment in medical patients. Gen Hosp Psych 31:123–130, 2009

Mergui J, Raveh D, Gropp C, et al: Prevalence and characteristics of cluster B personality disorder in a consultation-liaison psychiatry practice. Int J Psychiatry Clin Pract 19:65–70, 2015

Mickelson KD, Kessler RC, Shaver PR: Adult attachment in a nationally representative sample. J Pers Soc Psychology 73:1092–1106, 1997

Muskin PR, Haase EK: Personality disorders, in Textbook of Primary Care Medicine, 3rd Edition. Edited by Noble J (editor-in-chief). St Louis, CV Mosby, 2001, pp 458–464

Nash SS, Kent LK, Muskin PR: Psychodynamics in medically ill patients. Harv Rev Psychiatry 17:389–397, 2009

Oldham JM, Skodol AE: Charting the future of Axis II. J Pers Disord 14:17–29, 2000

Perkins DO, Davidson EJ, Leserman J, et al: Personality disorder in patients infected with HIV: a controlled study with implications for clinical care. Am J Psychiatry 150:309–315, 1993

Perry S, Viederman M: Management of emotional reactions to acute medical illness. Med Clin North Am 65:3–14, 1981

Quirk SE, Berk M, Chanen AM, et al: Population prevalence of personality disorder and associations with physical health comorbidities and health care utilization: a review. Personal Disord 7:136–146, 2016

Reuber M, Pukrop R, Bauer J, et al: Multidimensional assessment of personality in patients with psychogenic non-epileptic seizures. J Neurol Neurosurg Psychiatry 75:743–748, 2004

Rounsaville BJ, Kranzler HR, Ball S, et al: Personality disorders in substance abusers: relation to substance use. J Nerv Ment Dis 186:87–95, 1998

Sansone RA, Sansone LA: Chronic pain syndromes and borderline personality. Innov Clin Neurosci 9:10–14, 2012

Sansone RA, Sansone LA: The relationship between borderline personality and obesity. Innov Clin Neurosci 10:36–40, 2013

Sansone RA, Sansone LA: Personality disorders in the medical setting, in The American Psychiatric Publishing Textbook of Personality Disorders, Second Edition. Edited by Oldham JM, Skodol AE, Bender DS. Arlington, VA, American Psychiatric Publishing, 2014, pp 455–473

Sansone RA, Wiederman MW: Interference with wound healing: borderline patients in psychiatric versus medical settings. Prim Care Companion J Clin Psychiatry 11:271–272, 2009a

Sansone RA, Wiederman MW: Making medical situations worse: patient disclosures in psychiatric versus medical settings. J Med 2:169–171, 2009b

Sansone RA, Wiederman MW: Exercising an injury on purpose: relationships with borderline personality symptomatology. Prim Care Companion CNS Disord 15:PCC.12l01424, 2013

Sansone RA, Farukhi S, Wiederman MW: Disruptive behaviors in the medical setting and borderline personality. Int J Psychiatry Med 41:355–363, 2011

Skodol A: Overview of personality disorders. UpToDate. Last updated May 31, 2018. Available at: https://www.uptodate.com/contents/overview-of-personality-disorders. Accessed August 27, 2020.

Strain JJ, Grossman S: Psychological reactions to medical illness and hospitalization, in Psychological Care of the Medically Ill: A Primer in Liaison Psychiatry. New York, Appleton-Century-Crofts, 1975, pp 23–36

Torgersen S: Epidemiology, in The Oxford Handbook of Personality Disorders. Edited by Widiger TA. New York, Oxford University Press, 2012, pp 186–205

Uguz F, Ciçek E, Salli A, et al: Axis I and Axis II psychiatric disorders in patients with fibromyalgia. Gen Hosp Psychiatry 32:105–107, 2010

Wingfield T, McHugh C, Vas A, et al: Autoimmune encephalitis: a case series and comprehensive review of the literature. QJM 104:921–931, 2011

Wonderlich SA, Swift WJ, Slotnick HB, et al: DSM-III-R personality disorders in eating-disorder subtypes. Int J Eat Disord 9:607–616, 1990

CHAPTER 24

Personality Disorders in the Military Operational Environment

Ricky D. Malone, M.D., Col. (Ret.), M.C., U.S.A.
David M. Benedek, M.D., Col., M.C., U.S.A.

The unique aspects of military life—particularly in times of prolonged involvement in international conflict—may prove particularly challenging for persons with personality disorders (PDs). To the extent that PDs may be defined as pervasive, stable, and inflexible patterns of inner experience and behavior that deviate markedly from the expectations of an individual's culture (American Psychiatric Association 2013), it is evident that the patterns of behavior characterizing the various PDs would prove particularly maladaptive in a military operational environment requiring strict adherence to rules and regulations, limits on personal freedoms, life in harsh and austere environments, frequent and lengthy separations from usual sources of social support, repeated exposure to life-threatening situations, and the potential witnessing of sudden and severe injury or death. Impulsivity, disregard for safety of self or others, and lack of empathy or concern for the needs of others, all of which characterize Cluster B pathology, may compromise mission capability and lead to dangerous situations. The inability to take initiative or reluctance to engage in new activities and the lack of decisiveness observed in avoidant and dependent PDs also interfere with many

All opinions, interpretations, conclusions, and recommendations contained herein are those of the authors and should not be construed as representing the positions or policies of an author's institution including, but not limited to, the Uniformed Services University of the Health Sciences, the United States Department of Veterans Affairs, and the United States Department of Defense.

military occupational tasks. Finally, the emotional and behavioral consequences of difficulty developing and maintaining supportive social relationships experienced by those with Cluster A pathology often declare themselves in deployed environments where service members must live and work in close quarters with little privacy or personal space, often with communal sleeping and shower areas.

Perhaps less obvious is the notion that behaviors composing various PDs also deviate markedly from the expectations of a service member's organizational culture. Although there are certainly cultural differences among members of the U.S. Army, Navy, Air Force, and Coast Guard, all branches of the uniformed services espouse values of honor and integrity, trust for—and dedication to—fellow service members, personal sacrifice, courage, and devotion to duty (Halvorson 2010). While this often sounds like lofty rhetoric, successful members of the military must eventually internalize these values to varying degrees in order to survive the rigors of military life and the dangers of combat. Thus, dysfunctional patterns of inner experience and behavior, including disregard for regulations or social norms, mistrust of others, discomfort in the presence of others, intense feelings of abandonment, exploitation of others, impulsiveness, or inability to maintain interpersonal or occupational commitments, would most certainly deviate from the expectations of persons steeped in military culture. The vignettes throughout this chapter illustrate the idea that behaviors and affective states observed in persons with PDs may become even more apparent to fellow service members during times of occupational stress and may come to the attention of clinicians in a variety of ways, including self-referral, referral from other (i.e., non–mental health) care providers, or referral from military command. The following vignette illustrates how some of these personality traits may manifest in the military environment.

Case Example 1

Vanessa Jenkins, an 18-year-old National Guard private, completed basic training and began military occupational skill training as a medic. Shortly afterward, Private Jenkins presented to the mental health clinic with complaints of mood lability with frequent tearfulness and marked difficulty concentrating, stating that she had failed all of her tests on the first try but passed on the second. She reported that she had difficulty sleeping at night and subsequently suffered daytime somnolence that impaired her academic performance. Further history revealed that Private Jenkins had experienced a chaotic childhood, having been raised by her father since age 2 after he divorced her drug-abusing mother. She admitted to physical abuse during her elementary school years, sexual abuse at age 13, and emotional abuse for most of her life, but was reluctant to provide details. She had a history of self-mutilation but had not engaged in any self-injury recently. Ms. Jenkins had enlisted in the National Guard "pretty much on a whim" after an argument with her father about her lack of employment. She said she was following in her father's footsteps in an attempt to garner his approval and sought training as a medic in order to be in his unit when she returned to her home state after active duty training. Private Jenkins agreed with the psychiatrist that her personality was a "poor fit with the military" and that she joined mainly to please her father. She expressed that she would feel a sense of relief if the decision to leave the military was made for her rather than a result of her quitting or failing. In this case, a recommendation for administrative separation met her needs and avoided the potential for repeated failures in the ensuing months.

The U.S. military has long recognized that persons with behavioral or interpersonal impairments that are commonly manifested in PDs may be poorly suited for military duty. Both military culture and military regulations require that leaders must strive to correct the deficiencies in their service members and to rehabilitate behavior that is detrimental to occupational or social functioning within the military through mentoring, corrective training, or even nonjudicial punishment as determined by the unit commander after administrative investigation and review (i.e., an "Article 15" in the Army or a "Captain's Mast" in the Navy). Behavioral health care, ranging from medication management to individual and group supportive, psychoeducational, cognitive-behavioral, and, in some cases, intensive psychodynamic psychotherapy, is available to service members who seek treatment for mental disorders within a wide variety of treatment facilities on military bases and during deployment. However, in recognition of the traditional view of the ingrained and enduring nature of PD-related behaviors and the barriers to effective treatment of PDs imposed by occupational requirements of military service (e.g., ready access to weapons, frequent moves, short-notice deployment to locations without the full panoply of psychiatric resources), all branches of the military also promulgate regulations that allow for relatively expeditious *administrative* separation (without disability compensation, as opposed to *medical* separation) of service members with PDs. If identified prior to enlistment (i.e., through medical screening including review of pre-enlistment medical records), the diagnosis of PD serves as a bar to enlistment. Based on the traditional view that PDs have their onset in adolescence or early adulthood, the emergence of a PD diagnosis after enlistment is viewed, from a disability compensation standpoint, as the recognition of a condition that existed prior to enlistment. More recent studies suggesting that personality-disordered behavior may be more waxing and waning than enduring, or that personality disorders may emerge later in life, have cast some doubt on the presumption that a personality disorder existed prior to enlistment. Indeed, the recurrent nature of the stressors inherent to military life may precipitate episodes of decompensation rather than protect against them.

In this chapter we outline the limited data available on the prevalence of PDs in the U.S. military and discuss the limitations of these data. We then describe the manner in which individuals with PDs may come to the attention of military leaders and clinicians. After a description of the evolving regulations and processes for administrative disposition of service members with PD and the circumstances prompting recent changes, we conclude the chapter with a discussion of areas for further study pertaining to the treatment and management of service members with PDs.

Epidemiology of Personality Disorders in the U.S. Military

The U.S. military does not conduct comprehensive psychiatric or psychological screening on all persons entering active duty or such surveillance on any periodic basis after entry into active duty. Some specialized military occupations (e.g., Special Forces or recruiting duties) may use psychological screening for assessment and selection purposes, but these represent exceptions rather than the norm for military duty. Military accession standards preclude persons with a variety of medical illnesses, including chronic psychotic disorders, substance use disorders, and PDs, from enlistment, and documented histories of these illnesses serve as bars to initial enlistment. However, if such histories are not reported on enlistment applications or in medical records reviewed prior to enlistment, they may be missed. Therefore, prevalence rates for psychiatric diagnoses that do not necessarily come to clinical attention (including PDs) have not been clearly established.

As the military leadership has become increasingly concerned with the psychological burden associated with prolonged combat operations in Iraq and Afghanistan, systematic health surveillance efforts such as those conducted by the Mental Health Advisory Team have led to considerable data on the prevalence of psychiatric disorders in combat personnel. These studies have demonstrated significant increases in rates of diagnoses including major depression, posttraumatic stress disorder (PTSD), and substance use disorders at 3 months, 6 months, and 1 year following deployment, as well as increased prevalence of these disorders during deployment when compared with garrison or predeployment rates (Hoge et al. 2004). The Mental Health Advisory Team studies rely heavily on anonymous self-report questionnaires through which service members report symptoms experienced at the time of survey administration. Hence, they are not well suited for measuring prevalence of diagnoses best established by a longitudinally based clinical assessment, as may be desirable for PD diagnosis or diagnoses characterized by symptoms about which patients may lack insight and therefore lack capacity to self-report.

The military's increasing use of electronic data systems since the turn of the century, however, has provided unprecedented opportunity to conduct epidemiological research on health care utilization (Hoge et al. 2003). An initial systematic examination of military health care utilization databases showed that from 2000 to 2011, a total of 936,283 service members received at least one mental disorder diagnosis at a military treatment facility, and nearly half of these individuals had more than one (Armed Forces Health Surveillance Center 2012). Categories of mental disorder diagnosis for this analysis were ICD-9 (World Health Organization 1977) codes for adjustment disorders, alcohol abuse and dependence disorders, substance abuse and dependence disorders, anxiety disorders, PTSD, depressive disorders, PDs, schizophrenia, other psychoses, and other mental health disorders. Over this time period, rates of incident diagnosis of at least one mental disorder increased by approximately 65% (from 75,353 cases, or 5,387.1 cases/100,000 person-years, in 2000 to 129,678 cases, or 8,900.5 cases/100,000 person-years, in 2011). Not surprisingly, incidence rates of PTSD, anxiety disorders, depressive disorders, adjustment disorders, and other mental disorders generally increased during this time period (with adjustment disorders accounting for 85% of all incident diagnoses, and incidence rates of PTSD increasing approximately sixfold). However, over the entire period, relatively few incident diagnoses were attributable to PDs ($n=81,223$, or 4.5%). The incidence rate for the diagnostic category PD—which comprised all subtypes, including mixed—was generally stable at approximately 500 cases/100,000 person-years, and actually declined slightly over the period of study ($n=8,281$ in 2001; $n=4,110$ in 2011). Similarly stable patterns were observed for psychotic disorders and substance abuse and dependence disorders. A subsequent analysis of years 2007 through 2016 indicated that 853,060 service members had received any mental health diagnosis during this time frame, while 435,898 had received more than one diagnosis, and that the incidence rate for PD diagnosis generally continued to decline to a rate of 237/100,000 person-years in 2016 (Stahlman and Oetting 2018) (Figure 24–1). The fact that anxiety disorders and other mental health disorders were the categories seeing increased incidence rates during this time frame likely reflected increased recognition of subsyndromal PTSD and, perhaps, the utilization of other diagnostic codes in cases of behavior patterns consistent with repeated adjustment difficulties among those who presented for mental health evaluation.

These data are consistent with the notion that disorders whose diagnosis either requires temporal linkage to precipitating events (e.g., PTSD, adjustment disorders) or has been associated with exposure to stressful events (e.g., anxiety disorders, depressive disorders) would be expected to increase during times of heightened military operational tempo, increased deployment, and combat exposure. Although one might anticipate that substance use disorders would increase during such a period, it should be noted that general military orders imposed on all troops in the combat theater specifically preclude the use of alcohol, drastically reducing its availability and opportunities for abuse during deployments. From 2009 through 2016, the number of new alcohol or substance abuse diagnoses per year was on a declining trend for active duty service members, attributed in part to the education, prevention, and treatment programs developed over the past decade (Mendez 2018). Because epidemiological studies demonstrate stable rates of PD in the general U.S. population, the slight decrease in incidence rates of PD may also seem counterintuitive. However, the idea that a pattern of behavior and symptoms attributable to PD in times of peace and stability might be otherwise diagnostically accounted for in patients with significant histories of traumatic combat exposure seems plausible—particularly given the well-documented overlap of symptoms of PTSD and, in particular, Cluster B PDs (Bollinger et al. 2000). Other contributing factors might include an evolving and heightened degree of caution in rendering a diagnosis of PD, as reflected in recent changes to military policy requiring a higher level of scrutiny regarding such diagnoses in personnel with potential combat exposure in the preceding 2 years (U.S. Department of Defense 2019).

Clinical Presentation of Personality Disorders in the Military

Behavioral health care is available to members on active duty and their dependents as well as retirees through a worldwide network of tertiary medical centers, community hospitals, and ambulatory care facilities. In many instances, to facilitate access to care, military installations have established additional mental health–specific ambulatory care centers on bases that already housed behavioral health clinics within their general medical facilities. In addition to issues of access to care created by increased demand, well-described barriers to psychiatric care in military settings include stigma, concerns about impact of receiving care on one's career, concerns about the impact of the use of psychotropic medications on specific career assignments or deployment capability, and the challenges associated with finding the time to receive care (to attend appointments) in the context of a demanding workload (Hoge et al. 2004).

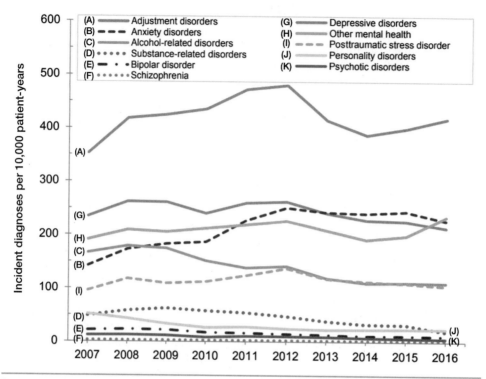

FIGURE 24–1. Annual incidence rates of mental health disorders, active component, U.S. Armed Forces, 2007-2016.

Source. Adapted from Stahlman and Oetting 2018.

Although service members with PDs may not necessarily seek treatment, in part because of lack of insight into the notion that their inner experience or behavior deviates from cultural norms, they may present to either primary care physicians or mental health specialists for assistance in times of emotional crisis (e.g., suicidal ideation when a deployment threatens the security of a romantic relationship, excessive anger or depressed mood after failing to receive a promotion). In other circumstances, maladaptive behaviors (e.g., impulsive aggression, substance misuse, disregard for direct orders, self-injurious acts) may be directly observed by commanders or reported by subordinates concerned for the safety of the service member. Others in the command may become concerned that a mental disorder may be jeopardizing a service member's ability to carry out his or her mission. Commanders, supervisors, or peers may certainly encourage fellow service members to seek mental health treatment in these circumstances. Considerable effort has been invested by the services in destigmatizing mental health care and promoting the concept that service members should actively encourage their colleagues to voluntarily seek treatment or counseling when such concerns arise.

Case Example 2

A 22-year-old female soldier failed to present for afternoon formation. Her barracks roommate reported having heard the service member arguing with her boyfriend on the phone just before formation, went back to the barracks to search for her roommate, and discovered she had impulsively lacerated her wrists. The service member was brought to the emergency room, where she told the emergency room physician that her boyfriend had broken up with her over the phone because "he knew I was going overseas for 6 months and didn't want to be tied down to me if I wasn't going to be close by." She noted, "Breakups are always hard for me; I get like this every time I think I am going to be alone again." The service member's commander referred the soldier for psychiatric evaluation. At her evaluation, the service member reported a history of impulsive behavior, stating she had joined the military "without really thinking about what it meant" in a futile attempt to preserve a previous relationship with another service member she met at a party weeks before. She also reported a pattern of unstable and intense interpersonal relationships, affective instability, chronic feelings of emptiness, suicidal behavior in the context of two previous romantic breakups, and that the prospect of deployment had her feeling, "I don't know, like maybe the Army is trying to cause me to lose control." The stress on interpersonal relationships and repeated periods of separation stemming from military deployments would overwhelm her limited psychological resources.

Case Example 3

While in Kuwait awaiting movement orders to assume a security mission in Iraq, a platoon of 25 soldiers was housed in a medium-sized tent, on cots approximately 18 inches apart. Members of the unit became particularly concerned about a new member of the unit, 20-year-old PFC Smith. PFC Smith politely declined all invitations to play cards, dominoes, or video games with others in the tent. Moreover, he chose not to join the others for meals or to watch movies, and shied away from all efforts to engage in spontaneously organized athletic or training activities, or even to include him in small talk. Finally, one member of the unit told his senior enlisted supervisor, "We're all worried about Smith. We don't think we can go into battle with this guy. He won't talk to us—how do we know he's got our back? The commander should have this guy checked out." The supervisor approached PFC Smith, reminded him of the importance of teamwork and team spirit to mission success, and told him that others were worried about him. Smith replied, "I'm fine. I don't see what the big deal is. I'm just kind of a loner. I don't need them, and they don't need me. We just need to do our jobs and get home." The supervisor encouraged PFC Smith to "do me a favor, and check in with the doctors in the combat stress center. I can't make you go, but if you do and nothing comes of it, I can tell the commander the docs think you are good to go." In this case, the supervisor appropriately encouraged self-referral rather than going immediately to a command-directed evaluation for the assessment of avoidant behavior that only became problematic in the close confines inherent in military deployments.

Military Administrative Policies Regarding Personality Disorders

Each branch of the service has developed regulations and instructions allowing for command-directed involuntary referral of service members for behavioral health evaluation on an emergent basis if, upon discussion with a mental health professional, there is reason to believe that a mental disorder has rendered a service member at imminent risk of self-harm or harm to others. These same regulations outline procedures for nonemergent command-directed involuntary referrals in situations where the commander believes mental disorder may be the cause of a decrement in job performance to the point of compromising a service member's fitness for duty or ability to carry out the missions unique to his or her military assignment and training. These regulations also outline various protections afforded to the service member under such circumstances, including the required credentials of the person conducting the evaluation, the right to be advised in advance and in writing of the reason for the referral, the right to counsel, and the avenue for appeal of any recommendations made as a result of such a referral (U.S. Department of Defense 2013). Such referrals may result in recommendations for the allowance of time for ongoing treatment or other accommodations to be made by the command, and may lead to the establishment of a diagnosis, which, if treatment is unsuccessful, may result in the initiation of procedures for medical or administrative discharge of the service member.

Regardless of whether service members present of their own accord, present at the encouragement of peers, or come to clinical attention by virtue of command-directed evaluation, appropriate treatment is initiated. In the case of physical illness, injury, or major mental disorders incurred while on active duty and considered sufficiently refractory to treatment to preclude further military service, the conditions leading to medical retirement (to include disability compensation) are articulated in Department of Defense Instruction 6130.03, "Medical Standards for Appointment, Enlistment, or Induction Into the Military Services" (U.S. Department of Defense 2018b). The procedures for disability processing, only after a member has received the maximum degree of medical benefit from acute treatment, are enumerated in Department of Defense Instruction 1332.18: "Disability Evaluation System" (U.S. Department of Defense 2018a).

Military policy and regulations have been devised to take into account the demands of ongoing military service. Historically, service regulations have addressed conditions that are considered *unsuitable* for military service but that do not necessarily render the service member *unfit* for military service (i.e., not amounting to disability). These include such conditions as enuresis and motion sickness, as well as behavioral conditions that would limit the person's ability to adapt to the demands of military service but not otherwise interfere with routine civilian life activities. Regulations allow for the administrative separation of soldiers demonstrating "a deeply ingrained maladaptive pattern of behavior of long duration that interferes with the Soldier's ability to perform duty" (U.S. Department of the Army 2016, p. 57). The diagnosis of a PD for the purpose of separation under these regulations may be made only by a psychiatrist or a licensed clinical psychologist. The clinician is advised that a recommendation for this course of action should follow only from a detailed history that supports the presence of long-standing maladaptive behavior and difficulties functioning in interpersonal relationships, rather than simply an adjustment reaction to current stressors (Diebold 1997). The individual must meet the diagnostic criteria for the specific PD or the relevant personality traits for a diagnosis of other specified or unspecified PD. Current regulations do not permit medical retirement (i.e., disability) for service members whose PD appears to emerge only after enlistment. However, policy allows for administrative separation on the basis of behavior (repeated adjustment difficulties) that may be a manifestation of the emergence of "late onset" personality disorder (see below).

Many of the larger military medical centers are able to offer treatments such as dialectical behavior therapy or other cognitive-behavioral therapies, both in groups and individually, to address maladaptive symptoms of PDs. Most treatment facilities are able to offer supportive counseling and psychodynamically based therapies. (See Chapters 12 through 15 in this volume for detailed discussions of psychotherapies that are effective in the treatment of PDs.)

Medication management for associated symptoms of affective dysregulation is also increasingly employed, even though such treatments represent off-label use and have only limited support in the literature. (See Chapter 17, "Pharmacological Management," in this volume for a detailed discussion of medications available for use with patients with PDs.) Nonetheless, the clinical utility of these treatments continues to be limited by their relatively long-term nature in many cases and the lack of availability in the deployed environment, where they are more likely to be needed because maladaptive behaviors increase in response to the additional stressors. The commanders' need to address problematic behaviors administratively and/or through disciplinary action will often result in separation before significant therapeutic improvement is possible.

The regulations further provide that even when a service member is diagnosed with a PD, a recommendation for administrative separation remains only a recommendation, with the final disposition determined by the commander only after "the Soldier has been counseled formally concerning deficiencies and has been afforded ample opportunity to overcome those deficiencies as reflected in appropriate counseling or personnel records" (U.S. Department of the Army 2016, p. 59). This guidance is in keeping with the special emphasis the military places on mentorship and leadership and is consistent with military values exhorting leaders to exhaust efforts to rehabilitate deficiencies in their subordinates before giving up on them. It may be in contradiction, however, to traditional theories that conceptualize PD as being a deeply ingrained and inflexible pattern of response, symptoms of which may become exacerbated under stress and may have low potential for significant change over time (Diebold 1997; Leroux 2014). Recent developments regarding the effectiveness of treatments targeting particularly maladaptive behaviors in PDs may render this guidance more salient in the future, providing the potential for increased successful rehabilitation.

Service regulations that address conditions considered unsuitable for military service (U.S. Department of the Air Force 2019; U.S. Department of the Army 2016; U.S. Department of the Navy 2018) are derived from U.S. Department of Defense (2019) policy. As previously noted, these include conditions such as motion sickness, enuresis, and sleepwalking, which would not generally be considered disabling but which could obviously be incompatible with the demands of military service. This category also includes adjustment disorders, which predictably are frequently comorbid with PDs in the military environment and also constitute a likely reason for presentation to clinical attention. Adjustment disorders are viewed as the manifestation of an inability to adapt to the stressors of military life, which may be situationally driven but also represent some degree of underlying predisposition, whether or not it rises to the level of a PD. If the clinician believes the predisposition is significant enough to make chronic or recurrent adjustment difficulties likely, this establishes the potential for administrative separation of the service member for the adjustment disorder without (or before) a diagnosis of PD, even when underlying characterological issues predominate. This option serves to decrease the impetus to prematurely diagnose a PD as a means of offering the individual administrative separation and to avoid the often-pejorative label that a PD diagnosis constitutes when in reality military enlistment may simply represent a poor match for the individual's psychological makeup. Theoretically, some persons whose character traits might serve well in combat but not in peacetime are lost to active duty through this process. Similarly, the external structure and discipline of routine military life in the absence of significant combat stressors might provide a protective environment to foster personal growth in some PDs with impairment in a sense of self or lack of independent goal-directedness. However, since military life is characterized by a repeated cycle of military deployment followed by garrison duty, traits that serve one well in only one setting but not the other equate to a poor match between psychological makeup and military duty.

Recent Policy Changes

In 2009, public concern arose about soldiers who had been administratively separated from the army for PD after combat tours in Iraq and Afghanistan. The potential injustice of soldiers being separated without medical or other benefits when symptoms of posttraumatic stress may have contributed to behavior problems led the U.S. Army Medical Command to develop policies assuring that those who had served combat tours would undergo screening for PTSD and traumatic brain injury. If subsequent clinical evaluation confirms clinically significant symptoms, such individuals are medically separated instead and thus retain benefits, even if comorbid PD complicates the clinical picture. In 2011, the Department of Defense revised its instruction to extend these safeguards to all of the military services; the instruction was last updated in 2019 (U.S. Department of Defense 2019). Recognizing the potential for other diagnoses, including those considered unsuitable but not disabling, this instruction extended these safeguards to administrative separations for adjustment disorders as well and requires comprehensive screening for mental health issues in addition to PTSD and traumatic brain injury.

In late 2011, concerns were raised about Medical Evaluation Boards, the first step in the disability process, for psychiatric conditions conducted at Madigan Army Medical Center at Joint Base Lewis-McChord in Washington State. These concerns eventually resulted in the establishment of the Army Task Force on Behavioral Health, chartered to conduct a comprehensive evaluation of the Disability Evaluation System in an effort to "review, assess and, where needed, improve behavioral health evaluations and diagnoses in the context of Disability Evaluation System" (Army Task Force on Behavioral Health 2013, p. 7). The task force made a number of recommendations regarding processes to improve the efficiency of the Disability Evaluation System, as well as the need to educate service members and clinicians regarding the diagnostic assessment process. The Department of Defense adopted many of these recommendations to standardize the evaluation process across all of the military services (U.S. Department of Defense 2018a). The goals of these changes are to enhance the comprehensiveness of the assessment process and to ensure careful evaluation of all symptoms, including behavioral changes that might stem from PD or adjustment disorder. Although specific guidelines about the conducting of evaluations were not made, the process allows these behavioral changes to be considered in a light that would be most beneficial to the service member in terms of potential disability compensation versus administrative separation.

Case Example 4

A 24-year-old specialist returned from a combat tour in Afghanistan, where his unit had been under attack several times. In one mission, the convoy he was traveling in struck a roadside improvised explosive device, destroying the vehicle in front of his and killing one of his friends. In the weeks following his redeployment, his wife noted that his previous jealous tendencies were now expressed in angry verbal outbursts whenever she returned from errands. She also noted that he was increasingly irritable and slept poorly, awakening in the night and thrashing about. When frustrated, he would strike her pet poodle, and he would frequently sit alone in their suburban backyard drinking beer and watching a campfire, in violation of a city ordinance against building fires in the neighborhood. She convinced him to go to the mental health clinic, where an evaluation additionally revealed a childhood history of conduct disorder, several legal detentions before age 18 that were expunged from his record, and an increase in speeding and reckless driving since his return. Because these behaviors had markedly increased since his deployment, he was offered treatment for posttraumatic stress and referred for a disability evaluation. In this instance symptoms resulted in a disability rating for PTSD rather than administrative separation, despite the presence of pre-existing antisocial personality traits or disorder that may have rendered the service member more vulnerable to PTSD.

Conclusion

Involvement in long-term combat operations necessitating frequent and prolonged deployment, disruption of families and other sources of social support, repeated exposures to harsh and intermittently life-threatening environments, and higher workloads for service members (even while in garrison) have resulted in a heightened awareness of the emotional and behavioral challenges confronting combat veterans. The military has invested considerable efforts in the development of better approaches to the assessment and management of PTSD, traumatic brain injury, and the interpersonal and occupational impairments that may result from these disorders. These efforts have also resulted in an increased awareness of the diagnostic overlap not only between these entities, but also with adjustment disorders and PDs, as each of these may manifest in patterns of maladaptive behavior that may only come to clinical attention with the added stressors of deployment and redeployment.

All branches of the military have historically recognized PDs as ingrained patterns of behavior developing in childhood or adolescence and blossoming in early adulthood. As such, these disorders have been viewed as having low probability for significant response to rehabilitative efforts in the context of the challenges inherent to military life and therefore as grounds for administrative separation in accordance with military regulations. These same regulations have always left room for commanders to retain service members with PDs and presumably allow or encourage these service members to avail themselves of treatment opportunities in the military. However, recent policy developments seem to suggest recognition that symptoms emerging in the aftermath of combat—which may have in the past been attributed to PD—should be considered in a diagnostic light that best promotes ongoing treatment either within the military system or through the disability system to provide the opportunity for continued treatment in the Veterans Affairs setting after medical, rather than administrative, discharge.

Further research is needed not only to focus diagnostic efforts but also to develop treatment approaches to behaviors that result in loss of fitness for further military duty. Treatments are needed that target impulsive behavior (including aggression), high-risk behaviors (including substance abuse), and affective instability, whether these behaviors result from PD, PTSD, or comorbid conditions. The extent to which recent advances in the treatment of PDs (e.g., dialectical behavior therapy for borderline PD) may allow for effective treatment in military operational environments must also be explored.

References

American Psychiatric Association: Diagnostic and Statistical Manual of Mental Disorders, 5th Edition. Arlington, VA, American Psychiatric Association, 2013

Armed Forces Health Surveillance Center: Mental disorders and mental health problems, active component, U.S. Armed Forces, 2000–2011. MSMR 19(6):11–17, 2012. Available at: www.afhsc.mil/viewMSMR?file=2012/v19_n06.pdf. Accessed August 27, 2013.

Army Task Force on Behavioral Health: Corrective Action Plan, January 2013. Available at: www.pdhealth.mil/army-task-force-behavioral-health-corrective-action-plan-january-2013. Accessed August 31, 2020.

Bollinger AR, Riggs DS, Blake DD, et al: Prevalence of personality disorders among combat veterans with posttraumatic stress disorder. J Trauma Stress 13:255–270, 2000

Diebold CJ: Military administrative psychiatry, in Principles and Practice of Military Forensic Psychiatry. Edited by Lande RG, Armitage DT. Springfield, IL, Charles C Thomas, 1997, pp 269–304

Halvorson A: Understanding the Military: The Institution, the Culture and the People, 2010. Working draft. Rockville, MD, Substance Abuse and Mental Health Services Administration, 2010. Available at: www.samhsa.gov/sites/default/files/military_white_paper_final.pdf. Accessed April 9, 2020.

Hoge CW, Messer SC, Engel CC, et al: Priorities for psychiatric research in the U.S. military: an epidemiological approach. Mil Med 68:182–185, 2003

Hoge CW, Castro CA, Messer SC, et al: Combat duty in Iraq and Afghanistan, mental health problems, and barriers to care. N Engl J Med 351:3–22, 2004

Leroux TC: U.S. military discharges and pre-existing personality disorders: a health policy review. Admin Policy Ment Health 42(6):748–755, 2014. Available at: https://blogs.uw.edu/brtc/files/2014/12/Leroux-2014-US-military-discharges-for-PDs.pdf. Accessed January 11, 2020.

Mendez BHP: Substance abuse prevention, treatment, and research efforts in the military. Congressional Research Service. In Focus, August 17, 2018. Available at https://fas.org/sgp/crs/natsec/IF10951.pdf. Accessed September 3, 2019.

Stahlman S, Oetting AA: Mental disorders and problems, active component, U.S. Armed Forces, 2007–2016. MSMR 25(3):2–11, 2018. Available at: https://health.mil/Reference-Center/Reports/2018/01/01/Medical-Surveillance-Monthly-Report-Volume-25-Number-3. Accessed January 11, 2020.

U.S. Department of the Air Force: Instruction (AFI) 36-3208: Administrative Separation of Airmen. Washington, DC, U.S. Department of the Air Force, 2019. Available at: https://static.e-publishing.af.mil/production/1/af_a1/publication/afi36-3208/afi36-3208.pdf. Accessed September 3, 2019.

U.S. Department of the Army: Active Duty Enlisted Administrative Separations (Army Regulation 635-200). Washington, DC, U.S. Department of the Army, 2016. Available at: https://armypubs.army.mil/epubs/DR_pubs/DR_a/pdf/web/AR635-200_Web_FINAL_18JAN2017.pdf. Accessed September 3, 2019.

U.S. Department of Defense: Instruction No 6490.04: Mental Health Evaluations of Members of the Military Services. Washington, DC, U.S. Department of Defense, 2013. Available at: www.esd.whs.mil/Portals/54/Documents/DD/issuances/dodi/649004p.pdf. Accessed August 29, 2019.

U.S. Department of Defense: Instruction No 1332.18: Disability Evaluation System. Washington, DC, U.S. Department of Defense, 2018a. Available at: www.esd.whs.mil/Portals/54/Documents/DD/issuances/dodi/133218p.pdf?ver=2018-05-24-133105-050. Accessed September 3, 2019.

U.S. Department of Defense: Instruction 6130.03: Medical Standards for Appointment, Enlistment, or Induction Into the Military Services. Washington, DC, U.S. Department of Defense, 2018b. Available at: www.esd.whs.mil/Portals/54/Documents/DD/issuances/dodi/613003p.pdf. Accessed August 29, 2019.

U.S. Department of Defense: Instruction No 1332.14: Enlisted Administrative Separations. Washington, DC, U.S. Department of Defense, 2019. Available at: www.esd.whs.mil/Portals/54/Documents/DD/issuances/dodi/133214p.pdf?ver=2019-03-14-132901-200. Accessed September 3, 2019.

U.S. Department of the Navy: Separation by Reason of Convenience of the Government—Medical Conditions Not Amounting to a Disability (MILPERSMAN 1900-120). Washington, DC, U.S. Department of the Navy, November 2018. Available at: www.public.navy.mil/bupers-npc/reference/milpersman/1000/1900Separation/Documents/1900-120.pdf. Accessed September 3, 2019.

World Health Organization: International Classification of Diseases, 9th Revision. Geneva, World Health Organization, 1977

PART V

Future Directions

CHAPTER 25

Translational Research in Borderline Personality Disorder

Christian Schmahl, M.D.
Sabine C. Herpertz, M.D.

In this chapter, we focus on two domains of borderline personality disorder (BPD) psychopathology—dysfunctions of social interaction and perceptual alterations (pain and dissociation)—to demonstrate that modern behavioral neuroscience methodology and translational approaches can be useful for understanding mechanisms underlying this psychopathology and ultimately help to improve therapy for patients with BPD. In these two domains, animal models are of particular value and can be used to better understand underlying disease constructs as well as for testing behavioral and pharmacological interventions. Animal models of research, however, are still in their infancy.

We provide an overview of dysfunctional social interaction in BPD, with a special focus on empathy and the role of oxytocin, with a short side trip to the field of antisocial personality disorder (ASPD). We then discuss disturbed pain processing and the role of pain in the context of emotion regulation in BPD. Closely related to this aspect of BPD, dissociation as a distinct feature of BPD has interesting parallels in animal research, as we outline at the end of this chapter.

Dysfunctions of Social Interaction

Impaired Interpersonal Functioning in BPD

Interpersonal dysfunction is the most prominent characteristic of personality disorders (PDs) in general, although its nature varies among the different types. Within the

Alternative DSM-5 Model for Personality Disorders (AMPD), moderate or greater impairment in interpersonal functioning is one of the two defining features of a personality disorder. Interpersonal functioning comprises empathy and intimacy. Empathy is the capacity to understand, appreciate, and tolerate others' experiences, motivations, and emotions; to take the perspective of others; and to understand or predict the effects of one's behavior on others. Intimacy describes the capacity to connect with others, to enjoy closeness, and to emphasize mutuality. From the view of translational research, interpersonal dysfunction has been best studied in BPD, although there has been additional research in the antisocial realm.

Impairments in interpersonal functioning have been discussed as being the best discriminators for the diagnosis of BPD (Gunderson et al. 2007; Modestin 1987; Zanarini et al. 1990), and longitudinal studies have shown the impact of interpersonal problems on BPD functioning over the long term (Gunderson et al. 2011; Zanarini et al. 2010). Intolerance of aloneness, long regarded as one of the central features of BPD resulting in dysfunctional attachment behaviors, typically is demonstrated as an oscillation between attention seeking and detached avoidance (Gunderson et al. 1996).

Gunderson and Lyons-Ruth (2008) emphasized "the fearful or highly reactive component of this interpersonal style that is probably the more distinctive and pathogenic component" (p. 23) and referred to this interpersonal style as the "interpersonal hypersensitivity" phenotype. Experimental studies point in particular to interpersonal threat hypersensitivity. Individuals with BPD tend to frequently experience interpersonal threat, making them ascribe resentment to others (Domes et al. 2008). In one study, adolescents with BPD exhibited difficulties in disengaging attention from threatening facial information during early stages of attention (Jovev et al. 2012). High rejection sensitivity, defined as the disposition to anxiously expect, readily perceive, and intensively react to rejection (Berenson et al. 2009), appears to be another facet of threat hypersensitivity, with individuals with BPD scoring highest on related measures (i.e., the Rejection Sensitivity Questionnaire and the Questionnaire on Thoughts and Feelings) compared with several other clinical samples or healthy control subjects (Staebler et al. 2011). Rejection hypersensitivity has also been targeted by using an experimental study design, the Cyberball (a ball-tossing computer game paradigm), which reliably provokes feelings of social exclusion (Staebler et al. 2011). In this study, patients with BPD exhibited a biased perception of exclusion; they felt excluded even when they were objectively included. They had more negative self-referential feelings and more negative feelings against others before the game started, and they reported resentments against others during the ball-tossing game, which increased when they were excluded. In a recently developed animal model for social rejection, rejected animals displayed higher emotional reactivity as well as decreased pain sensitivity, thus mirroring features of BPD (Schneider et al. 2014).

Unresolved attachment might lie at the core of BPD (Fonagy and Luyten 2009; see also Chapter 7, "Development, Attachment, and Childhood Experiences: A Mentalization Perspective," in this volume), so that patients with BPD show no coherent attachment style but instead demonstrate rapid shifts between avoidant and anxious attachment. Reflecting avoidant attachment, they pay little attention to or have low memory for positive social information (Domes et al. 2006b), and in response to their attachment needs, they show hyperreactivity to socially negative, potentially threatening, and even neutral stimuli in a neural network of the brain that has been implicated in aversion, withdrawal, or even defense responses (Vrticka and Vuilleumier 2012).

Although individuals with BPD demonstrated no deficits in facial emotion recognition for simple tasks (Domes et al. 2009), they did demonstrate impairment in complex tasks in assessing emotion recognition. For example, patients with BPD showed lower performance when integrated facial and prosodic stimuli were applied, but they showed normal ability to recognize isolated facial or prosodic emotions (Minzenberg et al. 2006). Contradicting the previous assumption of general hypersensitivity to facial emotions in patients with BPD, experimental data suggest subtle impairments in labeling accuracy accompanied by a bias toward negative emotions—that is, a tendency to interpret ambiguous faces in a more negative way (Arntz and Veen 2001; Wagner and Linehan 1999). Interestingly, when presentation times of facial cues were modified (von Ceumern-Lindenstjerna et al. 2010b), adolescent patients with BPD demonstrated stronger initial attention to brief visualization of negative facial expressions than did healthy adolescent comparison subjects, and when in a negative mood, the adolescents with BPD also showed difficulties in disengaging attention from negative facial expressions that were presented to them (von Ceumern-Lindenstjerna et al. 2010a). Consistent with the expectation that patients with BPD are prone to anger, participants rather specifically showed a bias toward the perception of anger in a study using ambiguous facial stimuli in the form of blends of basic emotions (Domes et al. 2008). In a study using visual event-related potentials, this bias was associated with enhanced amplitudes of the P100 and reduced amplitudes of the N170 and P300, suggesting alterations in very early visual, as well as deficient structural and categorical, processing of faces (Izurieta Hidalgo et al. 2016). In a study performed by Meyer et al. (2004), the anxious attachment style of patients with BPD was related to negative face appraisals, and particularly a tendency to rate faces as less friendly and more rejecting. Considering differences in the presentation times of facial stimuli across recent studies, Daros et al. (2013) claim that the increased arousal of patients with BPD may either lead to enhanced detection of subtle facial threat or hinder classification of fully displayed facial emotions in binding attentional resources by salient social cues. Studies in BPD that have applied functional neuroimaging to measure neuronal responses to negative facial emotions consistently indicate a bias toward emotionally negative or threatening social information, such as increased and prolonged amygdala responses (Donegan et al. 2003; Minzenberg et al. 2007), and thus support behavioral findings. Amygdala hyperactivity could be further specified by Koenigsberg and his group, who found deficient habituation not only in the amygdala (Koenigsberg et al. 2014) but also beyond, in the salience network comprising the anterior insula and the dorsal anterior cingulate cortex, when emotional pictures were repeatedly presented (Denny et al. 2018). Interestingly, Vrticka et al. (2008) showed that anxiously attached individuals—analogous to those with BPD—show amygdala hyperactivation in response to angry faces, which may reflect a tendency to experience enhanced distress in aversive, nonvalidating interpersonal situations.

Patients with BPD show a failure to synchronize their brain activity with those of others: In a hyperscanning context, dyads with one BPD patient exhibited reduced cross-brain neural coupling between the temporo-parietal junctions during a joint attention task compared with dyads of healthy controls (Bilek et al. 2017). Adaptive social interaction requires unbiased perception of social signals, as well as the ability to take the perspective of others and to exhibit empathy, and, thus, challenges an individual's capacity to couple one's brain activity with that of the interacting other. Empathy subsumes several facets (Decety and Moriguchi 2007): 1) a cognitive capacity to take the perspective of another person (i.e., cognitive empathy), 2) an affective response to another individual (i.e., affective empathy), and 3) a self-regulatory capacity that modulates a person's inner state. Thus, it is not sufficient to understand empathy as an affective experience of another person's emotional state; it also requires attribution of emotions to others independent of one's own mental state. This requires self-awareness, no confusion between self and other (reflections of functioning of the self, according to the AMPD), and a capacity to modulate one's own emotional states. Recently, a fourth facet of empathy—empathic concern or compassion, respectively—has been put forth, involving the tendency to care and provide helping support for others (Decety et al. 2015b; Kanske et al. 2017). Regarding patients with BPD, recognition of intentions and mental state reasoning capacities have been found to be compromised (Fonagy and Bateman 2006; Nemeth et al. 2018). Using self-report measures of cognitive empathy, such as the Interpersonal Reactivity Index (IRI; Davis 1983), several, although not all, authors found a diminished capacity for appropriate perspective taking in patients with BPD (Arntz et al. 2009; Guttman and Laporte 2000; Harari et al. 2010; New et al. 2012). Other studies testing for the capacity of patients with BPD to infer the mental states of others also suggest impairments of cognitive empathy using the faux pas task that challenges participants' capability to accurately infer thoughts and intentions of others (Harari et al. 2010). However, other authors did not find abnormal cognitive empathy using other theory of mind (ToM) tasks (Ghiassi et al. 2010).

In response to the critique that previous research studies have made use of stimulus material with low ecological validity, Dziobek et al. (2006) developed the Movie for the Assessment of Social Cognition (MASC). The MASC is a highly ecologically valid video-based test that presents social interactions among multiple characters and thereby assesses the viewer's capacity to identify social signals such as language, gestures, and facial expressions. Preißler et al. (2010) were the first to use this task in patients with BPD and found them to have impaired recognition of the feelings, thoughts, and intentions of others. Sharp et al. (2011) applied the MASC in work with a group of adolescents with BPD and reported impaired cognitive empathy in young subjects scoring high on borderline traits compared with those scoring low. According to this study, difficulties in cognitive empathy are especially characterized by a tendency to hypermentalize in social situations—that is, to show a distorted interpretation that goes beyond an interpretation warranted by the data. This tendency may not be specific to BPD but may be related to personality disorder psychopathology in general and may significantly contribute to interpersonal dysfunction (Normann-Eide et al. 2020). Interestingly, cognitive empathy was shown to correlate with self-report measures of emotion regulation, suggesting that high-arousal emotional states might interfere with cognitive empathy ability, as exemplified by the model of empathy proposed by Decety and Moriguchi (2007). However, in contrast to studies using the MASC to assess capacity to identify social signals, two studies provided evidence of a better and more rapid performance by patients with BPD in the Reading the Mind in the Eyes Test (RMET) (Barnow et al. 2012; Fertuck et al. 2009), which is reported to relate to mentalizing processes (but may relate to other psychological mechanisms, as discussed later in this section).

Empathy measurements that facilitate differentiation between cognitive and affective empathy suggest that a dissociation between these two facets is typical of individuals with BPD. Harari et al. (2010), using the IRI as a self-report questionnaire, as well as faux pas tasks, found that patients with BPD showed impaired performance in cognitive empathy and cognitive ToM measures but not impairment in affective aspects of empathy. In a study by New et al. (2012), "personal distress" as one aspect of affective empathy turned out to be even higher among patients with BPD than among healthy control subjects. However, when focusing on the IRI's Empathic Concern subscale, a measurement of compassion for others, New et al. (2012) found that patients with BPD did not differ from nonclinical controls. Dziobek et al. (2011) found that patients with BPD reported slightly lower values on the IRI, and they reported lower performance on both affective and cognitive empathy, when compared with nonclinical controls, on the Multifaceted Empathy Task (MET), reflecting the results of a more objective and ecologically valid instrument. The MET consists of photographs depicting people in emotionally charged situations. In the condition of affective empathy, subjects are instructed to label their own emotion in the context of another individual experiencing, for example, distress, whereas in the case of cognitive empathy, participants had to label the emotional state of others in a particular context.

Neurobiological data support the model that cognitive and affective empathy are distinct phenomena that rely on different neurocognitive circuits (Singer 2006). In a functional magnetic resonance imaging (fMRI) study using the MET, Dziobek et al. (2011) found that individuals with BPD exhibited worse performance than healthy control subjects on both cognitive and affective empathy. Neuronal activities were reduced in the left superior temporal sulcus during the cognitive empathy condition, whereas insular activity was enhanced in the emotional empathy condition, in the patients with BPD compared with the healthy controls. Interestingly, activation in the right middle insula was positively correlated with skin conductance responses, indicating increased arousal in the patients with BPD. Given that the tendency to experience personal distress in response to the suffering of others has been associated with middle insular activation in healthy subjects (Decety and Moriguchi 2007), this fMRI study was interpreted to reflect increased arousal and personal distress in patients with BPD due to deficient emotion regulatory processes in the interpersonal realm, hampering empathy processes.

Mier et al. (2013), applying an emotional ToM task, found higher neuronal activity in the amygdala but lower activity in the superior temporal sulcus and superior temporal gyrus together with lower activity in the inferior frontal gyrus in patients with BPD compared with nonclinical controls. In this study, subjects viewed facial stimuli with neutral, joyful, angry, and fearful expressions. Each facial expression was introduced by a different statement. In the emotional intention task (affective ToM), the participants had to indicate by button press whether or not the statement matched the picture of the person. This task, in which participants are instructed to identify the intentions of the presented persons, challenges ToM or mentalizing processes, mediated in the inferior prefrontal cortex as a premotor area and part of the "mirror" neuron system, with its activity being associated with the representation and mirroring of actions and intentions (Coricelli 2005; Iacoboni et al. 2005). Using the RMET, Barnow et al. (2012) also reported lower activity in mentalizing areas such as the right superior temporal gyrus and the right precuneus, as well as higher activity in the amygdala, in patients with BPD compared with controls. In a study by O'Neill and colleagues (2015), cognitive empathy again appeared to be particularly impaired in states of high emotional arousal, since functional connectivity between emotion regulation areas (e.g., anterior cingulate cortex) and the ToM network (temporo-parietal junction, middle cingulate cortex, and inferior parietal lobe) was found to be reduced in the resting state as well as during performance of ToM tasks.

Furthermore, higher activity in the mirror system (e.g., somatosensory cortex) and the posterior insula were found in patients with BPD compared with control subjects during viewing of others mourning (Sosic-Vasic et al. 2019). Automatic encoding of somatosensory and emotional aspects of experiences without self-awareness may result in increased emotional contagion and thus the failure to properly discriminate between one's feelings and those of others. High affective empathy as found in some, but not all, behavioral studies in BPD may be designated as emotional contagion due to exaggerated resonance with others' mental states tracing back to identity diffusion in BPD. This phenomenon may hinder the ability of individuals with BPD to experience compassion for others and cause them, instead, to be affected by their own emotions triggered through the emotions of others. In any case, higher-order metacognitive processes may fail to modulate the lower-level automatic emotional contagion.

In correspondence with the assumption of high automatic simulation (but low conscious mentalizing of the other's emotional states and intentions), patients with BPD exhibited higher activity of the musculus corrugator supercilii during viewing of negative facial stimuli such as anger, sadness, and disgust (Matzke et al. 2014) but lower electromyographic activity in the musculus levator labii in response to happy and surprised faces (i.e., faces that reflect emotional states rather distinct from the subjects' own).

Emotional simulation theory proposes that in social primates the mental states of others can be understood on the basis of one's own mental states (Gallese and Goldman 1998), encompassing an understanding of social situations that is immediate, automatic, and almost reflex-like. As Gallese (2007) notes, "This particular dimension of social cognition is embodied, in that it mediates between the multimodal experiential knowledge of our own lived body and the way we experience others" (p. 659). This basal mechanism is not related to higher cognitive functions, and it is less reliant on learned knowledge about social interactions (Frith and Frith 2006). The understanding of others' sensory experiences, rather, seems to rely on vicarious activation of somatosensory cortices in the observer. Humans activate their own motor, somatosensory, and nociceptive representations while perceiving the actions of others, and they activate representations of their own emotional states while observing others' emotions.

Social Cognition and Empathy in Psychopathy

In a meta-analysis of 20 studies on findings from antisocial subjects regarding the processing of human faces, Marsh and Blair (2008) reported a robust link between antisocial behavior and deficits in recognizing fearful expressions. Antisocial subjects also showed some deficits when processing sad faces; however, these responses were less prominent than responses to fearful faces, so that a specific, rather than a global, deficit in expression processing may be characteristic of individuals with ASPD. In functional neuroimaging studies, adolescents with early-onset, but not those with late-onset, conduct disorder exhibited reduced amygdala activation in response to sad faces when compared with neutral faces. However, adolescents with conduct disorder, independent of age at onset, showed diminished amygdala response to angry faces when compared with neutral faces (Fairchild et al. 2009; Passamonti et al. 2010), and this deficit has been associated with amygdala dysfunction of developmental origin. Additionally, the processing of fearful facial expressions has been studied in individuals with psychopathy, who showed poor fearful expression recognition as well as poor startle response, and thus a failure of aversive cues to prime normal defensive action (Blair et al. 2004; Patrick 1994). The co-occurrence of both deficiencies has been interpreted to reflect an amygdala-based fear simulation deficit that explains reduced fear response and is associated with an impairment in the capacity to identify the expresser's emotional state (Goldman and Sripada 2005; Lawrence and Calder 2004). More specifically, significantly reduced fractional anisotropy as an indirect measure of microstructural integrity, reported from diffusion tensor imaging, suggests that abnormal connectivity in the amygdala–orbitofrontal network may contribute to the neurobiological mechanisms underlying emotional detachment and impulsive antisocial behavior in psychopathy (Craig et al. 2009).

Regarding capabilities in ToM functions, psychopathic subjects have been shown to have unimpaired cognitive empathy. Psychopathic patients do well on a RMET, but they may perform this task by means of other mechanisms than those used by patients with BPD—namely, by cognitively adopting the perspective of others. In fact, subjects with ASPD or psychopathy, in particular, are probably good at perceiving others' intentions; however, they disregard the emotions of others. "The psychopath cannot simulate emotions he cannot experience, and must rely exclusively on cognitive inputs to his theory of mind mechanism" (Decety and Moriguchi 2007, p. 14). Emotional incapacity has been intensively investigated in males with psychopathic traits, but future research is needed to investigate whether a reliable emotional deficit is also true for psychopathic female offenders.

Studies in psychopathic offenders found reduced gray matter volumes in cortical areas related to empathic processing and moral judgment (i.e., in anterior rostral prefrontal cortex and temporal poles) (Gregory et al. 2012). Volume reductions were also found in midline cortical areas (Bertsch et al. 2013b) involved in the processing of self-referential information and self-reflection (i.e., the dorsomedial prefrontal cortex and posterior cingulate/precuneus) and in recognizing emotions of others (i.e., the postcentral gyrus). Consistent with these findings, the psychopathy scores of individuals who were instructed to perform moral compared with nonmoral decision-making processes were found to correlate with decreased activation in an area extending from the dorsolateral prefrontal cortex to the medial prefrontal cortex (Reniers et al. 2012). The authors suggested that moral decision making entails intact self-referential and mentalizing processing, which appears to be disrupted in psychopathic individuals. However, in the study by Bertsch et al. (2013b), reduced gray matter volumes in temporal poles, compared with those in healthy control subjects, were found not in those with ASPD and psychopathic traits but rather in criminal offenders with comorbid conditions of ASPD and BPD.

Individuals with ASPD exhibited enhanced activations in brain regions representing cognitive ToM (i.e., superior temporal sulcus, temporoparietal junction, precuneus, and the medial and ventrolateral prefrontal cortex) but decreased amygdala activation during a RMET; interestingly, this activation pattern correlated with psychopathy scores (Schiffer et al. 2017). When instructed to perform an affective ToM task, criminal offenders with psychopathy showed decreased activations in the amygdala, superior temporal sulcus, and inferior prefrontal cortex as well as lower functional connectivity between the amygdala and the superior temporal sulcus (Mier et al. 2014). Furthermore, higher psychopathy scores were correlated with lower neuronal activity in the anterior insula, dorsal anterior cingulate cortex, amygdala, and inferior frontal gyrus while subjects were labeling their emotions in response to emotional faces (Seara-Cardoso et al. 2016).

Decety and colleagues (2015b) were able to differentiate between affective sharing and empathic concern (i.e., compassion) in individuals with various degrees of psychopathy in a study using electroencephalography (EEG). Significant correlations with psychopathy in late (i.e., late positive potential), but not in early, components of processing are consistent with the assumption of abnormal top-down processes of appraisal that are needed to elicit other-oriented motivation for compassion rather than deficient automatic attentional bottom-up processes of perceiving others´ pain. The findings of this EEG study are consistent with data from fMRI studies (Decety et al. 2013; Meffert et al. 2013) indicating that psychopaths, when explicitly instructed to focus on social cues in images of others in pain, show activations of the emotional empathy circuit (anterior cingulate cortex and anterior insula) comparable to those of healthy volunteers, but exhibit abnormally low activity in the ventromedial prefrontal cortex, which is involved in compassion and moral decision making. This conclusion is also consistent with data from a large group of criminal offenders, showing that psychopaths are characterized by reduced activity in the superior temporal sulcus and temporo-parietal junction, the anterior cingulate cortex, and the dorsomedial prefrontal cortex when passively watching a harmful as opposed to a supportive social interaction, but show increased activity in the same brain areas when performing the explicit task of inferring the emotional state of the victim rather than the perpetrator (Decety et al. 2015a).

Social Dysfunction and the Role of Oxytocin

Oxytocin, the so-called prosocial hormone, plays a critical role in intimate relationships such as parenting and romantic relationships; oxytocin may also, to some degree, play a role in most meaningful interpersonal relationships. Oxytocin is synthesized in magnocellular neurons of the paraventricular and supraoptic nuclei of the hypothalamus, from which it is transported to the posterior pituitary, where it is released. Oxytocin receptors are especially prevalent in brain areas involved in social behaviors, including the bed nucleus of the stria terminalis, hypothalamic paraventricular nucleus, amygdala, ventral tegmental area, and nucleus accumbens. Interestingly, in rats, oxytocin neurons from the hypothalamic, paraventricular, and supraoptic nuclei project to a wide range of oxytocin receptors throughout forebrain structures, including the amygdala (Knobloch et al. 2012).

Oxytocin modulates the formation of social memories as well as the processing of social cues, such as facial expressions. A number of studies now shed light on the specific facial processes in which oxytocin is involved: oxytocin improves the recognition of emotions (Lischke et al. 2012) and enhances early attentional processing of selectively happy faces (Domes et al. 2013); it appears to enhance the recognition of emotional expressions in static (Di Simplicio et al. 2009; Guastella et al. 2010; Marsh et al. 2010) and dynamic (Fischer-Shofty et al. 2010) images of faces; and it improves emotion recognition by directing attention to salient facial features, such as the eyes (Gamer et al. 2010; Guastella et al. 2008), with better performance when the subject is instructed to "read" the emotional state of another from the eye region (Domes et al. 2006a). Interestingly, oxytocin application was associated with greater task-related pupil dilation, a finding that also suggests increased recruitment of attentional resources (Prehn et al. 2013). Furthermore, the latter study provides the first evidence that oxytocin promotes an attentional bias to positive social cues; in correspondence with these data, the intranasal administration of oxytocin was followed by increased ratings of trustworthiness and attractiveness of unfamiliar faces in a study of healthy volunteers by Theodoridou and colleagues (2009).

Oxytocin is thought not only to be involved in the attentional processing of salient social cues, such as facial expressions, but also to interact with rewards associated with social interactions. Dopaminergic neurons running from the ventral tegmental area to the nucleus accumbens are responsible for the active pathways facilitating the affiliation process. Interestingly, both areas are known to show a high density of oxytocin receptors and to interact with the dopamine system. One theory is that oxytocin enhances the hedonic value of social interactions by activating these areas that are rich in dopamine receptors. Anatomical and immunocytochemical studies have revealed that the receptor binding sites and neuronal fibers of oxytocin and dopamine exist in the same central nervous system regions, often in close apposition to each other (for a review, see Baskerville and Douglas 2010), with oxytocin-dopamine interactions within the nucleus accumbens and the ventral tegmental area probably being bidirectional. In addition, oxytocin may exert effects on dopamine release that mediate its effects on affiliation, social memory, and so on.

In rodent mothers, suckling and maternal cues (e.g., smell) related to their infants enhance maternal care at least in part by enhancing expression of oxytocin receptors in the nucleus accumbens and the ventral tegmental area. Interestingly, oxytocin has been shown to enhance the experience of attachment security in humans (Buchheim et al. 2009). Therefore, this effect may have early evolutionary primed roots: during early development, interpersonal eye contact plays a particular role in facilitating the development of dopaminergic-neuropeptidergic reward circuits that are later responsive to social cues (Skuse and Gallagher 2009). Therefore, oxytocin may promote interpersonal trust by, on the one hand, inhibiting the hypothalamic-pituitary-adrenal (HPA) axis and defensive behaviors and, on the other, activating dopaminergic reward circuits, enhancing the rewarding value of social encounters. Additionally, genetic studies suggest that in infants who carry the four-repeat variant of the dopamine receptor D_4 allele (*DRD4*) (which is associated with more efficient dopamine function), the reward value of maternal attachment cues may be enhanced so that the quality of parental cues may have greater implications for the child's development (Gervai et al. 2007).

Regarding BPD, Stanley and Siever (2010) explored the hypothesis that the neurobiological underpinnings of maladaptive interpersonal functioning may be related to systems mediating affiliation and affect regulation, which "shape the trajectory of interpersonal development in the context of the specific interpersonal environment" (p. 26). Recent oxytocin studies in individuals with BPD suggest reduced oxytocin concentrations in blood samples, even after controlling for estrogen, progesterone, and contraceptives (Bertsch et al. 2013c). Although plasma oxytocin correlated negatively with experiences of childhood trauma, in particular with emotional neglect and abuse, the results of mediation analyses did not support a simple model of oxytocin being a prominent mediator in the link between childhood trauma and BPD. Future studies are needed to further elucidate the relationships among oxytocin in plasma and cerebrospinal fluid, early adversity, attachment style, and adult interpersonal functioning. Recently published oxytocin challenge studies indicate that oxytocin decreases the stress response not only in healthy individuals (Heinrichs et al. 2001, 2003, 2009) but also in patients with BPD (Simeon et al. 2011). Using the Trier Social Stress Test, Simeon et al. (2011) found that intranasal oxytocin application was followed by a decrease of poststress dysphoria as well as of cortisol response in patients with BPD. In a study that applied a trust game in which the payoff is highest for both players in the case of successful cooperation, oxytocin was not found to uniformly facilitate trust and prosocial behavior in a gender-mixed sample of BPD individuals; rather, behavior depended on attachment style (Bartz et al. 2010). Although analyses did not find more trusting behavior in patients with BPD following oxytocin challenge, data revealed that this neuropeptide promoted actual cooperative behavior for anxiously attached but low avoidant individuals but impeded cooperative behavior for anxiously attached, intimacy-avoidant individuals. Oxytocin may facilitate interpersonal behavior by decreasing social threat hypersensitivity in BPD. Thereby, oxytocin was found to normalize amygdala activity in response to angry faces as well as associated abnormal eye gaze behavior such as more and faster initial fixation changes to the eyes of angry faces in women with BPD (Bertsch et al. 2013a). Furthermore, oxytocin decreased neuronal activity in the amygdala and insula during the processing of visual scenes, and it normalized the abnormal coupling between amygdala activity and gaze behavior in women with BPD (Lischke et al. 2017). However, research on the role of oxytocin in the etiology and neurobiology of BPD is still in its infancy (Herpertz and Bertsch 2015).

Perceptual Alterations

Pain and Nonsuicidal Self-Injury

Nonsuicidal self-injury (NSSI) is frequent in patients with BPD and involves phenomena such as cutting, burning, and head banging; these behaviors can usually be relatively clearly distinguished from suicidal behavior (Nock 2009). In patients with BPD, auto-aggression without suicidal intent is usually repetitive, has limited potential for serious or fatal physical harm, and involves a different spectrum of motives than suicidal or ambivalent auto-aggression (Brown et al. 2002; Favazza 1989; Herpertz 1995). There is robust evidence that patients with BPD use NSSI to achieve quick release from strong aversive inner tension (Brown et al. 2002; Favazza 1989; Herpertz 1995; Kleindienst et al. 2008; Leibenluft et al. 1987). Release from aversive inner tension via NSSI can be understood as a dysfunctional coping mechanism of patients with BPD when they try to regulate emotions (Favazza 1989; Paris 1995) and as being positively and negatively reinforced by intra- and interpersonal factors (Nock 2009; Hooley and Franklin 2018).

"Tension release" (Herpertz 1995) and relief or escape from emotions (Brown et al. 2002; Chapman et al. 2006; Kleindienst et al. 2008) are thought to be the predominant motives for NSSI, although several studies revealed that motives for NSSI in patients with BPD are complex and cannot be easily reduced to a single reason. NSSI is also used to terminate symptoms of dissociation such as derealization and depersonalization. Further motives include self-punishment, feeling physical pain, reducing anxiety and despair, emotion generation, controlling others, distraction, and preventing oneself from acting on suicidal feelings (Brown et al. 2002; Favazza 1989; Osuch et al. 1999; Shearer 1994).

Some limited understanding of the neurobiological underpinnings of NSSI is emerging. Self-injury in patients with BPD is clearly related to emotion dysregulation as well as disturbed pain processing. Several studies have demonstrated that self-injurious patients with BPD show reduced pain sensitivity in relation to emotional stress (Bohus et al. 2000; Ludascher et al. 2007; Schmahl et al. 2004). In the first study (Bohus et al. 2000), patients were investigated twice, under baseline conditions and during high levels of stress. Even under baseline conditions, pain sensitivity in the Cold Pressor Test was significantly lower in patients with BPD than in members of a healthy control group. During high levels of stress, the same patients revealed a further decrease in pain sensitivity in comparison to the baseline condition. The close correlation between aversive tension and pain sensitivity was also replicated on an interindividual level (Ludascher et al. 2007). Reduced pain sensitivity was confirmed using different methods of pain stimulation such as laser (Schmahl et al. 2004) or heat (Schmahl et al. 2006). A recent meta-analysis confirmed reduced pain sensitivity in persons with NSSI, most of them with disorders fulfilling BPD diagnostic criteria (Koenig et al. 2016).

It was also demonstrated that reduction of pain sensitivity is not related to a disturbance of the sensory-discriminative component of pain processing, but rather to an alteration in affective pain processing (Cardenas-Morales et al. 2011; Schmahl et al. 2004). Spatial discrimination of laser pain stimuli was not disturbed in spite of reduced subjective pain perception (Schmahl et al. 2004). Also, laser-evoked potentials including the P300 component as a measure of attentional processes were not reduced. This finding speaks for normal processing of pain from the periphery through the lateral pain pathway to the somatosensory cortex. In addition, a functional polymorphism (Val158Met) of the gene coding for catechol-O-methyltransferase distribution was found to be associated with cognitive neural pain processing in healthy persons but with affective neural pain processing in patients with BPD (Schmahl et al. 2012b).

In an attempt to test the influence of psychopathological states on pain sensitivity, Ludascher et al. (2009) compared patients who had not inflicted NSSI for at least 6 months with patients who showed ongoing NSSI. Sensitivity to pain, including laser and heat pain sensitivity, was measured in these two groups as well as in a healthy comparison group. Overall, a linear trend was found, with the BPD group that had terminated NSSI ranging halfway between the BPD group with ongoing NSSI and the healthy comparison group. These findings suggest that cessation of self-injurious behavior leads to a normalization of pain sensitivity in patients with BPD. In a similar study, patients with remitted BPD (three or fewer DSM-IV criteria met) had a pain sensitivity ranging between that of patients with active BPD and that of healthy control participants (Bekrater-Bodmann et al. 2015). Remitted patients also showed a reduction of urge for self-injury after a stress challenge and did not show the correlation between painfulness of an experimental stimulus and stress reduction usually found in patients with NSSI (Willis et al. 2018).

On a neural level, reduced pain sensitivity is related to the activation of an antinociceptive network of brain regions in patients with BPD. More specifically, tonic heat pain stimuli, with adjustment for individual pain sensitivity during an fMRI study, elicited higher activity in the dorsolateral prefrontal cortex together with reduced activity in the amygdala, perigenual anterior cingulate cortex, and posterior parietal cortex in patients with BPD compared with healthy age-matched control subjects (Schmahl et al. 2006).

As mentioned in the first paragraph of this section, painful stimuli—for example, in the context of NSSI—appear to play a decisive role in the dysfunctional attempts of patients with BPD to regulate emotions. As cognitive methods of emotion regulation such as reappraisal appear not to be successful in correcting prefrontal-limbic dysbalance in patients with BPD (Koenigsberg et al. 2009; Schulze et al. 2011), one can speculate that painful stimulation may have an effect on brain activation in regions related to emotion regulation. Indeed, thermal stimuli—independent of painfulness—led to a reduction of stress-induced amygdala hyperactivity (Niedtfeld et al. 2010). In this study, viewing of pictures to induce negative versus neutral affect was combined with thermal (painful and nonpainful) stimulation. Picture viewing led to increased activity in the amygdala and insula in patients with BPD compared with healthy control subjects; then, both nonpainful warm and painful hot stimuli were related to a reduction of these increased signals. In a later functional connectivity analysis, Niedtfeld et al. (2012) found that painful heat stimulation, but not nonpainful warm stimulation, following negative emotional pictures led to more negative coupling of amygdala with medial prefrontal cortex. This negative coupling, which can be associated with a normal inhibitory connection, was found to be present in healthy control participants during nonpainful warm stimulation. Taken together, findings from this study suggest that in patients with BPD, painful stimuli are necessary to restore inhibitory prefrontal-limbic connection. This may explain why patients need strong painful stimuli, as in the context of NSSI, to regulate their emotional arousal. After successful therapy, however, this mechanism appears to lose its function, as patients measured with this paradigm did not reveal amygdala deactivation by pain any longer, but rather showed a "healthy" amygdala activation (Niedtfeld et al. 2017).

From a perspective of experimental psychopathology (i.e., modeling of pathological behavior under laboratory conditions), several aspects of NSSI should be considered when studies on its neurobiological background are being designed. NSSI is a complex behavioral pattern that comprises—besides painful experience—other aspects such as tissue damage or seeing one's own blood flow. Modeling such a complex behavior under laboratory conditions is a difficult and challenging task. In a first attempt to investigate the role of tissue damage in the context of NSSI, Reitz et al. (2012) studied incision-induced pain in patients with BPD. (This study and all the following were approved by the appropriate institutional review board). In a pilot study, stress was first induced by mental arithmetic under time pressure and negative social feedback. Directly after this stress induction, the investigator made a small incision with a scalpel on the subject's forearm and then recorded subjective as well as objective (heart rate) measures of stress. The incision led to a decrease of aversive tension in patients with BPD but to a further increase of aversive tension in healthy controls. Heart rate in patients with BPD decreased after the incision, but not after a sham condition in which the skin was touched with the blunt end of the scalpel. Findings from an fMRI study confirmed tension release via incision and suggest that incision, but not the sham treatment, leads to a deactivation of the amygdala and a restoration of the typical post-stress connectivity pattern between amygdala and medial prefrontal cortex (Reitz et al. 2015).

Further studies have been undertaken to elucidate the role of tissue injury and seeing of blood in the context of NSSI. Interestingly, the reduction of stress levels after a pain stimulus occurs regardless of whether the pain stimulus is associated with tissue injury (Willis et al. 2017). For this purpose, incision was compared with an equally painful pressure stimulus, which was applied by means of a blade placed on the skin but not injuring it. Both stimuli led to a similar reduction of stress levels. In another study, stress relief with and without artificial blood (red-colored fluid with temperature and texture similar to real blood) was compared in the context of the application of the blade stimulus. In the first minutes after the painful stimulation, there was a tendency for a stronger decrease in stress levels in the blood condition as compared with the nonblood condition in the BPD group compared with healthy controls (HCs), and the BPD patients showed a significantly stronger decrease in urge for NSSI in the blood condition than the HC group (Naoum et al. 2016).

From a neurochemical point of view, the endogenous opioid system (EOS) appears to play an important role in the context of disturbed pain processing and NSSI (Bandelow et al. 2010; Stanley and Siever 2010). The EOS is assumed to be related to stress-induced analgesia as well as to dissociation in patients with BPD. Patients with BPD and NSSI had significantly lower levels of cerebrospinal fluid β-endorphin and met-enkephalin when compared with a non-NSSI group (Stanley et al. 2010), and an increase of salivary β-endorphin levels after self-injury could recently be demonstrated in a study using ambulatory assessment of real-life NSSI events (L.M. Stoerkel, A. Karabatsiakis, J. Hepp, et al.: "Salivary Beta-Endorphin in Non-suicidal Self-Injury: An Ambulatory Assessment Study," unpublished manuscript). NSSI and dissociation can be reduced by treatment with the opioid antagonist naltrexone (Bohus et al. 1999; Schmahl et al. 2012a; Sonne et al. 1996). One potential mechanism, besides blocking opioid-mediated positive reinforcement processes, is the reduction of stress-related dissociative symptoms by naltrexone, which reduces the need to terminate dissociative states by using NSSI. More research on the involvement of the EOS and its different components in NSSI and BPD is clearly warranted.

Dissociation

Dissociation is a ubiquitous phenomenon in psychiatric conditions (Lyssenko et al. 2018) and is composed of varying degrees of amnesia, depersonalization, derealization, and reduced sensory perception, including reduced pain sensitivity. In patients with BPD, dissociation is state-dependent and closely related to stress levels (Ludascher et al. 2007; Stiglmayr et al. 2008). Although dissociative states can be reliably assessed, the investigation of neurobiological processes underlying dissociative states is relatively new. Patients with dissociative identity disorder revealed markedly reduced volumes of hippocampus and, particularly, amygdala (Vermetten et al. 2006). On a neurophysiological level, reduced P300 amplitudes (Kirino 2006), altered magnetoencephalography-measured brain waves (Ray et al. 2006), and altered cortical excitability (Spitzer et al. 2004) have been associated with dissociative experiences in patients and healthy control subjects. A close correlation between pain sensitivity and dissociation levels has also been demonstrated experimentally (Ludascher et al. 2007, 2010). In these studies, dissociation was related to reduced pain sensitivity.

It has been suggested that dissociation constitutes an emotional overmodulation mode in response to the experience of (traumatic) stress as opposed to an emotional undermodulation mode with predominant intrusive symptoms, and that these two modes can also be segregated on a neurofunctional level (Lanius et al. 2010; Ludascher et al. 2010; Sierra and Berrios 1998). Particularly, overactivity of medial prefrontal brain regions with concomitant limbic down-regulation is thought to underlie dissociative psychopathology. Corroboration of these assumptions comes from several sources. Patients with BPD and high levels of dissociation had significantly lower startle responses compared with patients with low levels of dissociation (Ebner-Priemer et al. 2005). This finding may also be interpreted in light of reduced amygdala activity during dissociative states as suggested by Sierra and Berrios (1998). Results from a study investigating the influence of dissociation on emotional-cognitive processing lends further evidence for the model of emotional overmodulation; dissociation scores were negatively correlated with activity in amygdala, insula, and anterior cingulate cortex during emotional distraction while BPD subjects were performing a working memory task (Krause-Utz et al. 2012). This investigation was repeated using experimentally induced (script-driven imagery) dissociative states. Script-driven imagery is well suited to specifically inducing dissociation in patients with BPD (Ludascher et al. 2010). Individual situations eliciting dissociation are depicted for each patient. During the presentation of the script, higher values for dissociation as well as reduced pain sensitivity during induced dissociation were found (Ludascher et al. 2010). After script-induced dissociation, BPD patients again showed amygdala deactivation together with working memory impairment (Krause-Utz et al. 2018).

The results of a classical conditioning study highlight a potential negative side effect of dampened limbic, particularly amygdala, activity: a significant reduction of fear conditioning and emotional learning processes during dissociative states (Ebner-Priemer et al. 2009). When patients with BPD were retrospectively separated into two groups (those with dissociation during fear conditioning and those without), only those without dissociation revealed normal fear conditioning processes, whereas patients with dissociation did not show differential conditioning in terms of skin conductance responses or emotional valence coding.

Given the disturbance of emotional learning processes in relation to changes in limbic brain activity, it is not surprising to find a profound negative impact of dissociation on psychotherapy outcome, because most psychological treatments rely on basic learning processes to reach changes in psychopathology. In several psychiatric disorders, dissociation could be demonstrated to be a negative predictor of psychotherapy outcome (Rufer et al. 2006; Spitzer et al. 2007). In a study in patients with BPD, high baseline scores on the Dissociative Experience Scale predicted poor improvement after a 3-month course of dialectical behavior therapy, even after controlling for overall baseline symptom severity (Kleindienst et al. 2011).

The construct of dissociation has been derived from clinical experience as well as research in humans. There is to date no animal model for dissociation. Hence, animal research must rely on human analogues of this phenomenon. Translational research has to develop research designs to study these components in parallel in animals and humans.

Dissociation is a phylogenetically evolved, complex behavioral pattern with species-specific modifications. One possible analogue of dissociation in animals can be derived from behavioral research using fear-conditioning paradigms. The behavior systems approach views an animal as having a set of several genetically determined, prepackaged behaviors that it uses to solve particular functional problems. If the problem has to be solved immediately, the animal's behavioral repertoire becomes restricted to those genetically hardwired behaviors. This was outlined by Bolles (1970) in his *species-specific defense reaction* (SSDR) theory. When an animal is confronted by a natural environmental threat (e.g., a predator) or an artificial one (e.g., an electrical shock), its behavioral repertoire becomes restricted to its SSDRs. Freeze, fight, and flight are examples of SSDRs. The so-called defensive behavior system (Fanselow 1994) is organized by the imminence of a predator and can be divided into three stages: preencounter, postencounter, and circa-strike. *Preencounter* defensive behaviors include reorganization of meal patterns and protective nest maintenance, if an animal has to leave a safe nesting area. When the level of fear increases (e.g., because of actual detection of a predator), the *postencounter* defensive behavior mode becomes active. This mode includes multiple dimensions (Bohus et al. 1996; Fanselow 1994; Mayer and Fanselow 2003): 1) a motor component (freezing), 2) a sensory component (opiate analgesia), 3) an autonomic component (activity of the sympathetic and parasympathetic nervous systems), 4) an endocrinological component (HPA axis), and 5) an emotional component (anxiety). In the case of physical contact (e.g., the experience of pain), the animal engages in more active defenses, such as biting and jumping. This is an example of *circa-strike* behavior. Analogies between these types of animal behavior and dissociation in humans have been discussed (Nijenhuis and den Boer 2007).

In animals, critical anatomical structures for postencounter defensive behavior are the amygdala, the ventral periaqueductal gray (PAG), and the hypothalamus (for an overview, see Brandao et al. 2008). The amygdala has a central relay function or mediation of postencounter defensive behavior with important glutamatergic input from the thalamus to the lateral amygdala (Fanselow 1994). Furthermore, the central amygdala mediates transfer of information about the threat level to the ventral PAG, which in turn appears to mediate analgesia and freezing by opioidergic neurotransmission (Fanselow and Gale 2003; LeDoux 1992). The switch between freezing and more active behavioral patterns (fight, flight) appears to involve two parts of the PAG: whereas freezing is mediated by the ventral PAG, fight and flight responses involve the dorsal PAG (Brandao et al. 2008). Autonomic and endocrinological responses are mediated by connections of the amygdala with the hypothalamus (LeDoux et al. 1988). The exact localization of the emotional component is unclear but can be assumed to rely on amygdala–prefrontal cortex pathways (LeDoux 2002). Circa-strike behavior is mediated by the superior colliculus and the dorsolateral PAG, which receive nociceptive input from the spinal cord and the trigeminal nucleus (Blomqvist and Craig 1991). In phylogenetically more recent species, such as humans, these systems can be assumed to be usually controlled by higher cortical regions and to be activated under high levels of stress.

It can be hypothesized that dissociation is the representation of the postencounter defense mode in humans, comprising the same dimensions as described in animals but extended by an emotional-psychological component (depersonalization, derealization, and emotional numbness). In this model, self-destructive behavior, which can be observed frequently during dissociative states, such as in patients with BPD, may represent an analogue of the pain-induced switch of behavioral modes from postencounter to the circa-strike behavioral mode in a human being faced with high levels of aversive stress.

Conclusion

Research in the field of specific types of PDs, particularly BPD and ASPD, has significantly deepened the understanding of the nature of these disorders by applying methods of experimental psychopathology and neuroscience. Although affect regulation—the pathological trait of emotional lability, according to DSM-5 Section III, "Emerging Measures and Models"—is the functional domain that has been most intensively studied in PDs, recent research has focused on the interpersonal domain and on perception issues. Future studies should conflate these approaches by giving priority to detecting the unfavorable interaction between these domains. The AMPD in Section III of DSM-5 provides an elaborate classificatory approach to future studies in this field, making possible more homogeneous samples of patients to include in research studies. The evaluation of the degree and quality of impairment of interpersonal functioning (empathy and intimacy) will enable clinicians and researchers to profoundly describe interpersonal dysfunctioning in patients beyond nosological categorization and to identify its relation to brain dysfunctions and facilitate translational research.

Although animal models related to the complex psychopathology of PDs are still at the very beginning, they promise further advances in understanding gene × environment interactions and their epigenetic modulations in individuals prone to be highly vulnerable to adversity throughout their lives. Finally, translational research can contribute not only to clarifying the pathophysiology of PDs but also, based on a deepened understanding of treatment mechanisms, to developing innovative treatment options, whether in psychotherapy or pharmacological add-on treatments with substances that may enhance psychotherapeutic effects, such as oxytocin in the interpersonal realm.

References

Arntz A, Veen G: Evaluations of others by borderline patients. J Nerv Ment Dis 189:513–521, 2001

Arntz A, Bernstein D, Oorschot M, et al: Theory of mind in borderline and cluster-C personality disorder. J Nerv Ment Dis 197:801–807, 2009

Bandelow B, Schmahl C, Falkai P, et al: Borderline personality disorder: a dysregulation of the endogenous opioid system? Psychol Rev 117:623–636, 2010

Barnow S, Limberg A, Stopsack M, et al: Dissociation and emotion regulation in borderline personality disorder. Psychol Med 42:783–794, 2012

Bartz J, Simeon D, Hamilton H, et al: Oxytocin can hinder trust and cooperation in borderline personality disorder. Soc Cogn Affect Neurosci 6:556–563, 2010

Baskerville TA, Douglas AJ: Dopamine and oxytocin interactions underlying behaviors: potential contributions to behavioral disorders. CNS Neurosci Ther 16:92–123, 2010

Bekrater-Bodmann R, Chung BY, Richter I, et al: Deficits in pain perception in borderline personality disorder: results from the thermal grill illusion. Pain 156:2084–2092, 2015

Berenson KR, Gyurak A, Ayduk O, et al: Rejection sensitivity and disruption of attention by social threat cues. J Res Pers 43:1064–1072, 2009

Bertsch K, Gamer M, Schmidt B, et al: Oxytocin and reduction of social threat hypersensitivity in women with borderline personality disorder. Am J Psychiatry 170:1169–1177, 2013a

Bertsch K, Grothe M, Prehn K, et al: Volumetric differences between antisocial offenders with borderline personality disorder and antisocial offenders with psychopathic traits. Eur Arch Psychiatr Clin Neurosci 38:129–137, 2013b

Bertsch K, Schmidinger I, Neumann I, et al: Reduced plasma oxytocin levels in female patients with borderline personality disorder. Horm Behav 63:424–429, 2013c

Bilek E, Stossel G, Schafer A, et al: State-dependent cross-brain information flow in borderline personality disorder. JAMA Psychiatry 74:949–957, 2017

Blair RJR, Mitchell DG, Peschardt KS, et al: Reduced sensitivity to others' fearful expressions in psychopathic individuals. Pers Indiv Dif 37:1111–1122, 2004

Blomqvist A, Craig AD: Organization of spinal and trigeminal input to the PAG, in The Midbrain Periaqueductal Grey Matter: Functional, Anatomical, and Immunohistochemical Organization. Edited by Depaulis A, Bandler R. New York, Plenum, 1991, pp 345–363

Bohus B, Koolhaas JM, Korte SM, et al: Forebrain pathways and their behavioural interactions with neuroendocrine and cardiovascular function in the rat. Clin Exp Pharmacol Physiol 23:177–182, 1996

Bohus MJ, Landwehrmeyer GB, Stiglmayr CE, et al: Naltrexone in the treatment of dissociative symptoms in patients with borderline personality disorder: an open-label trial. J Clin Psychiatry 60:598–603, 1999

Bohus M, Limberger M, Ebner U, et al: Pain perception during self-reported distress and calmness in patients with borderline personality disorder and self-mutilating behavior. Psychiatry Res 95:251–260, 2000

Bolles RC: Species-specific defense reactions and avoidance learning. Psychol Rev 77:32–48, 1970

Brandao ML, Zanoveli JM, Ruiz-Martinez RC, et al: Different patterns of freezing behavior organized in the periaqueductal gray of rats: association with different types of anxiety. Behav Brain Res 188:1–13, 2008

Brown MZ, Comtois KA, Linehan MM: Reasons for suicide attempts and nonsuicidal self-injury in women with borderline personality disorder. J Abnorm Psychol 111:198–202, 2002

Buchheim A, Heinrichs M, George C, et al: Oxytocin enhances the experience of attachment security. Neuroendocrinology 34:1417–1422, 2009

Cardenas-Morales L, Fladung AK, Kammer T, et al: Exploring the affective component of pain perception during aversive stimulation in borderline personality disorder. Psychiatry Res 186:458–460, 2011

Chapman AL, Gratz KL, Brown MZ: Solving the puzzle of deliberate self-harm: the experiential avoidance model. Behav Res Ther 44:371–394, 2006

Coricelli G: Two-levels of mental states attribution: from automaticity to voluntariness. Neuropsychologia 43:294–300, 2005

Craig MC, Catani M, Deeley Q, et al: Altered connections on the road to psychopathy. Mol Psychiatry 14:946–953, 2009

Daros AR, Zakzanis KK, Ruocco AC: Facial emotion recognition in borderline personality disorder. Psychol Med 43:1953–1963, 2013

Davis MH: Measuring individual differences in empathy: evidence for a multidimensional approach. J Pers Soc Psychol 44:113–126, 1983

Decety J, Moriguchi Y: The empathic brain and its dysfunction in psychiatric populations: implications for intervention across different clinical conditions. Biopsychosoc Med 1:22, 2007

Decety J, Skelly LR, Kiehl KA: Brain response to empathy-eliciting scenarios involving pain in incarcerated individuals with psychopathy. JAMA Psychiatry 70:638–645, 2013

Decety J, Chen C, Harensk CL, Kiehl KA: Socioemotional processing of morally-laden behavior and their consequences on others in forensic psychopaths. Hum Brain Mapp 36:2015–2026, 2015a

Decety J, Lewis KL, Cowell JM: Specific electrophysiological components disentangle affective sharing and empathic concern in psychopathy. J Neurophysiol 114:493–504, 2015b

Denny B, Fan TJ, Fels S, et al: Sensitization of the neural salience network to repeated emotional stimuli following initial habituation in patients with borderline personality disorder. Am J Psychiatry 175:657–664, 2018

Di Simplicio M, Massey-Chase R, Cowen PJ, et al: Oxytocin enhances processing of positive versus negative emotional information in healthy male volunteers. J Psychopharmacol 23:241–248, 2009

Domes G, Heinrichs M, Michel A, et al: Oxytocin improves "mind-reading" in humans. Biol Psychiatry 61:731–733, 2006a

Domes G, Winter B, Schnell K, et al: The influence of emotions on inhibitory functioning in borderline personality disorder. Psychol Med 36:1163–1172, 2006b

Domes G, Czieschnek D, Weidler F, et al: Recognition of facial affect in borderline personality disorder. J Pers Disord 22:135–147, 2008

Domes G, Schulze L, Herpertz SC: Emotion recognition in borderline personality disorder: a review of the literature. J Pers Disord 23:6–19, 2009

Domes G, Steiner A, Porges SW, et al: Oxytocin differentially modulates eye gaze to naturalistic social signals of happiness and anger. Psychoneuroendocrinology 38:1198–1202, 2013

Donegan NH, Sanislow CA, Blumberg HP, et al: Amygdala hyperreactivity in borderline personality disorder: implications for emotional dysregulation. Biol Psychiatry 54:1284–1293, 2003

Dziobek I, Fleck S, Kalbe E, et al: Introducing MASC: a movie for the assessment of social cognition. J Autism Dev Disord 36:623–636, 2006

Dziobek I, Preissler S, Grozdanovic Z, et al: Neuronal correlates of altered empathy and social cognition in borderline personality disorder. Neuroimage 57:539–548, 2011

Ebner-Priemer UW, Badeck S, Beckmann C, et al: Affective dysregulation and dissociative experience in female patients with borderline personality disorder: a startle response study. J Psychiatr Res 39:85–92, 2005

Ebner-Priemer UW, Mauchnik J, Kleindienst N, et al: Emotional learning during dissociative states in borderline personality disorder. J Psychiatry Neurosci 34:214–222, 2009

Fairchild G, Van Goozen SH, Calder AJ, et al: Deficits in facial expression recognition in male adolescents with early onset or adolescence-onset conduct disorder. J Child Psychol Psychiatry 50:627–636, 2009

Fanselow MS: Neural organization of the defensive behavior system responsible for fear. Psychonomic Bulletin and Review 1:429–438, 1994

Fanselow MS, Gale GD: The amygdala, fear, and memory. Ann N Y Acad Sci 985:125–134, 2003

Favazza AR: Why patients mutilate themselves. Hosp Community Psychiatry 40:137–145, 1989

Fertuck EA, Jekal A, Song I, et al: Enhanced "Reading the Mind in the Eyes" in borderline personality disorder compared to healthy controls. Psychol Med 39:1979–1988, 2009

Fischer-Shofty M, Shamay-Tsoory SG, Harari H, et al: The effect of intranasal administration of oxytocin on fear recognition. Neuropsychologia 48:179–184, 2010

Fonagy P, Bateman AW: Mechanisms of change in mentalization-based treatment of BPD. J Clin Psychol 62:411–430, 2006

Fonagy P, Luyten P: A developmental, mentalization-based approach to the understanding and treatment of borderline personality disorder. Dev Psychopathol 21:1355–1381, 2009

Frith CD, Frith U: The neural basis of mentalizing. Neuron 50:531–534, 2006

Gallese V: Before and below "theory of mind": embodied simulation and the neural correlates of social cognition. Philos Trans R Soc Lond B Biol Sci 362:659–669, 2007

Gallese V, Goldman AI: Mirror neurons and the simulation theory of mind-reading. Trends Cogn Sci 2:493–501, 1998

Gamer M, Zurowski B, Büchel C: Different amygdala subregions mediate valence-related and attentional effects of oxytocin in humans. Proc Natl Acad Sci USA 107:9400–9405, 2010

Gervai J, Novak A, Lakatos K, et al: Infant genotype may moderate sensitivity to maternal affective communications: attachment disorganization, quality of care, and the DRD4 polymorphism. Soc Neurosci 2:307–319, 2007

Ghiassi V, Dimaggio G, Brüne M: Dysfunctions in understanding other minds in borderline personality disorder: a study using cartoon picture stories. J Psychother Res 20:657–667, 2010

Goldman AI, Sripada CS: Simulationist models of face-based emotion recognition. Cognition 94:193–213, 2005

Gregory S, Ffytche D, Simmons A, et al: The antisocial brain: psychopathy matters. Arch Gen Psychiatry 69:962–972, 2012

Guastella AJ, Mitchell PB, Dadds MR: Oxytocin increases gaze to the eye region of human face. Biol Psychiatry 63:3–5, 2008

Guastella AJ, Kenyon AR, Alvares GA, et al: Intranasal arginine vasopressin enhances the encoding of happy and angry faces in humans. Biol Psychiatry 67:1220–1222, 2010

Gunderson JG, Lyons-Ruth K: BPD's interpersonal hypersensitivity phenotype: a gene-environment-developmental model. J Pers Disord 22:22–41, 2008

Gunderson JG, Zanarini MC, Kisiel C: Borderline personality disorder, in DSM-IV Source Book, Section IV, Vol 2. Edited by Widiger TA, Frances AJ, Pincus HA, et al. Washington, DC, American Psychiatric Press, 1996, pp 717–733

Gunderson JG, Bateman A, Kernberg O: Alternative perspectives on psychodynamic psychotherapy of borderline personality disorder: the case of "Ellen." Am J Psychiatry 164:1333–1339, 2007

Gunderson JG, Zanarini MC, Choi-Kain LW, et al: Family study of borderline personality disorder and its sectors of psychopathology. Arch Gen Psychiatry 68:753–762, 2011

Guttman HA, Laporte L: Empathy in families of women with borderline personality disorder, anorexia nervosa, and a control group. Fam Process 39:345–358, 2000

Harari H, Shamay-Tsoory SG, Ravid M, et al: Double dissociation between cognitive and affective empathy in borderline personality disorder. Psychiatr Res 175:277–279, 2010

Heinrichs M, Baumgartner T, Ehlert U, et al: Effects of oxytocin and social support on psychoendocrine stress responsiveness in healthy men. Psychosom Med 63:149–150, 2001

Heinrichs M, Baumgartner T, Kirschbaum C, et al: Social support and oxytocin interact to suppress cortisol and subjective responses to psychosocial stress. Biol Psychiatry 54:1389–1398, 2003

Heinrichs M, von Dawans B, Domes G: Oxytocin, vasopressin, and human social behavior. Front Neuroendocrinol 30:548–557, 2009

Herpertz S: Self-injurious behaviour: psychopathological and nosological characteristics in subtypes of self-injurers. Acta Psychiatr Scand 91:57–68, 1995

Herpertz SC, Bertsch K: A new perspective on the pathophysiology of borderline personality disorder: a model of the role of oxytocin. Am J Psychiatry 172: 840-851, 2015

Hooley JM, Franklin JC: Why do people hurt themselves? A new conceptual model of nonsuicidal self-injury. Clinical Psychological Science 6:428–451, 2018

Iacoboni M, Molnar-Szakacs I, Gallese V, et al: Grasping the intentions of others with one's own mirror neuron system. PLoS Biol 3:e79, 2005

Izurieta Hidalgo NA, Oelkers-Ax R, Nagy K, et al: Time course of facial emotion processing in women with borderline personality disorder: an ERP study. J Psychiatry Neurosci 41:16–26, 2016

Jovev M, Green M, Chanen A, et al: Attentional processes and responding to affective faces in youth with borderline personality features. Psychiatry Res 199:44–50, 2012

Kanske P, Bockler A, Singer T: Models, mechanisms and moderators dissociating empathy and theory of mind. Curr Top Behav Neurosci 30:193–206, 2017

Kirino E: P300 is attenuated during dissociative episodes. J Nerv Ment Dis 194:83–90, 2006

Kleindienst N, Bohus M, Ludascher P, et al: Motives for nonsuicidal self-injury among women with borderline personality disorder. J Nerv Ment Dis 196:230–236, 2008

Kleindienst N, Limberger MF, Ebner-Priemer UW, et al: Dissociation predicts poor response to dialectical behavioral therapy in female patients with borderline personality disorder. J Pers Disord 25:432–447, 2011

Knobloch HS, Charlet A, Hoffmann LC, et al: Evoked axonal oxytocin release in the central amygdala attenuates fear response. Neuron 73:553–566, 2012

Koenig J, Thayer JF, Kaess M: A meta-analysis on pain sensitivity in self-injury. Psychol Med 46:1597–1612, 2016

Koenigsberg HW, Fan J, Ochsner KN, et al: Neural correlates of the use of psychological distancing to regulate responses to negative social cues: a study of patients with borderline personality disorder. Biol Psychiatry 66:854–863, 2009

Koenigsberg HW, Denny BT, Fan J, et al: The neural correlates of anomalous habituation to negative emotional pictures in borderline and avoidant personality disorder patients. Am J Psychiatry 171:82–90, 2014

Krause-Utz A, Oei NY, Niedtfeld I, et al: Influence of emotional distraction on working memory performance in borderline personality disorder. Psychol Med 42:2181–2192, 2012

Krause-Utz A, Winter D, Schriner F, et al: Reduced amygdala reactivity and impaired working memory during dissociation in borderline personality disorder. Eur Arch Psych Clin Neurosci 268:401–415, 2018

Lanius RA, Vermetten E, Loewenstein RJ, et al: Emotion modulation in PTSD: clinical and neurobiological evidence for a dissociative subtype. Am J Psychiatry 167:640–647, 2010

Lawrence AD, Calder AJ: Homologizing human emotions, in Emotion, Evolution, and Rationality. Edited by Evans D, Cruse P. Oxford, UK, Oxford University Press, 2004, pp 15–47

LeDoux JE: Emotion and the amygdala, in The Amygdala: Neurobiological Apects of Emotion, Memory, and Mental Dysfunction. Edited by Aggleton JP. New York, Wiley-Liss, 1992, pp 339–351

LeDoux JE: Synaptic Self: How Our Brains Become Who We Are. New York, Viking, 2002

LeDoux JE, Iwata J, Cicchetti P, et al: Different projections of the central amygdaloid nucleus mediate autonomic and behavioral correlates of conditioned fear. J Neurosci 8:2517–2529, 1988

Leibenluft E, Gardner DL, Cowdry RW, et al: The inner experience of the borderline self-mutilator. J Pers Disord 1:317–324, 1987

Lischke T, Berger C, Prehn C, et al: Intranasal oxytocin enhances emotion recognition from dynamic facial expressions and leaves eye-gaze unaffected. Psychoneuroendocrinology 37:475–481, 2012

Lischke A, Herpertz SC, Berger C, et al: Divergent effects of oxytocin on (para-)limbic reactivity to emotional and neutral scenes in females with and without borderline personality disorder. Soc Cogn Affect Neurosci 12:1783–1792, 2017

Ludascher P, Bohus M, Lieb K, et al: Elevated pain thresholds correlate with dissociation and aversive arousal in patients with borderline personality disorder. Psychiatry Res 149:291–296, 2007

Ludascher P, Greffrath W, Schmahl C, et al: A cross-sectional investigation of discontinuation of self-injury and normalizing pain perception in patients with borderline personality disorder. Acta Psychiatr Scand 120:62–70, 2009

Ludascher P, Valerius G, Stiglmayr C, et al: Pain sensitivity and neural processing during dissociative states in patients with borderline personality disorder with and without comorbid posttraumatic stress disorder: a pilot study. J Psychiatry Neurosci 35:177–184, 2010

Lyssenko L, Schmahl C, Weidner L, et al: Dissociation in psychiatric disorders—a meta-analysis of studies using the Dissociative Experience Scale. Am J Psychiatry 175:37–46, 2018

Marsh AA, Blair RJ: Deficits in facial affect recognition among antisocial populations: a meta-analysis. Neurosci Biobehav Rev 32:454–465, 2008

Marsh AA, Yu HH, Pine DS, et al: Oxytocin improves specific recognition of positive facial expressions. Psychopharmacology (Berl) 209:225–232, 2010

Matzke B, Herpertz SC, Berger C, et al: Facial reactions to emotional expressions in borderline personality disorder: a facial electromyography study. Psychopathology 47:101—110, 2014

Mayer EA, Fanselow MS: Dissecting the components of the central response to stress. Nat Neurosci 6:1011–1012, 2003

Meffert H, Gazzola V, den Boer JA, et al: Reduced spontaneous but relatively normal deliberate vicarious representations in psychopathy. Brain 136 (pt 8):2550–2562, 2013

Meyer B, Pilkonis PA, Beevers CG: What's in a (neutral) face? Personality disorders, attachment styles, and the appraisal of ambiguous social cues. J Pers Disord 18:320–336, 2004

Mier D, Lis S, Esslinger C, et al: Neuronal correlates of social cognition in borderline personality disorder. Soc Cogn Affect Neurosci 8:531–537, 2013

Mier D, Haddad L, Diers K, et al: Reduced embodied simulation in psychopathy. World J Biol Psychiatry 15:479–487, 2014

Minzenberg MJ, Poole JH, Vinogradov S: Adult social attachment disturbance is related to childhood maltreatment and current symptoms in borderline personality disorder. J Nerv Ment Dis 194:341–348, 2006

Minzenberg MJ, Fan J, New AS, et al: Fronto-limbic dysfunction in response to facial emotion in borderline personality disorder: an event-related fMRI study. Psychiatry Res 155:231–243, 2007

Modestin J: Counter-transference reactions contributing to completed suicide. Br J Med Psychol 60:379–385, 1987

Naoum J, Reitz S, Krause-Utz A, et al: The role of seeing blood in non-suicidal self-injury in female patients with borderline personality disorder. Psychiatry Res 246:676–682, 2016

Nemeth N, Matrai P, Hegyi P, et al: Theory of mind disturbances in borderline personality disorder: a meta-analysis. Psychiatry Res 270:143–153, 2018

New AS, Aan Het Rot M, Ripoll LH, et al: Empathy and alexithymia in borderline personality disorder: clinical and laboratory measures. J Pers Disord 26:660–675, 2012

Niedtfeld I, Schulze L, Kirsch P, et al: Affect regulation and pain in borderline personality disorder: a possible link to the understanding of self-injury. Biol Psychiatry 68:383–391, 2010

Niedtfeld I, Kirsch P, Schulze L, et al: Functional connectivity of pain-mediated affect regulation in borderline personality disorder. PLoS One 7:e33293, 2012

Niedtfeld I, Schmitt R, Winter D, et al: Pain-mediated affect regulation is reduced after dialectical behavior therapy in borderline personality disorder: a longitudinal fMRI study. SCAN 12:739–747, 2017

Nijenhuis ERS, den Boer JA: Psychobiology of traumatization and trauma-related structural dissociation of the personality, in Traumatic Dissociation: Neurobiology and Treatment. Edited by Vermetten E, Dorahy NJ, Spiegel D. Washington, DC, American Psychiatric Publishing, 2007, pp 219–236

Nock MK: Why do people hurt themselves? New insights into the nature and functions of self-injury. Curr Dir Psychol Sci 18:78–83, 2009

Normann-Eide E, Antonsen BRT, Kvarstein EH, et al: Are impairments in theory of mind specific to borderline personality disorder? J Pers Disord 34(6):827–841, 2020

O'Neill A, D'Souza A, Samson AC, et al: Dysregulation between emotion and theory of mind networks in borderline personality disorder. Psychiatry Res 231:25–32, 2015

Osuch EA, Noll JG, Putnam FW: The motivations for self-injury in psychiatric inpatients. Psychiatry 62:334–346, 1999

Paris J: Understanding self-mutilation in borderline personality disorder. Harv Rev Psychiatry 13:179–185, 1995

Passamonti L, Fairchild G, Goodyer IM, et al: Neural abnormalities in early onset and adolescence-onset conduct disorder. Arch Gen Psychiatry 67:729–738, 2010

Patrick CJ: Emotion and psychopathy: startling new insights. Psychophysiology 31:319–330, 1994

Prehn K, Schulze L, Rossmann S, et al: Effects of emotional stimuli on working memory processes in male criminal offenders with borderline and antisocial personality disorder. World J Biol Psychiatry 14:71–78, 2013

Preißler S, Dziobek I, Ritter K, et al: Social cognition in borderline personality disorder: evidence for disturbed recognition of the emotions, thoughts, and intentions of others. Front Behav Neurosci 4:182, 2010

Ray WJ, Odenwald M, Neuner F, et al: Decoupling neural networks from reality: dissociative experiences in torture victims are reflected in abnormal brain waves in left frontal cortex. Psychol Sci 17:825–829, 2006

Reitz S, Krause-Utz A, Pogatzki-Zahn EM, et al: Stress regulation and incision in borderline personality disorder—a pilot study modeling cutting behavior. J Pers Disord 26:605–615, 2012

Reitz S, Kluetsch R, Niedtfeld I, et al: Incision and stress regulation in borderline personality disorder: neurobiological mechanisms of self-injurious behaviour. Br J Psychiatry 207:165–172, 2015

Reniers RL, Corcoran R, Völlm BA, et al: Moral decision-making, ToM, empathy and the default mode network. Biol Psychol 90:202–210, 2012

Rufer M, Held D, Cremer J, et al: Dissociation as a predictor of cognitive behavior therapy outcome in patients with obsessive-compulsive disorder. Psychother Psychosom 75:40–46, 2006

Schiffer B, Pawliczek C, Muller BW, et al: Neural mechanisms underlying affective theory of mind in violent antisocial personality disorder and/or schizophrenia. Schizophr Bull 43:1229–1239, 2017

Schmahl C, Greffrath W, Baumgartner U, et al: Differential nociceptive deficits in patients with borderline personality disorder and self-injurious behavior: laser-evoked potentials, spatial discrimination of noxious stimuli, and pain ratings. Pain 110:470–479, 2004

Schmahl C, Bohus M, Esposito F, et al: Neural correlates of antinociception in borderline personality disorder. Arch Gen Psychiatry 63:659–667, 2006

Schmahl C, Kleindienst N, Limberger M, et al: Evaluation of naltrexone for dissociative symptoms in borderline personality disorder. Int Clin Psychopharmacol 27:61–68, 2012a

Schmahl C, Ludascher P, Greffath W, et al: COMT val158met polymorphism and neural pain processing. PLoS One 7:e23658, 2012b

Schneider P, Hannusch C, Schmahl C, et al: Adolescent peer-rejection persistently alters pain perception and CB1 receptor expression in female rats. Eur Neuropsychopharmacol 24:290–301, 2014

Schulze L, Domes G, Kruger A, et al: Neuronal correlates of cognitive reappraisal in borderline patients with affective instability. Biol Psychiatry 69:564–573, 2011

Seara-Cardoso A, Sebastian CL, Viding E, Roiser JP: Affective resonance in response to others' emotional faces varies with affective ratings and psychopathic traits in amygdala and anterior insula. Soc Neurosci 11:140–152, 2016

Sharp C, Pane H, Ha C, et al: Theory of mind and emotion regulation difficulties in adolescents with borderline traits. J Am Acad Child Adolesc Psychiatry 50:563–573, 2011

Shearer SL: Dissociative phenomena in women with borderline personality disorder. Am J Psychiatry 151:1324–1328, 1994

Sierra M, Berrios GE: Depersonalization: neurobiological perspectives. Biol Psychiatry 44:898–908, 1998

Simeon D, Bartz J, Hamilton H, et al: Oxytocin administration attenuates stress reactivity in borderline personality disorder: a pilot study. Psychoneuroendocrinology 36:1418–1421, 2011

Singer T: The neuronal basis and ontogeny of empathy and mind reading: review of literature and implications for future research. Neurosci Biobehav Rev 30:855–863, 2006

Skuse DH, Gallagher L: Dopaminergic-neuropeptide interactions in the social brain. Trends Cogn Sci 13:27–35, 2009

Sonne S, Rubey R, Brady K, et al: Naltrexone treatment of self-injurious thoughts and behaviors. J Nerv Ment Dis 184:192–195, 1996

Sosic-Vasic Z, Eberhardt J, Bosch JE, et al: Mirror neuron activations in encoding of psychic pain in borderline personality disorder. Neuroimage Clin 22:101737, 2019

Spitzer C, Willert C, Grabe HJ, et al: Dissociation, hemispheric asymmetry, and dysfunction of hemispheric interaction: a transcranial magnetic stimulation approach. J Neuropsychiatry Clin Neurosci 16:163–169, 2004

Spitzer C, Barnow S, Freyburger HJ, et al: Dissociation predicts symptom-related treatment outcome in short-term inpatient psychotherapy. Aust NZ J Psychiatry 41:682–687, 2007

Staebler K, Renneberg B, Stopsack M, et al: Facial emotional expression in reaction to social exclusion in borderline personality disorder. Psychol Med 41:1929–1938, 2011

Stanley B, Siever LJ: The interpersonal dimension of borderline personality disorder: toward a neuropeptide model. Am J Psychiatry 167:24–39, 2010

Stanley B, Sher L, Wilson S, et al: Non-suicidal self-injurious behavior, endogenous opioids and monoamine neurotransmitters. J Affect Dis 124:134–140, 2010

Stiglmayr CE, Ebner-Priemer UW, Bretz J, et al: Dissociative symptoms are positively related to stress in borderline personality disorder. Acta Psychiatr Scand 117:139–147, 2008

Theodoridou A, Rowe AC, Penton-Voak IS, et al: Oxytocin and social perception: oxytocin increases perceived facial trustworthiness and attractiveness. Horm Behav 56:128–132, 2009

Vermetten E, Schmahl C, Lindner S, et al: Hippocampal and amygdalar volumes in dissociative identity disorder. Am J Psychiatry 163:630–636, 2006

von Ceumern-Lindenstjerna IA, Brunner R, Parzer P, et al: Attentional bias in later stages of emotional information processing in female adolescents with borderline personality disorder. Psychopathology 43:25–32, 2010a

von Ceumern-Lindenstjerna I, Brunner R, Parzer P, et al: Initial orienting to emotional faces in female adolescents with borderline personality disorder. Psychopathology 43:79–87, 2010b

Vrticka P, Vuilleumier P: Neuroscience of human social interactions and adult attachment style. Front Hum Neurosci 6:212, 2012

Vrticka P, Andersson F, Grandjean D, et al: Individual attachment style modulates human amygdala and striatum activation during social appraisal. PLoS One 3:e2868, 2008

Wagner AW, Linehan MM: Facial expression recognition ability among women with borderline personality disorder: implications for emotion regulation? J Pers Disord 13:329–344, 1999

Willis F, Kuniss S, Kleindienst N, et al: The role of nociceptive input and tissue injury on stress regulation in borderline personality disorder. Pain 158:479–487, 2017

Willis F, Kuniss S, Kleindienst N, et al: Stress reactivity and pain-mediated stress regulation in remitted patients with borderline personality disorder. Brain Behav 8:e00909, 2018

Zanarini MC, Gunderson JG, Frankenburg FR: Cognitive features of borderline personality disorder. Am J Psychiatry 147:57–63, 1990

Zanarini MC, Frankenburg FR, Reich DB, et al: The 10-year course of psychosocial functioning among patients with borderline personality disorder and axis II comparison subjects. Acta Psychiatr Scand 122:103–109, 2010

Alternative DSM-5 Model for Personality Disorders

The current approach to personality disorders appears in Section II of DSM-5, and an alternative model developed for DSM-5 is presented here in Section III. The inclusion of both models in DSM-5 reflects the decision of the APA Board of Trustees to preserve continuity with current clinical practice, while also introducing a new approach that aims to address numerous shortcomings of the current approach to personality disorders. For example, the typical patient meeting criteria for a specific personality disorder frequently also meets criteria for other personality disorders. Similarly, other specified or unspecified personality disorder is often the correct (but mostly uninformative) diagnosis, in the sense that patients do not tend to present with patterns of symptoms that correspond with one and only one personality disorder.

In the following alternative DSM-5 model, personality disorders are characterized by impairments in personality *functioning* and pathological personality *traits*. The specific personality disorder diagnoses that may be derived from this model include antisocial, avoidant, borderline, narcissistic, obsessive-compulsive, and schizotypal personality disorders. This approach also includes a diagnosis of personality disorder—trait specified (PD-TS) that can be made when a personality disorder is considered present but the criteria for a specific disorder are not met.

General Criteria for Personality Disorder

General Criteria for Personality Disorder

The essential features of a personality disorder are

A. Moderate or greater impairment in personality (self/interpersonal) functioning.
B. One or more pathological personality traits.
C. The impairments in personality functioning and the individual's personality trait expression are relatively inflexible and pervasive across a broad range of personal and social situations.
D. The impairments in personality functioning and the individual's personality trait expression are relatively stable across time, with onsets that can be traced back to at least adolescence or early adulthood.
E. The impairments in personality functioning and the individual's personality trait expression are not better explained by another mental disorder.
F. The impairments in personality functioning and the individual's personality trait expression are not solely attributable to the physiological effects of a substance or another medical condition (e.g., severe head trauma).
G. The impairments in personality functioning and the individual's personality trait expression are not better understood as normal for an individual's developmental stage or sociocultural environment.

A diagnosis of a personality disorder requires two determinations: 1) an assessment of the level of impairment in personality functioning, which is needed for Criterion A, and 2) an evaluation of pathological personality traits, which is required for Criterion B. The impairments in personality functioning and personality trait expression are relatively inflexible and pervasive across a broad range of personal and social situations (Criterion C); relatively stable across time, with onsets that can be traced back to at least adolescence or early adulthood (Criterion D); not better explained by another mental disorder (Criterion E); not attributable to the effects of a substance or another medical condition (Criterion F); and not better understood as normal for an individual's developmental stage or sociocultural environment (Criterion G). All Section III personality disorders described by criteria sets, as well as PD-TS, meet these general criteria, by definition.

Criterion A: Level of Personality Functioning

Disturbances in **self** and **interpersonal** functioning constitute the core of personality psychopathology, and in this alternative diagnostic model they are evaluated on a continuum. Self functioning involves identity and self-direction; interpersonal functioning involves empathy and intimacy (see Table 1). The Level of Personality Functioning Scale (LPFS; see Table 2) uses each of these elements to differentiate five levels of impairment, ranging from little or no impairment (i.e., healthy, adaptive functioning; Level 0) to some (Level 1), moderate (Level 2), severe (Level 3), and extreme (Level 4) impairment.

Impairment in personality functioning predicts the presence of a personality disorder, and the severity of impairment predicts whether an individual has more than

---

TABLE 1.   **Elements of personality functioning**

Self:

1. *Identity:* Experience of oneself as unique, with clear boundaries between self and others; stability of self-esteem and accuracy of self-appraisal; capacity for, and ability to regulate, a range of emotional experience.

2. *Self-direction:* Pursuit of coherent and meaningful short-term and life goals; utilization of constructive and prosocial internal standards of behavior; ability to self-reflect productively.

Interpersonal:

1. *Empathy:* Comprehension and appreciation of others' experiences and motivations; tolerance of differing perspectives; understanding of the effects of one's own behavior on others.

2. *Intimacy:* Depth and duration of connection with others; desire and capacity for closeness; mutuality of regard reflected in interpersonal behavior.

---

one personality disorder or one of the more typically severe personality disorders. A moderate level of impairment in personality functioning is required for the diagnosis of a personality disorder; this threshold is based on empirical evidence that the moderate level of impairment maximizes the ability of clinicians to accurately and efficiently identify personality disorder pathology.

Criterion B: Pathological Personality Traits

Pathological personality traits are organized into five broad domains: Negative Affectivity, Detachment, Antagonism, Disinhibition, and Psychoticism. Within the five broad **trait domains** are 25 specific **trait facets** that were developed initially from a review of existing trait models and subsequently through iterative research with samples of persons who sought mental health services. The full trait taxonomy is presented in Table 3. The B criteria for the specific personality disorders comprise subsets of the 25 trait facets, based on meta-analytic reviews and empirical data on the relationships of the traits to DSM-IV personality disorder diagnoses.

Criteria C and D: Pervasiveness and Stability

Impairments in personality functioning and pathological personality traits are *relatively* pervasive across a range of personal and social contexts, as personality is defined as a pattern of perceiving, relating to, and thinking about the environment and oneself. The term *relatively* reflects the fact that all except the most extremely pathological personalities show some degree of adaptability. The pattern in personality disorders is maladaptive and relatively inflexible, which leads to disabilities in social, occupational, or other important pursuits, as individuals are unable to modify their thinking or behavior, even in the face of evidence that their approach is not working. The impairments in functioning and personality traits are also *relatively* stable. Personality traits—the dispositions to behave or feel in certain ways—are more stable than the symptomatic expressions of these dispositions, but personality traits can also change. Impairments in personality functioning are more stable than symptoms.

Criteria E, F, and G: Alternative Explanations for Personality Pathology (Differential Diagnosis)

On some occasions, what appears to be a personality disorder may be better explained by another mental disorder, the effects of a substance or another medical condition, or a normal developmental stage (e.g., adolescence, late life) or the individual's sociocultural environment. When another mental disorder is present, the diagnosis of a personality disorder is not made if the manifestations of the personality disorder clearly are an expression of the other mental disorder (e.g., if features of schizotypal personality disorder are present only in the context of schizophrenia). On the other hand, personality disorders can be accurately diagnosed in the presence of another mental disorder, such as major depressive disorder, and patients with other mental disorders should be assessed for comorbid personality disorders because personality disorders often impact the course of other mental disorders. Therefore, it is always appropriate to assess personality functioning and pathological personality traits to provide a context for other psychopathology.

Specific Personality Disorders

Section III includes diagnostic criteria for antisocial, avoidant, borderline, narcissistic, obsessive-compulsive, and schizotypal personality disorders. Each personality disorder is defined by typical impairments in personality functioning (Criterion A) and characteristic pathological personality traits (Criterion B):

- Typical features of **antisocial personality disorder** are a failure to conform to lawful and ethical behavior, and an egocentric, callous lack of concern for others, accompanied by deceitfulness, irresponsibility, manipulativeness, and/or risk taking.
- Typical features of **avoidant personality disorder** are avoidance of social situations and inhibition in interpersonal relationships related to feelings of ineptitude and inadequacy, anxious preoccupation with negative evaluation and rejection, and fears of ridicule or embarrassment.
- Typical features of **borderline personality disorder** are instability of self-image, personal goals, interpersonal relationships, and affects, accompanied by impulsivity, risk taking, and/or hostility.
- Typical features of **narcissistic personality disorder** are variable and vulnerable self-esteem, with attempts at regulation through attention and approval seeking, and either overt or covert grandiosity.
- Typical features of **obsessive-compulsive personality disorder** are difficulties in establishing and sustaining close relationships, associated with rigid perfectionism, inflexibility, and restricted emotional expression.
- Typical features of **schizotypal personality disorder** are impairments in the capacity for social and close relationships, and eccentricities in cognition, perception, and behavior that are associated with distorted self-image and incoherent personal goals and accompanied by suspiciousness and restricted emotional expression.

The A and B criteria for the six specific personality disorders and for PD-TS follow. All personality disorders also meet criteria C through G of the General Criteria for Personality Disorder.

Antisocial Personality Disorder

Typical features of antisocial personality disorder are a failure to conform to lawful and ethical behavior, and an egocentric, callous lack of concern for others, accompanied by deceitfulness, irresponsibility, manipulativeness, and/or risk taking. Characteristic difficulties are apparent in identity, self-direction, empathy, and/or intimacy, as described below, along with specific maladaptive traits in the domains of Antagonism and Disinhibition.

Proposed Diagnostic Criteria

A. Moderate or greater impairment in personality functioning, manifested by characteristic difficulties in two or more of the following four areas:

1. *Identity:* Egocentrism; self-esteem derived from personal gain, power, or pleasure.
2. *Self-direction:* Goal setting based on personal gratification; absence of prosocial internal standards, associated with failure to conform to lawful or culturally normative ethical behavior.
3. *Empathy:* Lack of concern for feelings, needs, or suffering of others; lack of remorse after hurting or mistreating another.
4. *Intimacy:* Incapacity for mutually intimate relationships, as exploitation is a primary means of relating to others, including by deceit and coercion; use of dominance or intimidation to control others.

B. Six or more of the following seven pathological personality traits:

1. *Manipulativeness* (an aspect of **Antagonism**): Frequent use of subterfuge to influence or control others; use of seduction, charm, glibness, or ingratiation to achieve one's ends.
2. *Callousness* (an aspect of **Antagonism**): Lack of concern for feelings or problems of others; lack of guilt or remorse about the negative or harmful effects of one's actions on others; aggression; sadism.
3. *Deceitfulness* (an aspect of **Antagonism**): Dishonesty and fraudulence; misrepresentation of self; embellishment or fabrication when relating events.
4. *Hostility* (an aspect of **Antagonism**): Persistent or frequent angry feelings; anger or irritability in response to minor slights and insults; mean, nasty, or vengeful behavior.
5. *Risk taking* (an aspect of **Disinhibition**): Engagement in dangerous, risky, and potentially self-damaging activities, unnecessarily and without regard for consequences; boredom proneness and thoughtless initiation of activities to counter boredom; lack of concern for one's limitations and denial of the reality of personal danger.
6. *Impulsivity* (an aspect of **Disinhibition**): Acting on the spur of the moment in response to immediate stimuli; acting on a momentary basis without a plan or consideration of outcomes; difficulty establishing and following plans.
7. *Irresponsibility* (an aspect of **Disinhibition**): Disregard for—and failure to honor—financial and other obligations or commitments; lack of respect for—and lack of follow-through on—agreements and promises.

Note. The individual is at least 18 years of age.

Specify if:
   With psychopathic features.

Specifiers

A distinct variant often termed *psychopathy* (or "primary" psychopathy) is marked by a lack of anxiety or fear and by a bold interpersonal style that may mask maladaptive behaviors (e.g., fraudulence). This psychopathic variant is characterized by low levels of anxiousness (Negative Affectivity domain) and withdrawal (Detachment domain) and high levels of attention seeking (Antagonism domain). High attention seeking and low withdrawal capture the social potency (assertive/dominant) component of psychopathy, whereas low anxiousness captures the stress immunity (emotional stability/resilience) component.

In addition to psychopathic features, trait and personality functioning specifiers may be used to record other personality features that may be present in antisocial personality disorder but are not required for the diagnosis. For example, traits of Negative Affectivity (e.g., anxiousness) are not diagnostic criteria for antisocial personality disorder (see Criterion B) but can be specified when appropriate. Furthermore, although moderate or greater impairment in personality functioning is required for the diagnosis of antisocial personality disorder (Criterion A), the level of personality functioning can also be specified.

Avoidant Personality Disorder

Typical features of avoidant personality disorder are avoidance of social situations and inhibition in interpersonal relationships related to feelings of ineptitude and inadequacy, anxious preoccupation with negative evaluation and rejection, and fears of ridicule or embarrassment. Characteristic difficulties are apparent in identity, self-direction, empathy, and/or intimacy, as described below, along with specific maladaptive traits in the domains of Negative Affectivity and Detachment.

Proposed Diagnostic Criteria

A. Moderate or greater impairment in personality functioning, manifested by characteristic difficulties in two or more of the following four areas:

1. *Identity:* Low self-esteem associated with self-appraisal as socially inept, personally unappealing, or inferior; excessive feelings of shame.
2. *Self-direction:* Unrealistic standards for behavior associated with reluctance to pursue goals, take personal risks, or engage in new activities involving interpersonal contact.
3. *Empathy:* Preoccupation with, and sensitivity to, criticism or rejection, associated with distorted inference of others' perspectives as negative.
4. *Intimacy:* Reluctance to get involved with people unless being certain of being liked; diminished mutuality within intimate relationships because of fear of being shamed or ridiculed.

B. Three or more of the following four pathological personality traits, one of which must be (1) Anxiousness:

1. *Anxiousness* (an aspect of **Negative Affectivity**): Intense feelings of nervousness, tenseness, or panic, often in reaction to social situations; worry about the negative effects of past unpleasant experiences and future negative possibilities; feeling fearful, apprehensive, or threatened by uncertainty; fears of embarrassment.

2. *Withdrawal* (an aspect of **Detachment**): Reticence in social situations; avoidance of social contacts and activity; lack of initiation of social contact.
3. *Anhedonia* (an aspect of **Detachment**): Lack of enjoyment from, engagement in, or energy for life's experiences; deficits in the capacity to feel pleasure or take interest in things.
4. *Intimacy avoidance* (an aspect of **Detachment**): Avoidance of close or romantic relationships, interpersonal attachments, and intimate sexual relationships.

Specifiers

Considerable heterogeneity in the form of additional personality traits is found among individuals diagnosed with avoidant personality disorder. Trait and level of personality functioning specifiers can be used to record additional personality features that may be present in avoidant personality disorder. For example, other Negative Affectivity traits (e.g., depressivity, separation insecurity, submissiveness, suspiciousness, hostility) are not diagnostic criteria for avoidant personality disorder (see Criterion B) but can be specified when appropriate. Furthermore, although moderate or greater impairment in personality functioning is required for the diagnosis of avoidant personality disorder (Criterion A), the level of personality functioning also can be specified.

Borderline Personality Disorder

Typical features of borderline personality disorder are instability of self-image, personal goals, interpersonal relationships, and affects, accompanied by impulsivity, risk taking, and/or hostility. Characteristic difficulties are apparent in identity, self-direction, empathy, and/or intimacy, as described below, along with specific maladaptive traits in the domain of Negative Affectivity, and also Antagonism and/or Disinhibition.

Proposed Diagnostic Criteria

A. Moderate or greater impairment in personality functioning, manifested by characteristic difficulties in two or more of the following four areas:
1. *Identity:* Markedly impoverished, poorly developed, or unstable self-image, often associated with excessive self-criticism; chronic feelings of emptiness; dissociative states under stress.
2. *Self-direction:* Instability in goals, aspirations, values, or career plans.
3. *Empathy:* Compromised ability to recognize the feelings and needs of others associated with interpersonal hypersensitivity (i.e., prone to feel slighted or insulted); perceptions of others selectively biased toward negative attributes or vulnerabilities.
4. *Intimacy:* Intense, unstable, and conflicted close relationships, marked by mistrust, neediness, and anxious preoccupation with real or imagined abandonment; close relationships often viewed in extremes of idealization and devaluation and alternating between overinvolvement and withdrawal.

B. Four or more of the following seven pathological personality traits, at least one of which must be (5) Impulsivity, (6) Risk taking, or (7) Hostility:
1. *Emotional lability* (an aspect of **Negative Affectivity**): Unstable emotional experiences and frequent mood changes; emotions that are easily aroused, intense, and/or out of proportion to events and circumstances.
2. *Anxiousness* (an aspect of **Negative Affectivity**): Intense feelings of nervousness, tenseness, or panic, often in reaction to interpersonal stresses; worry about

the negative effects of past unpleasant experiences and future negative possibilities; feeling fearful, apprehensive, or threatened by uncertainty; fears of falling apart or losing control.

3. *Separation insecurity* (an aspect of **Negative Affectivity**): Fears of rejection by—and/or separation from—significant others, associated with fears of excessive dependency and complete loss of autonomy.

4. *Depressivity* (an aspect of **Negative Affectivity**): Frequent feelings of being down, miserable, and/or hopeless; difficulty recovering from such moods; pessimism about the future; pervasive shame; feelings of inferior self-worth; thoughts of suicide and suicidal behavior.

5. *Impulsivity* (an aspect of **Disinhibition**): Acting on the spur of the moment in response to immediate stimuli; acting on a momentary basis without a plan or consideration of outcomes; difficulty establishing or following plans; a sense of urgency and self-harming behavior under emotional distress.

6. *Risk taking* (an aspect of **Disinhibition**): Engagement in dangerous, risky, and potentially self-damaging activities, unnecessarily and without regard to consequences; lack of concern for one's limitations and denial of the reality of personal danger.

7. *Hostility* (an aspect of **Antagonism**): Persistent or frequent angry feelings; anger or irritability in response to minor slights and insults.

Specifiers

Trait and level of personality functioning specifiers may be used to record additional personality features that may be present in borderline personality disorder but are not required for the diagnosis. For example, traits of Psychoticism (e.g., cognitive and perceptual dysregulation) are not diagnostic criteria for borderline personality disorder (see Criterion B) but can be specified when appropriate. Furthermore, although moderate or greater impairment in personality functioning is required for the diagnosis of borderline personality disorder (Criterion A), the level of personality functioning can also be specified.

Narcissistic Personality Disorder

Typical features of narcissistic personality disorder are variable and vulnerable self-esteem, with attempts at regulation through attention and approval seeking, and either overt or covert grandiosity. Characteristic difficulties are apparent in identity, self-direction, empathy, and/or intimacy, as described below, along with specific maladaptive traits in the domain of Antagonism.

Proposed Diagnostic Criteria

A. Moderate or greater impairment in personality functioning, manifested by characteristic difficulties in two or more of the following four areas:

1. *Identity:* Excessive reference to others for self-definition and self-esteem regulation; exaggerated self-appraisal inflated or deflated, or vacillating between extremes; emotional regulation mirrors fluctuations in self-esteem.

2. *Self-direction:* Goal setting based on gaining approval from others; personal standards unreasonably high in order to see oneself as exceptional, or too low based on a sense of entitlement; often unaware of own motivations.

     3. **Empathy:** Impaired ability to recognize or identify with the feelings and needs of others; excessively attuned to reactions of others, but only if perceived as relevant to self; over- or underestimate of own effect on others.

     4. **Intimacy:** Relationships largely superficial and exist to serve self-esteem regulation; mutuality constrained by little genuine interest in others' experiences and predominance of a need for personal gain.

B. Both of the following pathological personality traits:

     1. **Grandiosity** (an aspect of **Antagonism**): Feelings of entitlement, either overt or covert; self-centeredness; firmly holding to the belief that one is better than others; condescension toward others.

     2. **Attention seeking** (an aspect of **Antagonism**): Excessive attempts to attract and be the focus of the attention of others; admiration seeking.

Specifiers

Trait and personality functioning specifiers may be used to record additional personality features that may be present in narcissistic personality disorder but are not required for the diagnosis. For example, other traits of Antagonism (e.g., manipulativeness, deceitfulness, callousness) are not diagnostic criteria for narcissistic personality disorder (see Criterion B) but can be specified when more pervasive antagonistic features (e.g., "malignant narcissism") are present. Other traits of Negative Affectivity (e.g., depressivity, anxiousness) can be specified to record more "vulnerable" presentations. Furthermore, although moderate or greater impairment in personality functioning is required for the diagnosis of narcissistic personality disorder (Criterion A), the level of personality functioning can also be specified.

Obsessive-Compulsive Personality Disorder

Typical features of obsessive-compulsive personality disorder are difficulties in establishing and sustaining close relationships, associated with rigid perfectionism, inflexibility, and restricted emotional expression. Characteristic difficulties are apparent in identity, self-direction, empathy, and/or intimacy, as described below, along with specific maladaptive traits in the domains of Negative Affectivity and/or Detachment.

Proposed Diagnostic Criteria

A. Moderate or greater impairment in personality functioning, manifested by characteristic difficulties in two or more of the following four areas:

     1. **Identity:** Sense of self derived predominantly from work or productivity; constricted experience and expression of strong emotions.

     2. **Self-direction:** Difficulty completing tasks and realizing goals, associated with rigid and unreasonably high and inflexible internal standards of behavior; overly conscientious and moralistic attitudes.

     3. **Empathy:** Difficulty understanding and appreciating the ideas, feelings, or behaviors of others.

     4. **Intimacy:** Relationships seen as secondary to work and productivity; rigidity and stubbornness negatively affect relationships with others.

B. Three or more of the following four pathological personality traits, one of which must be (1) Rigid perfectionism:

1. ***Rigid perfectionism*** (an aspect of extreme **Conscientiousness** [the opposite pole of Disinhibition]): Rigid insistence on everything being flawless, perfect, and without errors or faults, including one's own and others' performance; sacrificing of timeliness to ensure correctness in every detail; believing that there is only one right way to do things; difficulty changing ideas and/or viewpoint; preoccupation with details, organization, and order.

2. ***Perseveration*** (an aspect of **Negative Affectivity**): Persistence at tasks long after the behavior has ceased to be functional or effective; continuance of the same behavior despite repeated failures.

3. ***Intimacy avoidance*** (an aspect of **Detachment**): Avoidance of close or romantic relationships, interpersonal attachments, and intimate sexual relationships.

4. ***Restricted affectivity*** (an aspect of **Detachment**): Little reaction to emotionally arousing situations; constricted emotional experience and expression; indifference or coldness.

Specifiers

Trait and personality functioning specifiers may be used to record additional personality features that may be present in obsessive-compulsive personality disorder but are not required for the diagnosis. For example, other traits of Negative Affectivity (e.g., anxiousness) are not diagnostic criteria for obsessive-compulsive personality disorder (see Criterion B) but can be specified when appropriate. Furthermore, although moderate or greater impairment in personality functioning is required for the diagnosis of obsessive-compulsive personality disorder (Criterion A), the level of personality functioning can also be specified.

Schizotypal Personality Disorder

Typical features of schizotypal personality disorder are impairments in the capacity for social and close relationships and eccentricities in cognition, perception, and behavior that are associated with distorted self-image and incoherent personal goals and accompanied by suspiciousness and restricted emotional expression. Characteristic difficulties are apparent in identity, self-direction, empathy, and/or intimacy, along with specific maladaptive traits in the domains of Psychoticism and Detachment.

Proposed Diagnostic Criteria

A. Moderate or greater impairment in personality functioning, manifested by characteristic difficulties in two or more of the following four areas:

1. ***Identity:*** Confused boundaries between self and others; distorted self-concept; emotional expression often not congruent with context or internal experience.
2. ***Self-direction:*** Unrealistic or incoherent goals; no clear set of internal standards.
3. ***Empathy:*** Pronounced difficulty understanding impact of own behaviors on others; frequent misinterpretations of others' motivations and behaviors.
4. ***Intimacy:*** Marked impairments in developing close relationships, associated with mistrust and anxiety.

B. Four or more of the following six pathological personality traits:

1. *Cognitive and perceptual dysregulation* (an aspect of **Psychoticism**): Odd or unusual thought processes; vague, circumstantial, metaphorical, overelaborate, or stereotyped thought or speech; odd sensations in various sensory modalities.
2. *Unusual beliefs and experiences* (an aspect of **Psychoticism**): Thought content and views of reality that are viewed by others as bizarre or idiosyncratic; unusual experiences of reality.
3. *Eccentricity* (an aspect of **Psychoticism**): Odd, unusual, or bizarre behavior or appearance; saying unusual or inappropriate things.
4. *Restricted affectivity* (an aspect of **Detachment**): Little reaction to emotionally arousing situations; constricted emotional experience and expression; indifference or coldness.
5. *Withdrawal* (an aspect of **Detachment**): Preference for being alone to being with others; reticence in social situations; avoidance of social contacts and activity; lack of initiation of social contact.
6. *Suspiciousness* (an aspect of **Detachment**): Expectations of—and heightened sensitivity to—signs of interpersonal ill-intent or harm; doubts about loyalty and fidelity of others; feelings of persecution.

Specifiers

Trait and personality functioning specifiers may be used to record additional personality features that may be present in schizotypal personality disorder but are not required for the diagnosis. For example, traits of Negative Affectivity (e.g., depressivity, anxiousness) are not diagnostic criteria for schizotypal personality disorder (see Criterion B) but can be specified when appropriate. Furthermore, although moderate or greater impairment in personality functioning is required for the diagnosis of schizotypal personality disorder (Criterion A), the level of personality functioning can also be specified.

Personality Disorder—Trait Specified

Proposed Diagnostic Criteria

A. Moderate or greater impairment in personality functioning, manifested by difficulties in two or more of the following four areas:

1. Identity
2. Self-direction
3. Empathy
4. *Intimacy*

B. One or more pathological personality trait domains OR specific trait facets within domains, considering ALL of the following domains:

1. **Negative Affectivity** (vs. Emotional Stability): Frequent and intense experiences of high levels of a wide range of negative emotions (e.g., anxiety, depression, guilt/shame, worry, anger), and their behavioral (e.g., self-harm) and interpersonal (e.g., dependency) manifestations.
2. **Detachment** (vs. Extraversion): Avoidance of socioemotional experience, including both withdrawal from interpersonal interactions, ranging from casual, daily interactions to friendships to intimate relationships, as well as restricted affective experience and expression, particularly limited hedonic capacity.

3. **Antagonism** (vs. Agreeableness): Behaviors that put the individual at odds with other people, including an exaggerated sense of self-importance and a concomitant expectation of special treatment, as well as a callous antipathy toward others, encompassing both unawareness of others' needs and feelings and a readiness to use others in the service of self-enhancement.
4. **Disinhibition** (vs. Conscientiousness): Orientation toward immediate gratification, leading to impulsive behavior driven by current thoughts, feelings, and external stimuli, without regard for past learning or consideration of future consequences.
5. **Psychoticism** (vs. Lucidity): Exhibiting a wide range of culturally incongruent odd, eccentric, or unusual behaviors and cognitions, including both process (e.g., perception, dissociation) and content (e.g., beliefs).

Subtypes

Because personality features vary continuously along multiple trait dimensions, a comprehensive set of potential expressions of PD-TS can be represented by DSM-5's dimensional model of maladaptive personality trait variants (see Table 3). Thus, subtypes are unnecessary for PD-TS, and instead, the descriptive elements that constitute personality are provided, arranged in an empirically based model. This arrangement allows clinicians to tailor the description of each individual's personality disorder profile, considering all five broad domains of personality trait variation and drawing on the descriptive features of these domains as needed to characterize the individual.

Specifiers

The specific personality features of individuals are always recorded in evaluating Criterion B, so the combination of personality features characterizing an individual directly constitutes the specifiers in each case. For example, two individuals who are both characterized by emotional lability, hostility, and depressivity may differ such that the first individual is characterized additionally by callousness, whereas the second is not.

Personality Disorder Scoring Algorithms

The requirement for any two of the four A criteria for each of the six personality disorders was based on maximizing the relationship of these criteria to their corresponding personality disorder. Diagnostic thresholds for the B criteria were also set empirically to minimize change in prevalence of the disorders from DSM-IV and overlap with other personality disorders, and to maximize relationships with functional impairment. The resulting diagnostic criteria sets represent clinically useful personality disorders with high fidelity, in terms of core impairments in personality functioning of varying degrees of severity and constellations of pathological personality traits.

Personality Disorder Diagnosis

Individuals who have a pattern of impairment in personality functioning and maladaptive traits that matches one of the six defined personality disorders should be diagnosed with that personality disorder. If an individual also has one or even several prominent traits that may have clinical relevance in addition to those required for the diagnosis (e.g., see narcissistic personality disorder), the option exists for these to be noted as specifiers. Individuals whose personality functioning or trait pattern is substantially different from that of any of the six specific personality disorders should be diagnosed with PD-TS. The individual may not meet the required number of A or B criteria and, thus, have a subthreshold presentation of a personality disorder. The individual may have a mix of features of personality disorder types or some features that are less characteristic of a type and more accurately considered a mixed or atypical presentation. The specific level of impairment in personality functioning and the pathological personality traits that characterize the individual's personality can be specified for PD-TS, using the Level of Personality Functioning Scale (Table 2) and the pathological trait taxonomy (Table 3). The current diagnoses of paranoid, schizoid, histrionic, and dependent personality disorders are represented also by the diagnosis of PD-TS; these are defined by moderate or greater impairment in personality functioning and can be specified by the relevant pathological personality trait combinations.

Level of Personality Functioning Scale

Like most human tendencies, personality functioning is distributed on a continuum. Central to functioning and adaptation are individuals' characteristic ways of thinking about and understanding themselves and their interactions with others. An optimally functioning individual has a complex, fully elaborated, and well-integrated psychological world that includes a mostly positive, volitional, and adaptive self-concept; a rich, broad, and appropriately regulated emotional life; and the capacity to behave as a productive member of society with reciprocal and fulfilling interpersonal relationships. At the opposite end of the continuum, an individual with severe personality pathology has an impoverished, disorganized, and/or conflicted psychological world that includes a weak, unclear, and maladaptive self-concept; a propensity to negative, dysregulated emotions; and a deficient capacity for adaptive interpersonal functioning and social behavior.

Self and *Interpersonal* Functioning Dimensional Definition

Generalized severity may be the most important single predictor of concurrent and prospective dysfunction in assessing personality psychopathology. Personality disorders are optimally characterized by a generalized personality severity continuum with additional specification of stylistic elements, derived from personality disorder symptom constellations and personality traits. At the same time, the core of personality psychopathology is impairment in ideas and feelings regarding self and interpersonal relationships; this notion is consistent with multiple theories of personality disorder and their research bases. The components of the Level of Personality Functioning Scale—identity, self-direction, empathy, and intimacy—are particularly central in describing a personality functioning continuum.

Mental representations of the self and interpersonal relationships are reciprocally influential and inextricably tied, affect the nature of interaction with mental health professionals, and can have a significant impact on both treatment efficacy and outcome, underscoring the importance of assessing an individual's characteristic self-concept as well as views of other people and relationships. Although the degree of disturbance in the self and interpersonal functioning is continuously distributed, it is useful to consider the level of impairment in functioning for clinical characterization and for treatment planning and prognosis.

Rating Level of Personality Functioning

To use the Level of Personality Functioning Scale (LPFS) (Table 2), the clinician selects the level that most closely captures the individual's *current overall* level of impairment in personality functioning. The rating is necessary for the diagnosis of a personality disorder (moderate or greater impairment) and can be used to specify the severity of impairment present for an individual with any personality disorder at a given point in time. The LPFS may also be used as a global indicator of personality functioning without specification of a personality disorder diagnosis, or in the event that personality impairment is subthreshold for a disorder diagnosis.

Personality Traits

Definition and Description

Criterion B in the alternative model involves assessments of personality traits that are grouped into five domains. A *personality trait* is a tendency to feel, perceive, behave, and think in relatively consistent ways across time and across situations in which the trait may manifest. For example, individuals with a high level of the personality trait of *anxiousness* would tend to *feel* anxious readily, including in circumstances in which most people would be calm and relaxed. Individuals high in trait anxiousness also would *perceive* situations to be anxiety-provoking more frequently than would individuals with lower levels of this trait, and those high in the trait would tend to *behave* so as to avoid situations that they *think* would make them anxious. They would thereby tend to *think* about the world as more anxiety provoking than other people.

Importantly, individuals high in trait anxiousness would not necessarily be anxious at all times and in all situations. Individuals' trait levels also can and do change throughout life. Some changes are very general and reflect maturation (e.g., teenagers generally are higher on trait impulsivity than are older adults), whereas other changes reflect individuals' life experiences.

Dimensionality of Personality Traits

All individuals can be located on the spectrum of trait dimensions; that is, personality traits apply to everyone in different degrees rather than being present versus absent. Moreover, personality traits, including those identified specifically in the Section III model, exist on a spectrum with two opposing poles. For example, the opposite of the trait of *callousness* is the tendency to be empathic and kind-hearted, even in circumstances in which most persons would not feel that way. Hence, although in Section III this trait is labeled *callousness,* because that pole of the dimension is the primary focus, it could be described in full as *callousness versus kind-heartedness.* Moreover, its oppo-

TABLE 2. Level of Personality Functioning Scale

| Level of impairment | SELF | | INTERPERSONAL | |
	Identity	Self-direction	Empathy	Intimacy
0—Little or no impairment	Has ongoing awareness of a unique self; maintains role-appropriate boundaries. Has consistent and self-regulated positive self-esteem, with accurate self-appraisal. Is capable of experiencing, tolerating, and regulating a full range of emotions.	Sets and aspires to reasonable goals based on a realistic assessment of personal capacities. Utilizes appropriate standards of behavior, attaining fulfillment in multiple realms. Can reflect on, and make constructive meaning of, internal experience.	Is capable of accurately understanding others' experiences and motivations in most situations. Comprehends and appreciates others' perspectives, even if disagreeing. Is aware of the effect of own actions on others.	Maintains multiple satisfying and enduring relationships in personal and community life. Desires and engages in a number of caring, close, and reciprocal relationships. Strives for cooperation and mutual benefit and flexibly responds to a range of others' ideas, emotions, and behaviors.
1—Some impairment	Has relatively intact sense of self, with some decrease in clarity of boundaries when strong emotions and mental distress are experienced. Self-esteem diminished at times, with overly critical or somewhat distorted self-appraisal. Strong emotions may be distressing, associated with a restriction in range of emotional experience.	Is excessively goal-directed, somewhat goal-inhibited, or conflicted about goals. May have an unrealistic or socially inappropriate set of personal standards, limiting some aspects of fulfillment. Is able to reflect on internal experiences, but may overemphasize a single (e.g., intellectual, emotional) type of self-knowledge.	Is somewhat compromised in ability to appreciate and understand others' experiences; may tend to see others as having unreasonable expectations or a wish for control. Although capable of considering and understanding different perspectives, resists doing so. Has inconsistent awareness of effect of own behavior on others.	Is able to establish enduring relationships in personal and community life, with some limitations on degree of depth and satisfaction. Is capable of forming and desires to form intimate and reciprocal relationships, but may be inhibited in meaningful expression and sometimes constrained if intense emotions or conflicts arise. Cooperation may be inhibited by unrealistic standards; somewhat limited in ability to respect or respond to others' ideas, emotions, and behaviors.

TABLE 2.   Level of Personality Functioning Scale (*continued*)

Level of impairment	SELF		INTERPERSONAL	
	Identity	Self-direction	Empathy	Intimacy
2—Moderate impairment	Depends excessively on others for identity definition, with compromised boundary delineation. Has vulnerable self-esteem controlled by exaggerated concern about external evaluation, with a wish for approval. Has sense of incompleteness or inferiority, with compensatory inflated, or deflated, self-appraisal. Emotional regulation depends on positive external appraisal. Threats to self-esteem may engender strong emotions such as rage or shame.	Goals are more often a means of gaining external approval than self-generated, and thus may lack coherence and/or stability. Personal standards may be unreasonably high (e.g., a need to be special or please others) or low (e.g., not consonant with prevailing social values). Fulfillment is compromised by a sense of lack of authenticity. Has impaired capacity to reflect on internal experience.	Is hyperattuned to the experience of others, but only with respect to perceived relevance to self. Is excessively self-referential; significantly compromised ability to appreciate and understand others' experiences and to consider alternative perspectives. Is generally unaware of or unconcerned about effect of own behavior on others, or unrealistic appraisal of own effect.	Is capable of forming and desires to form relationships in personal and community life, but connections may be largely superficial. Intimate relationships are predominantly based on meeting self-regulatory and self-esteem needs, with an unrealistic expectation of being perfectly understood by others. Tends not to view relationships in reciprocal terms, and cooperates predominantly for personal gain.

TABLE 2. Level of Personality Functioning Scale *(continued)*

Level of impairment	SELF		INTERPERSONAL	
	Identity	Self-direction	Empathy	Intimacy
3—Severe impairment	Has a weak sense of autonomy/ agency; experience of a lack of identity, or emptiness. Boundary definition is poor or rigid: may show overidentification with others, overemphasis on independence from others, or vacillation between these. Fragile self-esteem is easily influenced by events, and self-image lacks coherence. Self-appraisal is un-nuanced: self-loathing, self-aggrandizing, or an illogical, unrealistic combination. Emotions may be rapidly shifting or a chronic, unwavering feeling of despair.	Has difficulty establishing and/or achieving personal goals. Internal standards for behavior are unclear or contradictory. Life is experienced as meaningless or dangerous. Has significantly compromised ability to reflect on and understand own mental processes.	Ability to consider and understand the thoughts, feelings, and behavior of other people is significantly limited; may discern very specific aspects of others' experience, particularly vulnerabilities and suffering. Is generally unable to consider alternative perspectives; highly threatened by differences of opinion or alternative viewpoints. Is confused about or unaware of impact of own actions on others; often bewildered about peoples' thoughts and actions, with destructive motivations frequently misattributed to others.	Has some desire to form relationships in community and personal life, but capacity for positive and enduring connections is significantly impaired. Relationships are based on a strong belief in the absolute need for the intimate other(s), and/or expectations of abandonment or abuse. Feelings about intimate involvement with others alternate between fear/rejection and desperate desire for connection. Little mutuality: others are conceptualized primarily in terms of how they affect the self (negatively or positively); cooperative efforts are often disrupted due to the perception of slights from others.

TABLE 2. Level of Personality Functioning Scale *(continued)*

Level of impairment	SELF		INTERPERSONAL	
	Identity	Self-direction	Empathy	Intimacy
4—Extreme impairment	Experience of a unique self and sense of agency/autonomy are virtually absent, or are organized around perceived external persecution. Boundaries with others are confused or lacking. Has weak or distorted self-image easily threatened by interactions with others; significant distortions and confusion around self-appraisal. Emotions not congruent with context or internal experience. Hatred and aggression may be dominant affects, although they may be disavowed and attributed to others.	Has poor differentiation of thoughts from actions, so goal-setting ability is severely compromised, with unrealistic or incoherent goals. Internal standards for behavior are virtually lacking. Genuine fulfillment is virtually inconceivable. Is profoundly unable to constructively reflect on own experience. Personal motivations may be unrecognized and/or experienced as external to self.	Has pronounced inability to consider and understand others' experience and motivation. Attention to others' perspectives is virtually absent (attention is hypervigilant, focused on need fulfillment and harm avoidance). Social interactions can be confusing and disorienting.	Desire for affiliation is limited because of profound disinterest or expectation of harm. Engagement with others is detached, disorganized, or consistently negative. Relationships are conceptualized almost exclusively in terms of their ability to provide comfort or inflict pain and suffering. Social/interpersonal behavior is not reciprocal; rather, it seeks fulfillment of basic needs or escape from pain.

site pole can be recognized and may not be adaptive in all circumstances (e.g., individuals who, due to extreme kind-heartedness, repeatedly allow themselves to be taken advantage of by unscrupulous others).

Hierarchical Structure of Personality

Some trait terms are quite specific (e.g., "talkative") and describe a narrow range of behaviors, whereas others are quite broad (e.g., Detachment) and characterize a wide range of behavioral propensities. Broad trait dimensions are called *domains,* and specific trait dimensions are called *facets.* Personality trait *domains* comprise a spectrum of more specific personality *facets* that tend to occur together. For example, withdrawal and anhedonia are specific trait *facets* in the trait *domain* of Detachment. Despite some cross-cultural variation in personality trait facets, the broad domains they collectively comprise are relatively consistent across cultures.

The Personality Trait Model

The Section III personality trait system includes five broad domains of personality trait variation—Negative Affectivity (vs. Emotional Stability), Detachment (vs. Extraversion), Antagonism (vs. Agreeableness), Disinhibition (vs. Conscientiousness), and Psychoticism (vs. Lucidity)—comprising 25 specific personality trait facets. Table 3 provides definitions of all personality domains and facets. These five broad domains are maladaptive variants of the five domains of the extensively validated and replicated personality model known as the "Big Five," or Five Factor Model of personality (FFM), and are also similar to the domains of the Personality Psychopathology Five (PSY-5). The specific 25 facets represent a list of personality facets chosen for their clinical relevance.

Although the Trait Model focuses on personality traits associated with psychopathology, there are healthy, adaptive, and resilient personality traits identified as the polar opposites of these traits, as noted in the parentheses above (i.e., Emotional Stability, Extraversion, Agreeableness, Conscientiousness, and Lucidity). Their presence can greatly mitigate the effects of mental disorders and facilitate coping and recovery from traumatic injuries and other medical illness.

Distinguishing Traits, Symptoms, and Specific Behaviors

Although traits are by no means immutable and do change throughout the life span, they show relative consistency compared with symptoms and specific behaviors. For example, a person may behave impulsively at a specific time for a specific reason (e.g., a person who is rarely impulsive suddenly decides to spend a great deal of money on a particular item because of an unusual opportunity to purchase something of unique value), but it is only when behaviors aggregate across time and circumstance, such that a pattern of behavior distinguishes between individuals, that they reflect traits. Nevertheless, it is important to recognize, for example, that even people who are impulsive are not acting impulsively all of the time. A trait is a tendency or disposition toward specific behaviors; a specific behavior is an instance or manifestation of a trait.

Similarly, traits are distinguished from most symptoms because symptoms tend to wax and wane, whereas traits are relatively more stable. For example, individuals with higher levels of *depressivity* have a greater likelihood of experiencing discrete episodes of a depressive disorder and of showing the symptoms of these disorders, such as difficulty concentrating. However, even patients who have a trait propensity to *depressivity* typically cycle through distinguishable episodes of mood disturbance, and specific symptoms such as difficulty concentrating tend to wax and wane in concert with specific episodes, so they do not form part of the trait definition. Importantly, however, symptoms and traits are both amenable to intervention, and many interventions targeted at symptoms can affect the longer term patterns of personality functioning that are captured by personality traits.

Assessment of the DSM-5 Section III Personality Trait Model

The clinical utility of the Section III multidimensional personality trait model lies in its ability to focus attention on multiple relevant areas of personality variation in each individual patient. Rather than focusing attention on the identification of one and only one optimal diagnostic label, clinical application of the Section III personality trait model involves reviewing all five broad personality domains portrayed in Table 3. The clinical approach to personality is similar to the well-known review of systems in clinical medicine. For example, an individual's presenting complaint may focus on a specific neurological symptom, yet during an initial evaluation clinicians still systematically review functioning in all relevant systems (e.g., cardiovascular, respiratory, gastrointestinal), lest an important area of diminished functioning and corresponding opportunity for effective intervention be missed.

Clinical use of the Section III personality trait model proceeds similarly. An initial inquiry reviews all five broad domains of personality. This systematic review is facilitated by the use of formal psychometric instruments designed to measure specific facets and domains of personality. For example, the personality trait model is operationalized in the Personality Inventory for DSM-5 (PID-5), which can be completed in its self-report form by patients and in its informant-report form by those who know the patient well (e.g., a spouse). A detailed clinical assessment would involve collection of both patient- and informant-report data on all 25 facets of the personality trait model. However, if this is not possible, due to time or other constraints, assessment focused at the five-domain level is an acceptable clinical option when only a general (vs. detailed) portrait of a patient's personality is needed (see Criterion B of PD-TS). However, if personality-based problems are the focus of treatment, then it will be important to assess individuals' trait facets as well as domains.

Because personality traits are continuously distributed in the population, an approach to making the judgment that a specific trait is elevated (and therefore is present for diagnostic purposes) could involve comparing individuals' personality trait levels with population norms and/or clinical judgment. If a trait is elevated—that is, formal psychometric testing and/or interview data support the clinical judgment of elevation—then it is considered as contributing to meeting Criterion B of Section III personality disorders.

TABLE 3.   **Definitions of DSM-5 personality disorder trait domains and facets**

DOMAINS (Polar Opposites) and Facets	Definitions
NEGATIVE AFFECTIVITY (vs. Emotional Stability)	Frequent and intense experiences of high levels of a wide range of negative emotions (e.g., anxiety, depression, guilt/shame, worry, anger) and their behavioral (e.g., self-harm) and interpersonal (e.g., dependency) manifestations.
Emotional lability	Instability of emotional experiences and mood; emotions that are easily aroused, intense, and/or out of proportion to events and circumstances.
Anxiousness	Feelings of nervousness, tenseness, or panic in reaction to diverse situations; frequent worry about the negative effects of past unpleasant experiences and future negative possibilities; feeling fearful and apprehensive about uncertainty; expecting the worst to happen.
Separation insecurity	Fears of being alone due to rejection by—and/or separation from—significant others, based in a lack of confidence in one's ability to care for oneself, both physically and emotionally.
Submissiveness	Adaptation of one's behavior to the actual or perceived interests and desires of others even when doing so is antithetical to one's own interests, needs, or desires.
Hostility	Persistent or frequent angry feelings; anger or irritability in response to minor slights and insults; mean, nasty, or vengeful behavior. *See also* Antagonism.
Perseveration	Persistence at tasks or in a particular way of doing things long after the behavior has ceased to be functional or effective; continuance of the same behavior despite repeated failures or clear reasons for stopping.
Depressivity	*See* Detachment.
Suspiciousness	*See* Detachment.
Restricted affectivity (lack of)	The **lack of** this facet characterizes **low levels** of Negative Affectivity. *See* Detachment for definition of this facet.
DETACHMENT (vs. Extraversion)	Avoidance of socioemotional experience, including both withdrawal from interpersonal interactions (ranging from casual, daily interactions to friendships to intimate relationships) and restricted affective experience and expression, particularly limited hedonic capacity.
Withdrawal	Preference for being alone to being with others; reticence in social situations; avoidance of social contacts and activity; lack of initiation of social contact.
Intimacy avoidance	Avoidance of close or romantic relationships, interpersonal attachments, and intimate sexual relationships.
Anhedonia	Lack of enjoyment from, engagement in, or energy for life's experiences; deficits in the capacity to feel pleasure and take interest in things.
Depressivity	Feelings of being down, miserable, and/or hopeless; difficulty recovering from such moods; pessimism about the future; pervasive shame and/or guilt; feelings of inferior self-worth; thoughts of suicide and suicidal behavior.
Restricted affectivity	Little reaction to emotionally arousing situations; constricted emotional experience and expression; indifference and aloofness in normatively engaging situations.
Suspiciousness	Expectations of—and sensitivity to signs of—interpersonal ill-intent or harm; doubts about loyalty and fidelity of others; feelings of being mistreated, used, and/or persecuted by others.

TABLE 3.   Definitions of DSM-5 personality disorder trait domains and
            facets *(continued)*

DOMAINS (Polar Opposites) and Facets	Definitions
ANTAGONISM (vs. Agreeableness)	Behaviors that put the individual at odds with other people, including an exaggerated sense of self-importance and a concomitant expectation of special treatment, as well as a callous antipathy toward others, encompassing both an unawareness of others' needs and feelings and a readiness to use others in the service of self-enhancement.
Manipulativeness	Use of subterfuge to influence or control others; use of seduction, charm, glibness, or ingratiation to achieve one's ends.
Deceitfulness	Dishonesty and fraudulence; misrepresentation of self; embellishment or fabrication when relating events.
Grandiosity	Believing that one is superior to others and deserves special treatment; self-centeredness; feelings of entitlement; condescension toward others.
Attention seeking	Engaging in behavior designed to attract notice and to make oneself the focus of others' attention and admiration.
Callousness	Lack of concern for the feelings or problems of others; lack of guilt or remorse about the negative or harmful effects of one's actions on others.
Hostility	*See* Negative Affectivity.
DISINHIBITION (vs. Conscientiousness)	Orientation toward immediate gratification, leading to impulsive behavior driven by current thoughts, feelings, and external stimuli, without regard for past learning or consideration of future consequences.
Irresponsibility	Disregard for—and failure to honor—financial and other obligations or commitments; lack of respect for—and lack of follow-through on—agreements and promises; carelessness with others' property.
Impulsivity	Acting on the spur of the moment in response to immediate stimuli; acting on a momentary basis without a plan or consideration of outcomes; difficulty establishing and following plans; a sense of urgency and self-harming behavior under emotional distress.
Distractibility	Difficulty concentrating and focusing on tasks; attention is easily diverted by extraneous stimuli; difficulty maintaining goal-focused behavior, including both planning and completing tasks.
Risk taking	Engagement in dangerous, risky, and potentially self-damaging activities, unnecessarily and without regard to consequences; lack of concern for one's limitations and denial of the reality of personal danger; reckless pursuit of goals regardless of the level of risk involved.
Rigid perfectionism (lack of)	Rigid insistence on everything being flawless, perfect, and without errors or faults, including one's own and others' performance; sacrificing of timeliness to ensure correctness in every detail; believing that there is only one right way to do things; difficulty changing ideas and/or viewpoint; preoccupation with details, organization, and order. The *lack of* this facet characterizes *low levels* of Disinhibition.

TABLE 3.   **Definitions of DSM-5 personality disorder trait domains and facets** *(continued)*

DOMAINS (Polar Opposites) and Facets	Definitions
PSYCHOTICISM (vs. Lucidity)	Exhibiting a wide range of culturally incongruent odd, eccentric, or unusual behaviors and cognitions, including both process (e.g., perception, dissociation) and content (e.g., beliefs).
Unusual beliefs and experiences	Belief that one has unusual abilities, such as mind reading, telekinesis, or thought-action fusion; unusual experiences of reality, including hallucination-like experiences.
Eccentricity	Odd, unusual, or bizarre behavior, appearance, and/or speech; having strange and unpredictable thoughts; saying unusual or inappropriate things.
Cognitive and perceptual dysregulation	Odd or unusual thought processes and experiences, including depersonalization, derealization, and dissociative experiences; mixed sleep-wake state experiences; thought-control experiences.

Clinical Utility of the Multidimensional Personality Functioning and Trait Model

Disorder and trait constructs each add value to the other in predicting important antecedent (e.g., family history, history of child abuse), concurrent (e.g., functional impairment, medication use), and predictive (e.g., hospitalization, suicide attempts) variables. DSM-5 impairments in personality functioning and pathological personality traits each contribute independently to clinical decisions about degree of disability; risks for self-harm, violence, and criminality; recommended treatment type and intensity; and prognosis—all important aspects of the utility of psychiatric diagnoses. Notably, knowing the level of an individual's personality functioning and his or her pathological trait profile also provides the clinician with a rich base of information and is valuable in treatment planning and in predicting the course and outcome of many mental disorders in addition to personality disorders. Therefore, assessment of personality functioning and pathological personality traits may be relevant whether an individual has a personality disorder or not.

Index

*Page numbers printed in **boldface** type refer to tables and figures.*